IMPROVING OUTCOMES AND PREVENTING RELAPSE IN COGNITIVE-BEHAVIORAL THERAPY

Improving Outcomes and Preventing Relapse in Cognitive-Behavioral Therapy

Edited by
MARTIN M. ANTONY
DEBORAH ROTH LEDLEY
RICHARD G. HEIMBERG

THE GUILFORD PRESS
New York   London

©2005 The Guilford Press
A Division of Guilford Publications, Inc.
72 Spring Street, New York, NY 10012
www.guilford.com

Printed in the United States of America

This book is printed on acid-free paper.

Last digit is print number: 9   8   7   6   5   4   3   2   1

Library of Congress Cataloging-in-Publication Data

Improving outcomes and preventing relapse in cognitive-behavioral therapy /
edited by Martin M. Antony, Deborah Roth Ledley, Richard G. Heimberg.
    p. cm.
 Includes bibliographical references and indexes.
 ISBN 1-59385-197-9 (hardcover : alk. paper)
 1. Cognitive therapy.   I. Antony, Martin M.   II. Ledley, Deborah Roth.   III.
Heimberg, Richard G.
 RC489.C63I55 2005
 616.89′142—dc22

                                  2005016594

To Cynthia
—M. M. A.

To Gary
—D. R. L.

To Linda
—R. G. H.

About the Editors

Martin M. Antony, PhD, is Professor in the Department of Psychiatry and Behavioural Neurosciences at McMaster University. He is also Director of the Anxiety Treatment and Research Centre and Psychologist-in-Chief at St. Joseph's Healthcare in Hamilton, Ontario. Dr. Antony has published 15 books and more than 100 scientific papers and book chapters in the areas of cognitive-behavioral therapy and anxiety disorders; received early career awards from the Society of Clinical Psychology (American Psychological Association), the Canadian Psychological Association, and the Anxiety Disorders Association of America; and is a Fellow of the American and Canadian Psychological Associations. He is actively involved in clinical research on anxiety disorders and in teaching and education, and also maintains a clinical practice.

Deborah Roth Ledley, PhD, is Assistant Professor of Psychology in Psychiatry at the University of Pennsylvania School of Medicine, as well as a faculty member at the Center for the Treatment and Study of Anxiety at the University of Pennsylvania. Dr. Ledley's scholarly publications include scientific articles and book chapters on the nature and treatment of social phobia, obsessive–compulsive disorder, and other anxiety disorders. She is coauthor of *Making Cognitive-Behavioral Therapy Work: Clinical Process for New Practitioners*.

Richard G. Heimberg, PhD, is Professor of Psychology, Director of Clinical Training, and Director of the Adult Anxiety Clinic of Temple University. He is also past president of the Association for Advancement of Behavior Therapy. Dr. Heimberg is well known for his efforts to develop and evaluate cognitive-behavioral treatments for social anxiety, and has published more than 250 articles and chapters on social anxiety, the anxiety disorders, and related topics. He is coeditor or coauthor of several books, including *Social Phobia: Diagnosis, Assessment, and Treatment; Managing Social Anxiety: A Cognitive-Behavioral Therapy Approach; Generalized Anxiety Disorder: Advances in Research and Practice; Cognitive-Behavioral Group Therapy for Social Phobia: Basic Mechanisms and Clinical Strategies;* and *Making Cognitive-Behavioral Therapy Work: Clinical Process for New Practitioners*.

Contributors

Martin M. Antony, PhD, Anxiety Treatment and Research Centre, St. Joseph's Healthcare, and Department of Psychiatry and Behavioural Neurosciences, McMaster University, Hamilton, Ontario, Canada

Peter J. Bieling, PhD, Mood Disorders Program, St. Joseph's Healthcare, and Department of Psychiatry and Behavioural Neurosciences, McMaster University, Hamilton, Ontario, Canada

Jacqueline Carter, PhD, Eating Disorders Program, University Health Network, Toronto General Hospital, and Department of Psychiatry, University of Toronto, Toronto, Ontario, Canada

Yael Chatav, MA, Department of Psychology, University of Colorado at Boulder, Boulder, Colorado

Michelle G. Craske, PhD, Department of Psychology, University of California, Los Angeles, Los Angeles, California

Norah C. Feeny, PhD, Departments of Psychiatry and Psychology, Case Western Reserve University, Cleveland, Ohio

Edna B. Foa, PhD, Center for the Treatment and Study of Anxiety, University of Pennsylvania School of Medicine, Philadelphia, Pennsylvania

Martin E. Franklin, PhD, Center for the Treatment and Study of Anxiety, University of Pennsylvania School of Medicine, Philadelphia, Pennsylvania

Richard G. Heimberg, PhD, Department of Psychology, Temple University, Philadelphia, Pennsylvania

Dominic Lam, PhD, Department of Psychology, Institute of Psychiatry, King's College, London, United Kingdom

Deborah Roth Ledley, PhD, Center for the Treatment and Study of Anxiety, University of Pennsylvania School of Medicine, Philadelphia, Pennsylvania

Warren Mansell, DPhil, DClinPsy, Department of Psychological Medicine, Institute of Psychiatry, London, United Kingdom

Randi E. McCabe, PhD, Anxiety Treatment and Research Centre, St. Joseph's Healthcare, and Department of Psychiatry and Behavioural Neurosciences, McMaster University, Hamilton, Ontario, Canada

Traci McFarlane, PhD, Ambulatory Care for Eating Disorders, University Health Network, Toronto General Hospital, and Department of Psychiatry, University of Toronto, Toronto, Ontario, Canada

Margaret L. McKelvie, MA, Department of Psychology, University of Colorado at Boulder, Boulder, Colorado

Marion Olmsted, PhD, Ambulatory Care for Eating Disorders, University Health Network, Toronto General Hospital, and Department of Psychiatry, University of Toronto, Toronto, Ontario, Canada

Anushka Pai, BA, Center for the Treatment and Study of Anxiety, University of Pennsylvania School of Medicine, Philadelphia, Pennsylvania

David S. Riggs, PhD, Center for the Treatment and Study of Anxiety, University of Pennsylvania School of Medicine, Philadelphia, Pennsylvania

Frederick Rotgers, PsyD, Department of Psychology, Philadelphia College of Osteopathic Medicine, Philadelphia, Pennsylvania

Karen Rowa, PhD, Anxiety Treatment and Research Centre, St. Joseph's Healthcare, and Department of Psychiatry and Behavioural Neurosciences, McMaster University, Hamilton, Ontario, Canada

Zindel V. Segal, PhD, Centre for Addiction and Mental Health and Department of Psychiatry, University of Toronto, Toronto, Ontario, Canada

Laura Sharp, MS, Department of Psychology, Philadelphia College of Osteopathic Medicine, Philadelphia, Pennsylvania

Nicholas Tarrier, PhD, Academic Division of Clinical Psychology, University of Manchester, Manchester, United Kingdom

Allison M. Waters, PhD, School of Psychology, Griffith University, Gold Coast, Australia

Mark A. Whisman, PhD, Department of Psychology, University of Colorado at Boulder, Boulder, Colorado

Preface

Over the past few decades, effective psychological treatments have been developed for assessing and treating people who suffer from a wide range of psychological problems (Antony & Barlow, 2002; Barlow, 2001). However, relatively little attention has been paid to the individuals who do not benefit fully from current treatments or experience a return of their symptoms some time after treatment has ended. This book fills that gap by providing detailed suggestions for how to maximize treatment outcomes following cognitive-behavioral therapy (CBT), particularly with challenging patients, and how to prevent relapse and recurrence.

This volume is organized around particular syndromes, with chapters on each of the major anxiety disorders, depression, bipolar disorder, schizophrenia, alcohol use disorders, eating disorders, and couple distress. Each chapter begins with a brief overview of the problem and a description of standard, evidence-based psychological treatments. In addition, a review of the literature on predictors of outcome following CBT is provided, followed by a detailed, practical discussion of clinical strategies for overcoming obstacles and improving outcomes during treatment. Examples of topics covered in many of the chapters include dealing with comorbidity, enhancing motivation and readiness for change, augmenting CBT using other approaches, improving homework compliance, and adapting standard treatment protocols to particular types of clinical presentations.

Each chapter also includes a detailed discussion of the factors that contribute to relapse and recurrence once treatment has ended. Practical strategies for preventing a return of symptoms are also reviewed. Although the specific guidelines vary from chapter to chapter, examples of strategies covered include the use of maintenance therapy (either occasional CBT visits, medications, or self-help approaches), strategies for managing stress, and recommendations for maintaining healthy lifestyle habits, such as proper diet, exercise, and sleep. Each chapter ends with a case example illustrating these strategies with a particularly challenging client.

We would like to thank several individuals who helped make this book possible. First, thank you to David Grant, Sam Katerji, and Eli Swartz for assistance with editing several chapters. Thanks as well to Jim Nageotte and the staff at The Guilford Press, who were involved in shaping this project from the beginning and transforming the manuscript into the book you are reading now. Finally, thanks to the contributing authors for their outstanding work.

REFERENCES

Antony, M. M., & Barlow, D. H. (Eds.). (2002). *Handbook of assessment and treatment planning for psychological disorders.* New York: Guilford Press.

Barlow, D. H. (Ed.). (2001). *Clinical handbook of psychological disorders* (3rd ed.). New York: Guilford Press.

MARTIN M. ANTONY
DEBORAH ROTH LEDLEY
RICHARD G. HEIMBERG

Contents

1   Panic Disorder and Agoraphobia   1
    Randi E. McCabe and Martin M. Antony

2   Social Anxiety Disorder   38
    Deborah Roth Ledley and Richard G. Heimberg

3   Generalized Anxiety Disorder   77
    Allison M. Waters and Michelle G. Craske

4   Obsessive–Compulsive Disorder   128
    Martin E. Franklin, David S. Riggs, and Anushka Pai

5   Posttraumatic Stress Disorder   174
    Norah C. Feeny and Edna B. Foa

6   Depression   204
    Karen Rowa, Peter J. Bieling, and Zindel V. Segal

7   Bipolar Disorder   246
    Dominic Lam and Warren Mansell

8   Eating Disorders   268
    Traci McFarlane, Jacqueline Carter, and Marion Olmsted

9   Schizophrenia   306
    Nicholas Tarrier

10   Alcohol Use Disorders   348
     Frederick Rotgers and Laura Sharp

11   Couple Distress   380
     Mark A. Whisman, Margaret L. McKelvie, and Yael Chatav

     Author Index   409

     Subject Index   425

IMPROVING OUTCOMES AND PREVENTING RELAPSE IN COGNITIVE-BEHAVIORAL THERAPY

Panic Disorder and Agoraphobia

RANDI E. McCABE
MARTIN M. ANTONY

OVERVIEW OF THE DISORDER

Although panic attacks may occur in the context of any anxiety disorder, *unexpected* or "out of the blue" panic attacks are the central feature of panic disorder. Panic disorder is characterized by recurrent unexpected panic attacks involving a sudden onset of intense fear or discomfort that is accompanied by physical symptoms (e.g., palpitations, sweating, and shaking), cognitive symptoms (i.e., fear of dying, losing control, or going crazy), or both. These unexpected episodes of panic are associated with persistent concern about future attacks and worry about the meaning or consequences of attacks (that the panic may lead to a "catastrophic" outcome such as having a heart attack, fainting, loss of bowel control, etc.). In addition, panic attacks are often accompanied by behavioral change in response to the attacks such as avoiding certain activities or places or engaging in safety behaviors (e.g., only going out when accompanied or when carrying certain objects such as a mobile phone, water, or medication) (American Psychiatric Association, 2000). Data from the National Comorbidity Survey indicate a lifetime prevalence of 3.5% for panic disorder (Eaton, Kessler, Wittchen, & Magee, 1994).

Panic disorder is often accompanied by *agoraphobia*, which refers to anxiety about, or avoidance of, situations in which it may not be easy to escape or get help in the event of experiencing panic symptoms (American Psychiatric Association, 2000). Data from the National Comorbidity Survey indicate a lifetime prevalence of 1.5% for panic disorder with agoraphobia (Eaton et al., 1994). Typical situations that individuals with panic disorder fear or avoid include crowded places, grocery stores and shopping malls, public transportation, being home alone, driving in heavy traffic or on highways, movie theatres and arenas, airplanes, waiting in line, taking walks, restaurants, enclosed places (e.g., elevators), and open spaces (e.g., parks). Patterns of avoidance associated with agoraphobia are variable. Some individuals avoid just a few situations such as crowds and flying, whereas others avoid a much wider range of situations. It is common for individuals with moderate to severe agoraphobia to describe a "safe zone" or a certain radius around their home in which they feel comfortable. Travel outside this "safe zone" is particularly difficult if not completely avoided, especially if unaccompanied. Most individuals with panic disorder also report symptoms of agoraphobia (Eaton et al., 1994).

Panic disorder is more common in females than in males. For example, one study based on the National Comorbidity Survey found the lifetime occurrence of panic disorder was roughly two and one half times higher in females than in males (Eaton et al., 1994). Compared to men, women tend to have more severe and chronic forms of panic disorder with agoraphobia (Yonkers et al., 1998), increased agoraphobic avoidance symptoms (Turgeon, Marchand, & Dupuis, 1998), and increased respiration-related symptoms (difficulty breathing, feeling faint, and feeling smothered) during panic attacks (Sheikh, Leskin, & Klein, 2002).

Panic disorder is often a chronic condition (Keller et al., 1994) that is associated with significantly reduced quality of life (Keller et al., 1994), increased health care utilization (Klerman, Weissman, Ouellette, Johnson, & Greenwald, 1991), and high social and economic costs (Hofmann & Barlow, 1999).

Although there are a number of empirically supported treatment options for panic disorder, some individuals do not respond to treatment and for others, treatment leads only to a partial response (Rosenbaum, Pollack, & Pollack, 1996). Thus, we are challenged to continue to improve our current treatments and to further our understanding of the mechanisms underlying suboptimal treatment response and relapse following treatment. In the first part of this chapter, we provide an overview of empirically supported treatments, focusing specifically on cognitive-behavioral therapy and pharmacotherapy. We then review predictors of treatment outcome and relapse, highlighting barriers to successful treatment, and providing practical clinical strategies for improving response to cognitive-behavioral treatment and preventing recurrence of symptoms. In the final part of the chapter, we present a case to illustrate specific treatment challenges that often arise and how to overcome these obstacles to recovery.

OVERVIEW OF EMPIRICALLY
SUPPORTED TREATMENTS

Cognitive-behavioral therapy and pharmacotherapy are the only approaches to treating panic disorder that are well established, based on a large number of controlled studies.

Cognitive-Behavioral Therapy

Cognitive-behavioral therapy (CBT) is an empirically supported psycho-therapeutic intervention for panic disorder and is listed as a first-line treatment in practice guidelines for the treatment of panic disorder (e.g., American Psychiatric Association, 1998; Anxiety Review Panel, 2000). CBT approaches have tended to include various combinations of strategies, such as psychoeducation, cognitive restructuring, interoceptive exposure (i.e., exposure to feared symptoms), *in vivo* exposure (i.e., exposure to feared situations), and relaxation-based strategies (e.g., breathing retraining). Combined in any of a number of different ways, these strategies tend to be useful for reducing the frequency of panic, agoraphobic avoidance, and other features of panic disorder (for detailed review, see Antony & Swinson, 2000; Taylor, 2000).

There are a number of different CBT approaches to treating panic disorder that have been developed (for a review, see Margraf, Barlow, Clark, & Telch, 1993). For example, Clark et al. (1994, 1999) developed a cognitive-behavioral approach that focuses on cognitive restructuring and behavioral experiments to challenge catastrophic beliefs about physical sensations and phobic situations. In contrast, panic control treatment (PCT; Barlow & Craske, 2000) combines psychoeducation, breathing retraining, cognitive restructuring, interoceptive exposure, and *in vivo* exposure to the extent that agoraphobic avoidance is a problem (for a review, see Antony & McCabe, 2002). Sensation-focused intensive therapy (S-FIT; Heinrichs, Spiegel, & Hofmann, 2002) combines the active ingredients of PCT with exposure techniques for agoraphobia and relapse prevention strategies, along with a self-study workbook that may be applied in an intensive treatment format over 8 days or in a group over 3 months.

Regardless of the specific packaging of treatment strategies, CBT for panic disorder has demonstrated efficacy in research settings (e.g., Barlow, Gorman, Shear, & Woods, 2000). Although there is less known about the effectiveness of CBT for panic disorder outside the research setting, initial findings indicate a comparable treatment response in community mental health and other service-oriented settings (e.g., Wade, Treat, & Stuart, 1998). The length of treatment is typically 10–12 sessions. CBT leads to reductions in anxiety symptoms, anxious cognitions, agoraphobic avoidance, and depressive symptoms (e.g., Hahlweg, Fiegenbaum, Frank, Schroeder, & von Witzleben, 2001). CBT for panic disorder has also been found to improve physical health symptom ratings, independent from its impact on anxiety symptoms (Schmidt et al., 2003).

Pharmacotherapy

With respect to pharmacotherapy, treatment options include antidepressants, anxiolytics, and combined treatments (most commonly medication plus CBT). Selective serotonin reuptake inhibitors (SSRIs) are effective treatments for panic disorder and are also likely to help with certain comorbid disorders such as depression (den Boer & Slaap, 1998). SSRIs are recommended as drugs of first choice with a treatment period of 12–24 months and a slow discontinuation over a period of 4–6 months (Ballenger et al., 1998). Other medication options include certain tricyclic antidepressants (TCAs), other antidepressants (e.g., venlafaxine; Pollack et al., 1996), and high-potency benzodiazepines (for reviews, see Antony & Swinson, 2000; Roy-Byrne & Cowley, 2002; Weissman, 2002). A recent study comparing SSRIs to TCAs using an effect-size analysis indicated no significant differences with regard to efficacy or tolerability in short-term trials (Otto, Tuby, Gould, McLean, & Pollack, 2001).

Despite the number of medications that have demonstrated antipanic efficacy, relapse rates upon discontinuation are high (Ballenger, 1993; Toni et al., 2000), and between 20 and 40% of individuals do not respond to treatment (Slaap & den Boer, 2001). Predictors of nonresponse include longer duration of illness, greater pretreatment severity (e.g., more severe agoraphobic avoidance, higher panic frequency, and certain comorbid disorders), and personality disorders (for a review, see Slaap & den Boer, 2001). The physician's level of experience has also been associated with outcome (Gorman et al., 2003).

Cognitive-Behavioral Therapy versus Pharmacotherapy

Meta-analytic studies comparing treatment approaches indicate that pharmacological treatments, CBT, and combinations of these approaches are effective for reducing the symptoms of panic disorder both in the short term (van Balkom et al., 1997) and at follow-up (ranging from 1 month to 8 years) (Bakker, van Balkom, Spinhoven, Blaauw, & van Dyck, 1998). These studies also indicate greater dropout associated with pharmacotherapy than CBT (Bakker et al., 1998). For example, attrition rates in one meta-analytic study were 5.6%, 19.8%, and 22.0% for cognitive-behavioral treatments, pharmacological treatments, and combined cognitive-behavioral and pharmacological treatment, respectively (Gould, Otto, & Pollack, 1995).

Findings from meta-analytic studies comparing the relative and combined efficacy of pharmacological and cognitive-behavioral treatments for panic disorder are mixed. Some research indicates that antidepressants combined with *in vivo* exposure are more effective than cognitive-behavioral interventions alone for short-term (van Balkom et al. 1997) and long-term (Bakker et al., 1998) outcome, particularly for agoraphobic avoidance. Other studies indicate relatively few differences between CBT, medication, and their combination in acute treatment outcome (Barlow et al., 2000). However, in the long-term, cognitive-behavioral treatments appear to be more effective in maintaining treatment gains and preventing relapse than pharmacological treatments (Barlow et al., 2000; Gould et al., 1995).

Need for Strategies to Improve Treatment Response and Prevent Relapse

Despite the demonstrated efficacy of CBT interventions for panic disorder, there is still a need to improve treatment response, particularly in the long term, for a number of reasons.

Poor Initial Response to Treatment

Some treatment completers do not respond to CBT. For example, in one effectiveness trial, 87% of participants were panic-free at the end of treatment (Wade et al., 1998), indicating that more than 1 in 10 patients did not respond optimally. Furthermore, many people who are panic-free may continue to have significant agoraphobic avoidance, and indeed, this may be why they are panic-free (i.e., they do not have panic attacks because they avoid panic-related situations). In one study, 89% of treatment completers were identified as being panic-free at 1-year follow-up, although 28% continued to report significant agoraphobic concerns (Stuart, Treat, & Wade, 2000). The issue of what qualifies as good treatment response is particularly relevant for patients with moderate to severe agoraphobia. For example, Clark et al. (1994) found that 30% of patients who had received cognitive-behavioral therapy did not meet criteria for high end-state functioning (defined as zero panic attacks in the month preceding assessment and a clinical severity rating of less than or equal to 2 on scale from 0 to 8 or "very severely disturbing-disabling") at 15-month follow-up. Thus, additional treatment strategies are needed to target this group of patients.

Occurrence of Residual Symptoms during Follow-Up

Even if a good response to treatment is achieved, residual symptoms are common. In one study, one-third of a sample that had achieved a good response to treatment experienced persistent residual anxiety and somatic symptoms at 1-year follow-up (Corominas, Guerrero, & Vallejo, 2002). In addition, across a number of studies, a sizable percentage of individuals continue to report panic attacks at follow-up assessments: 17% at 6-month follow-up (Telch et al., 1993); 11% at 1-year follow-up (Stuart et al., 2000); and 13% at 2-year follow-up (Craske, Brown, & Barlow, 1991). Follow-up data beyond 2 years are almost nonexistent.

Fluctuating Course of Panic Disorder

The fluctuating course of panic disorder is not necessarily reflected in typical measures of outcome, as evidenced by the discrepancy between the percentage of panic-free patients (usually measured in the month preceding the assessment) and the percentage of patients meeting high end-state functioning criteria (e.g., Clark et al., 1994; Craske et al., 1991). For example, T. Brown and Barlow (1995) reported that 74.6% of their sample was panic-free 2 years after completing CBT, but only 57% met high end-state functioning criteria. This discrepancy may be due to the fact that most studies use cross-sectional methods that do not capture the fluctuating course of panic symptoms experienced by many patients following CBT for panic disorder (T. Brown & Barlow, 1995). For example, more than one-third of the sample classified as panic-free at 2-year follow-up reported experiencing panic attacks in the year preceding assessment (T. Brown & Barlow, 1995). In addition, 27% of participants who had completed a course of CBT for panic disorder sought out further treatment, although further treatment did not confer additional improvement (T. Brown & Barlow, 1995).

Attrition

A sizable proportion of individuals drop out of treatment. For example, Wade et al. (1998) reported a dropout rate of 26% among patients receiving treatment in a community mental health center. High rates of attrition may be particularly problematic in clinical service settings, compared to those in clinical research settings. Recall that Gould et al. (1995), in their meta-analysis of studies of the efficacy of CBT, reported that the average rate of attrition was only 5.6%.

Outcome Study Exclusion Criteria

Many patients who are characteristic of those seen in clinical settings are excluded from randomized controlled trials because of the presence of psychotic symptoms, bipolar disorder, organic conditions, substance use disorders, moderate to severe agoraphobic avoidance, concurrent or recent treatment, suicidality, or additional diagnoses in need of immediate treatment (e.g., depression). For example, in one review, the average inclusion rate for studies of the treatment of panic disorder was 36% (Westen & Morrison, 2001). These high exclusion rates may inflate the efficacy of CBT for panic disorder, raising questions about how well findings can be generalized to real-life treatment settings. In support of this view, Westen and Morrison (2001) found that exclusion rates were positively correlated with the percentage of patients included in the study who showed improvement (Westen & Morrison, 2001). However, a benchmarking study conducted in a community mental health clinic and using less stringent exclusion criteria yielded results similar to those obtained in research settings (Wade et al., 1998).

PREDICTORS OF TREATMENT OUTCOME

After a quarter century of research on predictors of response to CBT for panic disorder, findings are largely mixed, and there are few clear prognostic indicators. Different methodologies (e.g., different predictor variables and measurement tools), variations across studies in the CBT components used, and limited sample sizes make it difficult to draw consistent conclusions. This section reviews factors that have been investigated as possible predictors of outcome, both in the short and the long term.

Demographic Characteristics

Studies indicate that demographic variables are generally not predictive of treatment outcome (e.g., Sharp & Power, 1999). CBT for panic disorder appears to be effective regardless of age or gender. However, other important demographic variables such as cultural and ethnic background have yet to be adequately examined.

Personality and Personality Disorders

Although there are a few studies suggesting that personality variables are not predictive of treatment outcome (e.g., Massion et al., 2002), the majority indicate that personality pathology has a negative impact on the outcome of CBT for panic disorder (for a review, see Mennin & Heimberg, 2000). The presence of personality disorders has been associated with poorer outcome and slower progress in CBT for panic disorder (e.g., Keijsers, Hoogduin, & Schaap, 1994; Marchand, Goyer, Dupuis, & Mainguy, 1998). With regard to broad personality dimensions, higher levels of extraversion have been associated with improved outcome (Sharp & Power, 1999), and lower levels of extraversion predict higher rates of residual symptoms following successful treatment (Corominas et al., 2002).

Symptom Severity

The severity of the core features of panic disorder appears to be a strong prognostic indicator of outcome. Severity of agoraphobic complaints and catastrophic agoraphobic cognitions were both found to be significant predictors of poor treatment outcome (Keijsers et al., 1994). Lower levels of self-rated anxiety, lower panic frequency, lower levels of agoraphobic avoidance, and higher levels of social and occupational functioning at pretreatment have been related to improved treatment outcome (with CBT or fluvoxamine; Sharp & Power, 1999). In addition, change in anxiety sensitivity (particularly the physical concerns subscale of the Anxiety Sensitivity Index; Peterson & Reiss, 1993) is a significant predictor of symptom change following CBT treatment (Schmidt & Bates, 2003). Severity of symptoms is also a significant predictor of long-term outcome following CBT for panic disorder. Increased panic frequency, increased agoraphobic avoidance, and social maladjustment have been related to outcome at 6-month follow-up (Sharp & Power, 1999). Pretreatment severity of panic disorder has also been related to end-state functioning and panic-free status at 24-month follow-up after CBT for panic disorder (T. Brown & Barlow, 1995).

Therapist Qualities

Although therapist characteristics have been associated with treatment outcome (Huppert et al., 2001; Williams & Chambless, 1990), neither the quality of the therapeutic relationship (Keijsers et al., 1994) nor the patient's perception of the therapist (de Beurs, van Dyck, Lange, & van Balkom, 1995) appears to be a significant factor in treatment outcome. Evidence is mixed for the relationship of therapist experience and outcome, with some studies showing that therapist experience is related to outcome (Huppert et al., 2001) and other studies suggesting that it is not (Halhweg et al., 2001).

Depression

Evaluation of the impact of major depressive disorder on the outcome of CBT for panic disorder has been equivocal (for a review, see Mennin & Heimberg, 2000). Some studies indicate that depression has an adverse impact on outcome (e.g., Laberge, Gauthier, Côté, Plamondon, & Cormier, 1993). Comorbid major depression was associated with lower end-state functioning (Rief, Trenkamp, Auer, & Fichter, 2000) and poorer outcome 6 months following CBT (Sharp & Power, 1999). However, other studies indicate that individuals with major depressive disorder may be less likely to be panic-free immediately after treatment but not at follow-up (e.g., T. Brown, Antony, & Barlow, 1995). In addition, the response to treatment of individuals with panic disorder and depression is comparable to individuals with panic disorder without comorbid depression (Chudzik, McCabe, Antony, & Swinson, 2001; McLean, Woody, Taylor, & Koch, 1998; Rief et al., 2000).

Other Factors

Although pain symptoms are associated with higher levels of anxiety and mood symptoms in individuals with panic disorder, they have not been found to significantly affect response to CBT (Schmidt, Santiago, Trakowski, & Kendren, 2002). Other factors that do not appear to affect treatment outcome include the duration of the disorder (T. Brown & Barlow, 1995; Hahlweg et al., 2001), number of treatment sessions (Halhweg et al., 2001), marital dissatisfaction (Keijsers et al., 1994), perceived parental upbringing (de Beurs et al., 1995), and comorbidity with other anxiety disorders (T. Brown et al., 1995).

Other factors associated with treatment outcome include motivation for treatment (Keijsers et al., 1994), chronic life stress (Wade, Monroe, & Michelson, 1993), and expressed emotion among family members, such as emotional overinvolvement or hostility (Chambless & Steketee, 1999). Use of psychotropic medication during treatment (primarily benzodiazepines) has been associated with poorer outcome at 24-month follow-up (T. Brown & Barlow, 1995). However, recent evidence suggests that discontinuation of medication does not affect outcome following cognitive-behavioral therapy for panic disorder; nor does it lead to greater likelihood of relapse at 1-year follow-up (G. Brown, Bieling, Beck, Newman, & Levy, 2001).

Evidence for homework compliance as a predictor of treatment outcome is mixed. Some studies indicate a relationship between homework compliance and treatment outcome (e.g., Edelman & Chambless, 1993) and others do not (e.g., Woods, Chambless, & Steketee, 2002).

Predictors of Dropout

Initial studies examining motivation for change based on Prochaska and colleagues' continuum of readiness for therapeutic change, the stages-of-change model (Prochaska & DiClemente, 1992; Prochaska & Norcross, 1994), indicate that stage of change is a predictor of whether individuals complete treatment. In a preliminary study examining stages of change as predictors of response to CBT for panic disorder, individuals classified as being in one of the preaction stages (precontemplation, contemplation) were more likely to drop out of treatment than those in the action stage (Dozois, Westra, Collins, Fung, & Garry, 2004). Other research has found that level of motivation and level of education have small, yet significant, associations with dropout from CBT for panic disorder (Keijsers, Kampman, & Hoogduin, 2001).

Personality psychopathology and initial symptom severity do not appear to be associated with dropout from CBT (Keijsers et al., 2001). In a randomized controlled trial of panic disorder conducted by Grilo et al. (1998), dropout was associated with household income, negative treatment attitudes, less education, shorter length of previous treatment, increased anxiety sensitivity, decreased agoraphobic avoidance, and a coping style of seeking social support. Psychiatric comorbidity and personality style were not related to dropout.

COMMON TREATMENT OBSTACLES AND PRACTICAL STRATEGIES FOR IMPROVING OUTCOME

Based on our review of predictors of treatment outcome, this next section presents useful strategies for enhancing treatment success. Treatment strategies are organized around common obstacles that arise in the various stages of readiness to change (Prochaska & DiClemente, 1992) and when implementing the different treatment components.

Motivation

CBT strategies for panic disorder are based on the assumption that an individual is ready for change and willing to actively work in therapy. However, not all individuals who present for treatment are ready to actively engage in the therapy process. There may be a number of reasons for resistance to change including fear of change, fear of treatment strategies, and secondary benefits derived from symptoms (e.g., attention from family and decreased responsibility). Prochaska and DiClemente (1992) have articulated a series of stages of change based on their transtheoretical model: precontemplation, contemplation, preparation, action, and maintenance. Although this model was originally applied in the addictions field, it has proven to be useful in conceptualizing resistance to treatment and treatment failure in other areas as well (e.g., Dozois et al., 2004; Hasler, Delsignore, Milos, Buddeberg, & Schnyder, 2004). Applying this model to panic disorder may be useful for selecting appropriate treatment strategies and for working with the patient at his or her stage of change using motivational enhancement techniques (Miller & Rollnick, 2002) prior to CBT. Motivational enhancement techniques include validation of the patient's particular stage of change through expression of empathy, identifying discrepancies between the patient's goals and problem behaviors (e.g., avoidance), "rolling with resistance" by emphasizing personal control and approaching treatment as an experiment, and supporting self-efficacy by focusing on personal strengths and highlighting positives (for a review, see Miller & Rollnick, 2002).

In the *precontemplation* stage, an individual does not yet acknowledge that there is a problem. Although most individuals with panic disorder will acknowledge that they have a problem, they may not view the problem as having a psychological basis and, therefore, they may be unwilling to engage in psychotherapeutic interventions. Given that 10 of the 13 panic attack symptoms (e.g., heart palpitations, sweating, and dizziness) are physical in nature, it is not surprising that a number of individuals with panic disorder continue to believe that their symptoms have a physiological basis, despite medical tests to the contrary. Treatment strategies for individuals in the precontemplation stage of change include building a therapeutic alliance and raising awareness about the nature of anxiety and panic through psychoeducation and reflection on the individual's own personal experiences with panic.

In the *contemplation* stage, an individual is aware that there is a problem but is not ready to complete the steps necessary for treating the problem. A number of individuals with panic disorder who present for treatment may not be ready to engage in CBT for a variety of reasons, including fear of the treatment strategies (e.g., exposure to panic symptoms and to situations that the individual avoids), lack of time or commitment to treatment due to other priorities or stressors, and possible benefits of not changing (e.g., spouse does all the driving and manages the household). Treatment strategies for individuals in the contemplation stage of change include psychoeducation regarding the nature of anxiety and panic, exploration of the benefits and costs of engaging in treatment, and a thorough explanation of the treatment and how it works.

In the *preparation* stage, an individual is ready for action and is taking the initial steps necessary for change. At this point, treatment strategies include setting realistic goals and discussion of the treatment process and underlying rationale. In the *action* stage, an individual is ready to engage in active treatment strategies for symptom control, and this may be the best time to proceed with CBT for panic disorder. Once symptom control is achieved, a person may enter the *maintenance* stage. At this point, treatment strategies should focus on relapse prevention and preparing for potential setbacks or recurrence of anxiety and panic.

To assess motivation for treatment and to determine an individual's current stage of change, the University of Rhode Island Change Assessment Scale (URICA; McConnaughy, Prochaska, & Velicer, 1983) is a useful tool. The URICA is a brief, 32-item scale that assesses attitudes toward changing problem behaviors and four stages of change: precontemplation, contemplation, action, and maintenance. URICA scores may be used to select treatment strategies and also to measure outcome. Although the URICA has demonstrated reliability and validity in an alcoholism treatment population, researchers have only just begun to examine responses to this measure in anxiety-disordered individuals (e.g., Dozois et al., 2004).

Therapy Rationale

Explaining the rationale for CBT for panic disorder is a very important and critical activity at the initiation of therapy. It is at this point that the individual is first engaged in active treatment. It is important to explain the treatment procedures in a way that makes sense to the individual so that the active stage of treatment can begin. For treatment to be successful, the patient must "buy into" treatment. Explaining the treatment rationale using simple language to which he or she can relate is imperative. If the individual has doubts about the therapist, the treatment, or his or her ability to complete the treatment, therapy may end before it begins.

A number of obstacles may arise when explaining the therapy rationale. A common reaction that occurs when people are given information on the effectiveness of CBT for panic disorder is one of disbelief in the treatment strategies (e.g., "I know this works for others, but I really don't think it will work for me," or "I have lived with this so long and tried everything, so I don't see how this is going to be any different"). One intervention for addressing this obstacle follows Miller and Rollnick's (2002) "roll with resistance" strategy. Instead of engaging in a debate about the effectiveness of CBT, it is more useful to agree with the individual and normalize the ambivalent reaction (e.g., "I am not surprised that you feel that way. It is common for people to have difficulty believing that these strategies will be helpful") and then to roll with the resistance (e.g., "I realize that it is hard to imagine that this treatment approach will be helpful to you; the best thing to do is to keep an open mind and try the strategies as an experiment. In this way, you can see if they are helpful based on your own experience. When you think about how much your panic has interfered in your life, what do you have to lose by trying this approach? What do you possibly have to gain?") (for further strategies relating to the treatment rationale, see Addis & Carpenter, 2000).

If the patient raises doubts about the benefits of a psychological intervention for a problem that he or she perceives as being primarily biological (genetics, chemical imbalance in the brain, etc.), it can be useful to acknowledge the role that biology plays in the etiology and maintenance of panic disorder. In addition, the therapist can take this opportunity to discuss the interactions between biological and psychological functions and ways in which psychological interventions can influence biological processes. A useful analogy is that of weight control. Although weight and physical fitness are influenced by genetics and other biological processes, they can also be influenced by behavior. People who have a genetic predisposition to be anxious may have to work harder at managing their anxiety than people who are genetically predisposed to be calm, but that does not mean it cannot be done. In fact, the long-term data support psychological interventions for panic disorder over medication treatments, despite evidence supporting the contributions of biological factors to the disorder.

If an individual does not express reservations about the treatment, it does not mean that he or she does not have any. Often, individuals have doubts about the treatment but are hesitant to express them. Thus, it is important to specifically ask the individual about his or her understanding of the treatment rationale and whether there are any questions, concerns, or reservations (e.g., "Does this treatment make sense to you?" "How do you think this treatment applies to you? Can you tell me about any doubts or concerns that you may have about this treatment?" "Do you have any questions about anything that we have covered regarding the treatment and how it works?").

A major emphasis in CBT for panic disorder is on exposure to one's fears. This treatment component is typically scary for patients and may cause them to have second thoughts about engaging in treatment. A useful intervention for addressing patients' concerns about exposure is to normalize the concerns and to emphasize the gradual pace of treatment and the patient's personal control (e.g., "It makes sense that hearing about exposure sounds very scary for you. Before coming to treatment, most people cope with their anxiety by avoiding situations, and here I am suggesting that you do the opposite of avoid. Avoidance is a strategy that seems to work in the short term. However, avoidance does not work in the long term, or you would not be here today. Avoidance provides "short-term gain" for "long-term pain," whereas exposure involves learning to tolerate "short-term pain" for "long-term gain." Considering all the reasons that brought you in for help right now, do you think you might be willing to try this treatment?").

Treatment Goals

The next step in CBT for panic disorder is to establish realistic treatment goals. Although patients with panic disorder often express the desire for complete symptom elimination, such a goal is usually not realistic. Anxiety and fear are part of normal human experience, and most patients obtain only partial symptom relief following treatment. Thus, it is essential to have a discussion regarding what the patient will realistically get out of therapy. This may take place in the context of a discussion about the important roles that anxiety and fear play in our lives. Realistic therapy goals include learning new ways of responding to anxiety and panic (e.g., as uncomfortable physical sensations rather than harbingers of danger or catastrophe), developing a set of skills to manage symptoms, increasing one's tolerance of discomfort, and taking back control of one's life.

Psychoeducation

Psychoeducation in CBT for panic disorder involves increasing the patient's level of knowledge and awareness of the nature of anxiety and panic. One common risk associated with this treatment component is the therapist being drawn into doing all the talking, making it difficult to tell whether the patient fully understands the information provided. Thus the therapist should strive to:

- Make the psychoeducational portion of treatment more interactive and less didactic.
- Use a whiteboard, chalkboard, or easel to illustrate the CBT model of panic in a visual way.
- Ask frequent questions to assess the patient's level of understanding.
- Ask the patient for examples based on his or her personal experience that illustrate the concepts under discussion.
- Use in-session experiments.

Cognitive Strategies

Cognitive strategies for panic focus on examining the evidence for anxious thoughts with an emphasis toward shifting to more realistic ways of interpreting or perceiving triggers of anxiety and panic. A number of obstacles are commonly associated with this treatment component.

It is common for patients to view being anxious or having a panic attack as a defeat or failure. This response results in reduced motivation for treatment. To overcome this obstacle, episodes of anxiety or panic should be reframed as opportunities to learn and to practice newly acquired skills rather than as signs of defect or failure. The therapist should encourage patients to focus on what they did behaviorally in the situation (e.g., stayed in the mall despite feeling anxious) rather than on how they felt (e.g., whether they had a panic attack).

Another common obstacle is for patients to report that they do not have any thoughts (e.g., "The panic comes on so quick that I don't know what my thoughts are."). One strategy to overcome this challenge is to educate the patient on the automaticity of thoughts (e.g., "It is common for people to feel like they don't have any thoughts because emotional reactions can happen so quickly that they feel automatic") and then to focus on slowing things down the next time that the patient feels anxious to examine what triggered the anxious feelings and how he or she responded to them. Instead of reacting automatically, encourage the patient to practice taking a step back from the emotion and to observe feelings, thoughts, and behaviors in an analytical way. Have patients ask themselves questions to elicit their thoughts (e.g., "What was going through my mind right before I started feeling panicky?" "What am I afraid might happen?"). If the patient is having difficulty eliciting cognitions while sitting in the therapist's office, exposure to the feared situation may increase awareness of his or her anxious thoughts. If these suggestions are ineffective, it may be useful for the therapist to list some of the common thoughts that often arise among people with panic disorder to see whether any of these ring true for the patient.

For some people, the cognitive work may be difficult. Patients may continue to report that they have no thoughts despite repeated attempts to elicit them. Other people may be less cognitively minded. If this is the case, therapy should emphasize more simple, straightforward cognitive strategies (e.g., focusing on a small number of cognitive distortions, repeating key concepts within and between sessions, providing examples to illustrate important concepts, and using cue cards to counter common anxious thoughts). If the individual continues to have difficulty using the cognitive strategies, therapy should focus more on behavioral strategies, such as exposure. Behavioral strategies are powerful methods for changing cognitions.

Another common obstacle associated with cognitive techniques is that patients have difficulty believing the alternative, more realistic ways of thinking. It is common to hear, "I know rationally that my feared outcome will not happen but I still really *feel* that it will." One strategy to address this problem is to have patients externalize their anxiety. Rather than seeing anxiety as a sign of true danger that requires a response, anxiety can be conceptualized as stemming from "sneaky thoughts that try to trick you." It may also be helpful to have patients rate the level of their belief in the likelihood of the feared outcome on a 0–100 scale, *based on how they feel.* For example, an individual may know realistically that the chance of vomiting during a panic attack is about 0% based on his or her own experience (i.e., having had hundreds of panic attacks but not having vomited) but may still view the likelihood of vomiting as high based on the intensity of his or her fear. In these cases, behavioral strategies (e.g., exposure) are often useful for challenging patients' anxious predictions as well as illustrating that thoughts (i.e., "I could vomit") do not equal behavior (i.e., vomiting).

It may also complicate cognitive work if the patient describes thoughts in vague and general terms. A practical strategy to deal with this problem is to help patients articulate their thoughts in a very specific and precise manner.

For example, thoughts such as "I will panic" and "I need to get out of here" are vague, as the specific meaning of these thoughts to the individual (e.g., the feared consequence) is not clear. Thoughts should be elaborated so that the therapist is able to perceive the precise meaning of the thought for the patient (e.g., "I will panic and pass out in front of everyone" or "I need to get out of here or else I will lose control of my bowels and have an accident").

Given that one predictor of poorer treatment outcome is a tendency to have more severe catastrophic agoraphobic cognitions, improved response may depend on developing more realistic patterns of thinking. If an individual has trouble countering his or her anxious thoughts in a specific situation, it may be useful to develop a cue card with questions that he or she can ask to elicit evidence (e.g., "What is the worst thing that can happen in this situation?").

It is also helpful to emphasize that developing more realistic thinking does not happen overnight. Rather, it is a skill that takes repeated practice to build. In any situation, there are always a number of appraisals that can be made. It is an important goal of treatment to increase the patient's awareness of other appraisals beyond anxiety-based interpretations. Over time, these alternate appraisals will become easier to generate. As alternate appraisals are made, the anxious appraisal becomes less powerful.

Exposure Strategies

Situational and interoceptive exposure are central components of CBT for panic disorder. One obstacle that often arises in the context of exposure is patients' reluctance to confront feared situations and sensations. Presenting the rationale for exposure in a credible way is a critical first step for overcoming this obstacle. In addition, it is often useful to deal with anxiety about exposure exercises by breaking them down into more manageable tasks and taking steps more gradually (e.g., riding a bus with a friend before riding a bus alone). Huppert and Baker-Morissette (2003) emphasize the notion of *avoidance as a choice*. In this way, the patient's response can be reframed with an emphasis on personal control instead of being controlled by anxiety (e.g., "I can't take the bus" vs. "I am anxious about taking the bus and choose not to do so").

Despite repeated exposure practice, some patients may report that their fear does not decrease. This may be due to heightened stress in the person's life, practices that are too brief or too infrequent, catastrophic thinking that does not change as a result of exposure alone, or the presence of subtle safety behaviors (e.g., distraction) that prevent extinction of the fear. If a person's fear does not decrease over the course of treatment, these issues should be evaluated and addressed directly if they appear to be affecting the individual's progress.

In addition to distraction, subtle safety behaviors include carrying safe objects (e.g., medication, gum, water, and a paper bag to breathe into), seeking reassurance (e.g., about personal safety or the meaning of physical symptoms), checking (e.g., monitoring physical symptoms), maintaining contact with others (e.g., being accompanied by a safe person or carrying a mobile phone or pager), staying near exits or bathrooms, using alcohol or drugs, or controlling the environment (e.g., wearing short sleeve shirts in winter or not using the heater to control physical symptoms). Ideally, safety behaviors should be identified during the initial assessment. However, it is common for some behaviors to go undetected until part way through treatment because the patient is unaware of the behavior or the function of the behavior and how it may affect treatment. The therapist should be vigilant for any safety behaviors when reviewing exposure practices. Once identified, safety behaviors should be incorporated as therapy targets during exposure.

Breathing Retraining

One obstacle that sometimes arises with breathing retraining is that it can become relied on as a subtle avoidance strategy, thus interfering with the course of treatment. For example, a patient may use diaphragmatic breathing to avoid feeling anxious and thus perpetuate catastrophic thoughts about the consequences of anxiety and the need to engage in safety behaviors to reduce discomfort. Unless a patient clearly has a tendency to hyperventilate, breathing retraining is not considered a necessary therapeutic ingredient and can be excluded (Antony & Swinson, 2000; Schmidt et al., 2000). If breathing retraining is used, it should be in the context of reducing initial physical symptoms of hyperventilation, or as a way of managing general feelings of stress and anxiety, rather than to avoid experiencing anxiety or panic. If breathing retraining appears to be serving the latter function, it should be discontinued.

Homework Compliance

Homework is essential for transferring skills learned in treatment to real-life situations that the patient encounters and for ensuring successful treatment outcome. Predictors of homework compliance include age and employment status, with older and unemployed individuals complying more with homework (Schmidt & Woolaway-Bickel, 2000). Therapist ratings of homework compliance have been found to be significantly related to treatment outcome (Schmidt & Woolaway-Bickel, 2000). Homework noncompliance is an obstacle that may arise for many reasons. As illustrated in Table 1.1, troubleshooting strategies should be chosen according to the underlying reason for incompletion of homework.

   With regard to CBT outcome for panic disorder, evidence suggests that it is more important to focus on homework quality versus quantity (Schmidt & Woolaway-Bickel, 2000). Thus, the therapist should emphasize the need to do homework following the recommended guidelines (e.g., completing the same prolonged exposure practice repeatedly, ideally until one's fear has decreased)

TABLE 1.1. Troubleshooting Strategies for Managing Homework Noncompliance

Reason for homework noncompliance	Troubleshooting strategy
The patient does not understand the homework task.	• Review homework task including specific details. Complete a practice exercise or example monitoring form during the session. • Provide homework assignments in writing.
Exposure practice is too difficult.	• Break down practice into more manageable tasks. • Conduct therapist-assisted exposures. • Use a family member or friend as a helper.
There is no time to practice.	• Schedule practices during normal activities (e.g., drive to work instead of being driven by someone else). • Take a week off work to practice exposure full time. • Hire a babysitter to care for the children, thereby freeing up time for exposure practices. • Discuss priorities and motivation for treatment.
There is no opportunity to practice.	• Plan out homework practices in session. Have a backup plan in case the original plan falls through.
The patient lacks motivation to complete homework assignments.	• Use motivational enhancement strategies. Review benefits and costs of continuing with treatment vs. putting treatment on hold.
The assigned homework seems irrelevant.	• Review connection of homework to therapy goals. Have patient (rather than the therapist) generate homework task (for exposure).

rather than simply completing a large quantity of homework (e.g., completing seven brief exposures, each in a different situation).

Other Strategies for Improving Treatment Outcome

The outcome of CBT for panic disorder may be improved by increasing the length of treatment as well as the frequency of sessions. Including a family member may also be useful in treatment, particularly for exposures. It is also helpful to include a psychoeducation session for family members so they can learn to take a supportive role without accommodating or reinforcing symptoms or dependence. This session can also prepare family members for the change in roles within the family that may occur as the patient develops greater independence.

When panic disorder is complicated by the presence of medical conditions, treatment may need to be adapted accordingly. For individuals with medical conditions (asthma, diabetes, etc.) that produce symptoms that are similar to those associated with panic, therapy should help the patient to differentiate between the symptoms of panic and those of the complicating condition. Interoceptive exposures may also need to be modified depending on the medical condition. For example, an individual with panic disorder and emphysema will not be able to engage in hyperventilation, and it may not be advisable for a woman who is in the latter stages of pregnancy to jog vigorously on the spot to raise her heart rate. A team approach is required, in which the physician treating the medical condition is consulted to determine the safety and appropriateness of various interoceptive exposure exercises.

Treatment may also need to be adapted for particular presentations of symptoms. For example, for individuals with moderate to severe agoraphobia, the intensity or length of exposure sessions should be increased, *in vivo* therapist-assisted exposure should be utilized, and additional exposure sessions offered as needed (Stuart et al., 2000). If patients have severe agoraphobia to the point that they are housebound, initial treatment sessions may need to be done in the patient's home.

The presence of comorbid conditions (mood disorders, substance abuse, psychosis, personality disorders, etc.) may also require treatment modification. For example, preliminary findings indicate that a modified CBT protocol for treating panic disorder in patients with schizophrenia is effective (Hofmann, Bufka, Brady, Du Rand, & Goff, 2000). Hofmann and colleagues described a number of modifications made to enhance treatment outcome in schizophrenic patients, including repetition and simplification of the psychoeducation component of treatment, the use of "catch phrases" or coping statements during the cognitive restructuring component, simplification of monitoring forms, and frequent review of the instructions for completing monitoring forms. Additional modifications included simplifying multistep instructions into simple, single steps that were repeatedly reviewed and using simple questions about the material being covered to engage the patient's attention and to keep the patient on task. Finally, more time within sessions and an increased number of sessions were required to cover the basic components of CBT treatment, particularly when active psychotic processes were present. In general, the inclusion of CBT strategies to target the comorbid disorder may be necessary and relevant. In addition, it may be helpful to spend some time at the outset of treatment differentiating panic symptoms from symptoms related to comorbid disorders.

Comorbidity can also complicate the decision of which problem to focus on first during treatment. Typically, treatment initially targets the problem that is most impairing or distressing to the patient. However, if one problem appears to be causing the other (e.g., impairment from panic disorder leading to symptoms of depression), there is good reason to think that engaging the patient in treatment of the panic disorder symptoms will also lead to improvements in the secondary problems. If the comorbid condition is likely to inter-

fere with the treatment of panic disorder, it should be the initial target of clinical attention. For example, for an individual who manages anxiety by
drinking six to eight beers per day and who has on occasion come to treatment sessions intoxicated, a detoxification program may be needed prior to
initiating treatment for panic disorder. Once the drinking is under control and
CBT for panic disorder is initiated, monitoring of alcohol use should be incorporated into the treatment sessions. To our knowledge, there are no published
studies examining unified CBT protocols designed to target both panic disorder and comorbid conditions, although research is currently under way (e.g.,
Barlow, Allen, & Choate, 2004; McCabe, Chudzik, Antony, Bieling, &
Swinson, 2003).

CBT may also be combined with other treatments (e.g., medications) to
augment treatment response. For example, combining medication with CBT is
recommended if response to CBT is not optimal (Otto, Gould, & Pollack,
1994) or in the case of severe agoraphobia (van Balkom et al., 1997). Currently, there are no studies that address the best ways in which to sequence
treatments. In other words, little is known about whether it is best to start
with CBT, start with medication, or begin both treatments concurrently. Given
the long-term advantages of CBT over medication, we typically recommend
starting with CBT and later adding medication if needed.

In some cases, CBT is administered with another concurrent psychological treatment. For example, an individual with early abuse issues who attends
supportive therapy may be referred by his family doctor to receive CBT for
panic disorder. In such a case, it is important for both therapists to work as a
team to avoid any conflicts that may arise between the different therapeutic
approaches. For example, the supportive psychotherapist may recommend
that the patient minimize anxiety-provoking exposures if he or she believes
that the patient is not ready to confront feared situations. The supportive psychotherapist may inadvertently encourage the patient to avoid experiences
that arouse anxiety or discomfort, and this may contradict the approach of
the cognitive-behavioral therapist.

In some cases, medications may interfere with CBT. For example,
benzodiazepines may interfere with exposure practices by reducing situational
anxiety (Başoğlu, Marks, Kilic, Brewin, & Swinson, 1994). In such instances,
it may be necessary to use interoceptive exposure to bring on anxiety symptoms or incorporate into the treatment a schedule for reducing the use of
benzodiazepines. The latter option should be coordinated with the physician
prescribing the medication. In the case of multiple treating professionals, a
coordinated team approach to treatment is best. If a patient is too distressed
to engage in CBT, and symptoms are too severe, short-term use of a benzodiazepine may be warranted until other therapies take effect (Sturpe &
Weissman, 2002).

Treatment may also be optimized by using assessment tools to identify
targets for treatment and residual symptoms. There are a variety of validated
measures for assessing the core features of panic. Some of the common mea-

sures include the Panic Disorder Severity Scale (PDSS; Shear et al., 1997), the Mobility Inventory for Agoraphobia (MI; Chambless, Caputo, Jasin, Gracely, & Williams, 1985), the Agoraphobic Cognitions Questionnaire (ACQ; Chambless, Caputo, Bright, & Gallagher, 1984), and the Anxiety Sensitivity Index (ASI; Peterson & Reiss, 1993). These scales, and others, can be found in a sourcebook compiled by Antony, Orsillo, and Roemer (2001).

In addition to these standard panic measures, having patients rate their anxiety and avoidance levels on their exposure hierarchy (i.e., list of 10–15 feared situations rank-ordered in terms of difficulty) at the beginning of each therapy session is a useful tool for guiding treatment and for monitoring progress. Exposure hierarchy ratings have been shown to be sensitive to change following CBT for panic disorder and to correlate with clinical improvement assessed by standard panic measures (McCabe, Rowa, Antony, Swinson, & Ladak, 2001). Individualized hierarchies offer more detailed information about specific areas requiring further follow-up and form a basis for identifying posttreatment goals for maintenance and continuation of treatment gains.

Finally, treatment may need to be adapted for the age and developmental stage of the patient. Specifically designed CBT protocols for treating panic disorder in children, adolescents, and older adults should be used (for a review, see Taylor, 2000). In children, the clinical expression of panic disorder features may vary from that seen in adolescents and adults (for a review, see Ollendick, 1998). In addition, including the family in treatment is a major component in the treatment of children and younger adolescents (Craske, 1997).

PREDICTORS OF RELAPSE

Panic disorder with or without agoraphobia is characterized by a chronic course, with symptoms often remaining after treatment has ended (Weisberg, Machan, Dyck, & Keller, 2002), and with a significant risk of relapse (Faravelli, Paterniti, & Scarpato, 1995; Pollack & Smoller, 1995). For our purposes, relapse is defined as the return of symptoms of panic disorder following a period of remission such that full criteria for the disorder are once again met. Additional treatment seeking during follow-up among patients who initially responded well to treatment may also be seen as a marker of relapse. From a research perspective, relapse is operationalized in a variety of ways. For example, one study defined relapse as a return of panic attacks and an increase in the severity of the core symptoms of panic disorder such that they were clinically significant as indicated by a specific clinical severity rating (e.g., T. Brown & Barlow, 1995).

A number of factors have been investigated as possible predictors of relapse. In a study by Fava et al. (2001), patients with panic disorder and agoraphobia (n = 132) who were panic-free following 12 sessions of exposure therapy were assessed at posttreatment intervals ranging from 2 to 14 years (median was 8 years). Approximately a quarter of the sample (23%) had a relapse during the follow-up period, with 62.1% of patients remaining in remission after 10 years. Higher rates of relapse were predicted by a younger age, high pretreatment depression scores, residual agoraphobic avoidance following treatment, and concurrent use of medication (including benzodiazepines and antidepressants).

Despite the results from the Fava et al. (2001) study, findings regarding the use of medication during CBT treatment have been inconsistent. There is evidence that among those who are successfully treated with both a psychological treatment (CBT or relaxation training) and a pill (either alprazolam or placebo), attribution of outcome to the pill versus the psychological treatment is associated with increased risk of relapse (Başoğlu et al., 1994). In addition, research on combining CBT and imipramine for panic disorder indicates that combined CBT and medication does not significantly improve long-term outcome for panic disorder and may contribute to relapse when medication is discontinued (Barlow et al., 2000), relative to CBT plus placebo. However, there is also preliminary evidence that medication discontinuation does not contribute to relapse or reduce the effectiveness of cognitive strategies for panic disorder (G. Brown et al., 2001).

A number of other factors have also been investigated as possible predictors of relapse. Changes in anxiety sensitivity (i.e., the extent to which an individual is fearful of the sensations associated with panic attacks, as measured by the ASI physical concerns factor) was a significant predictor of outcome 6 months after group CBT, with a smaller degree of change associated with increased likelihood of relapse (Schmidt & Bates, 2003). This study replicated earlier findings regarding the relationship between anxiety sensitivity and relapse (Ehlers, 1995). In addition, Ehlers (1995) found that heightened heartbeat perception, which tends to be associated with panic disorder (van der Does, Antony, Barsky, & Ehlers, 2000), predicted relapse during the first year following treatment. Finally, T. Brown et al. (1995) found that individuals with comorbid diagnoses at 3-month follow-up were more likely to seek additional treatment in the 24-month period after CBT, compared to individuals with panic disorder without comorbid diagnoses (50% vs. 21.7%).

PRACTICAL STRATEGIES FOR PREVENTING RELAPSE

Based on the predictors of long-term outcome and relapse, there are a number of clinical interventions that may be useful for preventing relapse:

- Psychoeducation regarding relapse and the episodic nature of panic disorder should be incorporated in treatment (preparing the patient for possible setbacks) and combined with relapse prevention strategies aimed specifically at detailing an action plan for managing recurrence of symptoms.
- Additional treatment to eliminate residual agoraphobic avoidance may be useful. Strategies may include increasing the number of therapist-assisted

exposures or including a family member as a coach. It may also be helpful to explore the benefits (comfort) and costs (increased risk of relapse) of ending treatment when the patient continues to experience residual avoidance.

• Teach the patient how to identify and manage episodes of symptom recurrence. Early identification is key in controlling the magnitude of a setback.

• Prepare the patient for the possible recurrence of symptoms during times of stress. During these periods, it is important not to resume avoidance behaviors. A few booster sessions during times of stress may be useful if the patient's panic symptoms appear to be worsening.

• Schedule occasional follow-up visits to monitor panic disorder symptoms using a psychometrically sound measure (e.g., the PDSS; Shear et al., 1997), so any recurrence of symptoms is identified and targeted accordingly (Shear, Clark, & Feske, 1998).

• Discuss lifestyle factors that may increase vulnerability for relapse (e.g., diet, sleep, exercise, and stress management) and plan changes accordingly. For example, individuals with panic disorder often report that a lack of sleep or stress at work increases their susceptibility to anxiety and panic. Thus, ensuring good sleep hygiene and managing one's workload may be important protective factors.

• Create a plan for long-term use of CBT strategies (including self-help strategies).

• If a patient is receiving combined medication and CBT, incorporate discussion that promotes internal attribution for treatment gains (e.g., "The medication can't be doing everything or else it wouldn't be so hard to do exposures! Therefore, you are doing the real work—the medication just makes it a bit more manageable").

• Use CBT to assist in the discontinuation of medications (rather than trying to discontinue them without CBT). Research indicates that discontinuation from benzodiazepines and antidepressants results in a significant increase in anxiety symptoms (Rickels, Schweizer, Weiss, & Zavodnick, 1993). CBT facilitates benzodiazepine discontinuation (Otto et al., 1993), and preliminary data suggest that CBT may also help a patient to stop taking antidepressants (Schmidt, Woolaway-Bickel, Trakowski, Santiago, & Vasey, 2002).

• Incorporate booster sessions or a more structured form of continuation therapy following acute treatment. For example, one study found that an additional eight treatment sessions focusing on *Safety Behavior Fading* (education regarding safety behaviors, continued elimination of safety behaviors, and problem solving for overcoming safety behaviors) led to additional treatment gains compared to therapy that did not include continuation treatment (Telch, Smits, Sloan, & Powers, 2002).

CASE EXAMPLE

In this section, a case is presented of an individual with panic disorder who was particularly challenging to treat and who benefited only partially from treatment. This case description includes some discussion of the ways in which treatment might have been improved, given the opportunity. Mr. Carr was a 50-year-old man who presented to a specialty treatment clinic for assessment and treatment of his symptoms of anxiety.

Personal History

Mr. Carr lived with his wife of 20 years and two sons ages 15 and 17. He reported being happily married. He described his wife as very supportive and indicated having a good relationship with his children. He had been working as an office administrator in a large manufacturing company until he took a leave of absence due to bouts of dizziness. He had been off work for a year, during which time he had undergone numerous physical examinations to determine the cause of his dizzy spells. All physical findings were negative. His doctor informed him that he was suffering from vertigo and that anxiety may also be playing a role in his symptoms. Thus, he was referred for psychological assessment.

Presenting Problem

Mr. Carr described episodes of dizziness that occurred "out of the blue" in which the room would seem to spin around him and he had difficulty maintaining his balance. During the assessment, it became evident that Mr. Carr was experiencing unexpected panic attacks in addition to his vertigo. These panic attacks began in his early 20s but did not become significantly impairing or distressing until the past year, shortly after the onset of vertigo. During a panic attack, Mr. Carr would experience a racing heart, sweating, shaking, shortness of breath, dizziness, and concerns that he would pass out. In the past year, he had become increasingly worried about additional panic attacks. He had recently started to avoid a wide range of situations for fear of both a panic attack and vertigo, including driving more than 10 minutes from home, crowds, airplanes, and waiting in line. He stated that he felt especially uncomfortable outside his "comfort zone"—within 10 miles of his house. He also reported that he felt more comfortable in a public situation when accompanied by his wife, in case he needed help. Mr. Carr's symptoms were consistent with a diagnosis of panic disorder with agoraphobia. Mr. Carr denied any history of mood disorder, additional anxiety disorders, psychotic symptoms, somatoform disorder, eating disorder, or substance use disorder. Apart from vertigo, Mr. Carr did not report any difficulties with his physical health.

Treatment Recommendations

Mr. Carr was offered individual CBT for his panic disorder with agoraphobia. He was very interested and motivated for treatment. He was also offered a psychiatric consultation to review medication options but declined as he did not like the idea of taking medication. Mr. Carr had never received psycho-therapy for his difficulties in the past.

Treatment Progress and Challenges

Over the course of treatment, a number of therapeutic challenges arose. As treatment progress is described, these challenges are outlined, along with strategies used to overcome them.

Session 1

The first session focused on discussing Mr. Carr's experience with panic attacks and vertigo including anxiety-provoking physical sensations, common anxious thoughts and predictions, and behavioral reactions to anxiety including escape, avoidance, and safety cues. The overlap of vertigo symptoms and panic was also discussed. The cognitive-behavioral model of panic disorder and agoraphobia was introduced, and an exposure hierarchy was developed. Homework included monitoring the three components of anxiety (thoughts, physical sensations, and behaviors) whenever he felt anxious or experienced an episode of vertigo. Self-help readings were also assigned.

Session 2

The week was reviewed. Mr. Carr reported that most of the week went well, until he had two panic attacks while shopping in the mall during the days pre-ceding the second therapy session. Homework was reviewed, as was the mate-rial covered in Session 1. Mr. Carr's typical behavioral response to his panic was to escape from the situation, and he left the mall in response to both panic attacks. The role of cognitions in maintaining anxiety was reviewed (with a focus on Mr. Carr's two episodes of panic in the past week), and the concept of cognitive distortions was introduced. Mr. Carr reported that his main con-cern during his panic attacks was the possibility that he would be embarrassed in front of others. Homework included monitoring his anxious thoughts dur-ing episodes of anxiety or vertigo and identifying cognitive distortions. He also agreed to stay in the situation if he felt anxious and monitor the three components of his anxiety more closely.

Session 3

Mr. Carr reported two panic attacks over the week. In both instances, he stayed in the situation and practiced observing the three components of anxi-ety and focusing on his anxious thoughts. This session focused on strategies to challenge anxious thoughts with the goal of more balanced or realistic think-ing. Homework involved countering his anxious thoughts using cognitive monitoring forms.

Session 4

Upon reviewing his homework, Mr. Carr reported that he had discovered that his core fearful thought was of becoming dizzy. He found that he would monitor his body for dizziness and distract himself if he felt dizzy. He also indicated fearing an attack of vertigo. The session focused on exploring his fear of dizziness and examining his anxious predictions. Different countering strategies were discussed. In addition, the short- versus long-term usefulness of distraction was reviewed.

The presence of a medical symptom (vertigo) with no known cause or treatment presented a number of obstacles during the treatment. First, the dizziness that was associated with Mr. Carr's vertigo was similar to the dizziness he experienced during his panic attacks. Second, the presence of a diagnosed medical condition contributed to Mr. Carr's fears that something must be physically wrong with him and his belief that physical sensations are dangerous. To address these issues, the therapist also addressed Mr. Carr's beliefs about episodes of vertigo, emphasizing noncatastrophic interpretations:

MR. CARR: When I become dizzy, it feels like I am going to pass out and I have to sit down or else something bad could happen. How am I supposed to do exposures if I have an episode of vertigo?

THERAPIST: Have you ever had something very bad happen during an episode of vertigo?

MR. CARR: No, but almost. I always sit down so I don't pass out.

THERAPIST: So it sounds like it *feels* like something really terrible is going to happen, but based on your own experience it never has.

MR. CARR: Yes, but that is because I sit down.

THERAPIST: What do you think about trying an experiment where you don't sit down the next time that you feel dizzy? That way, you can test out your prediction that something bad will happen?

MR. CARR: I don't know . . . why would I want to do that?

THERAPIST: Although your strategy of sitting down each time you feel dizzy may work in the short term, what effect do you think it has in the long term? In other words, what is the long-term effect on your life of avoiding situations that might actually provide you with an opportunity to find out whether your dizziness is in fact dangerous?

MR. CARR: It is not working because I can no longer go anywhere or do anything the way I used to.

THERAPIST: OK, so if it is not working for you, do you think it might be worth trying the strategies that we are discussing here to see if they might work better for you? What do you have to lose?

MR. CARR: Not much, I guess. But what if I pass out?

THERAPIST: Well, why don't you try it first when you are at home? The next time you are dizzy, don't sit down. Instead, keep doing what you are doing at the time. When you do experience vertigo, how long does it last?

MR. CARR: A few minutes.

THERAPIST: OK, so for a few minutes you may feel extremely dizzy. Do you think you can manage that?

MR. CARR: I could try. But what if I pass out?

THERAPIST: Well, let's say the worst case scenario happens and you do pass out. What would happen?

MR. CARR: I would collapse.

THERAPIST: OK, and then what?

MR. CARR: I guess that eventually I would come to.

THERAPIST: And then what?

MR. CARR: I guess I would get up. I never really thought that far ahead.

THERAPIST: Good. Well, that is what I would like you to try. I want to examine what your anxious predictions are and then really test them out. That way, your predictions can be based on your own experience rather than on what you *feel* might happen.

Session 5

Mr. Carr had done well practicing carrying on with his activities when he felt dizzy. He stated that he did not pass out and, as he continued with a task despite feeling dizzy, the dizziness usually decreased over time. The session focused on reviewing the rationale for planned exposures as well as guidelines for their conduct. Mr. Carr planned to practice driving out of his "safe zone" and to continue challenging his anxious thoughts.

Session 6

Mr. Carr experienced an episode of vertigo shortly after the last session, and he decided not to do the driving exposures. He reported feeling discouraged and more anxious throughout the week. He stated that he had woken up feeling anxious almost every morning. The session focused on processing Mr. Carr's thoughts and feelings about how the week went and how therapy was progressing. Mr. Carr realized that his negative thoughts about himself (e.g., seeing himself as a failure because he was too anxious to do the driving exposure) were contributing to his feeling anxious and unsettled in the morning.

MR. CARR: I just couldn't do the driving exposure as we planned. I feel like a failure. Maybe this treatment won't work. I was so hopeful.

THERAPIST: Exposures are a very challenging part of treatment. Is it possible that the exposure we planned may have been too difficult, or do you really think that the difficulties you had are because you are a failure?

MR. CARR: Well, I do feel like a failure, but when you put it that way, I guess that maybe this was too difficult for me right now.

THERAPIST: It seems like the episode of vertigo that you had also played a role in making your planned exposure seem too challenging right now. What sort of thoughts were you having?

MR. CARR: Well, after I had the vertigo, I started to worry that I might have an episode when I was driving and I could get in an accident.

THERAPIST: So it sounds like the episode of vertigo triggered some powerful anxious thoughts.

MR. CARR: Yes. I guess that played a major role in my decision to not do the exposures.

THERAPIST: OK. So perhaps this week we should choose an exposure practice that feels more manageable to you. We should also examine the anxious predictions you were making. It sounds like you believe that it is pretty dangerous for you to drive because of your vertigo.

MR. CARR: Well, it is dangerous. I could have an accident and hurt someone.

THERAPIST: Have you ever had an episode of vertigo when you were driving?

MR. CARR: Yes, just once. Although I have felt dizzy lots of times.

THERAPIST: OK, and what happened?

MR. CARR: Well I was driving down a narrow hill and I felt very dizzy. I wanted to pull over but there was no shoulder to pull off on.

THERAPIST: So what did you do?

MR. CARR: Well, I had to keep driving, so I did. But it was terrible. I drove right home after that.

THERAPIST: And did the vertigo last the whole time you were driving?

MR. CARR: No. It just lasted about a minute when I was driving on the hill.

THERAPIST: OK. Taking into account what we have covered so far in our sessions, what do you think about this incident based on your own experience?

MR. CARR: Well, I guess I felt like something dangerous would happen. But when I look at it realistically, nothing bad did happen.

THERAPIST: So you were able to drive, despite the vertigo, and despite the other times when you felt dizzy.

MR. CARR: I guess that's true.

THERAPIST: What do these experiences tell you about your ability to drive when you are dizzy?

MR. CARR: Well, I guess I am able to drive safely. The dizziness did pass. But I still *feel* like something bad could happen.

THERAPIST: That's OK. Over time, and as you practice exposures, you will notice that your level of belief in the realistic interpretation of events will increase and your belief in the anxious interpretation of events will decrease. Let me ask you, what percentage of you believes that you can drive safely despite feeling dizzy?

MR. CARR: 30%.

THERAPIST: OK. That gives us a starting point. When you think about it, it makes sense that you feel anxious about driving if you believe that you are 70% unsafe. Most people would feel very anxious if they felt 70% unsafe about driving.

MR. CARR: I never thought about it that way, but that makes a lot of sense.

THERAPIST: So what do you think we will be working toward?

MR. CARR: I guess as I practice the exposures, the 30% belief I will be safe will increase, and the 70% belief I will be unsafe will decrease.

THERAPIST: Exactly. So what exposure would you like to practice this week?

Session 7

Mr. Carr had practiced driving on some hills over the week as well as continuing to walk when he had an episode of vertigo. He reported feeling quite exhausted from the exposures. The session focused on reviewing how his exposures went and reinforcing all the difficult work he was doing. His feelings of exhaustion were normalized and strategies were discussed to deal with the effects of exposure (e.g., planning exposures when he did not have to do something right afterward, letting his family know that he might be more irritable because of the exposures, and planning some fun activities to reward himself after exposure practices).

Session 8

Mr. Carr practiced a number of driving exposures as well as starting to do other activities he had previously avoided. The rationale for interoceptive exposure was introduced and symptom testing was conducted. Mr. Carr's homework was to practice spinning in a chair to expose himself to feelings of dizziness.

Session 9

Mr. Carr reported that his week was "terrible." He had attempted to practice the interoceptive exposure but it was too difficult. He felt discouraged and reported that his anxiety over the week was heightened and he found the driving exposures much more difficult than the previous week. The session focused on discussing Mr. Carr's expectations for recovery. He identified that one of his expectations was that he should be able to "handle anything without stress." This belief was explored and Mr. Carr realized that he was placing a lot of pressure on himself to do everything perfectly. Once these beliefs were examined, he indicated that he felt some relief. The difficulty of doing the interoceptive exposure practices was discussed in the context of striking at the core of his fear of physical sensations, and his feelings were normalized. He was encouraged to reframe his experience the past week as a normal bump in the recovery process rather than a treatment failure. An interoceptive exposure practice was conducted in session (spinning in a chair), and Mr. Carr agreed to practice the exercise in the coming week despite his anxiety.

Session 10

Mr. Carr reported that his week was much better. He practiced spinning in the chair once a day and was able to practice identifying and countering his anxious thoughts about dizziness. He also did a number of personal experiments to challenge his anxious thoughts. For example, he realized that he had been avoiding bending over to pick things up and instead would keep his head upright, bend at the knees, and lower himself slowly to prevent the onset of vertigo. Over the week, he had practiced purposely bending over with his head upside down to challenge these fears. However, Mr. Carr had not practiced the planned driving exposures. He stated that it was too difficult to plan them as he never knew how he would feel on the chosen day. If it was a "good day" he would be able to do the exposure, but if it was a "bad day" he would not. The session focused on discussing what a "bad day" meant (for Mr. Carr it meant waking up feeling anxious and dizzy) and why it is even more important to practice exposure on a "bad day." Mr. Carr stated firmly that he preferred to stick to just doing exposures as they arose. He liked the cognitive strategies and found them very useful. He did not wish to plan exposures in advance.

Session 11

Mr. Carr reported that his week went well. He had some episodes of anxiety but persisted at whatever he was doing despite his feelings. The idea of combining interoceptive exposure and situational exposure was introduced (e.g., making himself dizzy in a store). Mr. Carr agreed to try this over the week but did not want to plan it in advance. His return to work was also discussed.

Session 12

In this final session, Mr. Carr's gains in treatment were reviewed, with an emphasis on the obstacles he overcame, the goals he was able to reach, and the goals that he still needed to work toward. His reluctance to plan exposures was discussed in terms of increasing his vulnerability for relapse due to the persistence of his beliefs about not planning things on a "bad day." A plan was put in place for how Mr. Carr could respond to future episodes of anxiety, panic, or vertigo. A scheduled follow-up session was offered but Mr. Carr preferred not to schedule a session. Instead, he agreed to call if he needed a booster session in the future.

Treatment Outcome

Although Mr. Carr did make some significant gains in treatment, including reduced episodes of anxiety, panic, and dizziness, decreased avoidance, and decreased impairment and distress, treatment was considered only partially successful. Upon completion of treatment, Mr. Carr still had a significant level of anxiety sensitivity and some agoraphobic avoidance, particularly on days when he did not "feel well." Further, Mr. Carr was resistant to the idea of planned exposures and he declined a follow-up treatment session that would have provided an opportunity to check on his progress and ensure that his gains had been maintained.

Upon reviewing this case, a number of practical strategies emerged that might have enhanced outcome:

- Incorporating additional sessions involving (1) therapist-assisted exposure to driving situations and (2) combined interoceptive and situational exposure.
- Bringing Mr. Carr's wife into session to educate her about the CBT model of treatment, enlist her help as a coach during planned exposures, and reduce her tendency to accommodate his symptoms (e.g., when Mr. Carr was having a "bad day," his wife tended to do the driving).
- Once again, reviewing with Mr. Carr the possible benefits of adding in a medication (e.g., an SSRI).

CONCLUSION

Despite the availability of empirically supported treatment options for panic disorder, there are some individuals who not respond to treatment or who drop out of treatment prematurely. There are also a significant number of individuals who experience residual symptoms and relapse following treatment. Thus, the challenge is to continue to improve our current treatments and to examine factors underlying suboptimal treatment response and relapse. This chapter examined predictors of treatment response and relapse. Factors associated with treatment response included personality variables, symptom severity, anxiety sensitivity, therapist characteristics, depression, motivation for treatment, chronic life stress, expressed emotion in the family, and medication discontinuation. Factors unrelated to response included demographic characteristics, quality of the therapeutic relationship, perception of the therapist, pain symptoms, duration of the disorder, the number of treatment sessions, comorbid anxiety disorders, perceived parental upbringing, and marital dissatisfaction. Predictors of relapse included younger age, higher pretreatment depression, residual posttreatment agoraphobic avoidance, concurrent use of antidepressants, anxiety sensitivity, and heightened heartbeat awareness. In consideration of these factors, practical strategies were outlined aimed at improving outcome and preventing relapse. A case illustration was used to demonstrate various therapeutic challenges and treatment strategies.

REFERENCES

Addis, M. E., & Carpenter, K. M. (2000). The treatment rationale in cognitive behavioral therapy: Psychological mechanisms and clinical guidelines. *Cognitive and Behavioral Practice, 7*, 147–156.

American Psychiatric Association. (1998). Practice guideline for the treatment of patients with panic disorder. *American Journal of Psychiatry, 144*(Suppl. 5), 1–34.

American Psychiatric Association. (2000). *Diagnostic and statistical manual of mental disorders* (4th ed., text rev.). Washington, DC: Author.

Antony, M. M., & McCabe, R. E. (2002). Empirical basis of panic control treatment. *Scientific Review of Mental Health Practice, 1*, 189–194.

Antony, M. M., Orsillo, S. M., & Roemer, L. (Eds.). (2001). *Practitioner's guide to empirically-based measures of anxiety*. New York: Kluwer Academic/Plenum Press.

Antony, M. M., & Swinson, R. P. (2000). *Phobic disorders and panic in adults: A guide to assessment and treatment*. Washington, DC: American Psychological Association.

Anxiety Review Panel. (2000). *Ontario guidelines for the management of anxiety disorders in primary care*. Toronto, Ontario, Canada: Publications Ontario.

Bakker, A., van Balkom, A. J. L. M., Spinhoven, P., Blaauw, B. M. J. W., & van Dyck, R. (1998). Follow-up on the treatment of panic disorder with or without agoraphobia: A quantitative review. *Journal of Nervous and Mental Disease, 186*, 414–419.

Ballenger, J. C. (1993). Panic disorder: Efficacy of current treatments. *Psychopharmacology Bulletin, 29*, 477–486.

Ballenger, J. C., Davidson, J. R. T., Lecrubier, Y., Nutt, D. J., Baldwin, D. S., den Boer, J. A., Kasper, S., & Shear, M. K. (1998). Consensus statement on panic disorder from the International Group on Depression and Anxiety. *Journal of Clinical Psychiatry, 59*, 47–54.

Barlow, D. H., Allen, L. B., & Choate, M. L. (2004). Toward a unified treatment for emotional disorders. *Behavior Therapy, 35*, 205–230.

Barlow, D. H., & Craske, M. (2000). *Mastery of your anxiety and panic (MAP-3)*. Boulder, CO: Graywind.

Barlow, D. H., Gorman, J. M., Shear, M. K., & Woods, S. W. (2000). Cognitive-behavioral therapy, imipramine, or their combination for panic disorder: A randomized controlled study. *Journal of the American Medical Association, 283*, 2529–2536.

Başoğlu, M., Marks, I. M., Kilic, C., Brewin, C. R., & Swinson, R. P. (1994). Alprazolam

32   McCABE *and* ANTONY

and exposure for panic disorder with agoraphobia attribution of improvement to medication predicts subsequent relapse. *British Journal of Psychiatry, 164,* 652–659.

Brown, G. K., Bieling, P. J., Beck, A. T., Newman, C. F., & Levy, S. J. (2001). Cognitive therapy for panic disorder: The impact of medication discontinuation on symptoms. *Cognitive and Behavioral Practice, 8,* 240–245.

Brown, T. A., Antony, M. M., & Barlow, D. H. (1995). Diagnostic comorbidity in panic disorder: Effect on treatment outcome and course of comorbid diagnoses following treatment. *Journal of Consulting and Clinical Psychology, 63,* 408–418.

Brown, T. A., & Barlow, D. H. (1995). Long-term outcome in cognitive-behavioral treatment of panic disorder: Clinical predictors and alternative strategies for assessment. *Journal of Consulting and Clinical Psychology, 63,* 754–765.

Chambless, D. L., Caputo, G. C., Bright, P., & Gallagher, R. (1984). Assessment of fear of fear in agoraphobics: The Body Sensations Questionnaire and the Agoraphobic Cognitions Questionnaire. *Journal of Consulting and Clinical Psychology, 52,* 1090–1097.

Chambless, D. L., Caputo, G. C., Jasin, S. E., Gracely, E. J., & Williams, C. (1985). The Mobility Inventory for agoraphobia. *Behaviour Research and Therapy, 23,* 35–44.

Chambless, D. L., & Steketee, G. (1999). Expressed emotion and behavior therapy outcome: A prospective study with obsessive-compulsive and agoraphobic outpatients. *Journal of Consulting and Clinical Psychology, 67,* 658–665.

Chudzik, S. M., McCabe, R. E., Antony, M. M., & Swinson, R. P. (2001, November). *The effect of a comorbid mood disorder on treatment outcome for panic disorder.* Paper presented at the meeting of the Association for Advancement of Behavior Therapy, Philadelphia.

Clark, D. M., Salkovskis, P. M., Hackmann, A., Middleton, H., Anastasiades, P., & Gelder, M. (1994). A comparison of cognitive therapy, applied relaxation and imipramine in the treatment of panic disorder. *British Journal of Psychiatry, 164,* 759–769.

Clark, D. M., Salkovskis, P. M., Hackmann, A., Wells, A., Ludgate, J., & Gelder, M. (1999). Brief cognitive therapy for panic disorder: A randomized controlled trial. *Journal of Consulting and Clinical Psychology, 67,* 583–589.

Corominas, A., Guerrero, T., & Vallejo, J. (2002). Residual symptoms and comorbidity in panic disorder. *European Psychiatry, 17,* 399–406.

Craske, M. G. (1997). Fear and anxiety in children and adolescents. *Bulletin of the Menninger Clinic, 61*(Suppl. A), A4–A36.

Craske, M. G., Brown, T. A., & Barlow, D. H. (1991). Behavioral treatment of panic disorder: A two-year follow-up. *Behavior Therapy, 22,* 289–304.

de Beurs, E., van Dyck, R., Lange, A. & van Balkom, A. J. L. M. (1995). Perceived upbringing and its relation to treatment outcome in agoraphobia. *Clinical Psychology and Psychotherapy, 2,* 78–85.

den Boer, J. A., & Slaap, B. R. (1998). Review of current treatment in panic disorder. *International Clinical Psychopharmacology, 13*(Suppl. 4), S25–S30.

Dozois, D. J. A., Westra, H. A., Collins, K. A., Fung, T. S., & Garry, J. K. F. (2004). Stages of change in anxiety: Psychometric properties of the University of Rhode Island Change Assessment (URICA) Scale. *Behaviour Research and Therapy, 42,* 711–729.

Eaton, W. W., Kessler, R. C., Wittchen, H. U., & Magee, W. J. (1994). Panic and panic disorder in the United States. *American Journal of Psychiatry, 151,* 413–420.

Edelman, R. E., & Chambless, D. L. (1993). Compliance during sessions and homework in exposure-based treatment of agoraphobia. *Behaviour Research and Therapy, 23,* 35–44.

Ehlers, A. (1995). A 1-year prospective study of panic attacks: Clinical course and factors associated with relapse. *Journal of Abnormal Psychology, 104,* 164–172.

Faravelli, C., Paterniti, S., & Scarpato, A. (1995). 5-year prospective, naturalistic follow-up study of panic disorder. *Comprehensive Psychiatry, 39,* 271–277.

Fava, G. A., Rafanelli, C., Grandi, S., Conti, S., Ruini, C., Magelli, L., & Belluardo, P. (2001). Long-term outcome of panic disorder with agoraphobia treated by exposure. *Psychological Medicine, 31,* 891–898.

Gorman, J. M., Martinez, J. M., Goetz, R., Huppert, J. D., Ray, S., Barlow, D. H., Shear, M. K., & Woods, S. W. (2003). The effect of pharmacotherapist characteristics on treatment outcome in panic disorder. *Depression and Anxiety, 17,* 88–93.

Gould, R. A., Otto, M. W., & Pollack, M. H. (1995). A meta-analysis of treatment outcome for panic disorder. *Clinical Psychology Review, 15,* 819–844.

Grilo, C. M., Money, R., Barlow, D. H., Goddard, A. W., Gorman, J. M., Hofmann, S. G., Papp, L. A., Shear, M. K., & Woods, S. W. (1998). Pretreatment patient factors predicting attrition from a multicenter randomized controlled treatment study for panic disorder. *Comprehensive Psychiatry, 39,* 323–332.

Hahlweg, K., Fiegenbaum, W., Frank, M., Schroeder, B., & von Witzleben, I. (2001). Short- and long term effectiveness of an empirically supported treatment for agoraphobia. *Journal of Consulting and Clinical Psychology, 69,* 375–382.

Hasler, G., Delsignore, A., Milos, G., Buddeberg, C., & Schnyder, U. (2004). Application of Prochaska's transtheoretical model of change to patients with eating disorders. *Journal of Psychosomatic Research, 57,* 67–72.

Heinrichs, N., Spiegel, D. A., & Hofmann, S. G. (2002). Panic disorder with agoraphobia. In F. W. Bond & W. Dryden (Eds.), *Handbook of brief cognitive behaviour therapy* (pp. 55–76). London: Wiley.

Hofmann, S. G., & Barlow, D. H. (1999). The costs of anxiety disorders: Implications for psychosocial interventions. In N. E. Miller & K. M. Magruder (Eds.), *Cost-effectiveness of psychotherapy* (pp. 224–234). New York: Oxford University Press.

Hofmann, S. G., Bufka, L. F., Brady, S. M., Du Rand, C., & Goff, D. C. (2000). Cognitive-behavioral treatment of panic in patients with schizophrenia: Preliminary findings. *Journal of Cognitive Psychotherapy, 14,* 381–392.

Huppert, J. D., & Baker-Morissette, S. L. (2003). Beyond the manual: The insider's guide to Panic Control Treatment. *Cognitive and Behavioral Practice, 10,* 2–13.

Huppert, J. D., Bufka, L. F., Barlow, D. H., Gorman, J. G., Shear, M. K., & Woods, S. W. (2001) Therapists, therapist effects, and CBT outcome for panic disorder: Results from a multi-center trial. *Journal of Consulting and Clinical Psychology, 69,* 747–755.

Keijsers, G. P., Hoogduin, C. A., & Schaap, C. P. D. R. (1994). Prognostic factors in the behavioral treatment of panic disorder with and without agoraphobia. *Behavior Therapy, 25,* 689–708.

Keijsers, G. P., Kampman, M., & Hoogduin, C. A. (2001). Dropout prediction in cognitive behavior therapy for panic disorder. *Behavior Therapy, 32,* 739–749.

Keller, M. B., Yonkers, K. A., Warshaw, M. G., Pratt, L. A., Golan, J., Mathews, A. O., White, K., Swots, A., Reich, J., & Lavori, P. (1994). Remission and relapse in subjects with panic disorder and panic with agoraphobia: A prospective short-interval naturalistic follow-up. *Journal of Nervous and Mental Disease, 182,* 290–296.

Klerman, G. L., Weissman, M. M., Ouellette, R., Johnson, J., & Greenwald, S. (1991). Panic attacks in the community: Social morbidity and health care utilization. *Journal of the American Medical Association, 265,* 742–746.

Laberge, B., Gauthier,, J. G., Côté, G., Plamondon,, J., & Cormier, H. J. (1993). Cognitive-behavioral therapy of panic disorder with secondary major depression: A preliminary investigation. *Journal of Consulting and Clinical Psychology, 61,* 1028–1037.

Marchand, A., Goyer, L. R., Dupuis, G., & Mainguy, N. (1998). Personality disorders and the outcome of cognitive-behavioral treatment of panic disorder with agoraphobia. *Canadian Journal of Behavioural Science, 30,* 14–23.

Margraf, J., Barlow, D. H., Clark, D. M., & Telch, M. J. (1993). Psychological treatment of panic: Work in progress on outcome, active ingredients, and follow-up. *Behaviour Research and Therapy, 31,* 1–8.

Massion, A. O., Dyck, I. R., Shea, M. T., Phillips, K. A., Warshaw, M. G., & Keller, M. B. (2002). Personality disorders and time to remission in generalized anxiety disorder, social phobia, and panic disorder. *Archives of General Psychiatry, 59,* 434–440.

McCabe, R. E., Chudzik, S., Antony, M. M., Bieling, P. J., & Swinson, R. P. (2003). *A randomized clinical trial examining the effectiveness of a cognitive behavioral treatment intervention specifically designed to treat major depression with comorbid panic disorder.* Unpublished data.

McCabe, R. E., Rowa, K., Antony, M. M., Swinson, R. P., & Ladak, Y. (2001, July). *The exposure hierarchy as a measure of cognitive and behavioral change, treatment progress and efficacy.* Paper presented at the World Congress of Behavioural and Cognitive Therapies, Vancouver, British Columbia.

McConnaughy, E. A., Prochaska, J. O., & Velicer, W. F. (1983). Stages of change in psychotherapy: Measurement and sample profiles. *Psychotherapy: Theory, Research and Practice, 3,* 368–375.

McLean, P. D., Woody, S., Taylor, S., & Koch, W. J. (1998). Comorbid panic disorder and major depression: Implications for cognitive-behavioral therapy. *Journal of Consulting and Clinical Psychology, 66,* 240–247.

Mennin, D. S., & Heimberg, R. G. (2000). The impact of comorbid mood and personality disorders in the cognitive-behavioral treatment of panic disorder. *Clinical Psychology Review, 20,* 339–357.

Miller, W. R., & Rollnick, S. (2002). *Motivational interviewing* (2nd ed.). New York: Guilford Press.

Ollendick, T. H. (1998). Panic disorder in children and adolescents: New developments, new directions. *Journal of Clinical Child Psychology, 27,* 234–245.

Otto, M. W., Gould, R. A., & Pollack, M. H. (1994). Cognitive-behavioral treatment of panic disorder: Considerations for the treatment of patients over the long term. *Psychiatric Annals, 24,* 307–315.

Otto, M. W., Pollack, M. H., Sachs, G. S., Reiter, S. R., Meltzer-Brody, S., & Rosenbaum, J. F. (1993). Discontinuation of benzodiazepine treatment: Efficacy of cognitive-behavioral therapy for patients with panic disorder. *American Journal of Psychiatry, 140,* 1485–1490.

Otto, M. W., Tuby, K. S., Gould, R. A., McLean, R. Y., & Pollack, M. H. (2001). An effect-size analysis of the relative efficacy and tolerability of serotonin selective reuptake inhibitors for panic disorder. *American Journal of Psychiatry, 158,* 1989–1992.

Peterson, R. A., & Reiss, S. (1993). *Anxiety Sensitivity Index Revised Test Manual.* Worthington, OH: IDS.

Pollack, M. H., & Smoller, J. W. (1995). The longitudinal course and outcome of panic disorder. *Psychiatric Clinics of North America, 18,* 785–801.

Pollack, M. H., Worthington III, J. J., Otto, M. W., Maki, K. M., Smoller, J. W., Manfro, G. G., Rudolph, R., & Rosenberg, J. F. (1996). Venlafaxine for panic disorder: Results form a double-blind, placebo-controlled study. *Psychopharmacology Bulletin, 32,* 667–670.

Prochaska, J. O., & DiClemente, C. C. (1992). The transtheoretical model of change. In J. C. Norcross & M. R. Goldfried (Eds.), *Handbook of psychotherapy integration* (pp. 300–334). New York: Basic Books.

Prochaska, J. O., & Norcross, J. C. (1994). *Systems of psychotherapy: A transtheoretical analysis.* Pacific Grove, CA: Brooks/Cole.

Rickels, K., Schweizer, E., Weiss, S., & Zavodnick, S. (1993). Maintenance drug treatment for panic disorder. II. Short-term and long-term outcome after drug taper. *Archives of General Psychiatry, 50,* 61–68.

Rief, W., Trenkamp, S., Auer, C., & Fichter, M. M. (2000). Cognitive behavior therapy in panic disorder and comorbid major depression. *Psychotherapy and Psychosomatics, 69,* 70–78.

Rosenbaum, J. F., Pollack, M. H., & Pollack, R. A. (1996). Clinical issues in the long-term treatment of panic disorder. *Journal of Clinical Psychiatry, 57,* 44–48.

Roy-Byrne, P. P., & Cowley, D. S. (2002). Pharmacological treatments for panic disorder, generalized anxiety disorder, specific phobia, and social anxiety disorder. In P. E. Nathan & J. M. Gorman (Eds.), *A guide to treatments that work* (2nd ed., pp. 337–365). London: Oxford University Press.

Schmidt, N. B., & Bates, M. J. (2003). Evaluation of a pathoplastic relationship between anxiety sensitivity and panic disorder. *Anxiety, Stress and Coping: An International Journal, 16,* 17–30.

Schmidt, N. B., McCreary, B. T., Trakowski, J., Santiago, H., Woolaway-Bickel, K., & Ialongo, N. (2003). Effects of cognitive-behavioral treatment on physical health status in patients with panic disorder. *Behavior Therapy, 34,* 49–63.

Schmidt, N. B., Santiago, H., Trakowski, J., & Kendren, J. M. (2002). Pain in patients with panic disorder: Relation to symptoms, cognitive characteristics and treatment outcomes. *Pain Research Management, 7,* 134–141.

Schmidt, N.B., & Woolaway-Bickel, K. (2000). The effects of treatment compliance on outcome in cognitive-behavioral therapy for panic disorder: Quality versus quantity. *Journal of Consulting and Clinical Psychology, 68,* 13–18.

Schmidt, N. B., Woolaway-Bickel, K. Trakowski, J., Santiago, H., Storey, J., Koselka, M., & Cook, J. (2000). Dismantling cognitive-behavioral treatment for panic disorder: Questioning the utility of breathing retraining. *Journal of Consulting and Clinical Psychology, 68,* 417–425.

Schmidt, N. B., Woolaway-Bickel, K. Trakowski, J., Santiago, H., & Vasey, M. (2002). Antidepressant discontinuation in the context of cognitive behavioral treatment for panic disorder. *Behaviour Research and Therapy, 40,* 67–73.

Sharp, D. M., & Power, K. G. (1999). Predicting treatment outcome for panic disorder and agoraphobia in primary care. *Clinical Psychology and Psychotherapy, 6,* 336–348.

Shear, M. K., Brown, T. A., Barlow, D. H., Money, R., Sholomskas, D. E., Woods, S. W., Gorman, J. M., & Papp, L. A. (1997). Multicenter Collaborative Panic Disorder Severity Scale. *American Journal of Psychiatry, 154,* 1571–1575.

Shear, M. K., Clark, D., & Feske, U. (1998). The road to recovery in panic disorder: Response, remission, and relapse. *Journal of Clinical Psychiatry, 59,* 4–8.

Sheikh, J. I., Leskin, G. A., & Klein, D. F. (2002). Gender differences in panic disorder: Findings from the National Comorbidity Survey. *American Journal of Psychiatry, 159,* 55–58.

Slaap, B. R., & den Boer, J. A. (2001). The prediction of nonresponse to pharmaco-therapy in panic disorder: A review. *Depression and Anxiety, 14,* 112–122.

Stuart, G. L., Treat, T. A., & Wade, W. A. (2000). Effectiveness of an empirically based treatment for panic disorder delivered in a service clinic setting 1–year follow-up. *Journal of Consulting and Clinical Psychology, 68,* 506–512.

Sturpe, D. A., & Weissman, A. M. (2002). What are effective treatments for panic disorder? *Journal of Family Practice, 51,* 743.

Taylor, S. (2000). *Understanding and treating panic disorder: Cognitive-behavioural approaches.* New York: Wiley.

Telch, M. J., Lucas, J. A., Schmidt, N. B., Hanna, H. H., Jaimez, T. L., & Lucas, R. A. (1993). Group cognitive-behavioral treatment of panic disorder. *Behaviour Research and Therapy, 31,* 279–287.

Telch, M. J., Smits, J. A. J., Sloan, T. B., & Powers, M. B. (2002, November). *Safety behavior fading in the treatment of panic disorder: Work in progress.* Paper presented at the meeting of the Association for Advancement of Behavior Therapy, Reno, NV.

Toni, C., Perugi, G., Frare, F., Mata, B., Vitale, B., Mengali, F., Rechhia, M., Serra, G., & Akiskal, H. S. (2000). A prospective naturalistic study of 326 panic-agoraphobic patients treated with antidepressants. *Pharmacopsychiatry, 33,* 121–131.

Turgeon, L., Marchand, A., & Dupuis, G. (1998). Clinical features in panic disorder with agoraphobia: A comparison of men and women. *Journal of Anxiety Disorders, 12,* 539–553.

van Balkom, A. J. L. M., Bakker, A., Spinhoven, P. H., Blaauw, B. M. J. W., Smeenk, S., & Ruesink, B. (1997). A meta-analysis on the treatment of panic disorder with or without agoraphobia. *Journal of Nervous and Mental Disease, 185,* 510–516.

van der Does, A. J. W., Antony, M. M., Barsky, A. J., & Ehlers, A. (2000). Heartbeat perception in panic disorder: A re-analysis. *Behaviour Research and Therapy, 38,* 47–62.

Wade, S. L., Monroe, S. M., & Michelson, L. K. (1993). Chronic life stress and treatment outcome in agoraphobia with panic attacks. *American Journal of Psychiatry, 150,* 1491–1495.

Wade, W. A., Treat, T. A., & Stuart, G. L. (1998). Transporting an empirically supported treatment for panic disorder to a service clinic setting: A benchmarking strategy. *Journal of Consulting and Clinical Psychology, 66,* 231–239.

Weisberg, R. B., Machan, J. T., Dyck, I. R., & Keller, M. B. (2002). Do panic symptoms during periods of remission predict relapse of panic disorder? *Journal of Nervous and Mental Disease, 190,* 190–197.

Weissman, A. M. (2002). What are effective treatments for panic disorder? *Journal of Family Practice, 51,* 743.

Westen, D., & Morrison, K. (2001). A multidimensional meta-analysis of treatments for depression, panic, and generalized anxiety disorder an empirical examination of the status of empirically supported therapies. *Journal of Consulting and Clinical Psychology, 59,* 875–899.

Williams, K. E., & Chambless, D. L. (1990). The relationship between therapist characteristics and outcome of *in vivo* exposure treatment for agoraphobia. *Behavior Therapy, 21,* 111–116.

Woods, C. M., Chambless, D. L., & Steketee, G. (2002). Homework compliance and be-
    havior therapy outcome for panic with agoraphobia and obsessive compulsive dis-
    order. *Cognitive Behaviour Therapy, 31,* 88–95.
Yonkers, K. A., Zlotnick, C., Allsworth, J., Warshaw, M., Shea, T., & Keller, M. B.
    (1998). Is the course of panic disorder the same in women and men? *American Jour-
    nal of Psychiatry, 155,* 596–602.

2

Social Anxiety Disorder

DEBORAH ROTH LEDLEY
RICHARD G. HEIMBERG

OVERVIEW OF THE DISORDER

Social anxiety disorder (also known as social phobia) is characterized by "a marked or persistent fear of social or performance situations" (American Psychiatric Association, 1994, p. 411). People with the disorder worry that they will do or say something in such situations that will elicit negative evaluation from others. Another concern of people with social anxiety disorder is that they will exhibit physical symptoms (e.g., blushing, shaking, sweating, etc.) in social or performance situations that will lead others to assume that they are extremely anxious to the exclusion of other, more benign interpretations (Roth, Antony, & Swinson, 2001).

People with social anxiety disorder can be fearful of a wide range of situations (Holt, Heimberg, Hope, & Liebowitz, 1992), from the near ubiquitous fear of public speaking to fear of other social and performance situations like initiating and maintaining conversations, doing things in front of other people (e.g., writing, eating, and drinking), speaking with authority figures (e.g., bosses), or making requests of others (e.g., asking others to change their behavior or asking for a raise at work). Individuals with social anxiety disorder who fear many social and performance situations are referred to as having the generalized type of social anxiety disorder, while persons with fears of a more limited nature (e.g., they fear only public speaking) are said to have non-generalized social anxiety disorder. Persons with generalized social anxiety disorder tend to have more severe social anxiety symptoms and suffer greater impairment than those with more discrete fears (Heimberg, Holt, Schneier, Spitzer, & Liebowitz, 1993).

Most people experience anxiety in some social or performance situations. In fact, some degree of social anxiety is adaptive, motivating us to prepare for a presentation at work or for a job interview or to be on our best behavior on a first date or when meeting new people at a party. The factor that distinguishes people with social anxiety disorder from those with more normative levels of social anxiety is the level of distress that they experience in social situations and the degree of impairment in social, educational, and occupational functioning that is associated with this distress, which can be significant (e.g., Antony, Roth, Swinson, Huta, & Devins, 1998; Schneier et al., 1994). In the National Comorbidity Survey (NCS), a diagnosis of social anxiety disorder was negatively related to educational attainment and income, and rates of social anxiety disorder were significantly higher in people who, at the time they were surveyed, were not working or in school (Magee, Eaton, Wittchen, McGonagle, & Kessler, 1996). Anecdotally, many clinicians who work with this population note that their clients are grossly underemployed given their intelligence and abilities. In the social realm, persons with social anxiety disorder are less likely to be married than people without the disorder (Schneier, Johnson, Hornig, Liebowitz, & Weissman, 1992) and suffer impairment in their romantic relationships and friendships (Schneier et al., 1994; Whisman, Sheldon, & Goering, 2000). These impairments in functioning illuminate the importance of learning how to best treat social anxiety disorder and how to ensure that those with the disorder will continue to function well once treatment is over.

OVERVIEW OF EMPIRICALLY SUPPORTED TREATMENTS

Psychosocial Approaches: Overview of Cognitive-Behavioral Therapy

The psychosocial approach that has gained the most empirical support for the treatment of social anxiety disorder is cognitive-behavioral therapy (CBT). CBT for social anxiety disorder most commonly includes three primary components: in-session exposures, cognitive restructuring, and homework assignments (see Heimberg & Becker, 2002). *In-session exposures* are designed to help patients face social and performance situations in which they experience distress and/or situations that they avoid completely. *Cognitive restructuring* (CR) involves helping patients to become more aware of their thoughts, examine these thoughts to see if they are dysfunctional, and, for those that are, engage in a process of reframing. The goal of CR is to help patients view the world in a less biased, more accurate way so that they do not see danger lurking in every corner of the social world (Heimberg, 2002). *Homework assignments* involving both *in vivo* exposures and self-administered CR are also a crucial part of CBT. The primary goal of homework is to have patients apply what they have learned in therapy to their "real lives" and to develop a belief that they can manage situations that previously seemed insurmountable.

Many patients with social anxiety disorder experience physiological symptoms of anxiety in anticipation of and during social situations. Both exposures (in-session and *in vivo*) and CR may serve to reduce physiological arousal. Because physiological arousal is a natural response to perceived threat, the reduction of the amount of threat perceived should be directly correlated with reduction in the amount of physiological arousal. However, some CBT programs for social anxiety disorder directly target physiological arousal with the techniques of *relaxation training* (e.g., alternating muscle tension and relaxation, diaphragmatic breathing, and relaxing imagery). Relaxation for social anxiety disorder is most effective when taught as an applied skill that can be employed by the patient in stressful situations (Öst, Jerremalm, & Johansson, 1981; see Öst, 1987, for a review of applied relaxation techniques). In fact, there is little evidence that relaxation training without this applied focus is any more effective than a control group, and it should not be used in the treatment of social anxiety disorder (Rodebaugh, Holaway, & Heimberg, 2004).

Another technique often used in the treatment of social anxiety disorder is *social skills training* (SST). SST is premised on the assumption that patients with social anxiety disorder lack skills like making good eye contact and initiating conversations and that their anxiety results from the negative feedback that they receive in the social world because of these deficits. In SST, the therapist typically models appropriate skills, and the patient practices the skills in "behavioral rehearsals" and receives corrective feedback from the therapist. Patients are then instructed to apply their newly learned skills in real-life situations as homework assignments.

Heimberg's Cognitive-Behavioral Group Therapy

Controlled trials have been carried out on various CBT programs for social anxiety disorder that include some combination of the aforementioned components. The most studied CBT program for social anxiety disorder is cognitive-behavioral group therapy (CBGT; Heimberg & Becker, 2002). CBGT is typically administered to groups of five to six patients in 12 weekly sessions, lasting approximately 2½ hours. Ideally, groups are led by one male and one female therapist, affording opportunities for a range of in-session exposures. In sessions 1–2, patients are educated about social anxiety, with greatest emphasis placed on delineating the cognitive-behavioral view of the maintenance of social anxiety disorder (Rapee & Heimberg, 1997) and on what must be done to modify dysfunctional thoughts and behaviors. Patients are also taught CR and are given the opportunity to practice these skills and receive feedback from the therapists. Thereafter, therapists lead patients through in-session exposure exercises that are tailored to their own unique concerns. Exposures are preceded and followed by therapist-directed CR exercises and patients are coached in adaptive thinking during the exposure itself. At the end of each session, a homework assignment is negotiated with each patient. Homework typically consists of exposures to real life situations and patient-directed pre- and postexposure CR, helping patients learn to be their own therapists. As treatment proceeds, patients confront increasingly anxiety-provoking situations and are also helped to explore the core beliefs that underlie their difficulties with social anxiety.

Foa's Comprehensive Cognitive-Behavioral Therapy

Foa and her colleagues developed comprehensive cognitive-behavioral therapy (CCBT; Foa, Franklin, & Kozak, 2001; Franklin, Jaycox, & Foa, 1999). CCBT is based on CBGT but also includes a social skills training component. To accommodate this added component, treatment is administered for 14, rather than for 12, sessions. The SST component consists of structured exercises that teach specific social skills to patients. The goal is to help patients perform more effectively in a range of social situations and thereby be reinforced for their behavior from those with whom they interact. The SST exercises include both verbal and nonverbal skills such as initiating conversations and making appropriate eye contact. At the beginning of treatment, patients' baseline social performance is assessed, they are given a rationale for why they should modify certain behaviors, and they are educated about the behavior to be learned. After a particular behavior or skill is demonstrated by the therapist, patients have a chance to try it out. SST role plays are typically quite brief and are followed by immediate feedback and positive reinforcement from the therapists. Immediately following this feedback, patients engage in the role play again, repeating this iterative process until the patient can perform the skill well. CCBT also includes longer exposures in the vein of CBGT, but prior to each exposure, the patient and therapists identify some specific social skills to target during the exposure and the patient is given the opportunity to rehearse them before the exposure begins.

Other investigators have also developed treatment programs that include a social skills training component. For example, social effectiveness therapy, developed by Turner, Beidel, Cooley, and Woody (1994), was found effective in an open trial with 13 patients and was also found to have good long-term efficacy (Turner, Beidel, & Cooley-Quille, 1995).

While group treatment certainly holds appeal for the treatment of social anxiety disorder, it can be logistically difficult to implement, particularly in clinical settings in which it can take a long time to gather a sufficient number of appropriate patients to form a group. With this in mind, CBGT has been adapted for individual therapy format, both by Heimberg and his colleagues (Hope, Heimberg, Juster, & Turk, 2000) and by other individuals (Lucas & Telch, 1993; Öst, Sedvall, Breitholtz, Hellström, & Lindwall, 1995). CCBT has also recently been adapted to individual format (Huppert, Roth, & Foa, 2003).

Clark's Cognitive Therapy

Most recently, Clark and his colleagues have developed a cognitive therapy program for social anxiety disorder, also carried out in individual therapy format (Clark, 2001). Clark's cognitive therapy (CT) is quite different from existing programs, particularly in its emphasis on the importance of self-focused attention and safety behaviors in the maintenance of social anxiety disorder. Because persons with social anxiety disorder are so concerned with how they are coming across to others, their attention tends to become increasingly focused on the self rather than on what is actually going on in the social situation. Furthermore, to decrease the likelihood that negative outcomes will occur in social situations, persons with social anxiety disorder engage in "safety behaviors" (i.e., behaviors that the person believes will reduce the probability of negative social consequences). For example, a patient who fears being judged negatively for blushing might wear heavy makeup and a turtleneck sweater all year round so that people will not notice this symptom. Similarly, a patient who fears that her hands will shake so much at a party that she will spill her drink might grip her glass very tightly and hold it with both hands. The paradox of safety behaviors, however, is that they can actually increase the likelihood that feared outcomes will occur. For example, by gripping the glass tightly, the latter patient might cause her arms to shake more, increasing the likelihood of spilling the drink. Clark's treatment is premised on the notion that patients must learn to shift attention outward and drop their safety behaviors in order to change their experiences in social situations and their beliefs about themselves.

The treatment begins with the therapist and patient deriving a model of social anxiety that is idiosyncratic to the patient's unique concerns. In deriving the model, the patient begins to see the detrimental effect of self-focused attention and safety behaviors. The point is most clearly made though during an experiment in which the patient performs a role play under two conditions: (1) while focusing inward and using safety behaviors and (2) while focusing outward and dropping safety behaviors. Patients are asked to make predictions before each role play and thereafter evaluate the accuracy of their predictions. Typically, patients come to see that (1) self-focus and use of safety behaviors are actually associated with more anxiety, not less; and (2) basing their assessment of how they performed in social situation on how they remember *feeling*, rather than on what actually happened, leaves them with a distorted view of how they come across to others (Clark, 2001).

Once this framework is set, patients engage in behavioral experiments (similar to exposures), always being mindful of shifting focus of attention and dropping safety behaviors. As with the initial experiment, patients continue to make predictions before each behavioral experiment and evaluate the accuracy of those predictions once the experiment concludes. Use is also made of video feedback (described in more detail later) to further correct the distorted images that patients have of how they come across to others. Standard CT techniques can be employed to help patients deal with anticipatory anxiety and postevent processing and with assumptions about the self that do not shift when behavioral experiments provide disconfirmatory evidence.

Pharmacotherapy

Medications are also frequently used to treat social anxiety disorder. The commonly accepted "first line" treatments for social anxiety disorder are the selective serotonin reuptake inhibitors (SSRIs), such as paroxetine and sertraline. These medications tend to yield relatively good outcomes, with mild side effects and low risk of overdose, and several controlled studies and meta-analyses support their efficacy (see Blanco et al., 2003; Davidson, 2003). Interestingly, two recent studies have suggested that the SSRI fluoxetine might not be particularly effective in the treatment of social anxiety disorder. In a study comparing Clark's CT, fluoxetine, and pill placebo (Clark et al., 2003), the CT group showed outcomes superior to the fluoxetine and placebo groups, which did not differ from one another. In a double-blind, placebo controlled study, Kobak, Greist, Jefferson, and Katzelnick (2002) also failed to find a difference between fluoxetine and placebo. Further research must be done to see if fluoxetine is perhaps less effective in the treatment of social anxiety disorder than other SSRIs.

Other drugs affecting various neurotransmitter systems have been less researched than the SSRIs. There has been some preliminary support for the use of venlafaxine, a serotonin and norepinephrine reuptake inhibitor (e.g., Altamura, Pioli, Vitto, & Mannu, 1999), but placebo-controlled trials with this drug are yet to be published. One study (Pande et al., 1999) has shown gabapentin, a medication used to treat seizures, to be more effective than placebo in the treatment of social anxiety disorder, but these findings must be replicated before conclusions about the effectiveness of the drug can be drawn.

While the monamine oxidase inhibitors (MAOIs), like phenelzine, are very effective for social anxiety disorder (Blanco, Antia, & Liebowitz, 2002), patients who take them must adhere to strict dietary restrictions, avoiding any foods, beverages, and medications containing tyramine; if they do not, they are at increased risk for an acute surge in blood pressure, with potentially serious effects. Given this risk, MAOIs are used only after other medications (SSRIs, benzodiazepines, venlafaxine, etc.) have proven ineffective for a given patient. The reversible MAOIs, (e.g., moclobemide and brofaromine) do not require the same dietary restrictions as traditional MAOIs, but there are drawbacks to this class of medication too. First, they are not widely available—brofaromine has been taken off the market, and moclobemide is not available in the United States. Furthermore, the data are mixed, with some studies showing reversible MAOIs to be superior to placebo (Versiani et al., 1992) and some showing no difference from placebo (Noyes et al., 1997; Oosterbaan, van Balkom, Spinoven, van Oppen, & van Dyck, 1998; Schneier et al., 1998).

The other class of medication to receive the most attention for the treatment of social anxiety disorder is the benzodiazepines. Although studies with the benzodiazepine clonazepam have yielded very positive results (e.g., Davidson et al., 1993), studies of other benzodiazepines (e.g., alprazolam) have been less promising (Gelernter et al., 1991). Benzodiazepines are frequently prescribed but must be administered with adequate supervision because of their abuse potential and their sometimes difficult withdrawal effects (e.g., the phenomenon of rebound anxiety on withdrawal from alprazolam).

Are Treatments for Social Anxiety Disorder Efficacious?

There is now ample evidence to suggest that CBT for social anxiety disorder produces superior outcomes to no treatment or control psychotherapies (see reviews by Rodebaugh et al., 2004; Zaider & Heimberg, 2003). Meta-analysis has been used to compare the various components of treatment that fall under the CBT umbrella. Taylor (1996) compared patients who received CR alone, SST, exposure alone, or CR plus exposure to either wait-list control groups or to patients who received placebo treatments (either pill placebo or a control psychotherapy). All variants of CBT were more effective than wait-list controls. Although none of the CBT components differed from one another, only CR plus exposure was significantly more effective than placebo control treatments. Other meta-analyses (e.g., Gould, Buckminster, Pollack, Otto, & Yap, 1997) and a dismantling study (Hope, Heimberg, & Bruch, 1995) suggest that exposure is an essential component of CBT for social anxiety disorder and that the inclusion of formal CR does not necessarily improve outcomes.

Studies have also examined the differential efficacy of CBT and medication in the treatment of social anxiety disorder. Unfortunately, some of these studies (e.g., Clark & Agras, 1991; Turner, Beidel, & Jacob, 1994) have used medications that were not found to differ from placebo in other studies, calling into question the utility of their findings. Two studies, however, deserve mention. In a large multisite study (Heimberg et al., 1998), CBGT was compared to the MAOI phenelzine. The study included two control treatments: educational supportive therapy (a control psychotherapy) and pill placebo. At the end of the 12-week study, CBGT and phenelzine had both yielded superior outcomes to the control treatments and did not differ from one another. Although patients who received phenelzine improved somewhat more quickly than those who received CBGT, the CBGT group was less likely to relapse during a 6-month follow-up period (Liebowitz et al., 1999). In the recent aforementioned study, Clark et al. (2003) compared their cognitive therapy for social anxiety disorder to fluoxetine and pill placebo. The group that received CT yielded better outcomes than the other two groups, which did not differ from one another.

Meta-analyses have also shed light on the relative efficacy of CBT and pharmacotherapy for social anxiety disorder (Federoff & Taylor, 2001; Gould et al., 1997). In both meta-analyses, CBT and pharmacotherapies were roughly equivalent in the treatment of social anxiety disorder. Interestingly, in the meta-analysis by Federoff and Taylor (2001), the benzodiazepines were the only class of drug significantly superior to CBT, but this was based on a small number of studies of the benzodiazepines. Therefore, the decision to use benzodiazepines as a sole treatment for social anxiety disorder must be weighed against their limitations.

In recent years, focus has been placed on whether combining pharmacotherapy and CBT yields better outcomes than using either monotherapy alone (Foa, Franklin, & Moser, 2002). Two major combined treatment studies have been completed (Heimberg et al., 1998, compared CBGT to phenelzine to a combination of both; Davidson et al., 2004, compared CCBT to fluoxetine to a combination of both). The studies yielded mixed findings, with one showing some support for the use of combined treatment over monotherapies (Heimberg, 2003), and the other finding monotherapies to be as effective as combined treatments (Davidson et al., 2004).

To summarize, effective treatments for social anxiety disorder are available. While CBT and medication yield similar outcomes, medication tends to work slightly faster, and CBT tends to have better long-term efficacy (Liebowitz et al., 1999). As we learn more about social anxiety disorder and revise our treatments based on the most up-to-date knowledge, it is possible that CBT will yield superior outcomes to medication alone (Clark et al., 2003). While strong evidence does not exist at this time supporting the use of combined treatment over monotherapies, further research on the issue is needed.

Despite the availability of effective treatments for social anxiety disorder, there is certainly room for improvement. While patients most definitely improve, many are still quite symptomatic at the end of treatment. Furthermore, although treatment leads to improvements in quality of life, patients who successfully complete CBT for social anxiety disorder still have much poorer quality of life than individuals who have no psychological disorder (Eng, Coles, Heimberg, & Safren, 2001). With established treatments now in existence, it is important to consider how to improve outcomes, in terms of both social avoidance and distress and level of social and occupational functioning.

PREDICTORS OF TREATMENT OUTCOME

Two features of social anxiety disorder have been examined as possible moderators of treatment outcome—subtype of social anxiety disorder and the presence of avoidant personality disorder (APD). Individuals with generalized social anxiety disorder tend to be a more impaired group than those with nongeneralized social anxiety disorder, calling into question whether they might also respond less well to treatment. Data suggest that patients with generalized social anxiety disorder improve during treatment to the same degree as do patients with nongeneralized social anxiety disorder, but because they tend to be more impaired at the beginning of treatment, it is more difficult for them to reach a high level of end-state functioning by the time treatment ends. It is possible that with longer or more intense treatment, patients with generalized social anxiety disorder could reach the same level of end-state functioning as those with nongeneralized social anxiety disorder (see Brown, Heimberg, & Juster, 1995).

APD, which is diagnosed in about 60% of patients with generalized social anxiety disorder (Heimberg, 1996), has also been examined as a possible moderator of treatment outcome. Some studies have shown that the presence of APD (or features of it) impedes treatment (e.g., Chambless, Tran, & Glass, 1997; Feske, Perry, Chambless, Renneberg & Goldstein, 1996). However, other studies that have taken subtype of social anxiety disorder into account, have found APD to be unrelated to outcome (e.g., Brown et al., 1995; Hope, Herbert, & White, 1995). In fact, despite APD's status as a chronic and stable (Axis II) disorder, Brown et al. (1995) found that 47% of patients with social anxiety disorder and a comorbid diagnosis of APD before treatment no longer qualified for a diagnosis of APD after a brief cognitive-behavioral treatment. A comorbid diagnosis of social anxiety disorder and APD might represent social anxiety disorder of great severity; as social anxiety disorder symptoms improve, the characteristics of APD appear to abate (Heimberg, 1996).

Other potential moderators of treatment outcome have also been explored. Although the data have not been wholly consistent, there is reasonable evidence to suggest that treatment expectancy, homework compliance, and pretreatment depression are related to treatment outcome (see Hofmann, 2000b). With respect to treatment expectancy, two studies (Chambless et al., 1997; Safren, Heimberg, & Juster, 1997) found that patients who expected to benefit from CBGT and who believed the treatment to be credible did better in therapy than did patients who started treatment with more negative expectations. Data have also shown that homework compliance plays an important role in outcome, with patients who are more compliant evidencing more gains immediately following treatment in one study (Leung & Heimberg, 1996) and at 6-month follow-up in another study (Edelman & Chambless, 1995).

In Chambless et al.'s (1997) study, the best predictor of treatment outcome was pretreatment level of depression, with more depressed patients making fewer gains in treatment than less depressed patients. In contrast, Erwin, Heimberg, Juster, and Mindlin (2002) found that patients with social anxiety disorder with comorbid depression made improvements similar to those achieved by patients with social anxiety disorder alone or with a comorbid anxiety disorder. However, because higher pretreatment levels of depression were associated with higher levels of pretreatment social anxiety, the more depressed patients also evidenced more severe levels of social anxiety following treatment. Interestingly, they were no longer more depressed than the other groups after treatment, despite their greater social anxiety.

Another recent study (Erwin, Heimberg, Schneier, & Liebowitz, 2003) examined the impact of patients' experience of anger on the outcome of cognitive-behavioral treatment for social anxiety disorder. Patients who experienced anger more frequently, were more quick-tempered, and were more likely to perceive unfair treatment by others were less likely to complete a 12-session course of CBGT. Among treatment completers, those who experienced more extreme anger and who managed their anger by suppressing its expression (possibly for fear of negative evaluation by group therapists and other group members) responded less favorably to CBGT.

To summarize, it appears that positive expectancies for treatment and homework compliance are positively related to treatment outcome and severity of social anxiety disorder and anger suppression are predictive of negative outcome. The generalized subtype of social anxiety disorder, the presence of APD, and the presence of comorbid depression are all associated with greater severity of social anxiety symptoms. Although patients with these characteristics improve in treatment, they complete treatment with more severe social anxiety symptoms because they also start treatment with more severe social anxiety symptoms. As noted, these patients might require longer or more intense treatment, or in the case of depression or anger, some alterations to treatment aimed at improving outcomes (see Erwin et al., 2003; Huppert et al., 2003).

PRACTICAL STRATEGIES FOR IMPROVING OUTCOME

Typical Obstacles in Implementing Treatment and Strategies for Overcoming Them

Given that the greatest fear of patients with social anxiety disorder is social interactions, it is important to consider how difficult it can be for individuals with social anxiety disorder to seek out treatment and to become engaged in it once they do so. Many patients with social anxiety disorder avoid talking on the telephone (particularly with strangers), making it very difficult for them to call and inquire about treatment. If they are able to come in for an evaluation, taking the next step and sharing personal information with a stranger can be just as difficult. In a study by Olfson et al. (2000), the vast majority of people with social anxiety disorder recognized that they had an anxiety disorder, but a major barrier to their seeking treatment was fear of what others might think or say.

With this in mind, it is of utmost importance to put potential patients at ease when they first call to inquire about treatment. It can be very comforting for patients to hear that their concerns are similar to those of other patients. If patients want to set up an appointment, it can also be very useful to make sure that they have all the information that they need before hanging up. Because they may be too anxious to ask (or because anxiety might lead them to forget to ask), patients should be told where to come for their appointment, how to get there, and what to bring with them. Patients might be reluctant to call back to ask for clarification for fear that they will be judged negatively even before their first appointment.

When patients do come in for an evaluation, it is best to acknowledge their potential discomfort right away. For example, a clinician can say, "It can be very difficult for patients to come in here and share personal things. I want you to know that I am not here to judge or evaluate you. Rather, I hope that we can spend some time today figuring out what is causing problems for you and how we can best help you."

Once an evaluation is under way, clinicians can take added steps to put patients at ease. For example, they can say, "Yes, a lot of our patients fear going on dates," or "It's very common for people who blush to worry that others will think they are odd," or "Yes, feelings of depression quite commonly come along with social anxiety." Although clinicians should not make patients feel like their problems are so "normal" that they do not warrant attention, it is most often the case that patients with social anxiety disorder feel comforted hearing that they are not alone and that the clinician is not judging them negatively for the difficulties they are having.

After the evaluation, the next step is to present treatment options. The decision to begin CBT can be frightening for patients with social anxiety disorder. They may have avoided social situations that cause them distress for many years. The idea of purposefully putting themselves in these situations as a means of feeling less anxious can seem radical. There are a number of ways to help patients feel more at ease with exposure-based treatments. First, it can be very helpful to normalize their reactions. Second, they should be told that they will be given some helpful tools prior to doing exposures. These tools include education about social anxiety disorder, a framework from which to understand social anxiety disorder and how to treat it, and specific strategies to manage their anxiety as they experience it. Finally, patients can be told that exposures are typically done gradually. In many treatment programs, the therapist and the patient build a hierarchy that consists of a list of feared situations, each of which is assigned a rating of how anxious it makes the patient feel. The hierarchy serves as a roadmap for treatment, with early exposures involving less anxiety-evoking items and later exposures involving items that are further up the hierarchy. The increased self-efficacy and shift in beliefs that are gained from earlier exposures help patients to feel more confident about confronting more difficult situations.

Another roadblock to treatment that can be encountered concerns the format of treatment. It inherently makes sense to conduct treatment for social anxiety disorder in a group format. However, many patients are frightened of group therapy, and when group treatment is the only option, clinicians must know how to deal with patients' reluctance. A good strategy is to tell patients that although the group encapsulates exactly what they fear (e.g., casual interaction before the group begins, sharing personal information, and doing things in front of other people), it allows them to try out these things in the safe, therapeutic environment. Heimberg and Becker (2002) have identified a number of other advantages of group treatment, including learning that others have similar problems, the opportunity to learn from other members of the group, and encouragement through observation of others' successes.

Clinicians should be ever mindful of the role that social anxiety can play in patients' ability to successfully engage in treatment. Patients may repeatedly cancel the first session or miss a session during which a difficult exposure is scheduled. Some patients begin missing sessions for no apparent reason. It can then be helpful to directly ask patients if social anxiety is interfering with their ability to engage in treatment. For example, in the case of a patient who misses consecutive sessions or who misses a session in which a difficult exposure was planned, the therapist can call and ask, "Were you feeling nervous about doing that exposure we planned?" Knowing these reactions are common can make patients feel more comfortable discussing them and working with the therapist to get the treatment back on track.

Typical Obstacles in Psychoeducation and Strategies for Overcoming Them

Some CBT programs for social anxiety disorder begin with a psychoeducational component. Psychoeducation might include providing patients with information about social anxiety disorder (prevalence rates, etiological factors, etc.; see Heimberg & Becker, 2002), teaching them the cognitive-behavioral approach to understanding and treating social anxiety disorder (Heimberg & Becker, 2002), or building with them an idiosyncratic model that helps them to understand what maintains their own social anxiety (Clark, 2001; Huppert et al., 2003).

Psychoeducation can be very beneficial when done properly. All too often, however, therapists lapse into lecture mode, wanting to move through the material efficiently and get to the "meat" of the treatment. This is a mistake that can negatively affect outcome, particularly for patients with social anxiety disorder. Some patients wait years to come for treatment and, without exception, are quite anxious during their first few sessions. As in any social situation, they worry about saying the right thing and making a good impression. They also typically feel quite alone and worry that the therapist will not understand them or will discount their problems as unimportant or beyond help.

The psychoeducational portion of treatment can be very beneficial in dispelling these beliefs. Rather than lecturing, psychoeducation should be done in an interactive manner, asking patients how various concepts apply to them. This helps them to feel as if the therapist is trying to understand them and makes them feel as if the treatment will be tailored to their unique concerns. As they gradually start to share information, they will become less anxious and will also learn that the therapist will not evaluate them negatively. Instead, the therapist should be encouraging and supportive, letting patients know that their concerns are very similar to those experienced by other patients with social anxiety disorder.

On the other hand, therapists should also be mindful that questions can sometimes leave socially anxious patients feeling uncomfortable and scrutinized. Clark (2001) suggests using a whiteboard during early sessions, for example, when deriving an idiosyncratic model of the patient's social anxiety.

Patients can feel more comfortable sharing information early in treatment when the therapists' eyes are not directly on them but on a whiteboard, chalk-board, or easel instead.

Typical Obstacles in Cognitive Restructuring and Strategies for Overcoming Them

Some CBT programs teach CR in a structured way prior to getting started with exposures. Patients are taught to identify their automatic thoughts, see how these thoughts affect their feelings and behaviors, and reframe thoughts that are dysfunctional or irrational. They are also taught how they can apply CR in the context of stressful social situations. In CBGT (Heimberg & Becker, 2002), patients engage in preprocessing before each in-session exposure. For example, a patient who is going to have a conversation with another person might believe, "I won't have anything to say." The patient is encouraged to evaluate this thought (e.g., "Will I really have *nothing* to say?" or "Have I ever been in a situation before where I had absolutely nothing to say?") and to reframe it (e.g., "I will likely have at least a few things to say"). They are also taught to keep a rational thought (called the "rational response") in mind dur-ing the exposure. Following exposures, patients are encouraged to engage in postprocessing during which they evaluate the validity of their predictions about the exposure. Following from this example, the patient might be asked whether he actually had nothing to say, what topics he talked about, how it was for him to talk about those topics, whether the other person introduced additional topics and he was able to converse about them, the percentage of the conversation he was silent, and so on.

One of the biggest obstacles that can come up during CR is that patients have a difficult time identifying what they think during stressful social situa-tions. Patients are generally not accustomed to "grabbing" their anxious thoughts but can become quite adept at doing so if they are asked the "right" questions. Heimberg and Becker (2002) recommend questions like, "What did you think might happen in that situation?" or "What were you worried about?" A problem can arise when patients have avoided a situation for a long time—it becomes difficult to know exactly what they fear. One solution is to have patients enter a stressful social situation and identify their automatic thoughts once they are in it.

Another problem that can arise with CR is that therapists and patients can get into verbal arguments about patients' thoughts. Therapists, typically wanting to help patients, can fall into the trap of trying to convince patients that their beliefs are "wrong" (e.g., saying to a patient who fears she will have nothing to say, "Of course you'll have things to say!") This strategy is highly counterproductive. First, patients can feel undermined and criticized—certainly problematic for the socially anxious patient who walks through life feeling this way. Second, it is unlikely that patients will actually learn much. Lasting cognitive changes come about when patients arrive at new ways of thinking through their own efforts.

Some patients are simply not good at identifying their thoughts and working through the process of CR. However, it is still essential that patients learn to use their experiences during in-session and *in vivo* exposures as a means of changing their beliefs. As such, it is extremely helpful to have patients make predictions prior to exposures and evaluate those predictions thereafter. A good way of getting at the latter is to ask patients, "What did you learn from that exposure?" Even without formal CR, a patient who fears he will have nothing to say during a conversation will likely be able to say at the end of the exposure, "I had a lot more to say than I had expected."

Typical Obstacles in Exposure Therapy and Strategies for Overcoming Them

Helping Patients Understand the Rationale for Exposures

As already noted, exposures are an essential component of CBT for social anxiety disorder. It is not unusual for patients to feel hesitant about doing in-session or *in vivo* exposures or to refuse to do them completely. Therefore, before moving on to ways to maximize the usefulness of exposures, it is first important to discuss how to "sell" patients on the importance of doing exposures at all. The most important thing for patients to understand is the role that avoidance plays in social anxiety. Avoidance can present itself in two ways: either complete avoidance of particular social situations or subtle avoidance, in which patients enter social situations but engage in subtle strategies or safety behaviors to prevent the occurrence of feared outcomes. Both forms of avoidance most certainly are "effective" in the short term, making patients feel less anxious. In the long run, however, avoidance perpetuates anxiety. Patients never learn that they capable of managing social situations, even without the use of safety behaviors. The only way for patients to gain this sense of self-efficacy and competence is through direct experience. Once patients understand this connection between anxiety and avoidance, they might benefit from keeping a motivating phrase in mind such as "Invest anxiety in a calmer future" (Hope, Heimberg, Juster, & Turk, 2000, p. 9). Such phrases serve to remind them that it is okay, and actually desirable, to feel anxious during exposures because it means that they are working on the exact situations that cause them difficulties.

With this said, many patients do not believe that they will feel less anxious as they more frequently engage in feared social situations. Again, it is a good idea to explain the rationale to them of repeated exposures. From an extinction perspective, with repeated exposures, patients will gradually come to feel less anxious in social situations. Furthermore, with repeated exposures, the beliefs that patients hold are likely to change. Specifically, they will come to see that the outcomes they fear are far less likely to occur than they expect, and that if they do occur, they are far less costly than they expect. In other words, repeated exposure reduces both the perceived probability and the cost of feared outcomes of social situations (Foa et al., 2001). When patients come to see that feared outcomes are unlikely, and less costly if they do occur, they will feel more comfortable entering previously avoided or distressing situations.

An important caveat bears mention here. Early in treatment, the therapist should be cautious of trying to *convince* patients that these changes will occur. A better alternative is to encourage the patient to take the stance of a scientist. It is fine for patients to hypothesize that exposures will not work for them as long as they are open to trying and then reevaluating their predictions once they have made some attempts. Therapists can say, "I've seen exposure therapy work for many other patients, and I really hope it works for you too. But we just won't know until we try. So, why don't we keep an open mind and see how it is working as we go along?" Most patients are receptive to this scientific stance and are appreciative of being permitted to come to conclusions based on their own experiences.

Planning Exposures

Once patients understand the rationale for exposures, they must work with the therapist to decide what exposures to do. As we have already discussed, a hierarchy of feared situations is often made that serves as a roadmap for treatment. Patients are asked to rate each hierarchy item according to how much distress it causes, using a standard metric called the Subjective Units of Discomfort Scale (SUDS) that ranges from 0 (no anxiety at all) to 100 (the most anxiety the patient can imagine). Rank-ordering items allows patients to confront their feared situations in a gradual way, using successes from lower-rated items to increase confidence in confronting items higher on the hierarchy.

An excellent way to generate items for the hierarchy is to use a tool such as the Liebowitz Social Anxiety Scale (LSAS; Liebowitz, 1987), the most commonly used clinician-administered measure of social anxiety. The LSAS inquires about 24 social and performance situations that can be problematic for socially anxious individuals. Patients are asked to rate the degree of distress they experience in each situation and the degree to which they have avoided each situation in the past week. In some situations, the LSAS might have been administered during the assessment process before treatment commenced. It can then be used as a reference for creating the hierarchy. If it was not administered once treatment begins, the scale items can be used more informally to generate ideas.

To be most effective, hierarchies should be sufficiently detailed, taking into account variables that might make situations easier or more difficult. For example, the LSAS includes the item, "Giving a party." While creating the hierarchy, patients should be asked for more detail about what they fear about that situation. This might result in more than one hierarchy item, such as "Having some close family members over for my husband's birthday," "Hosting a birthday party for my child," and "Hosting a party for my husband's work colleagues." Although all these items involve hosting people in one's home, they might elicit very different levels of anxiety for the patient.

Effective hierarchies should include items with a range of SUDS ratings. The first exposure should involve a situation that elicits moderate anxiety (a SUDS rating of 40 or 50)—patients might feel uncomfortable but are unlikely to feel so uncomfortable that they would have to flee from the room in fear. The goal is for the first exposure experience to be a positive one in which they see that their feared consequences are unlikely to occur or are not particularly costly if they do. A hierarchy that only includes items ranging from SUDS of 90 to 100 does not give the therapist any place to start. If patients can only generate items with high SUDS, the therapist should work hard to come up with some items that evoke less anxiety but are still meaningful to the patient.

At times, patients generate a number of hierarchy items but none with high SUDS ratings. This does not happen often, but if it does, therapists should spend some time exploring the reasons behind it. Some patients may intentionally leave items with high SUDS off the hierarchy, thinking that they would be impossible to master. If patients acknowledge having excluded items for this reason, the therapist should encourage them to place these items on the hierarchy anyway. Patients should be helped to see that these items might not be as daunting as they expect once they progress up the hierarchy and have successes with lower-rated items.

A final point about hierarchies deserves mention. Therapists can at times be tempted to put items on the hierarchy that *they* see as important in getting over social anxiety. For example, most individuals with social anxiety disorder fear giving speeches, and a therapist might believe that the hierarchies of all patients should include "giving a speech." The best way to engage patients in treatment is to make them feel as if the therapy is tailored to their own unique concerns and designed with their goals in mind. Consider a patient who is a stay-at-home mom, who might return to her previous work as a receptionist when her children start school. This patient is unlikely to have to make a formal speech in the foreseeable future, so time spent on formal public speaking would not be time well spent. Rather, this patient might want to practice speaking up at meetings because she expects to go to meetings of the Parent–Teachers Association at her children's school. This might be a small part of her treatment, however, with more focus placed on having casual conversations with other parents, hosting gatherings at her home, and so on. There is no point in forcing patients to put items on their hierarchies that are not relevant to them, especially as CBT is a time-limited treatment and every session is valuable.

Teaching Patients to "Be" in Social Situations in a New Way

Most patients with social anxiety disorder put themselves into social situations quite regularly but continue to experience difficulties with social anxiety. Recent research suggests that the way that patients behave in social situations likely serves to maintain their social anxiety over time. As such, over the course of treatment, patients must be taught to *be* in social situations in a different way.

Cognitive-behavioral models of social anxiety disorder emphasize the idea that when patients are in stressful social situations, they tend to focus on themselves rather than other aspects of the social situation (Clark & Wells, 1995; Rapee & Heimberg, 1997). Unfortunately, the self-images held by persons with social anxiety disorder tend to be very negative (e.g., Hackmann, Clark, & McManus, 2000). It would be reasonable to expect that by focusing on negative self-images when in social situations, persons with social anxiety disorder open themselves up to all sorts of negative outcomes. Support for this notion has been found in recent studies in which participants were told to purposely hold a negative self-image in their minds when they were in a mock social situation (e.g., Hirsch, Clark, Mathews, & Williams, 2003; Spurr & Stopa, 2003). As compared to when they are told to focus on a less negative self-image, holding their typical self-image (a very negative one) in mind led persons with social anxiety disorder to feel more anxious, rate their anxiety symptoms as more noticeable, and rate their performance more poorly. Furthermore, holding a very negative self-image had an impact on the judgment of objective assessors, who perceived participants more negatively in this condition than when they were told to hold a less negative self-image in their minds (Hirsch et al., 2003). In other words, being self-focused can increase the likelihood of negative evaluation, exactly the outcome that persons with social anxiety disorder fear.

Another detrimental effect of being self-focused is that persons with social anxiety disorder come away from social situations with inaccurate information (Rapee & Heimberg, 1997). They tend to be overly attuned to negative feedback, causing them to miss out on potentially positive feedback like smiles or nods (Veljaca & Rapee, 1998). Furthermore, being self-focused leads them to come away from situations with memories of how they think they came across (how they looked in their minds' eye), rather than on how they actually came across to others. These negative and distorted images that are held in memory are likely to have an impact on their willingness to enter social situations again in the future (e.g., Coles, Turk, & Heimberg, 2002; Coles, Turk, Heimberg, & Fresco, 2001; Hackmann et al., 2000).

Taken together, these studies suggest that it is crucially important to help patients shift their focus of attention outward in social situations. In the context of treatment, this means that therapists must give instructions to this effect in order to increase the effectiveness of exposures. This is best demonstrated in a study by Wells and Papageorgiou (1998), in which persons with social anxiety disorder were asked to engage in a number of tasks from their hierarchies either without specific instructions, after having been given the rationale for doing exposures based on the habituation model (i.e., with repeated exposure to the situation, anxiety will decrease), or after having been instructed to focus externally rather than focusing inward on the self. Instructions to take an external focus resulted in greater decrements in anxiety and negative beliefs about the self than the other conditions. Studies have also shown that even when patients are not specifically instructed to shift focus of attention, such a shift tends to occur over the course of treatments that include repeated exposures to feared social situations (e.g., Hofmann, 2000a; Woody, Chambless & Glass, 1997).

Collecting Useful Information during the Exposure

In addition to learning to shift one's focus of attention and drop safety behaviors, it is essential that exposures are set up so that patients actually learn something from doing them. A number of things can be done to facilitate a good learning experience. Two of these activities can be done prior to the exposure: having patients formulate predictions about what will happen during the exposure and helping patients to set behavioral goals for the exposure. During the exposure, information must be collected that helps patients evaluate their predictions and assess whether they met their goals. To this end, video feedback and feedback from confederates (other people who take part in the exposure) or other members of a therapy group can further enhance patients' learning experience.

An exposure is perhaps most effective when patients are asked to formulate very specific predictions about what they expect will happen (Clark, 2001; Huppert et al., 2003). Patients should be asked how anxious they expect to feel (on a scale from 0–100) and also to make predictions about the consequences that they fear. For many patients, their initial prediction will be quite elusive, such as "I'll look anxious" or "I'll do something stupid." The clinician must help the patient to formulate a clearer, more easily measurable prediction. For example, a patient who is very fearful of her hands shaking while trying to drink from a glass at a cocktail party might predict that there is a 90% probability that she will spill her drink. Similarly, a patient who is scared of drawing a blank during a casual conversation might predict that he will be unable to respond to any questions asked of him. These are very easy predictions to evaluate once the exposure is over.

Another tool that can be used when preparing for exposures is to have patients set specific behavioral goals (Heimberg & Becker, 2002). As with predictions, it is important that patients' goals be objective, measurable, and based on observable behavior rather than anxiety. Patients should be encouraged to enter situations regardless of how anxious they feel. In the foregoing examples, the patient who was nervous about spilling might set the goal, "I am going to have a soft drink at the party," and the patient who was nervous about casual conversation might set the goal, "I am going to ask the other person three questions and say three things about myself." Setting goals such as these lends structure to the exposure experience and introduces a better basis for evaluating success or failure than how the patient *felt*.

One of the best tools that can then be used to evaluate predictions and goals is video feedback. Many patients with social anxiety disorder will initially be averse to being taped, particularly if they are going to have to watch themselves. This can be framed as part of their social anxiety disorder, and patients should be helped to see that video feedback is meant to help them shift their beliefs about the image they are portraying to others, rather than an opportunity to scrutinize themselves and pick out their flaws. When exposures are being taped, it is essential that the picture captures the data that will be important when processing the exposure. For example, if the patient is worried about people noticing her hands shake, her hands must be in the picture. Also, if it is feasible, the picture should also capture the other people who are involved in the exposure. This can be particularly beneficial if patients have specific predictions about others' reactions (e.g., "When I talk, people will be so bored that they'll yawn and gaze off into space) or assume that symptoms (e.g., blushing) or behaviors (e.g., saying "um") that they exhibit are very unusual or much worse than those exhibited by others. By watching themselves and another person on the tape, patients with social anxiety disorder might be surprised to see that other people also blush or say "um" during conversations. In addition to making a videotape of the exposure, another very useful tool is to gather feedback from the people who participated in the exposure or from observers in a group therapy setting. The feedback that is collected should be very specific, aimed at evaluating the predictions that patients made about the exposure.

Processing the Exposure

Once the exposure is over, it is time to process it. This is perhaps the most important part of in-session exposures—possibly even more important than the exposure itself. The idea of postprocessing is to use all the tools available (e.g., predictions, goals, video, and participant ratings) to help the patients experience a shift in their beliefs.

Different treatment programs do different things during postprocessing. In CBGT (Heimberg & Becker, 2002) and individual CBT based on the same model (Hope et al., 2000), patients are asked if they accomplished their goals and, if they did not, what stood in their way. Finding out the latter can be useful fodder for future exposures. Patients are also asked to reflect on their cognitions. Specifically, they are asked whether the automatic thoughts that they expected actually occurred, whether they experienced any new automatic thoughts, and whether their rational response was helpful. Throughout exposures, patients are asked for the SUDS ratings every minute—during the postprocessing, they are asked to examine their pattern of SUDS during the exposure and make some sense of it (see Heimberg & Becker, 2002, for some typical patterns of SUDS ratings). Finally, patients are asked to rerate their belief in their initial automatic thoughts and in the rational response, with the intention that following the exposure, patients will believe less strongly in their negative thoughts and more strongly in their rational response. Patients are also asked at the end of the postprocessing to summarize what they have learned and how they can apply the lesson to their everyday life.

In Clark's (2001) treatment and individual CCBT (Huppert et al., 2003), the focus in postprocessing is on evaluating predictions. Patient should be asked to rate how anxious they actually were during the exposure, as well as to evaluate their specific predictions (e.g., "Did you spill your drink?" and "Were there large gaps of silence where you had nothing to say?"). Often, patients end up feeling less anxious during exposures than they expected, and they recognize that their feared consequences were much less likely to occur than they had predicted. Confederate feedback and feedback from fellow group therapy patients can add to the message. These individuals typically rate patients much better than patients would have expected, often do not notice feared symptoms (e.g., shaky hands, blushing), and even when feared consequences do occur, typically have much different interpretations than patients would expect them to have. For example, if a patient spills her drink, the confederate might say, "I felt badly that she spilled her drink. I did that once at a party too, and I was pretty embarrassed" or "I didn't think much of it at all. I just got a napkin and helped to clean it up." Such responses are in stark contrast to the prediction of the patient with social anxiety disorder who might think that if she spills a drink, people will think she is incompetent and not worthy of their friendship.

A problem that quite often occurs during postprocessing is discounting. When an exposure goes well, patients often attribute it to some external source like luck or the kindness of the other people involved ("He was just being nice"). It is very important for therapists to help patients see their contribution to the success of the exposure. They can be asked to reflect on what they were doing differently during the exposure (i.e., that they would not have done before treatment) that might have contributed to the positive outcome. For example, they might be able to say that they were trying to shift their attention outward or that that they were really trying to respond to questions with more than one-word answers. If patients discount in-session exposures as "artificial," they can be assigned the same exposure for homework. In this way, patients will see that they can manage in the "real world" as well, where people are not as invested in their success.

Video feedback can also be used during postprocessing, and one of its greatest strengths is that it is not particularly open to discounting. The purpose of video feedback is for patients to get a less biased picture of how they come across to others in social situations. Clark (2001) distinguishes between the "felt sense" and what *actually* happens in social situations. Socially anxious patients typically come away from situations judging themselves on how they *felt* in the situation. They assume that because they felt anxious, they must have looked anxious and performed badly. Video feedback can be used to help them see what actually happens in social situations—that is, what other people see—so that they come away from situations with more accurate information. It is then more likely that patients will feel an increased sense of self-efficacy and will start feeling more confident about entering social situations.

As with exposures, the way in which patients are instructed to carry out video feedback is very important. As we have already noted, the purpose of video feedback is not for patients to find fault with themselves. Rather, they are instructed to make predictions about what they will see and then to watch the video as an objective observer would. One nice way to explain this to patients is to tell them to pretend they are watching someone across the room at a party or watching a person in a movie. The importance of instructions for video feedback was demonstrated in a study by Harvey, Clark, Ehlers, and Rapee (2000). In this study, half of the participants were simply asked to view a tape of themselves giving a speech. The other half were asked about their expectations of what they would see before the tape was played. This manipulation, termed "cognitive preparation," was meant to illuminate for participants the discrepancy between their felt sense of how they looked during the speech and how they actually looked. While all participants rated their performance more positively after they had seen the tape than before, this difference was, in fact, significantly greater for participants who had received cognitive preparation. Kim, Lundh, and Harvey (2002) replicated and extended these findings, showing that cognitive preparation not only enhanced video feedback but also had implications for future speeches. Participants who received cognitive preparation had more positive reactions when asked to give a second speech and were less worried about it than participants who had not received cognitive preparation, suggesting that a corrected self-image had a very positive effect. Video feedback appears to be most effective when there is indeed a discrepancy between the patient's evaluation of his or her behavior and other people's evaluations (Rodebaugh & Chambless, 2002).

Once the postprocessing of one exposure is complete, it is the job of the clinician to decide where to go next with the treatment. One thing to keep in mind is that patients must learn to transfer what they have learned in session to their real lives outside therapy. If a patient asked a confederate out on a date during the in-session exposure, an appropriate homework assignment would be to ask someone out in real life. While in-session exposures are very useful, the most powerful learning experiences for patients with social anxiety disorder are those that come outside sessions. Although it would be unrealistic to hope that every exposure works out perfectly, patients should understand that simply *trying* things is useful. If a patient asks someone on a date and the person says "no," the patient should recognize that simply asking is a major improvement over doing nothing at all.

In moving from session to session, the hierarchy provides general direction, but each exposure also informs subsequent exposures. For example, one patient completed a few exposures that involved casual conversations with another person. She became quite comfortable with the conversations once they got going, but she had an extremely difficult time initiating these conversations. Therefore, in subsequent sessions, the patient was asked to initiate brief conversations with a several people, rather than engaging in a whole conversation with one person.

Methods of Improving Homework Compliance

As we have just noted, it is very important for patients to apply what they have learned to life outside therapy. Homework assignments in social anxiety disorder treatment can include reading psychoeducational material, doing self-monitoring, and, almost without exception, *in vivo* exposures and self-administered CR. The best way to sell the importance of homework to patients is to tell them that research has demonstrated that there is a positive relationship between homework compliance and outcome in treatment for social anxiety disorder (Edelman & Chambless, 1995; Leung & Heimberg, 1996). The more that patients practice being in social situations, the easier it will become—similar to learning any other new skill like a language or a sport.

There are numerous ways that homework compliance can be improved in the treatment of social anxiety disorder (see Huppert, Roth, & Foa, in press). First, it is essential that homework assignments are realistic and reasonable. Although an assignment should be selected that requires a patient to confront a feared situation, it should not be so anxiety provoking that a patient would have to leave in the middle. The goal, of course, is that the patient has success experiences, particularly early in treatment. It is important to remember that patients with social anxiety disorder might be reluctant to tell a therapist that a homework assignment is too difficult, so therapists should ask and should be open to patients' ideas for alterations. On a related note, patients should be involved in designing their homework assignments, particularly in the later stages of treatment. When patients select their own assignment, it has greater meaning for them, and they will likely be more motivated to follow through than if the therapist simply prescribes it. Therapists should always begin the session by checking in about homework and helping patients to process the experiences that they had.

Therapists who work with patients with a range of anxiety disorders often feel that it is more difficult to set up exposures for social anxiety disorder patients than for patients with other anxiety disorders. The complication with exposures for social anxiety disorder is that they invariably involve other people. Some patients with social anxiety disorder have very few social contacts at all. Even those who have contacts might be reluctant to change the nature of the interactions that they currently have. For example, a mother of small children might have always simply said "hello" to other mothers at school and at sporting events but avoided any further interaction with them. It can then be very difficult to ask another mother if she wants to have lunch or if she would like to plan a play date for the children. Due to the nature of the disorder, patients with social anxiety disorder worry that taking interactions to that next level might be construed by others as being odd or inappropriate.

With these issues in mind, it is not enough to just assign homework. Patients must be helped to formulate a plan to actually carry out the exposure. A person with very few social contacts might be encouraged to join a group or a club for people who share his interests. Getting this in motion might involve helping the patient to find listings of clubs in the community and planning what he should ask when he makes his initial phone calls to various groups (when does the group meet, how much does it cost, etc.) There will likely be many opportunities for exposures along the way (e.g., phone calls) before a patient actually starts to establish social connections. For patients who have some connections but worry about making a "next step," CR can be used to help patients overcome this barrier to progress. For example, the mother mentioned previously could be asked how she would feel if one of the other mothers asked her to lunch or asked her and her son over for a play date. Encouraging patients to put themselves in someone else's shoes can be a very effective way of correcting distorted thoughts and, with a more rational frame of mind, can spur patients into action.

Adding Social Skills Training as a Means of Improving Outcomes

As noted earlier, researchers have examined the utility of adding SST to traditional CBT programs. The question of whether SST is necessary in the treatment of social anxiety disorder has been discussed frequently in the literature. Some (e.g., Clark & Wells, 1995; Rapee & Heimberg, 1997) believe that most patients with social anxiety disorder have appropriate social skills but that their social anxiety interferes in their ability to function well in social situations. Others (e.g., Foa et al., 2001) believe that some patients with social anxiety disorder do lack social skills and need specific instruction and practice to acquire the skills that they lack.

Despite all the discussion about whether patients with social anxiety disorder lack social skills, little research has been done on whether SST is a useful addition to existing CBT programs. Recently, Herbert et al. (in press) completed a study in which patients with generalized social anxiety disorder were randomly assigned to receive 12 sessions of CBGT administered with SST or without SST. Patients who received CBGT with SST were significantly more likely to respond to treatment, reported experiencing less social anxiety, and came across as less anxious during behavior tests. Herbert's group also did a benchmarking study (Herbert, Rheingold, & Goldstein, 2002), comparing a 6-week CBGT program that included SST to the standard 12-week CBGT program used in other studies. They found their briefer treatment that included SST to be as effective as longer treatment programs that did not include SST.

In sum, preliminary evidence suggests that adding SST to existing CBT programs might improve outcomes. That the addition of SST improves outcomes, however, does not necessarily mean that patients had deficits in the first place. It is certainly possible that the perception of being more skilled leads to greater reductions in social anxiety or that SST contains aspects of exposure that may themselves be therapeutic. Future research on this issue should compare CBT with and without SST in the context of a placebo-controlled or wait-list trial and should also try to determine whether SST leads to a true acquisition of new skills or to a change in patients' perceptions of the skills that they have.

Walker (2003) is taking a slightly different approach, focusing on treatment that teaches persons with social anxiety disorder specific interpersonal skills, more broadly defined than specific social skills, such as eye contact or voice volume. In his treatment, patients are taught how to meet people who could eventually become friends or romantic partners (e.g., joining clubs and attending church or synagogue) and how to nurture casual relationships to become closer relationships. Although data are not yet available on the efficacy of these strategies, they are likely valuable additions to existing treatments for social anxiety disorder, particularly in light of the finding that even patients who respond well to treatment continue to report relatively poor, though much improved, quality of life (Eng et al., 2001).

ADAPTING TREATMENTS FOR
CHILDREN AND ADOLESCENTS

In contrast to the controversy about social skills deficits in socially anxious adults, it is generally agreed that socially anxious children do exhibit such deficits (Beidel, Turner, & Morris, 1999). As such, SST is considered an essential part of treatment (Beidel, Turner, & Morris, 2000; Spence, Donovan, & Brechman-Toussaint, 2000). A unique component of the SST that is used in CBT programs for children with social anxiety disorder is peer generalization (Beidel et al., 2000). Following SST, children with social anxiety disorder join a group of nonanxious peers for a social activity. This allows anxious children to try out their new skills in a naturalistic setting and to observe (and, ideally, model) the behavior of nonanxious children. Recently, promising preliminary results have also been found for a school-based social anxiety disorder treatment program (Masia, Klein, Storch, & Corda, 2001) that affords improved ability to generalize treatment gains to the natural environment and which also allows for the incorporation of peer support and teacher assistance into the treatment package.

Albano, Marten, Holt, Heimberg, and Barlow (1995) evaluated a cognitive-behavioral group treatment specifically designed to address social anxiety in adolescents (CBGT-A), based on Heimberg's CBGT for adults (Heimberg & Becker, 2002). For four out of five adolescents, criteria were no longer met for social anxiety disorder after 16 sessions of CBGT-A. Hayward et al. (2000) conducted a controlled trial of CBGT-A with a sample of 35 adolescent females who were randomly assigned to either CBGT-A or a no-treatment control group. The percentage of adolescents who no longer met criteria for social anxiety disorder was significantly higher in the CBGT-A group than in the control condition.

Treatment gains were also maintained by children receiving both CBGT-A (Albano et al., 1995) and Social Effectiveness Training for Children (Beidel et al., 2000) at 1-year and 6-month follow-up assessments, respectively. However, in the study by Hayward et al. (2000), differences between CBGT-A and the control condition were no longer significant at the 1-year follow-up assessment.

ADAPTING TREATMENTS FOR
PARTICULAR PRESENTATIONS

Many patients with social anxiety disorder fear that they will exhibit physical symptoms of anxiety like blushing, shaking, or sweating. Others fear that they will have a panic attack during social situations, making it difficult for them to function. Treatments can be adapted to patients with both of these types of concerns. In the case of patients who fear exhibiting particular physical symptoms, video and confederate feedback can first be employed to help patients to see that (1) their physical symptoms are likely less noticeable than they think and (2) even if their symptoms are noticed, people are unlikely to make negative judgments because of them. Once patients come to see these two points, exposures can be set up in which these symptoms are purposefully exacerbated. Clark (2001) calls this "interrogating the environment" (p. 422). Patients who fear sweating can wear a very warm shirt on a hot day or purposefully put circles of water under their arms; those who fear blushing can wear blush on their cheeks to make them very red; those who fear shaking can make their hands purposefully shake. Patients can then monitor the reactions of others either through video feedback, through confederate feedback, or in the natural environment. Even in these "extreme" situations, patients are often very surprised to see that people do not notice their symptoms, or that if they do, they think very little about them.

For patients who fear having panic attacks during social situations, exposures early in treatment will often show them that these attacks are much less likely than they think, particularly when they shift their attention outward, thereby becoming less aware of physical symptoms. If patients continue to believe that they would not be able to function if they were to have an attack, interoceptive exposure exercises used in the treatment of panic disorder (McCabe & Antony, Chapter 1, this volume) can be used to induce panic symptoms prior to doing an exposure. For example, if a patient fears having an attack while making a speech, he can be asked to hyperventilate or run up and down stairs before the speech. By doing this, patients show themselves that they can function despite uncomfortable physical symptoms.

Adjustments to treatment are sometimes necessary for patients with nongeneralized social anxiety disorder, particularly those with fears of public speaking. In clinical settings where confederates are not available to serve as an audience, patients should be encouraged to attend Toastmasters or a public speaking class so that they can have opportunities for appropriate exposures. We have seen some patients who are not particularly anxious doing speeches in the clinic setting but who have a great deal of anxiety at work. These patients can benefit from some of the treatment techniques by audiotaping feared situations at work like conference calls, giving reports at meetings, or making formal presentations. Small recorders, like those used to tape lectures, can be used inconspicuously. Although audiotapes do not provide visual feedback, patients will be able to examine their beliefs about the quality of their speech.

Finally, patients who fear very unrealistic consequences in social situations or who are worried about the long-term consequences of having social anxiety (ending up alone, with no friends, spouse, job, etc.) might benefit from imaginal exposure because these types of fears are very hard to "test out" in the context of *in vivo* exposures. Foa's group (see Huppert et al., 2003) has been experimenting with this technique, having had much success with imaginal exposure in the treatment of both obsessive–compulsive disorder and posttraumatic stress disorder (Foa & Wilson, 2001; Foa & Rothbaum, 1998).

ADAPTING TREATMENTS FOR COMORBIDITY

According to the NCS (Magee et al., 1996), social anxiety disorder is associated with a high degree of comorbidity. The most common co-occurring disorder in patients with social anxiety disorder is depression, followed by alcohol dependence. Unfortunately, patients with these comorbid diagnoses are typically excluded from large treatment outcome studies, leaving gaps in our knowledge of the functional relationship between the disorders and whether depression or substance use has a negative impact on treatment outcome. If the presence of these additional disorders does have a detrimental effect on treatment outcome for social anxiety disorder, possible adjustments to existing treatments must be explored in order to improve outcomes for these particularly impaired patients. For example, CCBT includes a module specifically designed to address comorbid depression (see Huppert et al., 2003). In CCBT, behavioral activation and cognitive therapy, empirically supported techniques used in the treatment of depression, are interwoven into treatment for social anxiety disorder. Use of these techniques is meant to improve motivation and increase hopefulness, both of which are likely important for retaining patients in treatment and helping them to achieve a good outcome. The findings of Erwin et al. (2003) suggest that a similar approach may be useful among socially anxious patients who have problems with anger management.

COMBINING COGNITIVE-BEHAVIORAL THERAPY WITH MEDICATIONS

As noted previously, there is a lack of empirical support at the current time for using combined CBT and medication rather than either medication or CBT alone. However, because individual patients may respond differently to each available strategy (medication alone, CBT alone, and combined treatment), it would be worthwhile to discover ways of predicting who is likely to respond to one approach versus another.

In the future, different strategies for combining treatments should also be examined. In studies of combined treatment to date, treatments have been administered concurrently, calling into question whether the first portion of CBT was carried out before the medication had even taken effect. Future studies should examine whether different strategies for combining medications may yield more optimal outcomes (e.g., having a medication lead-in for 4–6 weeks before CBT commences) and whether combined treatments should be given to all patients or just to those who partially respond to a monotherapy (e.g., augmenting CBT with medication in partial CBT responders or augmenting medication with CBT for partial medication responders).

PREDICTORS OF RELAPSE AND RECURRENCE

Very little has been written on predictors of relapse and recurrence in patients who have been treated for social anxiety disorder. Clinical experience sheds some light on factors that might be important. It is likely that the best predictor of relapse is avoidance. This can include both overt avoidance or reverting back to subtle avoidance strategies or safety behaviors when in anxiety-provoking social situations. When patients begin to avoid social situations, they reinforce the notion that they cannot manage them, and it becomes progressively more difficult to confront them. It can be difficult for patients to regularly confront feared situations, especially those that come up very infrequently (e.g., giving speeches). As we outline in the next section, therapists must help patients plan for ways that they can continue to work on feared situations once treatment is over, even if the situations do not frequently occur.

Another likely predictor of relapse is difficulty with generalization. It is impossible in time-limited treatments to do exposures to every situation that patients fear and to take into account the different variables that could make each situation more or less anxiety provoking. Patients must understand that the principles of treatment can be applied to *any* social situation. If they have not conquered all their feared situations during therapy, or if new feared situations arise, they must be prepared to apply what they have learned in treatment. Patients who avoid situations because they believe that they do not have the tools to manage them will likely begin having difficulties with social anxiety again.

STRATEGIES FOR PREVENTING
RELAPSE AND RECURRENCE

Although we have no strong data about predictors of relapse, strategies for preventing relapse are thought to be an important component of CBT programs for social anxiety disorder. Two essential strategies are helping patients to form reasonable expectations for the future and helping patients to feel confident about the skills they acquired during treatment and their abilities to apply these skills once treatment is over.

It is important that patients are helped to formulate a realistic picture of what life will be like for them after therapy. Although we certainly do not want to be pessimistic with clients, it would be unrealistic to tell them that once therapy ends, they will be gregarious and outgoing all the time, in all situations. Most patients with social anxiety disorder (and most people without social anxiety disorder!) will feel somewhat anxious in some social situations throughout their lives, even after a very successful course of treatment. As long as patients do not start avoiding social situations, or using subtle avoidance strategies to manage situations that they do enter, there is nothing wrong with feeling a bit of anxiety. If patients understand that they will continue to feel anxious from time to time, they will not be surprised or disappointed when it happens. What is most important is that they remember to judge the outcome of situations on what they *did*, rather than on how they *felt*. It is also very important for patients to view anxiety-provoking situations as opportunities to try out their new skills rather than as signs of failure.

Another excellent way to prevent relapse is to make sure that patients know that they have the skills required to maintain their gains, and even to make further progress, once therapy is over. It is typically impossible for persons with social anxiety disorder to accomplish all their goals by the end of therapy, particularly if they include things like making new friends, meeting a romantic partner, or getting a new job. Rather, patients need to continue working on their own to accomplish these goals. The best way to help patients feel that they can do this is to communicate throughout therapy that a goal is for patients to become their own therapists. This can be accomplished by having patients take a progressively more active role in planning in-session exposures and devising homework assignments. Some patients will be reluctant to do this, fearing negative evaluation from the therapist. Patients should be directly told that the therapist is not out to judge them but, rather, to help them to acquire the skills they need to get past their social anxiety—not only during therapy but also once it is over.

In addition to taking a progressively more active role in the treatment, patients must also be encouraged to seize upon opportunities that come up naturally in their day-to-day lives. For example, someone who usually keeps to herself at work should start having lunch or coffee with coworkers. Patients who do well in treatment, and those who continue to make gains once treatment is over, tend to be those who seize every opportunity they can to work on their social anxiety. Therapists should keep in mind that doing this is the antithesis of how socially anxious individuals typically manage their lives (i.e., via avoidance). As such, it is essential that therapists emphasize the importance of this shift throughout therapy and provide ample reinforcement to patients whenever they do seize the moment.

To get patients to see that they have acquired skills during therapy that can be applied to a broad range of situations, "social anxiety quizzes" can be used near the end of treatment. By this point in therapy, patients are typically less reluctant to be "tested" by the therapist and are actually excited to demonstrate their newly acquired knowledge. They can either be asked how they would deal with hypothetical situations that might come up in their own lives (e.g., "What would you do if your new job involved giving a weekly report at a staff meeting and you were really anxious about it?") or how they would advise another socially anxious person (e.g., "If you were a therapist, what would you tell a patient who was very nervous about giving a toast at his brother's wedding?") These quizzes show patients that they have acquired skills that can be applied to a whole range of social situations. Furthermore, if patients say that they have no idea how to deal with particular situations or get an answer to the social anxiety quiz "wrong," therapists will see gaps in their knowledge that can be addressed before therapy ends.

It is also helpful near the end of therapy to take of stock of what was accomplished and to set goals for the future. In terms of taking stock, patients can be asked to articulate their accomplishments in therapy (Hope et al., 2000). They can also review their hierarchy and assign new SUDS ratings. After successful therapy, most (if not all) SUDS ratings will have decreased. It is not enough though to simply make these ratings. Rather, patients should be asked why such significant changes occurred. Patients should be able to say that it was because their behaviors changed and, along with this, so did their beliefs about their abilities to function in the social world. Sometimes, patients will also recognize that the situations they confronted most frequently were the ones that showed the largest decrease in anxiety. This reinforces for patients the importance of frequently confronting feared situations.

In addition to looking back on the successes of therapy, it is important to set goals for the future because it will be impossible to accomplish every goal during a time-limited therapy (Hope et al., 2000). The therapist should make clear to patients that it is normal to not fully accomplish all their goals and should help patients set some goals that they can accomplish on their own by specified time intervals after therapy has ended (e.g., goals for 2 weeks, 1 month, 3 months, 6 months, and 1 year after treatment). They can also discuss how to accomplish these goals, dealing with any potential roadblocks that might stand in the way of success. For example, if a patient wants to meet a romantic partner, he might decide that within 2 weeks of completing treatment, he is going to join a dating service and that within 1 month, he would like to go on at least one date. Within 3 months, he might want to broaden his social activities if the dating service is not working out. This might involve getting involved in a group at church or joining a health club. Although it would be unrealistic to set a deadline for being in a romantic relationship, it is certainly reasonable to set goals for getting into social situations where accomplishing this ultimate goal is more likely.

Another excellent way to reduce the risk of relapse is to deal with small lapses as they arise, rather than waiting for full-blown relapse to occur. This is best accomplished through a few booster sessions or through a quick phone call or e-mail to the therapist. Unfortunately, due to the nature of social anxiety, patients with social anxiety disorder can feel reluctant to solicit help when they need it. They might fear negative judgment or worry that their difficulties will make the therapist feel badly about his or her own skills. With this in mind, socially anxious patients should actually be encouraged to be in touch. They should leave therapy with the sense that it is the norm to have periodic booster sessions and that a few booster sessions to help them over a rough patch is far better than ignoring problems and relapsing. One of our patients who had done very well in therapy came in for one booster session before a medical school interview. The session included some CR as well as a mock interview. The patient left the session recognizing that he had the skills he needed to manage this situation and also appreciating that some anxiety before a medical school interview was completely normal. This was of course a far better outcome than avoiding the interview and failing to realize his dreams of going to medical school.

CASE EXAMPLE

Peter was a 19-year-old college junior. His mother arranged for him to come in for an assessment because he was too anxious to use the telephone. He arrived at the appointed time and was visibly anxious, looking down throughout most of the assessment and providing short responses to questions. Peter reported fearing all social situations. Although he attended classes and would speak up if required for his grade (e.g., having a conversation in a language class), he avoided virtually everything else. He had no friends on campus, had never spoken to a professor, and even felt nervous doing day-to-day tasks like paying for his lunch in the cafeteria or asking for help with finding a book in the bookstore or library.

Peter's main concern was that his intense anxiety would get in the way of his performance. For example, when faced with initiating conversations, Peter believed that his anxiety would get in the way of him "knowing" what to say. Once Peter got past this initial anxiety, he then worried that he would come across to others as "odd." When probed, Peter explained that he had very different interests from other college students. Rather than liking sports and going out to bars, Peter liked going to art museums, seeing classical music concerts, and reading literature. He believed that if people knew what his interests were, they would perceive him to be "snobby" and "highbrow" and would not want to be friends with him. This then extended to a fear of always being alone, without friends or romantic relationships. Peter felt quite hopeless about making changes in his life, and this was congruent with an additional diagnosis of major depressive disorder.

Despite his severe presentation, Peter agreed to begin treatment. In the first session of treatment, Peter and his therapist developed a model to understand the maintenance of his social anxiety, and the therapist oriented Peter to the treatment program. Specifically, Peter was introduced to the idea that shifting his focus of attention and dropping safety behaviors might lead to more success and a greater sense of enjoyment in social situations. Given the presence of comorbid depression, Peter and his therapist also spent some time discussing the relationship between depression and social anxiety, and activity monitoring was assigned for the upcoming week.

When Peter came in for his next session, he seemed dejected and his depression had worsened. In doing the activity monitoring, Peter realized that he had very little in his life besides the simple day-to-day routines like going to class and eating meals. He explained that doing the homework made him feel hopeless about treatment, and he was wondering whether there was any chance that he could make improvements. The therapist helped Peter to see how social anxiety and depression were both getting in the way of his being more active and also how scheduling more pleasant activities would likely help his mood. She also told Peter that the goal of treatment would be to gradually add more social activities to his week, which would be positive for his social anxiety and would also have a positive impact on his mood. For the remainder of the session, Peter and his therapist worked on activity planning for the upcoming week, taking care not to schedule activities that Peter would not be able to accomplish because of his social anxiety. They decided that he would start a book he had been looking forward to reading, rent some movies, and go for some walks in the city. Cognitive therapy techniques were also used to help Peter examine the belief that his situation was hopeless.

Peter came in the following week having done a few of the scheduled activities, but he was still feeling depressed and hopeless. When patients come in for a session feeling this way, it can be tempting for the therapist to spend more time discussing these beliefs with the patient. In Peter's case, the therapist decided to progress to the treatment of Peter's social anxiety disorder. She believed that the best way to "convince" Peter that there was hope and that he could make changes was to show him through *doing*.

With this goal in mind, the rest of the session involved Peter's first in-session exposure. In this exposure, Peter had a casual conversation with a member of the clinic staff, making his first attempt to shift attention outward and drop his safety behaviors. Peter tried very hard to attend to the back-and-forth flow of the conversation, saying what first came to mind instead of trying to "filter" what he was going to say or saying very little so that the conversation would end sooner. Ratings were collected from the confederate and video feedback was used. Although Peter judged himself very harshly, the conversation went better than he had predicted and he also thought that he looked better on the video than he thought he would. The confederate found the conversation to be enjoyable, despite judging Peter to be quite anxious. When Peter was asked what he learned during this exposure, he said, "Maybe looking anxious doesn't translate into complete disaster."

Over the next few sessions, the same exposure was repeated with different confederates. Although Peter continued to judge himself harshly, his ratings improved each week. He was quite surprised to see how shifting his focus of attention could make him feel more "present" in the conversation and less anxious about his performance. With this being said, Peter continued to be a very challenging patient. His depression colored his judgments, causing him to put a negative spin on even the most positive feedback. Furthermore, he continued to be very avoidant outside sessions. His lack of activity—both nonsocial and social—appeared to be perpetuating his problems with social anxiety and depression.

After the fifth session of therapy, Peter went home for the 3-week winter break. He returned to school even more dejected than he had been, having spent 3 weeks seeing no one but his family, whom he reported to be highly critical and emotionally withdrawn. The therapist suggested to Peter that the start of the new semester could be seen as an opportunity to "turn over a new leaf," really trying to apply what he was doing in sessions to the "real world." Although extremely hesitant, Peter agreed to a very specific homework assignment for the upcoming week—to speak to one fellow student in each of his classes, to say something in each class (e.g., ask or answer a question), and to call the therapist each day to report how these exposures went. The phone calls served as both an exposure (Peter was anxious about the use of the telephone) and an opportunity to "troubleshoot" about homework right away, rather than waiting a whole week to find out that the assignment was too difficult. Peter phoned the day after this session, reporting that he had failed miserably—he had not spoken at all in class. When the therapist probed, it turned out that the class was being held in a room too small for the number of students so Peter had to sit on the floor and the teacher spent the whole time encouraging students to drop the class. The therapist commended Peter for phoning and helped him to see how extenuating circumstances made it difficult for him to complete the assigned work. The therapist then did not hear from Peter for the rest of the week.

When Peter came in for his next session, he explained that he had not spoken to anyone in his classes because he did not know how to initiate conversations. This was an issue that had come up in his earlier exposures—Peter would be so anxious at the beginning of an exposure that he "froze" and had to wait for the other person to start talking. He also explained that he did not call to check in with the therapist because he was worried that she would judge him negatively for not doing the homework. The therapist emphasized to Peter that she was not there to judge him, but rather was there to help him so that a whole week would not go by without his experiencing some success with his treatment. In this session, focus was placed on initiating conversations—Peter and the therapist walked through the clinic initiating conversations with several different people, and Peter had a very positive experience with this exercise. While he predicted that each conversation would last "zero seconds" because he would be unable to get a conversation going, each lasted between 5 and 10 minutes, leaving Peter quite amazed. He was sent home with the same homework as had been assigned the previous week.

At this point in treatment, Peter made a turn. He started to speak up in class, said hello to fellow students (which invariably turned into a lengthier interaction), and phoned the therapist each day to check in. As treatment continued, Peter progressed up his hierarchy, working on returning items to stores, asking for help from clerks, ordering food in the cafeteria, and going to movies on his own. Peter also joined a college political organization and the Young Friends of his local opera company. Peter became more adept at keeping his attention focused outward rather than being pulled into a state of self-focused attention. He also stopped using safety behaviors completely, coming to see through experience that they did more harm than good. Even with these significant changes, treatment continued to be a challenge for Peter. Often, when he first did an exposure, he simply *went* to a place (e.g., like a meeting or lecture) but did not engage with any other people. It took repeated exposures for Peter to finally speak to somebody. Furthermore, it was a constant challenge for the therapist to help Peter stop discounting every success that he had.

At the end of 16 sessions of treatment, Peter's mood and social anxiety had improved significantly. Criteria for depression were no longer met, but he continued to have moderately severe social anxiety. Over the course of treatment, however, he made some friends in his classes and the opera group. This afforded him the opportunity to continue working on his social anxiety while also maintaining a level of activity that would hopefully protect him from a relapse of his depression. In the final treatment sessions, Peter and his therapist completed a goal-setting worksheet, on which Peter articulated goals to achieve in the next month, 6 months, and 1 year. This worksheet provided Peter with the structure he would need to continue working on his social anxiety and depression with the skills that he had learned in therapy. When his therapist followed up with Peter 6 months later, his social anxiety had decreased further. He was talking in class regularly and had continued to forge friendships with people he had met during the time he was in therapy. He had also recently asked a woman on a date, something he had never done before. Interestingly, the woman had declined Peter's invitation, but he had been able to deal with his feelings of disappointment and had even shared these feelings with one of his new friends. Peter explained to his therapist that he was pleasantly surprised to see that sharing something potentially embarrassing with a friend did not result in his being judged negatively—in fact, it turned out to be beneficial. His friend told him that this woman was renowned for turning down dates and, in turn, offered to introduce Peter to a female friend of his. This introduction was to take place later that week, and although Peter felt nervous about it, he said that there was no chance that he would avoid it. Rather, like he had virtually every day since finishing treatment, he would use his CBT skills to help him through this challenging, but exciting, social situation.

CONCLUSION

We have come a long way since Liebowitz, Gorman, Fyer, and Klein (1985) termed social anxiety disorder "the neglected anxiety disorder" (p. 729). Since then, models have been developed to understand the maintenance of social anxiety disorder and how best to treat it (Clark & Wells, 1995; Rapee & Heimberg, 1997). Existing treatments that are grounded in cognitive-behavioral principles have yielded impressive effects, both immediately after treatment and in the long run. However, many patients who complete treatment for social anxiety disorder still evidence social anxiety symptoms and report impairments in their social and occupational functioning. This suggests that there still is room for improvements in our approach to treatment, which should result in improved outcomes for patients.

Recently, researchers have started to implement such improvements. Frameworks for understanding the maintenance of social anxiety disorder have been refined (Clark, 2001; Foa et al., 2001; Turk, Lerner, Heimberg, & Rapee, 2001), the way in which exposures are carried out has been improved (e.g., Clark, 2001; Hope et al., 2000), and new techniques like video feedback with cognitive preparation have been introduced that seem to contribute to superior outcomes (Harvey et al., 2000). As research continues with these novel approaches, we will undoubtedly learn to improve outcomes for patients with social anxiety disorder.

It is also essential that we start examining outcomes for more complex groups of patients. At this time, we know little about how the presence of co-occurring depression or substance use affects treatment outcome. Studies must be performed to see if these comorbid conditions do in fact have a detrimental effect on outcome, and if they do, special treatments must be developed that target both social anxiety and associated symptoms.

REFERENCES

Albano, A. M., Marten, P. A., Holt, C. S., Heimberg, R. G., & Barlow, D. H. (1995). Cognitive-behavioral group treatment for social phobia in adolescents: A preliminary study. *Journal of Nervous and Mental Disease, 183,* 649–656.

Altamura, A. C., Pioli, R., Vitto, M., & Mannu, P. (1999). Venlafaxine in social phobia: A study in selective serotonin reuptake inhibitor non-responders. *International Clinical Psychopharmacology, 14,* 239–245.

American Psychiatric Association. (1994). *Diagnostic and statistical manual of mental disorders* (4th ed.). Washington, DC: Author.

Antony, M. M., Roth, D., Swinson, R. P., Huta, V., & Devins, G. M. (1998). Illness intrusiveness in individuals with panic disorder, obsessive–compulsive disorder, or social phobia. *Journal of Nervous and Mental Disease, 186,* 311–315.

Beidel, D. C., Turner, S. M., & Morris, T. L. (1999). Psychopathology of childhood social phobia. *Journal of the American Academy of Child and Adolescent Psychiatry, 38,* 643–650.

Beidel, D. C., Turner, S. M., & Morris, T. L. (2000). Behavioral treatment of childhood social phobia. *Journal of Consulting and Clinical Psychology, 68,* 1072–1080.

Blanco, C., Antia, S. X., & Liebowitz, M. R. (2002). Pharmacological treatment of social anxiety disorder. *Biological Psychiatry, 51,* 109–120.

Blanco, C., Schneier, F. R., Schmidt, A., Blanco-Jerez, C.-R., Marshall, R. D., Sanchez-Lacày, A., & Liebowitz, M. R. (2003). Pharmacological treatment of social anxiety disorder: A meta-analysis. *Depression and Anxiety, 18,* 29–40.

Brown, E. J., Heimberg, R. G., & Juster, H. R. (1995). Social phobia subtype and avoidant personality disorder: Effect on severity of social phobia, impairment, and outcome of cognitive-behavioral treatment. *Behavior Therapy, 26,* 467–486.

Chambless, D. L., Tran, G. Q., & Glass, C. R. (1997). Predictors of response to cognitive-behavioral group therapy for social phobia. *Journal of Anxiety Disorders, 11,* 221–240.

Clark, D. B., & Agras, W. S. (1991). The assessment and treatment of performance anxiety in musicians. *American Journal of Psychiatry, 148,* 598–605.

Clark, D. M. (2001). A cognitive perspective on social phobia. In W. R. Crozier & L. E. Alden (Eds.), *International handbook of social anxiety: Concepts, research and interventions relating to the self and shyness* (pp. 405–430). Chichester, UK: Wiley.

Clark, D. M., Ehlers, A., McManus, F., Hackmann, A., Fennell, M., Campbell, H., Flower, T., Davenport, C., & Louis, B. (2003). Cognitive therapy vs fluoxetine in generalized social phobia: A randomized placebo controlled trial. *Journal of Consulting and Clinical Psychology, 71,* 1058–1067.

Clark, D. M., & Wells, A. (1995). A cognitive model of social phobia. In R. G. Heimberg, M. R. Liebowitz, D. A. Hope, & F. R. Schneier (Eds.), *Social phobia: Diagnosis, assessment, and treatment* (pp. 69–93). New York: Guilford Press.

Coles, M. E., Turk, C. L., & Heimberg, R. G. (2002). The role of memory perspective in social phobia: Immediate and delayed memories for role-played situations. *Behavioural and Cognitive Psychotherapy, 30,* 415–425.

Coles, M. E., Turk, C. L., Heimberg, R. G., & Fresco, D. M. (2001). Effects of varying levels of anxiety within social situations: Relationship to memory perspective and attributions in social phobia. *Behaviour Research and Therapy, 39,* 651–665.

Davidson, J. R. T. (2003). Pharmacotherapy of social phobia. *Acta Psychiatrica Scandinavica, 108*(Suppl. 417), 65–71.

Davidson, J. R. T., Foa, E., Huppert, J., Keefe, F., Franklin, M., Compton, J., Zhao, N., Connor, K., Lynch, T., & Gadde, K. (2004). Fluoxetine, comprehensive cognitive behavioral therapy (CCBT) and placebo in generalized social phobia. *Archives of General Psychiatry, 61,* 1005–1013.

Davidson, J. R. T., Potts, N., Richichi, E., Krishnan, R., Ford, S. M., Smith, R., & Wilson, W. H. (1993). Treatment of social phobia with clonazepam and placebo. *Journal of Clinical Psychopharmacology, 13,* 423–428.

Edelman, R. E., & Chambless, D. L. (1995). Adherence during sessions and homework in cognitive-behavioral group treatment of social phobia. *Behaviour Research and Therapy, 33,* 573–577.

Eng, W., Coles, M. E., Heimberg, R. G., & Safren, S. A. (2001). Quality of life following cognitive behavioral treatment for social anxiety disorder: Preliminary findings. *Depression and Anxiety, 13,* 192–193.

Erwin, B. A., Heimberg, R. G., Juster, H. R., & Mindlin, M. (2002). Comorbid anxiety and mood disorders among persons with social anxiety disorder. *Behaviour Research and Therapy, 40,* 19–35.

Erwin, B. A., Heimberg, R. G., Schneier, F. R., & Liebowitz, M. R. (2003). Anger experience and anger expression in social anxiety disorder: Pretreatment profile and predictors of attrition and response to cognitive-behavioral treatment. *Behavior Therapy, 34,* 331–350.

Fedoroff, I. C., & Taylor, S. T. (2001). Psychological and pharmacological treatments of social phobia: A meta-analysis. *Journal of Clinical Psychopharmacology, 21,* 311–324.

Feske, U., Perry, K. J., Chambless, D. L., Renneberg, B., & Goldstein, A. (1996). Avoidant personality disorder as a predictor for treatment outcome among generalized social phobics. *Journal of Personality Disorders, 10,* 174–184.

Foa, E. B., Franklin, M. E., & Kozak, M. J. (2001). Social phobia: An information processing perspective. In S. Hofmann & P. M. DiBartolo (Eds.), *From social anxiety to social phobia: Multiple perspectives* (pp. 268–280). Needham Heights, MA: Allyn & Bacon.

Foa, E. B., Franklin, M. E., & Moser, J. (2002). Context in the clinic: How well do CBT and medications work in combination? *Biological Psychiatry, 52,* 987–997.

Foa, E. B., & Rothbaum, B. O. (1998). *Treating the trauma of rape: Cognitive-behavioral therapy for PTSD.* New York: Guilford Press.

Foa, E. B., & Wilson, R. (2001). *Stop obsessing: How to overcome your obsessions and compulsions* (2nd ed.). New York: Bantam.

Franklin, M. E., Jaycox, L. H., & Foa, E. B. (1999). Social phobia: Social skills training. In M. Hersen & A. Bellack (Eds.), *Handbook of comparative treatments for adult disorders* (2nd ed., pp. 317–339). New York: Wiley.

Gelernter, C. S., Uhde, T. W., Cimbolic, P., Arnkoff, D. B., Vittone, B. J., Tancer, M. E., & Bartko, J. J. (1991). Cognitive-behavioral and pharmacological treatments for social phobia: A controlled study. *Archives of General Psychiatry, 48,* 938–945.

Gould, R. A., Buckminster, S., Pollack, M. H., Otto, M. W., & Yap, L. (1997). Cognitive-behavioral and pharmacological treatment for social phobia: A meta-analysis. *Clinical Psychology: Science and Practice, 4,* 291–306.

Hackman, A., Clark, D. M., & McManus, F. (2000). Recurrent images and early memories in social phobia. *Behaviour Research and Therapy, 38,* 601–610.

Harvey, A. G., Clark, D. M., Ehlers, A., & Rapee, R. M. (2000). Social anxiety and self-impression: Cognitive preparation enhances the beneficial effects of video feedback following a stressful social task. *Behaviour Research and Therapy, 38,* 1183–1192.

Hayward, C., Varady, S., Albano, A. M., Thienemann, M., Henderson, L., & Schatzberg, A. F. (2000). Cognitive-behavioral group therapy for social phobia in female adolescents: Results of a pilot study. *Journal of the American Academy of Child and Adolescent Psychiatry, 39,* 721–726.

Heimberg, R. G. (1996). Social phobia, avoidant personality disorder, and the multiaxial conceptualization of interpersonal anxiety. In P. Salkovskis (Ed.), *Trends in cognitive and behavioural therapies* (pp. 43–62). Sussex, UK: Wiley.

Heimberg, R. G. (2002). Cognitive-behavioral therapy for social anxiety disorder: Current status and future directions. *Biological Psychiatry, 51,* 101–108.

Heimberg, R. G. (2003, March). *Cognitive-behavioral and psychotherapeutic strategies for social anxiety disorder.* Paper presented at the annual meeting of the Anxiety Disorders Association of America, Toronto, Ontario, Canada.

Heimberg, R. G., & Becker, R. E. (2002). *Cognitive-behavioral group therapy for social phobia: Basic mechanisms and clinical strategies.* New York: Guilford Press.

Heimberg, R. G., Holt, C. S., Schneier, F. R., Spitzer, R. L., & Liebowitz, M. R. (1993). The issue of subtypes in the diagnosis of social phobia. *Journal of Anxiety Disorders, 7,* 249–269.

Heimberg, R. G., Liebowitz, M. R., Hope, D. A., Schneier, F. R., Holt, C. S., Welkowitz, L., Juster, H. R., Campeas, R., Bruch, M. A., Cloitre, M., Fallon, B., & Klein, D. F. (1998). Cognitive-behavioral group therapy versus phenelzine in social phobia: 12-week outcome. *Archives of General Psychiatry, 55,* 1133–1141.

Herbert, J. D., Gaudiano, B. A., Rheingold, A. A., Myers, V. H., Dalrymple, K., & Nolan, E. M. (in press). Social skills training augments the efficacy of cognitive behavioral group therapy for social anxiety disorder. *Behavior Therapy.*

Herbert, J. D., Rheingold, A. A., & Goldstein, S. G. (2002). Brief cognitive-behavioral group therapy for social anxiety disorder. *Cognitive and Behavioral Practice, 9,* 1–8.

Hirsch, C. R., Clark, D. M., Mathews, A., & Williams, R. (2003). Self-images play a causal role in social phobia. *Behaviour Research and Therapy, 41,* 909–921.

Hofmann, S. G. (2000a). Self-focused attention before and after treatment of social phobia. *Behaviour Research and Therapy, 38,* 717–725.

Hofmann, S. G. (2000b). Treatment of social phobia: Potential mediators and moderators. *Clinical Psychology: Science and Practice, 7,* 3–16.

Holt, C. S., Heimberg, R. G., Hope, D. A., & Liebowitz, M. R. (1992). Situational domains of social phobia. *Journal of Anxiety Disorders, 6,* 63–77.

Hope, D. A., Heimberg, R. G., & Bruch, M. A. (1995). Dismantling cognitive-behavioral group therapy for social phobia. *Behaviour Research and Therapy, 33,* 637–650.

Hope, D. A., Heimberg, R. G., Juster, H., & Turk, C. L. (2000). *Managing social anxiety: A cognitive-behavioral therapy approach (Client Workbook).* San Antonio, TX: Psychological Corporation.

Hope, D. A., Herbert, J. D., & White, C. (1995). Diagnostic subtype, avoidant personality disorder, and efficacy of cognitive behavioral group therapy for social phobia. *Cognitive Therapy and Research, 19,* 285–303.

Huppert, J. D., Roth, D. A., & Foa, E. B. (2003). Cognitive behavioral treatment of social phobia: New advances. *Current Psychiatry Reports, 5,* 289–296.

Huppert, J., Roth, D. & Foa, E. B. (in press). Using homework in behavioral therapy. *Journal of Psychotherapy Integration* [Special Issue: Integrating Between Session Homework Activities into Different Psychotherapies].

Kim, H.-Y., Lundh, L.-G., & Harvey, A. (2002). The enhancement of video feedback by cognitive preparation in the treatment of social anxiety. A single session experiment. *Journal of Behavior Therapy and Experimental Psychiatry, 33,* 19–37.

Kobak, K. A., Greist, J. H., Jefferson, J. W., & Katzelnick, D. J. (2002). Fluoxetine in social phobia: A double-blind, placebo-controlled pilot study. *Journal of Clinical Psychopharmacology, 22,* 257–262.

Leung, A. W., & Heimberg, R. G. (1996). Homework compliance, perceptions of control, and outcome of cognitive-behavioral treatment of social phobia. *Behaviour Research and Therapy, 34,* 423–432.

Liebowitz, M. (1987). Social phobia. *Modern Problems of Pharmacopsychiatry, 22,* 141–173.

Liebowitz, M. R., Gorman, J. M., Fyer, A. J., & Klein, D. F. (1985). Social phobia: Review of a neglected anxiety disorder. *Archives of General Psychiatry, 42,* 729–736.

Liebowitz, M. R., Heimberg, R. G., Schneier, F. R., Hope, D. A., Davies, S., Holt, C. S.,

Goetz, D., Juster, H. R., Lin, S.-L., Bruch, M. A., Marshall, R., & Klein, D. F. (1999). Cognitive-behavioral group therapy versus phenelzine in social phobia: Long-term outcome. *Depression and Anxiety, 10*, 89–98.

Lucas, R. A., & Telch, M. J. (1993, November). *Group versus individual treatment of social phobia.* Paper presented at the annual meeting of the Association for Advancement of Behavior Therapy, Atlanta, GA.

Magee, W. J., Eaton, W. W., Wittchen, H.-U., McGonagle, K. A., & Kessler, R. C. (1996). Agoraphobia, simple phobia, and social phobia in the National Comorbidity Survey. *Archives of General Psychiatry, 53*, 159–168.

Masia, C. L., Klein, R. G., Storch, E. A., & Corda, B. (2001). School-based behavioral treatment for social anxiety disorder in adolescents: Results of a pilot study. *Journal of the American Academy of Child and Adolescent Psychiatry, 40*, 780–786.

Noyes, R., Moroz, G., Davidson, J. R. T., Liebowitz, M. R., Davidson, A., Siegal, J., Bell, J., Cain, J. W., Curlick, S. M., Kent, T. A., Lydiard, R. B., Mallinger, A. G., Pollack, M. H., Rapaport, M., Rasmussen, S. A., Hedges, D., Schweitzer, E., & Uhlenhuth, E. H. (1997). Moclobemide in social phobia: A controlled dose-response trial. *Journal of Clinical Psychopharmacology, 17*, 247–254.

Olfson, M., Guardino, M., Struening, E., Schneier, F. R., Hellman, F., & Klein, D. F. (2000). Barriers to treatment of social anxiety. *American Journal of Psychiatry, 157*, 521–527.

Oosterbaan, D. B., van Balkom, A. J. L. M., Spinhoven, P., van Oppen, P., & van Dyck, R. (1998). *Cognitive therapy versus moclobemide in social phobia: A controlled study.* Unpublished manuscript, Department of Psychiatry and Institute for Research in Extramural Medicine, Vrije University, Amsterdam, The Netherlands.

Öst, L. G. (1987). Applied relaxation: Description of a coping technique and review of controlled studies. *Behaviour Research and Therapy, 25*, 397–409.

Öst, L. G., Jerremalm, A., & Johansson, J. (1981). Individual response patterns and the effects of different behavioral methods in the treatment of social phobia. *Behaviour Research and Therapy, 19*, 1–16.

Öst, L. G., Sedvall, H., Breitholtz, E., Hellstrøm, K., & Lindwall, R. (1995, July). *Cognitive-behavioral treatment for social phobia: Individual, group and self-administered treatment.* Paper presented at the triannual meeting of the World Congress of Behavioural and Cognitive Therapies, Copenhagen, Denmark.

Pande, A. C., Davidson, J. R., Jefferson, J. W., Janney, C. A., Katzelnick, D. J., Weisler, R. H., Greist, J. H., & Sutherland, S. M. (1999). Treatment of social phobia with gabapentin: A placebo-controlled study. *Journal of Clinical Psychopharmacology, 19*, 341–348.

Rapee, R. M., & Heimberg, R. G. (1997). A cognitive-behavioral model of anxiety in social phobia. *Behaviour Research and Therapy, 35*, 741–756.

Rodebaugh, T. L., & Chambless, D. L. (2002). The effects of video feedback on the self-perception of speech anxious participants. *Cognitive Therapy and Research, 26*, 629–644.

Rodebaugh, T. L., Holaway, R. M., & Heimberg, R. G. (2004). The treatment of social anxiety disorder. *Clinical Psychology Review, 24*, 883–908.

Roth, D. A., Antony, M. M., & Swinson, R. P. (2001). Interpretations for anxiety symptoms in social phobia. *Behaviour Research and Therapy, 39*, 129–138.

Safren, S. A., Heimberg, R. G., & Juster, H. R. (1997). Client expectancies and their relationship to pretreatment symtomatology and outcome of cognitive-behavioral group treatment for social phobia. *Journal of Consulting and Clinical Psychology,* 65, 694–698.

Schneier, F. R., Goetz, D., Campeas, R., Fallon, B., Marshall, R., & Liebowitz, M. R. (1998). Placebo-controlled trial of moclobemide in social phobia. *British Journal of Psychiatry, 172,* 70–77.

Schneier, F. R., Heckelman, L. R., Garfinkel, R., Campeas, R., Fallon, B. A., Gitow, A., Street, L., Del Bene, D., & Liebowitz, M. R. (1994). Functional impairment in social phobia. *Journal of Clinical Psychiatry, 55,* 322–331.

Schneier, F. R., Johnson, J., Hornig, C. D., Liebowitz, M. R., & Weissman, M. M. (1992). Social phobia: Comorbidity and morbidity in an epidemiologic sample. *Archives of General Psychiatry, 49,* 282–288.

Spence, S. H., Donovan, C., & Brechman-Toussaint, M. (2000). The treatment of childhood social phobia: The effectiveness of a social skills training-based cognitive-behavioural intervention with and without parental involvement. *Journal of Child Psychology and Psychiatry and Allied Disciplines, 41,* 713–726.

Spurr, J. M., & Stopa, L. (2003). The observer perspective: Effects on social anxiety and performance. *Behaviour Research and Therapy, 41,* 1009–1028.

Taylor, S. (1996). Meta-analysis of cognitive-behavioral treatments for social phobia. *Journal of Behavior Therapy and Experimental Psychiatry, 27,* 1–9.

Turk, C. L., Lerner, J., Heimberg, R. G., & Rapee, R. M. (2001). An integrated cognitive-behavioral model of social anxiety. In S. G. Hofmann & P. M. DiBartolo (Eds.), *From social anxiety to social phobia: Multiple perspectives* (pp. 281–303). Needham Heights, MA: Allyn & Bacon.

Turner, S. M., Beidel, D. C., Cooley, M. R., & Woody, S. R (1994). A multicomponent behavioral treatment for social phobia: Social effectiveness therapy. *Behaviour Research and Therapy, 32,* 381–390.

Turner, S. M., Beidel, D. C., & Cooley-Quille, M. R. (1995). Two-year follow-up of social phobics treated with Social Effectiveness Therapy. *Behaviour Research and Therapy, 33,* 553–555.

Turner, S. M., Beidel, D. C., & Jacob, R. G. (1994). Social phobia: A comparison of behavior therapy and atenolol. *Journal of Consulting and Clinical Psychology, 62,* 350–358.

Veljaca, K., & Rapee, R. M. (1998). Detection of negative and positive audience behaviours by socially anxious subjects. *Behaviour Research and Therapy, 36,* 311–321.

Versiani, M., Nardi, A. E., Mundim, F. D., Alves, A. A., Liebowitz, M. R., & Amrein, R. (1992). Pharmacotherapy of social phobia: A controlled study of moclobemide and phenelzine. *British Journal of Psychiatry, 161,* 353–360.

Walker, J. (2003, March). *Bringing the interpersonal into cognitive-behevaior therapy for social anxiety disorder.* Paper presented at the meeting of the Anxiety Disorders Association of America, Toronto, Ontario, Canada.

Wells, A., & Papageorgiou, C. (1998). Social phobia: Effects of external attention on anxiety, negative beliefs, and perspective taking. *Behavior Therapy, 29,* 357–370.

Whisman, M., Sheldon, C., & Goering, P. (2000). Psychiatric disorders and dissatisfaction with social relationships: Does type of relationship matter? *Journal of Abnormal Psychology, 109,* 803–808.

Woody, S. R., Chambless, D. L., & Glass, C. R. (1997). Self-focused attention in the treatment of social phobia. *Behaviour Research and Therapy, 35,* 117–129.

Zaider, T. I., & Heimberg, R. G. (2003). Nonpharmacologic treatments for social anxiety disorder. *Acta Psychiatrica Scandinavica, 108*(Suppl. 417), 72–84.

3

Generalized Anxiety Disorder

ALLISON M. WATERS
MICHELLE G. CRASKE

OVERVIEW OF THE DISORDER

Diagnostic criteria for generalized anxiety disorder (GAD) are met by as many as 5% of the population at some point during their lifetime (Kessler et al., 1994), with studies demonstrating that GAD causes considerable interference and psychosocial impairment (Massion, Warshaw, & Keller, 1993; Roy-Byrne & Katon, 1997; Wittchen, Zhao, Kessler, & de Boer, 1994). Many more individuals experience subclinical symptoms of GAD that although not sufficient to warrant a GAD diagnosis, still cause some degree of distress and interference in daily life. GAD is a chronic, self-perpetuating condition that rarely remits on its own (Yonkers, Warshaw, Massion, & Keller, 1996).

The central feature of GAD is excessive anxiety and worry across a number of life domains, and GAD is the disorder for which anxiety cues are the least circumscribed. Anxiety and worry are maintained by pervasive anxious processes that continuously drive the detection and interpretation of potential threats in many different areas (Craske, 2003a). As a consequence of such diffuse and apparently uncontrollable negative reactivity across an unpredictable range of situations, individuals with GAD may perceive themselves as being permanently anxious and "out of control" (Chorpita, 2001), and indeed, many individuals with GAD report their worry as being uncontrollable (Craske, Rapee, Jackel, & Barlow, 1989). Thus, the central domain of threat for GAD may be uncontrollable negative reactivity itself, with such excessive negative affect eroding the perception of oneself as being competent in managing life effectively (Craske, 2003a). This perception of personal ineffectiveness may lead, in turn, to more distress and negative affect and, thus, a self-perpetuating cycle of GAD.

GAD can be diagnosed in both adults and children, although most re-search to date has focused on adults. Females are far more likely than males to report symptoms meeting GAD criteria in both epidemiological and clinical populations, and scores on measures of trait anxiety also are typically higher in females (e.g., Blazer, George, & Hughes, 1991; Rapee, 1991; Wittchen et al., 1994). Moreover, in contrast to other anxiety disorders (e.g., panic disor-der) that tend to have clear onsets and more acute presentations, individuals with GAD may well have suffered from their symptoms for much of their lives and often describe a slow progressive onset of their GAD symptoms dating back to childhood (Anderson, Noyes, & Crowe, 1984; Rapee, 1985).

Since becoming a diagnostic category in the *Diagnostic and Statistical Manual of Mental Disorders* (DSM) in 1980, GAD has had a rather colorful history. As a residual category in DSM-III (American Psychiatric Association, 1980), GAD was diagnosed only if criteria for another Axis I disorder were not met, and was defined as the presence of continuous generalized anxiety for at least 1 month, accompanied by at least three of four symptoms includ-ing motor tension, autonomic hyperactivity, apprehensive expectation, and vigilance and scanning. The diagnostic criteria were revised in DSM-III-R (American Psychiatric Association, 1987) to reflect evidence that many indi-viduals reported generalized worry and apprehension beyond that accounted for by an Axis I disorder (Barlow & Di Nardo, 1991). Thus, no longer a resid-ual category, GAD was defined in DSM-III-R as the presence of excessive or unrealistic worry in two or more areas not related to another Axis I disorder, persisting for a period of at least six months, and accompanied by 6 out of 18 symptoms clustering into categories representing motor tension, autonomic hyperactivity, and vigilance and scanning.

In line with the difficulty that individuals with GAD experience in con-trolling the worry process compared to nondisordered individuals, (e.g., Abel & Borkovec, 1995; Borkovec, 1994; Borkovec, Shadick, & Hopkins, 1991; Craske, Rapee, et al., 1989), the key features of GAD were again redefined in DSM-IV (American Psychiatric Association, 1994) as excessive and uncon-trollable worry about a number of life events or activities persisting for at least 6 months. Furthermore, collective support for the motor tension and the vigi-lance symptom clusters (e.g., Hazlett, McLeod, & Hoehn-Saric, 1994; Hoehn-Saric, McLeod, & Zimmerli, 1989), but not the autonomic hyperactivity symptom cluster in distinguishing GAD from other anxiety disorders de-scribed in DSM-III-R (e.g., Brown, Marten, & Barlow, 1995), led to the DSM-IV definition including at least three of six associated symptoms from the motor tension and the vigilance clusters only. The DSM-IV criteria for GAD also require that the anxiety and worry not be better accounted for by another Axis I disorder; not occur exclusively during the course of a mood disorder, psychotic disorder, or developmental disorder; and not be bought about by a substance or a general medical condition. Finally, the anxiety or worry must cause distress or interference in functioning for a DSM-IV GAD diagnosis to be assigned. Thus, although GAD is not considered a residual category in

DSM-IV, GAD continues to be defined in the context of other mental disorders. To a large extent, such diagnostic rigor reflects the controversy concerning whether GAD is a distinct diagnostic category (e.g., Brown, Barlow, & Liebowitz, 1994), given the high rates of comorbidity with other anxiety and mood disorders (e.g., Brawman-Mintzer et al., 1993; Brown & Barlow, 1992; Massion et al., 1993).

In fact, studies have found GAD to be the most frequently assigned additional diagnosis for clients who have another anxiety or mood disorder (Brown, Campbell, Lehman, Grisham, & Mancill, 2001)—findings that Barlow and colleagues (e.g., Brown, Barlow, & Liebowitz, 1994) use to support the argument that GAD is a "basic" anxiety disorder and that the propensity to worry and to feel apprehensive is characteristic to varying degrees of most other anxiety disorders. Other researchers have argued that GAD may in fact resemble high levels of trait anxiety (Rapee, 1991), and that the features of GAD represent vulnerability markers in etiological models of emotional disorders in general (Clark, Watson, & Mineka, 1994). For example, because GAD loads largely on the higher-order construct of negative affect (Brown, Chorpita, & Barlow, 1998), which in turn, is common to all the anxiety and mood disorders, the features of GAD have been argued to represent predispositional vulnerabilities for the development of other anxiety and mood disorders (Brown, Barlow, & Liebowitz, 1994; Craske, 2003a). Regardless of the diagnostic and theoretical underpinnings of GAD, the high prevalence rates and considerable impact that features of this disorder have on the lives of many individuals points to the need for effective treatments.

In this chapter, we first review the literature on empirically supported treatments for GAD. We begin with a review of the literature on psychological approaches to treatment, which demonstrates the relative efficacy of cognitive-behavioral treatments (CBT), as well as pharmacological approaches. We then discuss factors that affect CBT outcome and strategies for maximizing client improvement. Relapse and recurrence of GAD are then discussed and practical strategies for their prevention are reviewed. Consideration also is given to how CBT treatments for GAD can be adapted based on individual differences and for older and younger clients. Finally, we describe the treatment of a 45-year-old female client with GAD whose case highlights some of the important issues discussed in this chapter.

OVERVIEW OF EMPIRICALLY SUPPORTED TREATMENTS

Evidence-Based Psychological Treatments

In accordance with diagnostic criteria and empirical evidence to date, treatment for GAD should target the major features of excessive, uncontrollable worry and associated muscle tension (Hazlett et al., 1994; Hoehn-Saric et al., 1989) and restricted autonomic activity (Borkovec & Hu, 1990; Borkovec, Lyonfields, Wiser, & Diehl, 1993; Hoehn-Saric et al., 1989). In a recent review of 13 controlled treatment outcome studies for GAD, Borkovec and Ruscio (2001) concluded that cognitive-behavioral approaches are more efficacious than wait-list control conditions (e.g., Barlow, Rapee, & Brown, 1992) and are more efficacious than nonspecific treatment conditions (e.g., Borkovec & Costello, 1993), at least in adults up to 55 years of age. However, whereas some studies comparing components of CBT with complete treatment packages have reported multicomponent packages to be more effective (e.g., Butler, Fennell, Robson, & Gelder, 1991), others have found individual CBT components and comprehensive packages to be comparable (e.g., Barlow et al., 1992; Borkovec, 2002). Thus, it remains unclear which components are active and necessary for effective treatment of GAD.

Of the studies with demonstrated efficacy, treatment components have typically included psychoeducation, early identification of anxiety triggers and self-monitoring (Overholser & Nasser, 2000), applied relaxation (Öst, 1987), cognitive restructuring (Borkovec & Costello, 1993; Borkovec et al., 1987), and some form of exposure to internal or external precipitants of worry (Borkovec & Costello, 1993; Craske, Street, & Barlow, 1989; Stanley, Beck, & Glassco, 1996). In this section, we review each of these components.

Psychoeducation

Many clients with GAD gain some initial reassurance through educational explanations about anxiety and its treatment. The three components of anxiety (i.e., physiological, cognitive, and behavioral) and the application of the three-system model to the client's symptoms are included in psychoeducation. The client learns about the nature of anxiety in terms of "fight or flight" reactions in order to normalize the physiological basis of anxiety and to highlight how anxiety is adaptive and useful at moderate levels and on a sporadic basis. Anxiety is explained as being problematic when it occurs too frequently or at excessive levels, with the rationale of treatment being to help the client learn to cope with anxiety and keep it at a manageable level rather than to eliminate anxiety completely. The client is informed about the role of worry—that although it might seem that worrying helps one feel more in control, it actually leads to enhanced distress and avoidance, which, in turn, reinforces the worry process because of the belief that worrying prevented feared outcomes from occurring. The client is informed about how anxiety develops and is maintained in terms of relevant information obtained about his or her own history.

Self-Monitoring

During the initial stages of treatment, clients are asked to record on a self-monitoring form the situations in their daily lives (whether external or internal) that trigger anxiety responses, and the internal cues (cognitive and somatic) that signal the initiation of an anxiety response. When introduced to self-monitoring, the client is given a self-monitoring form like the one depicted in Figure 3.1 and the therapist explains each component on the form. To facilitate the client's understanding of self-monitoring, he or she is instructed in session to either imagine a stressful or anxiety-provoking event or to recall a recent episode of worry and anxiety (e.g., invited to a party where I didn't know many people) and to record responses on the self-monitoring form. The client is asked to record the thoughts (e.g., "I won't be able to think of anything to say"), images and feelings (e.g., nervous and afraid), and somatic sensations (e.g., felt sick in the stomach) associated with the triggering event. Next, the client records how he or she reacted in the situation based on these thoughts and sensations (e.g., decided not to go to the party), and to examine how his or her reaction influenced subsequent perceptions about the triggering event (e.g., "meeting new people makes me anxious") and about him- or herself (e.g., "I'm so hopeless").

The client is instructed that self-monitoring of anxious triggers and responses should continue between sessions with the rationale being that the more skilled the client becomes in recognizing early-warning signs of anxiety, the earlier he or she can intervene with learned cognitive and behavioral strategies. Furthermore, self-monitoring continues throughout treatment to provide a record of change in anxiety levels as treatment progresses. The therapist reviews the client's self-monitoring at the commencement of each session and provides corrective feedback on the quality of the monitoring and the learning that has taken place.

Relaxation Training

As clients with GAD often experience elevated muscle tension and reduced flexibility of autonomic functioning (e.g., Hoehn-Saric & McLeod, 1988; Hoehn-Saric et al., 1989; Thayer, Friedman, & Borkovec, 1996), training in relaxation techniques can be clinically useful. The most common forms of relaxation training include progressive muscle relaxation (e.g., Bernstein, Borkovec, & Hazlett-Stevens, 2000) and techniques such as relaxation imagery, meditation, and a variety of paced breathing exercises. The client is first taught relaxation techniques in session and is then instructed to practice these

Date/Time	Triggering event	Thoughts	Sensations: physical and emotional	Behavioral urges and action taken	Anxiety level (0 to 100)
8:50 a.m., 8/4/2004	Running late for appointment	"They will think I am irresponsible"	Sweating; heart racing; nervous	Call and cancel the appointment	85

FIGURE 3.1. Client ongoing self-monitoring form depicting components for monitoring anxious triggers, thoughts, sensations, and behavioral urges.

techniques at least twice a day at home to increase his or her ability to achieve a relaxed state. In addition, the client is encouraged to use relaxation techniques as soon as anxiety cues are detected (e.g., muscle tension), during stressful events, and as frequently during the day as possible even when the client is not anxious (Öst, 1987). The purpose of applied relaxation is for a state of relaxation, rather than tension, to become the client's predominant tonic state as well as to help the client develop the capability to effectively manage acute episodes of anxiety. Moreover, given the tendency of clients with GAD to be locked in future-oriented patterns of worrisome behavior, applied relaxation training also can help promote a state of "present-moment awareness" or the capability to remain focused on present experiences and sensations (Borkovec & Ruscio, 2001).

Cognitive Therapy

Because GAD involves exaggerated perceptions of future threat and excessive worry that catastrophic events will occur, cognitive therapy is a central component of treatment for GAD and is aimed at helping clients recognize the link between these patterns of thinking and their anxiety. In introducing cognitive therapy, considerable care is given to helping the client understand that *interpretations* of situations rather than the situations themselves are responsible for elevated anxiety (Brown, O'Leary, & Barlow, 2001). The connection between thoughts and anxiety is highlighted through examples provided by the therapist and through examples drawn from the client's monitoring of anxiety-provoking events (e.g., running late for an appointment) and the associated thoughts and self-statements (e.g., "They'll think I'm irresponsible"). The first goal is to help the client see how he or she perceives situations to be dangerous and threatening. Next, the client is encouraged to recognize how thinking about situations in such a manner causes a range of emotional (e.g., anxious) and physical (e.g., heart racing and perspiring) responses and behavioral urges (e.g., "I'll phone to cancel the appointment") to occur. Thus, the client is taught to understand that anxiety reactions are the result of thinking about situations in a worrisome, catastrophic manner.

   In addition to identifying the actual content of anxiety-related thoughts, a central goal of cognitive therapy is to help the client recognize the types of cognitive errors included in his or her anxious thoughts. The therapist will provide the client with examples highlighting the distinction between the various cognitive distortions (see later) and the client is encouraged to examine the types of thinking errors he or she has committed during self-monitored anxiety-provoking events. Common errors of thinking (as reviewed by Beck, Emery, & Greenberg, 1985) that are particularly relevant for clients with GAD include the following:

   1. *Probability overestimation*—the tendency to overestimate the likelihood of a negative event occurring (e.g., "I will not be able to think of

anything to say, my friend will think I am stupid, she will never invite me to lunch with her friends again, and I will always be alone").

2. *Catastrophizing*—perceiving the situation to be intolerable, unmanageable, and beyond one's ability to cope (e.g., "This is terrible, I cannot cope with this").

3. *"All-or-nothing"* or *"black-and-white" thinking*—seeing things in rigid and inflexible "either-or" terms (e.g., "I am not worthwhile unless I am completely competent or successful in everything I do").

4. Personalizing—assuming inappropriate personal responsibility for events and circumstances. (e.g., "I am anxious because I am a weak person").

5. *Jumping to conclusions*—drawing extreme negative conclusions about things, often without sufficient information (e.g., "They are 15 minutes late. They have been in a bad car accident").

6. *Overgeneralizing*—inappropriately using the outcome of one event to judge other unrelated events (e.g., "I made such a fool of myself at the last staff meeting that I'll never be able to give a talk in front of others ever again").

It also is important that the client becomes aware of recurrent, underlying themes or rules reflecting core underlying beliefs (Newman, 2000). The client may often hold prescriptive rules that govern his or her behavior in relation to particular worries (e.g., "I should always be on time"). Such rules are misguidedly intended to prevent underlying beliefs about oneself from "rising to the surface" and becoming evident to others (e.g., "If I am not punctual all the time, people will know I'm useless").

Unhelpful negative thoughts, cognitive distortions, and rules and beliefs are targeted through various strategies designed to enable the client to examine the accuracy of his or her interpretations and predictions and to learn to replace inaccurate thoughts with more realistic, evidence-based thoughts. Because inaccurate negative thoughts may seem automatic and difficult to dismiss, the client's ability to engage in more flexible styles of thinking will require repeated, systematic countering—both in and out of the therapy session. In countering anxious thoughts, the client learns to view his or her thoughts as "hypotheses" to be tested rather than as absolute facts, and to either accept or reject these thoughts depending on the available supporting or negating evidence. The client learns to challenge anxious thinking by considering all available evidence when examining the accuracy of his or her thoughts and beliefs (e.g., "I rarely run late and I competently fulfill many responsibilities such as work and caring for my family"), by learning to view the situation from other perspectives (e.g., "when someone else runs late, I don't think they are irresponsible"), and to consider the consequences of allowing oneself to become distressed by the situation ("I will be flustered and stressed when I finally arrive").

Importantly, the client is instructed to act on the new evidenced-based alternative interpretations and to "test out" inaccurate thoughts and perceptions by engaging in behaviors that are "opposite" to his or her negative threat-related thoughts. For example, if the client's interpretation of running late for an appointment is to phone and cancel the appointment—an avoidant strategy for coping with the situation—the client is encouraged to "do the opposite" and instead to arrive late for the appointment. In this way, the client begins to acquire evidence that his or her most feared outcomes (i.e., "They will think I am irresponsible and will want nothing to do with me") frequently do not happen and that the effects of feeling anxious do not last forever and are manageable. Thus, through a process of identifying, challenging and changing inaccurate, danger-laden thoughts and rules, and by accruing evidence by engaging in behaviors that both disconfirm unhelpful cognitions and support the new alternatives, alteration to the client's core underlying beliefs can be achieved.

Worry Imagery Exposure

Based on conceptualizations of the nature of pathological worry as a means of avoiding intense negative affect and somatic arousal (e.g., Borkovec & Hu, 1990; Mennin, Heimberg, Turk, & Fresco, 2002), worry imagery exposure (e.g., Craske, Barlow, & O'Leary, 1992) involves systematic exposure to fear images attached to the client's two or three principal domains of worry. This exercise is designed to help the client with GAD to tolerate fear and to learn to habituate to fearful images as well as to provide additional opportunities for the implementation of cognitive strategies after each image. The client first identifies and hierarchically orders the fearful images associated with the core domains of worry beginning with the least anxiety-provoking worry. For example, for a client who worries about his or her work performance, imagery may include being laughed at by colleagues, being assigned new responsibilities, and making a mistake. Imagery training commences with the client first focusing on pleasant or neutral scenes and then shifts to the client vividly evoking the first fearful image as if it were actually occurring. In one version of exposure, the client holds the worry image for at least 25–30 minutes and then generates as many possible alternatives as they can to the worst possible outcome (Craske et al., 1992). In coping desensitization (e.g., Borkovec & Costello, 1993), cognitive restructuring techniques and relaxation skills are incorporated into the imagery. When the client experiences only a mild level of anxiety despite several attempts to vividly hold the image in mind, he or she is instructed to move on to the next image. When the therapist is confident the client is capable of completing the worry imagery exposure without assistance from the therapist, the exercise may be assigned as homework.

Other Strategies

Although the aforementioned techniques are the core components of most CBT approaches to GAD, other additional components may include *time management training, goal setting* (e.g., Brown et al., 2001), *problem solving* (e.g., Meichenbaum & Jaremko, 1983), and *worry behavior prevention* (e.g., Craske, Rappe, et al., 1989). As many clients with GAD may feel overwhelmed and pressured by stressors and obligations, time management training and goal setting are particularly useful for helping the client to focus his or her attention on the matters at hand rather than becoming preoccupied with worrisome patterns that prevent the accomplishment of tasks. Relatedly, as the client with GAD may have difficulty defining and resolving various challenges of daily life, problem-solving skills provide the client with skills for identifying problems and generating possible solutions.

Worry behavior prevention stems from research demonstrating that worry in GAD is often associated with some form of corrective, preventive, or ritualistic behavior (e.g., Craske, Rapee, et al., 1989; Schut, Castonguay, & Borkovec, 2001). For example, the client who is concerned about personal safety may always ring the doorbell before entering the house to let the burglar know he or she has arrived home so that the burglar can leave the house. Worry prevention behaviors are negatively reinforcing for clients in that they typically result in a temporary reduction in anxiety. However, in the long term, these behaviors are thought to contribute to the maintenance of anxiety. Worry behaviors are addressed in therapy by having the client record the frequency of each behavior, refrain from engaging in the worry behavior, and perhaps engage in an alternative behavior instead. Prior to performing the prevention exercise, the therapist elicits the client's expectations about what is likely to happen when he or she does not engage in the worry behavior (i.e., "There could be someone inside the house and I could get hurt"). After the worry behavior prevention exercise is completed, the therapist assists the client in comparing the outcome with his or her initial expectation (i.e., "There was no-one in the house"). This technique is employed for each identified worry behavior.

Summary

While CBT techniques appear to hold considerable promise for treating GAD and are recommended as the preferred form of psychotherapy for the disorder (e.g., Ballenger et al., 2001), relative to success rates for other anxiety disorders, CBT for GAD has produced modest and disappointing gains, and GAD remains the least successfully treated anxiety disorder (Brown, Barlow, & Liebowitz, 1994). For example, clinical improvement rates between 38 and 63% for GAD lag considerably behind treatment improvement rates for other anxiety disorders, such as panic disorder, which achieves improvement rates between 80 and 85%. In a comprehensive review of the GAD treatment literature, Barlow, Raffa, and Cohen (2002) argued that such modest treatment gains may reflect the fact that specific techniques to target key features of GAD have been missing from GAD treatment studies because, until the release of DSM-III-R, the key features of GAD had not been well defined. Another limitation is that GAD treatments have not been based on coherent cognitive models of GAD and, specifically, have not directly targeted mechanisms underlying problematic worry—the central feature of GAD (Wells, 1999). Indeed, Öst and Breitholtz (2000) argued that there are few, if any, GAD treatments that are designed specifically for GAD features, and that are based on empirically driven theory regarding the development and maintenance of GAD. Rather, these authors point out that most treatments for GAD, such as cognitive therapy and applied relaxation, for example, were originally developed for depression (cognitive therapy) and panic disorder or phobias (applied relaxation).

In summary, although CBT is the psychological treatment of choice for GAD, advances in the understanding and treatment of this disorder have been limited compared with those for other anxiety disorders. A significant proportion of GAD clients are not helped by CBT or continue to experience significant residual symptoms after treatment. Such modest gains have led researchers and practitioners to consider factors that may contribute to the lower success rates from CBT for GAD, and we discuss these factors later in this chapter.

Evidence-Based Pharmacological Treatments

Four main classes of pharmacological treatments have been examined in randomized controlled studies of GAD: benzodiazepines, buspirone, hydroxyzine, and antidepressants. Neuroleptics also have been used in pharmacological treatment of GAD, although few controlled studies support their effectiveness (Gale & Oakley-Browne, 2000) and the populations studied had mixed diagnoses. Furthermore, neuroleptics can be associated with tardive dyskinesia even in low doses, and in the absence of clinical evidence to support their effectiveness, neuroleptics are not recommended as first-line treatment for GAD (Ballenger et al., 2001).

Benzodiazepines

Although benzodiazepines (e.g., lorazepam and diazepam) have been examined in numerous double-blind treatment studies of GAD, and have tended to be popular in clinical practice, the role of these medications as first-line treatments for GAD is questionable given the chronic nature of the disorder and the need for appropriate long-term treatment (Ballenger et al., 2001). Furthermore, GAD is frequently comorbid with other anxiety and depressive disorders for which benzodiazepines are not desirable (Roy-Byrne & Cowley, 2002). Benzodiazepines may also be problematic if previous drug abuse or alcoholism is indicated, as well as for long-term use, due to the potential for tolerance and withdrawal reactions. Moreover, despite being one of the most frequently prescribed medications for anxiety in older adults, particularly for GAD, benzodiazepines are associated with falls, lack of coordination, and memory problems in the elderly.

Benzodiazepines appear only to be the first-choice treatment for acute episodes of anxiety, as distinct from GAD, because their rapid effects are useful for producing immediate symptom relief. For acute episodes (e.g., 4–6 weeks), benzodiazepines have been found to be superior to a placebo in most (e.g., Borison, Albrecht, & Diamond, 1990; Boyer & Feighner, 1993; Rickels, Schweizer, DeMartinis, Mandos, & Mercer, 1997), but not all, double-blind treatment studies (e.g., Pecknold et al., 1989; Ross & Matas, 1987). However, Ballenger et al. (2001) emphasize that physicians in general practice may fail to distinguish between an acute anxiety state and the ongoing anxiety disorder of GAD and overprescribe benzodiazepines, which may lead to inappropriate long-term use due to the rapid symptom relief that clients experience. Benzodiazepines may be particularly effective for somatic anxiety symptoms (Rickels et al., 1982), and it is notable that dose escalation is rare in GAD clients without a history of substance abuse (Rickels, Case, Downing, & Fridman, 1986). However, side effects may include sedation, psychomotor retardation, anterograde amnesia (Lucki, Rickels, & Geller, 1986), and tolerance, although clients with GAD may be less vulnerable than clients with panic disorder to experience withdrawal symptoms (Klein, Colin, Stolk, & Lenox, 1994).

Buspirone

This drug has been shown in several double-blind studies to be comparable to benzodiazepines for acute treatment of GAD (e.g., Rickels et al., 1982). In comparison to benzodiazepines, buspirone has a delayed (2–4 weeks) onset of action, may affect cognitive symptoms more than physical symptoms (Feighner & Cohn, 1989; Rickels et al., 1982), and has the advantage of being nonsedating and without evidence of tolerance or withdrawal symptoms. Common side effects include nausea, dizziness, and headaches. However, a lack of efficacy when comorbid conditions are present prevents buspirone from being recommended as a first-line treatment (Ballenger et al., 2001).

Hydroxyzine

The use of hydroxyzine is similar to that of benzodiazepines. However, although hydroxyzine does not cause dependence, it may have a sedating effect at the commencement of treatment (Roy-Byrne & Cowley, 2002). This drug has been shown to be superior to placebo for treating individuals with GAD, although side effects were more common in the treatment group than in the placebo group (Ferreri, Hantouche, & Billardon, 1994). Hydroxyzine is indicated for rapid reduction of acute anxiety states, but given the absence of demonstrated efficacy with depression, panic disorder, social phobia, or obsessive–compulsive disorder, this drug is not a recommended first-line treatment (Ballenger et al., 2001).

Antidepressants

In more recent years, antidepressants such as venlafaxine, imipramine, trazodone, and paroxetine have been shown in several double-blind treatment studies to be effective for treating GAD, with the most pronounced effects on psychic symptoms (e.g., Davidson, DuPont, Hedges, & Haskins, 1999; Gelenberg et al., 2000; Hoehn-Saric, McLeod, & Zimmerli, 1988). Furthermore, trials in clients with depression and comorbid anxiety suggest that some antidepressants, such as fluoxetine (Versiani et al., 1999), fluvoxamine (Houck, 1998), and amitriptyline (Versiani et al., 1999), hold promise as treatments for generalized anxiety.

Taken together, these studies suggest that antidepressants (particularly imipramine, venlafaxine, and paroxetine) are promising treatments for GAD. On the basis of such evidence, antidepressants are recommended as the first-line psychopharmacological treatment for GAD because of their safety, tolerability, and effectiveness, particularly given the high rates of comorbidity (Ballenger et al., 2001).

Comparing Psychological and Pharmacological Treatments

Several studies have compared the relative benefits of benzodiazepines, buspirone, and CBT in the treatment of GAD. Studies comparing diazepam (a benzodiazepine), CBT, and placebo, either alone or in combination for the treatment of GAD, have shown that outcome measures at posttreatment and at 6-month follow-up were superior for treatments involving CBT either alone or in combination with diazepam (e.g., Power, Simpson, Swanson, & Wallace, 1990a, 1990b). Moreover, whereas CBT produced the greatest long-term effects on anxiety reduction, diazepam in conjunction with CBT resulted in the earliest treatment gains.

Studies examining the efficacy of buspirone combined with psychological therapy (i.e., including psychoeducation, relaxation therapy, and cognitive therapy) and placebo therapy in the treatment of GAD revealed that all groups showed significant improvement after 8 weeks compared to baseline, although dropout rates were significantly higher in participants assigned to buspirone (Bond, Wingrove, Curran, & Lader, 2002). Thus, whereas CBT approaches to the treatment of GAD may be superior for producing long-term treatment gains, a combined approach may be the most appropriate for producing rapid, short-term symptom relief, particularly for clients suffering from moderate to severe GAD (Powers et al., 1990a; Schweizer & Rickels, 1996).

FACTORS AFFECTING OUTCOME FOLLOWING TREATMENT AND STRATEGIES FOR MAXIMIZING IMPROVEMENT

As discussed, a number of treatments may be associated with significant reduction of GAD symptoms. However, GAD remains a difficult disorder to treat effectively, and there is certainly room for improvement in GAD treatment outcome. Given that success rates from CBT for GAD lag behind those for many of the other anxiety disorders, with approximately 4 of every 10 clients undergoing CBT not making clinically significant improvements (Brown, Barlow, & Liebowitz, 1994), we discuss factors associated with current treatment approaches for GAD that may affect treatment outcome. Furthermore, for each variable reviewed, we discuss strategies for the therapist to help maximize client improvement.

Client Variables

Comorbidity

As discussed earlier in this chapter, GAD rarely occurs in isolation. Over 90% of individuals with GAD assessed in community samples report a history of some other psychological disorder in their lives and over 75% of individuals with a current principal diagnosis of GAD having other co-occurring anxiety or mood disorders (Brawman-Mintzer et al., 1993; Brown & Barlow, 1992; Massion et al., 1993; Wittchen et al., 1994). Thus, one characteristic of GAD that may be particularly influential on the process of treatment is the high rate of comorbidity.

It is thought that the high rate of co-occurring disorders associated with GAD may, in part, explain why studies have noted only modest treatment gains following CBT or pharmacological interventions (Brown et al., 2001). Although a few studies have examined the impact of co-occurring disorders on treatment outcome for GAD (e.g., Borkovec, Abel, & Newman, 1995; Durham, Allan, & Hackett, 1997; Sanderson, Beck, & McGinn, 1994), the results have been mixed and more empirical attention is required in this area. Nevertheless, from a clinical perspective, coexisting psychological disorders must be addressed in treatment planning given that the presence of these additional disorders are likely to have an impact on the effectiveness of CBT for GAD.

A challenge for the therapist when the client presents with multiple disorders is determining what to focus on first and how to plan treatment. Such decisions should be based on a thorough understanding of the client's entire diagnostic profile obtained from the initial assessment. A major consideration should be the severity and degree of impairment and distress caused by the various disorders and whether the different disorders play a role in maintaining each one another (Craske, 2003b). For example, if features of depression, such as lack of energy, feelings of worthlessness, and loss of pleasure and interest in usual activities, reinforce worries about personal ineffectiveness and incompetence, then the depressive features will need to be addressed during the initial stages of treatment.

It also is important to consider which of the presenting problems the client perceives to be the most impairing and distressing. Initial treatment success may be more likely if the client is focused on an area that is personally meaningful to him or her. Furthermore, when the co-occurring problems are other anxiety disorders, mastery over one domain of anxiety is more likely to lead, in turn, to positive treatment effects generalizing to other domains of fear and anxiety (Craske, 2003b). The therapist should encourage the client to choose an area of concern that has been the most distressing and disabling for at least the last month, rather than picking an issue that may only have been relevant over the past day or two (Craske, 2003b). Because some clients with GAD may have difficulty determining which domain of concern is the most distressing and impairing, the following strategies can be used:

1. Instruct the client to list his or her main domains of anxiety (e.g., GAD and panic disorder).
2. Ask the client to rate the extent of distress currently experienced in relation to each domain, using a 0–100 rating scale.
3. Ask the client to rate how much interference is currently experienced in relation to each domain, using a 0–100 rating scale.
4. Rank-order the different domains of worry based on the client's ratings of interference and distress within each domain of worry.
5. Check with the client that he or she is in agreement with focusing treatment on the domain rated as the most distressing and impairing (Craske, 2003b).

Another useful strategy for assessing the client's perception of what causes the most distress and impairment is to ask, "If you could receive treatment for only one of these problems, which problem would you choose?" Once the initial focus of treatment is determined, the therapist should encourage the client to remain focused on one area at a time—unless a crisis arises—in order to gain the most benefit from treatment (Craske, 2003b). The client should be informed that even if it feels as if the targeted area is no longer problematic, it is more effective to complete the entire course of CBT for that particular area than to terminate focus too soon. A useful analogy for highlighting the importance of completing one domain of concern at a time is that of taking a course of penicillin—it is necessary to take the full course even though the initial symptoms of infection have disappeared in order to prevent the illness from re-occurring in the future.

Stressful Life Events

The emergence of stressful life events during the course of therapy can be problematic for clients with GAD, given that worry and the associated features of GAD can be made worse by stress. An increase in stressful events can make it difficult for the client to attend sessions on a regular basis and may lead to noncompliance with homework and to an inability to give sufficient time and effort to implementing cognitive and behavioral strategies. In such cases, it can be challenging to maintain the appropriate balance between focusing on treatment goals and attending to the client's current difficulties. Emphasizing treatment goals too strongly when the client may not have the time or energy to devote to them can lead to failed attempts at achieving these goals, which in turn, may lead to dropout from treatment. On the other hand, an overemphasis on current life stressors can block treatment progress all together and cloud the purpose of CBT, which is a time-limited, goal-directed intervention (Beck & Emery, 1979). To prevent attrition while still maintaining the focus on treatment goals, the impact of the client's stressors should be discussed in session and an agreement reached about what can be achieved given the context of the client's current circumstances. Furthermore, a small amount of time (e.g., 5–10 minutes) at the commencement of each session can be devoted to discussing the client's current stressors, and, where appropriate, the client should be encouraged to employ techniques learned in treatment to these stressful events.

Interpersonal Functioning

Another factor thought to contribute to the lower success rates of CBT for GAD is that individuals with GAD may experience elevated levels of interpersonal difficulties (Borkovec, Newman, Pincus, & Lytle, 2002). Enhanced interpersonal problems have been found to be associated with poorer rates of clinical change in GAD symptomatology after treatment and failure to maintain treatment gains at follow-up assessment (Borkovec et al., 2002). Moreover, interpersonal problems have been found not only to reduce the effectiveness of CBT for GAD but also to be resistant to change following treatment with CBT (Borkovec et al., 2002). Along similar lines, Durham et al. (1997) found that although being married or cohabitating afforded a much greater probability of improvement and a much decreased probability of relapse, the benefits obtained by individuals with GAD were moderated by the *quality* of these relationships—tension and friction in the relationship were strongly associated with a reduced likelihood of improvement. To that end, it is notable that in studies of factors predicting the clinical course of GAD, poorer interpersonal functioning (particularly in spousal and family relationships) was associated with diminished likelihood of remission (Yonkers, Dyck, Warshaw, & Keller, 2000).

It has been argued that many of the interpersonal problems experienced by individuals with GAD stem from their tendency to continually focus on and avoid perceived potential threats, including the possibility of not being liked by others (Newman, 2000). Such avoidance is thought to lead individuals with GAD to become withdrawn, self-absorbed, and distracted in interpersonal contexts (Newman, 2000). By subtly avoiding potential threats in these contexts, individuals with GAD may fail to recognize the impact of their behavior on others. Such interpersonal behavior may lead, in turn, to others developing an unfavorable impression of the individual.

Because interpersonal difficulties may be among the factors contributing to lower success rates of CBT for GAD (Borkovec et al., 2002), acquiring a thorough understanding of the client's interpersonal functioning may be important for treatment planning. Useful information to obtain from the client includes how comfortable he or she feels with self-disclosure and expression of emotions, how he or she handles receiving perceived criticism from others, what his or her beliefs are about forming close relationships with others ("If I don't get too close, others will have no reason to dislike me," "If I let others get to know me, they will find out that I really am stupid"), and whether the client tends to avoid interpersonal situations. If the initial assessment indicates that the client experiences difficulty in interpersonal contexts, and it is thought that this difficulty plays a role in maintaining chronic worry and underlying concerns about personal ineffectiveness (Craske, 2003a), then interpersonal functioning may be usefully targeted during the early stages of treatment.

For the client whose interpersonal functioning contributes to the maintenance of GAD symptoms, a useful strategy, proposed by Newman (2000), is for the client to keep a diary of interpersonal interactions as a formal component of GAD treatment. The purpose of the diary is to help the client identify and alter problematic interpersonal avoidance. Examples of such avoidance include unwillingness to express emotional vulnerability to others, avoidance of becoming aware of how one may directly contribute to negative responses from others, and avoidance of interpersonal behavior change (Newman, 2000). The diary elicits information about the response the client hoped to receive from the other person, what he or she was afraid would happen, what action the client actually engaged in during the situation, and how the other person responded to the client's actions. By examining the recorded patterns of interpersonal behavior with the client, this form of self-monitoring helps the client to see how his or her interpersonal behavior (i.e., avoidance) is driven by fears (e.g., of being disliked or harmed by others) and to understand the consequences that stem from this style of interpersonal functioning (Newman, 2000). Importantly, the client should be encouraged to generate alternative ways of thinking about interpersonal situations and to put these alternatives into practice through the use of miniexperiments. Such experiments should be directed at situations the client avoids so that his or her "hypotheses" about what will happen can be tested (e.g., "If I refuse to do something someone asks of me, they will dislike me forever"). Continued use of the interpersonal interactions diary throughout treatment can provide important information for assessing the effectiveness of the treatment approach on interpersonal functioning.

Treatment Variables

Noncompliance with Self-Monitoring

A common obstacle in CBT treatment for GAD is noncompliance—both with self-monitoring and with other treatment strategies. Because self-monitoring is introduced early in treatment, compliance with these procedures can be a good initial indication of the client's motivation and commitment to treatment.

Initiating Compliance. One obstacle to initial compliance with self-monitoring and homework is the positive beliefs that clients with GAD typically hold about worry. Clients with GAD often maintain the view that worrying prepares them for, or protects them from, perceived threats and ultimately prevents feared events from happening. Noncompliance with self-monitoring may occur early in treatment when the client does not accept the idea that paying *more attention* to symptoms by self-monitoring the triggers and consequences of anxious sensations is likely to be useful (Newman, 2000).

It is important during the initial stages of treatment that the therapist provide a clear introduction to the principles of CBT and illustrate how self-monitoring and homework are integral components of the approach. In doing so, the therapist can make several points, including the following:

- That the purpose of self-monitoring is to develop a nonjudgmental self-awareness of oneself, whereby the client adopts a "personal scientist" approach to observing his or her reactions.
- How *objective* versus *subjective* self-monitoring lessens distress, increases understanding of emotional reactions, and enhances a sense of personal control.
- How subjective monitoring involves affect and catastrophic judgments about one's ongoing state, and that it is monitoring in a subjective manner that can make it seem like self-monitoring will enhance GAD symptoms. By contrast, objective monitoring is observing oneself "from a distance" in a nonjudgmental manner.
- Providing concrete examples of subjective versus objective monitoring, such as "I feel very anxious and I don't think I can go to work today" versus "my heart is racing and my palms are sweating, and one of my thoughts is that I won't be able to go to work today." In the first example illustrating subjective monitoring, an affective label has been assigned (i.e., "I feel very anxious") and a judgment about the meaning of this affective state has been made (i.e., "I won't be able to go to work today"). By contrast, the example of objective monitoring simply describes the sensations experienced with no emotion-laden interpretations assigned to these experiences.

In addition to drawing the distinction between objective and subjective monitoring, the therapist can introduce a set of exercises in session to reinforce learning to self-monitor objectively. The therapist can instruct the client to simply be aware of sensations, thoughts, and then feelings without judging their appropriateness or meaning but simply noticing their occurrence. In addition, the therapist can propose the analogy of the client sitting on a park bench and simply taking note of the people passing by. The following exercises, derived and modified by Craske (2003b) from mindfulness-based meditation approaches (e.g., Kabat-Zinn, 1994), can be introduced to help the client grasp the skill of observing oneself in a nonjudgmental, objective manner:

1. To promote awareness of physical sensations, ask the client to engage in a 2-minute exercise of body scanning, focusing on sensations in the feet and the hands. Ask the client to simply take note of all the sensations in his or her feet and hands (e.g., the tightness of shoelaces and hands resting on the armchair) without making judgments about these sensations.
2. To raise awareness of thoughts in a nonjudgmental manner, ask the client to engage in a 2-minute exercise of being posed the question, "What would it mean if you were to become the Statue of Liberty?" and note all the thoughts that come to mind.
3. To raise awareness of objectively monitoring sensations, thoughts and behavioral urges, have the client engage in a 2-minute exercise of being shown one positive and one negative pictorial image and noticing the different sensations (emotional and physical), thoughts (e.g., "That is cute" and "That is disgusting"), and behavioral urges (e.g., to smile and to look away) elicited by each picture.
4. To help the client apply these skills to personally meaningful situations, ask the client to engage in a 2-minute exercise of imagining a mildly to moderately anxiety-provoking situation relevant to the client's domains of worry and noticing physical and emotional sensations, thoughts, and behavioral urges.

For each exercise, the client is encouraged to state any descriptive words, visual images, or pictures that come to mind during this process (Craske, 2003b). Corrective feedback is given on whether the client was noting thoughts, sensations, or behavioral urges from a nonjudgmental, objective standpoint versus a subjective, affect-laden perspective. These exercises should be repeated in session as many times as is necessary for the client to become competent in self-monitoring in an objective manner. The client is then instructed to repeat these exercises at least three times before the next session. It may be useful for the therapist to help the client identify two or three mildly to moderately anxiety-provoking scenarios to monitor during homework exercises. The self-monitoring form depicted in Figure 3.1 can be used when completing these homework tasks and then reviewed at the commencement of each session.

Maintaining Compliance. A further complication with self-monitoring compliance is ensuring that the client persists with this task throughout treatment, a complication not necessarily unique to treatment of GAD. One reason for noncompliance with ongoing self-monitoring is that this procedure is not explained well to the client. When ongoing self-monitoring is first introduced, it is important that the therapist explains each of the components on the self-monitoring form (see Figure 3.1), describes clearly when self-monitoring should occur, and checks that the client understands what is involved. To help consolidate understanding, the therapist should ask the client to use the self-monitoring form in session to record any sensations, thoughts, and behaviors that occur during the most recent episodes of anxiety so that the therapist can give corrective feedback where appropriate. As in the monitoring exercises described earlier, it should be emphasized that the goal of ongoing self-monitoring is for the client to observe his or her responses *from a distance* rather than to judge emotional responding (Craske, 2003b). Thus, when introducing ongoing self-monitoring, it will be important for the therapist to effectively manage the session plan to allow sufficient time to discuss ongoing self-monitoring.

A further obstacle to ongoing self-monitoring is that the client does not persist with this task because monitored events have not consistently been reviewed and reinforced by the therapist at each session. Thus, it is important that the therapist routinely reviews self-monitoring progress across the course of treatment. Making homework review the first item on the agenda for each treatment session is a useful strategy for ensuring that self-monitoring is reinforced.

Noncompliance with self-monitoring homework may also occur because the client simply forgets to complete self-monitoring or because there is not enough time to complete the task. To deal with this problem, the therapist can help the client build reminders into his or her daily activities. For example, the client can be instructed to place reminder notes in locations that are likely to be seen, such as by the phone, refrigerator, computer, or television (Newman, 2000). The client also can be encouraged to ask a family member or friend to prompt him or her to complete self-monitoring exercises. In cases in which self-monitoring is not possible during the day (e.g., due to work commitments), an alternative can be for the client to place the self-monitoring forms beside his or her bed and to record anxiety-provoking situations that occurred during the day before going to sleep (Brown et al., 2001). If the latter strategy is thought to invoke worry and rumination prior to the client going to sleep, the forms could instead be placed in another prominent location the client routinely sees, such as next to the lounge chair or desk.

Issues That Arise When Using Cognitive Strategies

As discussed earlier, cognitive and perceptual change through treatment is important for achieving both initial and long-term gains from CBT. However, obstacles may be encountered when implementing cognitive techniques with clients with GAD. Some of these obstacles may concern client expectations about the results from cognitive strategies being immediate, or the client may have difficulty with particular aspects of cognitive restructuring, such as identifying automatic thoughts, recognizing cognitive errors, countering anxious thoughts, and generating and testing out alternatives through positive action.

Such obstacles may be due, at least in part, to particular cognitive characteristics of individuals with GAD, such as their tendency to engage in excessive rumination about particular events and to be locked in inflexible, future-oriented patterns of thinking.

However, despite that cognitive strategies are an important component of treatment for GAD, it has been argued that one reason for the modest treatment gains of CBT for GAD is that previous cognitive approaches have primarily focused on challenging the content of tangible stressors and problems of daily life, rather than focusing on metacognitive processes that underlie worrying itself (Wells, 1999). Such underlying processes include the positive (e.g., worrying helps me prepare for things) and negative beliefs (e.g., worry is uncontrollable and dangerous) that clients hold about their worry (Wells, 1999). In this section, we review strategies for dealing with obstacles associated with implementing cognitive techniques with clients with GAD as well as strategies for targeting metacognitive processes that underlie worrying.

Expecting Immediate Results. One common obstacle to cognitive restructuring is that the client with GAD may expect that cognitive techniques will produce an immediate reduction in anxiety symptoms (Leahy, 2002). If the client's expectation is that change (or a decrease in subjective anxiety) will be immediate, he or she may cease trying when things do not change immediately, thereby reinforcing the belief that anxiety is permanent and resistant to change. In introducing cognitive restructuring, the therapist should make it clear that the reduction of anxious symptoms is not the first goal of cognitive therapy. Instead, it should be emphasized that this procedure is intended to correct *distorted thinking* about the negative emotional states of chronic worry and the associated features of GAD, and that in doing so, the symptoms of GAD will eventually subside. It may therefore be useful to encourage the client to adopt a "work in progress" perspective regarding treatment and to consider the process of change in treatment to be like learning any other new skill, such as driving a car or riding a bike, in that change will occur with time, through continued practice and generalization. The therapist may need to repeatedly emphasize this "work in progress" perspective throughout treatment, particularly during the early stages when the client's distress is likely to be the strongest.

Obstacles to Identifying and Pursuing Thoughts. Some clients with GAD may have difficulty recognizing the content of specific cognitions or, once identified, may be reluctant to pursue anxious thoughts due to fear that this will exacerbate worry and associated GAD symptoms. When first introducing the idea of identifying danger-laden thoughts, the therapist should explain how detecting one's thoughts can be challenging because cognitions are "automatic" and may occur so rapidly in certain situations that they may be outside the client's awareness (Beck & Emery, 1979). In addition, the client must become clearly aware of the kinds of self-statements being made in particular situations and must learn to pursue his or her thoughts until arriving at the specific content or prediction that is creating the anxiety (Beck & Emery, 1979). To proceed no further than "surface-level" self-statements, such as "this is terrible—anything could have happened," serves to maintain or intensify anxiety by virtue of the catastrophic, unproductive nature of these thoughts.

To assist clients who experience difficulty with identifying thoughts, the therapist should explain that just like learning any other new skill, the identification of self-statements will become better with practice and that thoughts can usually be identified with careful questioning and observation of oneself. Moreover, because the client may first notice mood changes or physical sensations before recognizing what he or she was thinking in anxious situations, the therapist can instruct the client to regularly monitor his or her physical and emotional state so that the client becomes skilled in detecting early internal and external cues of anxiety. The client can be encouraged to regularly monitor mood state by periodically asking him- or herself questions, such as "how am I feeling right now," and can become more efficient in noting early physical cues of anxiety by regularly conducting "body scans" for signs of tension and anxiety. At times when clients recognize feeling anxious and worried, they can be instructed to "play back" in their mind the details of the situation they were just in before noticing feeling anxious and to ask themselves what that situation signaled to them or what they were thinking about at that time.

For example, Mark was a college student riding the bus on the way home from classes when he noticed feeling a vague sense of dread, an uneasiness in the stomach, and the fact that he was gripping the handles of his bag tightly. Mark played back in his mind the last few minutes of the bus ride, recalling salient memories and events, and recognized that he had begun feeling anxious after noticing a student from his class studying on the bus. Mark then asked himself, "What did that student studying signal to me?" and "What did it mean to me that he was studying?" Mark recognized that he had said to himself, "I should be studying too." Rather than stopping at this surface level of self-questioning, knowing that this kind of self-statement is likely to maintain worry and associated features, Mark continued to pursue the specific details by asking himself, "What does it say about me that I am not studying?" and he recognized that it signaled to him that he is "lazy." At this point, having uncovered the underlying cognition causing his anxiety (i.e., "I am lazy"), Mark then employed cognitive countering techniques (see later) to shift his thinking to be more realistic and more productive. Thus, by initially paying careful attention to his ongoing emotional state and physical sensations, and by being able to "play back" in his mind the events of the past few minutes, Mark was able to identify the stimulus that had triggered the surface-level anxious cognitions, and through the use of careful questioning, he was able to reveal the underlying thoughts that caused his anxiety.

The therapist can assist a client who experiences difficulty with identifying thoughts by having him or her play back recent episodes of anxiety in session and then guide him or her through the use of personal questioning techniques to identify underlying anxious cognitions. An alternative is to use an imagined scenario relevant to the client's domains of worry to practice the self-observation and questioning techniques. The therapist can also encourage the client to develop a list of prompts to help facilitate personal question asking, including "What would it mean if . . . ?," "What do you picture happening . . . ?," "What would it signal to me if . . . ?," and "What does it say about me that . . . ?" (Craske, 2003b).

Obstacles to Recognizing Cognitive Errors. When the client is skilled in identifying his or her thoughts in anxious situations, another complication can be that the client has difficulty recognizing errors of thinking. Being able to accurately recognize cognitive distortions can be helpful to clients with GAD because these individuals are likely to make interpretive errors, such as "probability overestimation," "catastrophizing," and "all-or-nothing thinking." A useful strategy for helping the client to routinely examine his or her thoughts for evidence of cognitive errors is to build this process into self-monitoring. In Figure 3.1, we demonstrate how the client's monitoring includes recording the thoughts, sensations, and behavioral urges associated with anxiety-provoking situations. After the client is competent in recognizing his or her anxious thoughts and the idea of cognitive errors has been introduced, the client can be provided with a new monitoring form containing an additional column for recording the type of cognitive error reflected in anxious thoughts. Finally, when the therapist reviews the client's self-monitoring progress at the commencement of each session, corrective feedback should be provided about the client's progress in recognizing the type of cognitive errors being committed.

Obstacles to Countering Thoughts and Generating Alternatives. Several obstacles may arise when helping the client with GAD to challenge worrisome thoughts and beliefs. One such obstacle can be that individuals can be very skilled at countering alternative evidence and logical interpretation because they are so often engaged in repetitive verbal activity aimed at anticipating and generating possible negative future outcomes (Newman, 2000). Therefore, the therapist can potentially get caught in a no-win debate with the client about the relative costs and benefits of various alternative perspectives. To avoid this, the therapist should emphasize that a central goal of countering is to learn to recognize that there are numerous ways of interpreting the same situation (in addition to the one the client rigidly holds on to) and to accept that there is no single "right" way of perceiving an event (Newman, 2000). Furthermore, the therapist should focus on identifying which of the alternatives the client has generated are the most adaptive and direct the client's attention to how these alternatives can be put into action.

Relatedly, because countering is a primary method for "decatastrophizing" events that the client views as negative (e.g., "making a mistake is terrible"), another obstacle can be that the client simply cannot appreciate how such an event can be viewed in any way other than negative and cata-strophic. To deal with this type of resistance, the therapist should emphasize that the basis for countering is not about critically evaluating whether an event is in fact negative and undesirable. Rather, the therapist can help the cli-ent recognize that it is the *severity of the consequences* stemming from the event that the client is viewing catastrophically (e.g., "They will think I am useless" and "I could lose my job") and that it is these catastrophic conse-quences that are the target of countering and critical evaluation (Craske, 2003b). Thus, the therapist should encourage the client to focus on the conse-quences of the event that is perceived as negative and emphasize that counter-ing techniques are directed toward the emotional and behavioral responses to the event versus the event itself. In addition, the therapist should emphasize the messages that (1) specific catastrophic events are unlikely (e.g., getting fired for making a mistake); and that (2) anxiety and related symptoms and their effects (e.g., sense of dread) are time-limited and manageable. The thera-pist should also reinforce the notion of the client adopting a "personal scien-tist" approach by questioning and "testing out" catastrophic thoughts rather than simply accepting them. For example, clients who interpret making a mis-take as being catastrophic could test out their hypotheses that others will think they are "useless" by specifically engaging in conversation with cowork-ers and objectively examining the reaction of others for evidence and counter-evidence of this interpretation.

Another obstacle to effective countering and self-questioning can be that the client with GAD may find it difficult to engage in flexible thinking pat-terns in order to generate alternative perspectives to his or her strongly held beliefs (Newman, 2000). To deal with this problem, the therapist can instruct the client to generate both positive and negative alternative self-statements for a number of ambiguous situations. Scenarios the therapist can present to the client may include the following:

1. Being ignored by a work colleague.
2. Completing a document at work without checking it over.
3. Arriving at a party or a friend's house later than expected.
4. Attending a meeting without having prepared for it.
5. Husband or wife is late arriving to meet you.

For each scenario, clients are instructed to use a pie chart to generate as many alternative interpretations as they can, listing their own initial interpre-tation as one piece of the pie chart. See the example in Figure 3.2, developed by Craske (2003b), as an example of using the pie chart to generate alterna-tive interpretations about what it means to be ignored by a work colleague. The therapist can then ask the client to consider what sources of information can be used to determine the accuracy of each interpretation (e.g., past experi-ence with this individual and objective information known about the other person and how he or she interacts with others) and to compare the various sources to his or her own mood or emotion as a source of judgment. Thus, similar to assisting the client to engage in objective versus subjective self-monitoring, the aim in generating alternative interpretations is to help the client identify alternatives that are objective and nonjudgmental rather than emotion-laden and subjective.

Another obstacle can be that although the client with GAD may well generate alternative thoughts and accept the logic of them, he or she may not "feel" that these alternatives are as believable as the original anxious thoughts. As a result, clients may be reluctant to take positive behavioral action consistent with these new alternatives. As Newman (2000) explains, clients with GAD may have played their catastrophic thoughts over and over so many times in their mind that this way of thinking is the only way that seems real to them. Furthermore, as individuals with GAD may well have had very few positive thoughts and images, any positive alternative may seem foreign and unbelievable (Newman, 2000).

One method for dealing with this problem is to emphasize the importance of taking action despite these concerns, rather than simply accepting the emotional appraisal of the situation. Thus, the therapist can introduce the client to the idea of conducting "mini-experiments" in which he or she "tests out" alternative interpretations in relatively neutral, benign situations and then simply "seeing what happens" (Craske, 2003b). In this way, clients are exposed to situations in which they may acquire disconfirming evidence of their old perspectives and supporting evidence for new ways of thinking. Thus, the therapist should emphasize the role of personal experience as being the most effective way of changing belief systems. Furthermore, it is important to

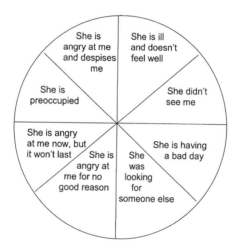

FIGURE 3.2. Example of a pie chart, developed by Craske (2003b), used to assist clients in generating alternative perspectives for interpreting situations. In this example, the therapist and client generate alternative reasons for being ignored by a coworker.

emphasize that the intention of mini-experiments is not only to improve the client's tolerance of emotional distress but to gather independent evidence that disconfirms misappraisals. The therapist should have the client begin with experiments that are practical, can be feasibly carried out, and are only mildly to moderately anxiety provoking. The client is instructed to list the exact feared outcome that is being tested and his or her hypothesis about what will happen. Examples of mini-experiments include the following:

Task	Hypothesis to be tested
Invite a friend over when I have purposely left the house a little untidy.	They will comment on my sloppiness.
Purposely arrive 5 minutes late to a meeting.	They will refuse to meet with me.
Drop the children off at school without checking on them until I pick them up.	They will be kidnapped.

The specific details of the mini-experiment are discussed in session, such as when the client will perform the mini-experiment and what tasks need to be completed in order for the mini-experiment to be conducted (e.g., dirty dishes are placed in the sink and on the coffee table before a friend comes over). At the following session, the therapist reviews the outcome of the mini-experiment, establishes whether the feared outcome occurred, and reinforces disconfirmation of the client's initial misappraisal based on the evidence obtained from the mini-experiment. New mini-experiments are then designed, building on what was learned from the last hypothesis-testing experiment.

Metacognitive Processes. The first step in addressing metacognitive processes in GAD is for the client to understand that GAD is characterized by a tendency to worry about worrying itself (e.g., "worrying will make me go crazy,") and to learn to challenge these negative underlying beliefs about worry. Metaworries first chosen for modification should be those concerning the dangerousness and uncontrollability of worry. Wells (1997) developed numerous strategies to help target these beliefs. Metaworries concerning the dangers of worrying can be challenged by reviewing the evidence and counterevidence in support of such appraisals. In most cases, even though the client may have subjectively felt distressed and troubled during episodes of worry, there is typically no objective evidence of the dangers of worrying (e.g., the client will never have actually fainted or had a heart attack in response to worrying). Thus, the client should be encouraged to examine the objective evidence regarding the dangers of worrying and to recognize that it is the catastrophic interpretation about the consequences of worrying and the associated distress that leads to the perception that he or she will "go crazy" from worrying. To further highlight that worrying—although unpleasant—will not result in objectively dangerous consequences (e.g., going crazy or losing one's mind), behavioral experiments involving increased worrying can be used, such as the client deliberately worrying more about a problem and purposely trying to lose control. Furthermore, to maximize disconfirmation during these experiments, the client should be instructed not to engage in thought control strategies (e.g., distraction) or other behaviors that reduce the risk of loss of control.

When the client's negative metabeliefs about the dangerousness of worrying have been targeted, beliefs concerning the uncontrollability of worrying should then be addressed. One strategy is to instruct the client to review episodes in which his or her worry was interrupted by conflicting demands such as, for example, when a friend unexpectedly came by to visit. Through these examples, the client should be encouraged to recognize that control over worry was achieved when attention was drawn away from the content of worry and directed to other matters. Evidence about the controllability of worry also can be highlighted through behavioral experiments in which the client postpones worrying until a specified time each day. In addition, the contradiction between negative and positive beliefs about worry should be emphasized. For example, if a client believes that worrying helps to protect him or her from perceived dangers and facilitates coping (i.e., positive beliefs about worry), these beliefs should be contrasted with the negative belief that worrying may cause a nervous breakdown (Wells, 1999). Challenging these disparate ideas can help to reduce the strength of the client's positive and negative beliefs about worrying. Finally, as the strength of these beliefs begins to loosen, behavioral experiments in the form of exposure sessions (whether real or imagined) to avoided situations should be introduced so that the client acquires personal experience of disconfirmed beliefs.

Positive beliefs about worry should next be targeted by having the client review the advantages and disadvantages of worrying and questioning the validity of these beliefs (e.g., questioning how worrying actually protects oneself from perceived dangers). In addition, the client should be instructed to engage in activities normally associated with worrying while deliberately increasing and decreasing worry and to examine whether worry improved or impaired performance or coping outcomes (Wells, 1997). If worrying helps performance, then suspension of worrying for several days should result in poorer coping whereas increased worrying should enhance coping. To maximize the effects of experiments of this type, what is meant by coping and what would constitute reduced or improved coping should be defined in observable and testable terms (e.g., not calling one's partner or children to check on their safety, arriving on time to appointments, and not canceling social engagements; Wells, 1997).

Relaxation Training

Some clients report that they cannot relax, that relaxation is not working for them, or that they cannot bring themselves to practice relaxation. Clients with

GAD also may report finding it hard to maintain attentional focus during relaxation, particularly given the tendency for these individuals to engage in future-oriented patterns of worrisome behavior (Borkovec & Ruscio, 2001). It is generally assumed that the obstacles to benefiting from relaxation-based treatments are related either to psychological factors or a lack of practice.

One psychological reason clients may have for difficulty with relaxation is that they feel too tense to relax. In this case, the client is describing the very symptom that needs treating as a reason for not relaxing. The therapist should emphasize that such tension reflects that the client has not experienced a state of relaxation for a long time and that although it may take a little longer than expected, a state of relaxation can be achieved with continued practice.

Another reason for difficulty with relaxation can be that the client is unable to maintain focus during relaxation training. The client should be encouraged to recognize that although thoughts will occur during the silence of relaxation, it is important not to respond to them. Moreover, drawing from the literature on acceptance-based conceptualizations of GAD (e.g., Roemer & Orsillo, 2002), when the client notices his or her attention has shifted away from the focus of relaxation, he or she should be encouraged to simply shift attention back to the relaxation exercise in a nonjudgmental, accepting manner rather than to elaborate on distracting thoughts and to respond emotionally.

Other reasons for noncompliance with relaxation may include the client feeling that relaxation is a waste of time or that it is impossible to find the place or the time to relax. The client should be encouraged to accept that like many other therapies (e.g., physiotherapy and radiotherapy), treatment takes time and it is necessary to actively participate in treatment to obtain maximum benefits. The client also should be encouraged to be flexible. If it is impossible to put aside 20 minutes for relaxation, 10 minutes will be useful. Furthermore, if the client cannot find a suitable place at home to complete relaxation exercises, a nearby park may be suitable. Finally, relaxation should not be scheduled when the client would rather be doing something else (e.g., during lunch time, when he or she would rather be meeting friends for lunch).

Some clients may discontinue relaxation because they believe they are not getting anything out of it. To address this issue, the therapist should point out that impatience is a key feature of tension and anxiety and is therefore an indicator that continued practice is necessary. Thus, the client should be encouraged to set long-term goals for relaxation rather than monitoring day-to-day progress.

Although relaxation exercises are intended to reduce levels of tension and anxiety, it is not uncommon for some clients to experience an increase in anxiety as they learn to relax and release tension. Referred to as "relaxation-induced anxiety" (e.g., Heide & Borkovec, 1983), this state of increased anxiousness can pose an obstacle to successful implementation of relaxation training because the client may interpret this initial increase in arousal in response to relaxation training as a sign that his or her anxiety is uncontrollable and impermeable even to anxiety treatment. The therapist should be particularly watchful for signs of relaxation-induced anxiety in clients with comorbid panic disorder (Cohen, Barlow, & Blanchard, 1985).

The therapist can normalize the client's experience by explaining that many individuals experience relaxation-induced anxiety when first undertaking formal relaxation exercises and that this is simply the result of the client having been unable to achieve a relaxed state for a long time. It also should be explained that anxiety about relaxation can stem from positive beliefs about worry (e.g., "worrying makes me feel safe"), and that "letting go" of such vigilance through relaxation may initially seem dangerous and anxiety provoking. The therapist should emphasize that this initial increase in anxiety is not dangerous and that these feelings indicate that the client is coming into contact with his or her body and noticing sensations that may have been kept in check for many years. Moreover, it is important that the client persist with relaxation exercises so that he or she acquires evidence that the initial anxiety does indeed subside. The therapist can instruct the client to attempt relaxation exercises in a gradual, stepwise manner starting with short durations of relaxation and progressively extending the sessions until he or she is able to reach increasingly deeper levels of relaxation without experiencing anxiety (Heide & Borkovec, 1983). For clients who experience high levels of relaxation-induced anxiety, it may be beneficial for the client to initially undertake relaxation exercises only in session until he or she feels confident in completing these exercises alone. At that point, relaxation training at home can be formalized through the use of a weekly timetable listing how frequently relaxation sessions should be performed, with the duration of the sessions increasing in a manner agreed on with the client. To avoid possible noncompliance, the therapist should review progress with relaxation training at each session and specifically inquire about the client's experience of relaxation-induced anxiety.

Worry Imagery Exposure

The purpose of worry imagery exposure is to help the client with GAD learn to tolerate negative affect and somatic sensations and to habituate to fearful images that may be motivating worry (Brown et al., 2001). In addition, worry imagery exposure provides additional opportunities for the client to apply cognitive restructuring strategies learned thus far in treatment. Perhaps the biggest obstacle when conducting worry imagery exposure is the occasional tendency for worry imagery not to elicit sufficient levels of anxiety during initial exposures (Brown et al., 2001). Numerous reasons may explain this phenomenon, but the most common reasons include (1) the imagery not being vivid enough, (2) the images being too vague and lacking definition, (3) the images not adequately tapping into the relevant domains of fear, (4) the client utilizing some kind of coping strategy during the imagery (e.g., cognitive restructuring and relaxation techniques), and (5) the client covertly avoiding full images related to the worry (Brown et al., 2001; Craske, 2003b).

Another obstacle that occasionally arises is that the client does not habituate to the imagery cues despite repeated exposure. Several reasons may account for this problem, including the client covertly avoiding exposure to the fear as his or her anxiety levels increase, failing to maintain the image during the course of exposure by attention shifting, and using an exposure duration that is too short (Brown et al., 2001; Craske, 2003b).

In dealing with these problems, an important initial step in the application of worry imagery exposure is to ensure that the client possesses a thorough understanding about the rationale and purpose of the exercise. It is important that the therapist emphasize that for worry imagery exposure to be effective, the client must fully experience his or her anxiety and must not make efforts to minimize or avoid sensations (Craske et al., 1992). In particular, the client may try not to think of the worst feared outcome or may allow his or her thoughts to wander during the procedure. The therapist should point out that although distraction from anxious thoughts or feelings may relieve anxiety in the short term, distraction may reinforce the client's view that certain thoughts and images are to be avoided and is therefore an ineffective long-term strategy (Craske et al., 1989).

To help ensure the client achieves clear vivid images that adequately tap into the relevant fear domains, a worry imagery form can be utilized (see Figure 3.3). The client is asked to record the main fears associated with each worry domain (e.g., safety of my husband and children) and to describe a recent example from each worry domain in as much detail as possible. The therapist should prompt the client to be as specific about features of the examples as possible (e.g., "My husband was 20 minutes late arriving home from work. I was suppose to go to a meeting, but I just couldn't leave the house until he arrived. Ten minutes after he should have been home, I called his cell phone but there was no answer which really made me worry that he was in an accident"). Next, the client should be encouraged to rate the degree of distress evoked by each example using a 0–100 scale, and to then rank-order these images from the least anxiety-provoking to the most anxiety-provoking situation. Care should be taken to ensure the client rank-orders the examples appropriately because attempts to avoid complete exposure to a particularly strong image may occur if the client confronts such an image too early into exposure.

Before starting each imagery session, the client should be prompted to describe the specific details of the event to help consolidate a specific and well-defined image. During worry imagery exposure, the therapist should monitor the client's nonverbal behavior for evidence of the utilization of coping strategies, such as paced breathing or muscle relaxation. Furthermore, it is important that the client's subjective anxiety ratings be systematically collected during the exposures using a 0–100 rating scale (both during session and during homework), as these ratings will provide a useful indication of progress and potential problems (Brown et al., 2001).

Occasionally, the client may experience difficulty with generating alterna-

Domain of Worry	Degree of Distress (0 to 100)	Rank Order
Domain 1: _____ Recent example: _____ _____ _____		
Domain 2: _____ Recent example: _____ _____ _____		
Domain 3: _____ Recent example: _____ _____ _____		

FIGURE 3.3. Worry Imagery Form.

tives to the worst feared outcome. This difficulty may be the result of the client being in the initial stages of learning to apply cognitive countering techniques or it may indicate a strong belief conviction associated with the particular domain of worry (Brown et al., 2001). When problems of this nature are noted, the therapist may need to initially suggest possible alternative perspectives for the client. However, once the client has grasped the concept of generating alternatives, the therapist should avoid providing these suggestions for the client.

Nonspecific Treatment Factors

Important nonspecific factors influencing treatment outcome for GAD include the client's beliefs about the appropriateness of the offered treatment (i.e., treatment credibility) and his or her expectancy that therapy will help (Borkovec & Ruscio, 2001). A useful method for monitoring the client's expectations and satisfaction with treatment is having the client complete a short questionnaire like the one depicted in Figure 3.4 at the commencement of each session. The therapist should review the client's ratings and address any evidence of dissatisfaction or low expectations of treatment efficacy.

Therapist competence in the use of cognitive-behavioral techniques, a thorough understanding of current models of worry and GAD, and appropriate nonspecific qualities such as communication of trust and empathy, logical reasoning skills, and the ability to tailor techniques to individuals are also critical variables for influencing treatment outcome (Brown et al., 2001).

Adapting Treatment for Different Populations

Previous research suggests that the likelihood of poorer response to CBT for GAD may be influenced by a range of individual difference factors, including being of older age, having the disorder for a long duration, using psychotropic medications, and having past experience with psychological and pharmacological treatments (e.g., Biswas & Chattopadhyay, 2001; Butler, 1993; Durham & Allan, 1993; Seivewright, Tyrer, & Johnson, 1998). In fact, recent studies with older adults suggest that these factors may work hand-in-hand to influence treatment outcome. For instance, Wetherell, Gatz, and Craske (2003) suggested that their smaller treatment effect with older adults with GAD compared to those reported in studies with younger participants may, in part, reflect that the older participants had experienced their anxiety symptoms for an average of almost 30 years, 40% were taking psychotropic medications, and almost 90% had previous experience with psychological or medication treatment. Together with the fact that many clients report experiencing their symptoms, to varying extents, for as long as they can remember (Rapee, 1985), these findings suggest that older clients may be more resistant to GAD treatment, at least as these treatments are offered in their present form.

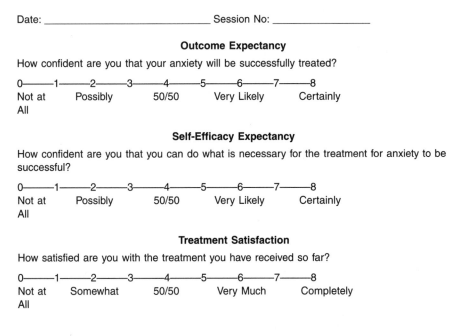

FIGURE 3.4. Client Expectations and Satisfaction Form.

In working with older clients with GAD, it is important that the therapist develop a sound understanding of the type of treatments the client has received in the past and how he or she responded to these various approaches. It is important to determine which components of past treatments the client found beneficial as well as the reasons why various treatment approaches were discontinued so that these factors can be taken into account in treatment planning.

Based on findings from treatment outcome studies, older clients with GAD may benefit from interventions including CBT approaches in combination with supportive psychotherapy and opportunities for self-disclosure and reflection of feelings (Stanley et al., 1996; Wetherell et al., 2003). Moreover, it has been suggested that tailoring the standard CBT group treatment package to include more interactive elements may enhance treatment outcome for older adults with GAD given that these individuals may be lonely or socially isolated (Wetherell et al., 2003). Furthermore, the addition of learning and memory aids, such as homework reminder calls and weekly reviews of all concepts and techniques learned, may hold promise for improving treatment outcome with older adults with GAD and accompanying cognitive impairment (Mohlman et al., 2003).

Children with GAD represent another population with whom the therapist may confront challenges. Although anxiety is a common, fluctuating, and transitory experience in childhood (Last, Perrin, Hersen, & Kazdin, 1996), anxiety in children and adolescents may increase in intensity, becoming chronic and developmentally disabling. Indeed, anxiety disorders are the most prevalent type of psychological disorder experienced by children and teenagers (Bernstein & Borchardt, 1991), and therapeutic studies have shown that children with anxiety symptoms virtually always present with some combination of GAD, separation anxiety disorder, and social phobia (Kendall, 1994). Moreover, for those children who experience clinical levels of anxiety, the prognosis appears to be poor, with studies indicating that childhood anxiety may be chronic and enduring (e.g., Keller et al., 1992).

Much like treatment studies with adults, CBT for anxiety disorders in children consists of six essential components: psychoeducation, somatic management, cognitive restructuring, problem solving, exposure, and relapse prevention. The most widely disseminated CBT protocol for childhood anxiety is Philip Kendall's *Coping Cat Program* (Kendall, Kane, Howard, & Siqueland, 1990). This protocol is appropriate for 7–16-year-old youth with GAD, separation anxiety disorder, and social phobia. Individual and group treatment manuals are available with adaptations for greater involvement of family members having demonstrated efficacy (Barrett, Dadds, & Rapee, 1996; Barrett, Duffy, Dadds, & Rapee, 2001; Spence, Donovan, Brechman-Toussaint, 2000). Indeed, although children with GAD, separation anxiety disorder and social phobia are often treated together, the results of treatment studies indicate that between 64% and 70.3% of treated children no longer met diagnostic criteria for an anxiety disorder by the end of treatment, with these results maintained at 12-month and 3-year follow-up (Kendall & Southam-Gerow, 1996). However, the success rates appear to be higher (e.g., 95.6%) when CBT is combined with family management training (Barrett et al., 1996). Moreover, the higher success rates of CBT for anxiety disorders in children, including GAD, as compared to the success rates from studies with adults (e.g., Brown, Barlow, & Liebowitz, 1994) and the elderly (e.g., Wetherell et al., 2003) are consistent with the view that GAD may be more difficult to treat the longer the client has suffered with this disorder.

Research is ongoing in the area of treatment for childhood anxiety disorders given that factors such as the degree of impairment experienced by the child, developmental level, and the degree of parental anxiety or psychopathology all warrant consideration and may affect the outcome of the child's treatment (Barrett et al., 1996; Howard & Kendall, 1996). Similarly, although recent evidence suggests that medications are effective for treating anxiety in children (e.g., Compton et al., 2001; Ryan, Siqueland, & Rickels, 2001), studies examining the relative efficacy of CBT, medication, and their combination are necessary.

It is now well accepted that the involvement of families in the treatment of childhood anxiety disorders is important. Although there are no clear guidelines for determining how much parents should be involved, more active parental involvement is recommended if (1) the child or adolescent is seriously impaired by anxiety or comorbidity, (2) the child is young in age or developmental level, and (3) the parents or other family members engage in behavior that accommodates the child's anxiety (Velting, Setzer, & Albano, 2004). By contrast, circumstances in which less active parental involvement is suggested includes (1) if the parents are themselves compromised by anxiety or other comorbid conditions, and (2) if the client is a teenager, so that he or she can be given the opportunity to assume self-responsibility (Velting et al., 2004).

In addition to determining the extent of involvement of the child's family in treatment, the therapist needs to consider the child's developmental level. The average age of onset for GAD in children is approximately 8.8 years (Weiss & Last, 2001). Thus, in younger children for whom limitations on cognitive processes are more pronounced, greater emphasis on behavioral approaches, such as hierarchical exposure and relaxation training, together with strong familial involvement (given the role of early attachment figures in the young child's life) may be a more logical approach. However, as children become more capable of expressing thoughts and fears with increasing age, a stronger emphasis on cognitive techniques is warranted when working with older children and adolescents. From a practical standpoint, working with youth during the middle childhood years as opposed to during adolescents is often easier because children are generally more amenable to treatment, their parents are usually easier to engage, and school-based interventions are easier to implement (Barrett, 2000).

Unfortunately, there are few treatment protocols developed specifically for adolescents, although one anxiety treatment protocol, the FRIENDS program, has been designed to respond to this need (Barrett, Lowry-Webster, & Holmes, 1998). One challenge for the therapist working with an adolescent is determining whether to treat him or her as a young adult or an older child. In general, the therapist should aim to make an early assessment of the adolescent's developmental level and to tailor the approach to each adolescent accordingly. Other obstacles can be that adolescents may feel embarrassed to be receiving treatment, may deny having such problems, and may be resistant to treatment efforts. To deal with this, the therapist should carefully address the adolescent's reluctance early in treatment and reassure him or her about confidentiality. The therapist also should encourage the adolescent to discuss his or her concerns about treatment and employ problem-solving techniques to help the adolescent weigh the advantages and disadvantages of treatment. It also may be beneficial to set small, short-term goals with the adolescent, such as committing to the first three or four sessions or learning the first component of treatment, such as psychoeducation, and then reviewing how he or she feels about treatment at that time.

Summary

In summary, although many clients with GAD benefit from CBT, there is a significant number who do not make substantial improvements after receiving treatment with this approach. Although systematic research is required to identify factors that contribute to the lower treatment outcomes rates for GAD, we have reviewed several variables that may affect treatment outcome. Some clients with GAD may present with more complex diagnostic profiles, more elevated levels of interpersonal difficulty, or they may be more affected by stress in their daily lives—factors that may need to be addressed during treatment in addition to targeting the key GAD features of worry and associated symptoms. Furthermore, the application of standard cognitive therapy techniques with clients with GAD may be challenging given the nature of worrisome cognitive processes, such as rigid inflexible thinking patterns and the tendency to be engaged in repetitive verbal activity and to delay behavioral action through rumination and indecisiveness. Moreover, treatment outcome may be improved with greater emphasis given to targeting metaworry and the positive and negative beliefs that underlie and maintain problematic worry. Taken together, the various factors that may have an impact on treatment outcome for GAD indicate that a thorough diagnostic and functional assessment is required for each presenting client and that the treatment plan and the specific interventions included be tailored to the key features of GAD (i.e., worry itself) and to the unique characteristics of the particular client rather than to a large number of strategies being applied to all individuals with a diagnosis of GAD (Antony, 2002; Craske, 2003a). In the next section, we review variables that may lead to relapse and recurrence of GAD and we discuss strategies that may help in their prevention.

RELAPSE AND RECURRENCE IN GENERALIZED ANXIETY DISORDER AND STRATEGIES FOR PREVENTION

It is well documented that GAD tends to be a chronic condition that waxes and wanes over time (e.g., Ballenger et al., 2001). Although the long-term effects of treatment are largely unknown, a few studies shed some light on factors that may increase the likelihood of relapse and recurrence after treatment.

Client Variables

Although more empirical research is required to determine the impact of comorbid disorders on the treatment of GAD, some evidence suggests that the presence of co-occurring Axis I disorders may be predictive of relapse after treatment for GAD (e.g., Durham et al., 1997). However, it is thought not to be the absolute *severity* of presenting comorbid problems but, rather, the more complex clinical presentation that makes the achievement of long-term treatment gains for GAD more difficult when co-occurring disorders are present (Durham et al., 1997). However, beyond the predictive value of comorbid disorders for the long-term outcome of GAD treatment, marital status, and the extent of tension and disharmony in the marital relationship in particular, has been found to be a powerful predictor of relapse (Durham et al., 1997). Such findings are loosely consistent with the work of Borkovec and colleagues (e.g., Borkovec et al., 2002) who found that failure to maintain treatment gains after CBT for GAD was predicted by heightened interpersonal problems. Although partner support during treatment has not been empirically assessed in outcome studies for GAD, the finding that marital problems and interpersonal difficulties may be predictive of relapse after treatment for GAD suggests that inclusion of the client's partner or a close relative or friend may enhance GAD treatment outcomes in the long term.

An exacerbation of GAD symptomatology after treatment also can be triggered by a number of other factors not necessarily unique to GAD. For instance, the client may discontinue regular practice and application of CBT techniques or simply get out of the habit of using CBT techniques without the regular input from the therapist (Newman, 2000). It also may be the case that going through a particularly stressful period may exacerbate a client's GAD symptomatology, leading to relapse. In these cases, the client may benefit from several follow-up sessions to become reacquainted with the techniques learned earlier during treatment and to help deal with current stressors.

Several individual difference factors, such as being of older age and having received psychiatric treatment in the past (e.g., Durham et al., 1997; Wetherell et al., 2003), also have been found to increase the likelihood of relapse in GAD. In addition to lower initial improvement rates, treatment outcome studies have shown that the percentage of older adults no longer meeting diagnostic criteria for GAD at follow-up is lower than in studies with younger adults, although these results may not necessarily reflect relapse but simply failure to improve (e.g., Wetherell et al., 2003). Conceivably, GAD may be more difficult to treat in older clients because these individuals have a longer history than younger clients of enduring unpredictable and uncontrollable negative reactivity in response to a wider range of accumulated threat cues, which in turn, has lead to more entrenched negative beliefs about worry (i.e., worry is abnormal and dangerous) and a stronger perception that one's anxiety is uncontrollable and impermeable to change (Craske, 2003a).

Treatment Variables

Although more research is required to determine factors associated with treatment of GAD that predict relapse following treatment, it would appear that the occurrence of cognitive and perceptual change through treatment is important for promoting durable improvements. For example, whereas several cognitive and behavioral strategies (e.g., applied relaxation, cognitive therapy) tend to be superior to wait-list and nondirective treatment conditions at posttreatment and at follow-up (e.g., Butler et al., 1991), participants whose treatment included cognitive therapy tended to be doing better at 6- and 12-month follow-up than those clients who did not receive this treatment (e.g., Borkovec & Costello, 1993; Butler et al., 1991).

Strategies for Treatment

Because of the chronic, waxing and waning nature of GAD, it is important that the long-term management of the disorder is integrated into treatment. After the client has made initial successful change in his or her ability to manage worry and anxiety, relapse prevention strategies should be introduced to ensure that the changes are maintained over time. Thus, rather than leaving relapse prevention to the end of therapy, skills for preventing relapse should be built in alongside the development of other skills such as relaxation, cognitive therapy, and worry exposure (e.g., Overholser & Nasser, 2000). Core components of relapse prevention include psychoeducation during treatment about relapse and recurrence, identifying and confronting potential high-risk situations for relapse, strengthening existing skills, and preparing for temporary setbacks.

Through psychoeducation during treatment, the client learns to expect that temporary setbacks will occur and to view such setbacks as opportunities for continued learning and improvement rather than as a relapse or the return of full GAD symptoms (e.g., Gorski & Miller, 1982). The client should be helped to develop a list of personal warning signs so that these lapses do not turn into relapses (Gorski & Miller, 1982). These warning signs may be cognitive (e.g., noticing recurring and persistent worries about a particular topic), somatic (e.g., having difficulty falling to sleep at night), or environmental (e.g., an upcoming exam).

The client should also develop a list of high-risk situations that have typically elicited anxiety responses in the past. However, rather than the client simply waiting for these high-risk problems to occur, new coping options for dealing with these situations are explored and practiced in session and the client is encouraged to actively seek out and confront these situations (Overholser & Nasser, 2000). During treatment, each confrontation is reviewed in session, and the client is taught to reflect on his or her ability to handle the situation in terms of (1) what strategies worked well in the past, and (2) what could be done differently the next time the situation is encountered.

In addition to building the aforementioned relapse prevention strategies into therapy, the client is reminded of the importance of effective problem solving (Brown et al., 2001) and time management (Meichenbaum & Jaremko, 1983) for preventing lapses, particularly if he or she is feeling pressured and overwhelmed by obligations and commitments. Finally, given the chronic nature of GAD, it may be useful to schedule follow-up visits, at least initially, rather than to have clients return for additional sessions when problems have already set in.

Psychopharmacological Approaches to Relapse Prevention

As discussed earlier, some antianxiety medications have proven efficacy for acute GAD treatment (e.g., Rickels et al., 1982), although GAD symptoms sometimes recur after the acute phase of drug therapy has ended (e.g., Rickels et al., 1986). In addition, the chronicity and high risk of recurrence makes either maintenance or intermittent drug therapy an attractive option for some individuals with GAD, particularly when the higher initial cost (both in terms of money and time) makes psychotherapy prohibitive (Schweizer & Rickels, 1996). However, in the long term, CBT may be more cost-effective than pharmacotherapy, due to the relatively higher rate of relapse following discontinuation from pharmacotherapy than following CBT. Furthermore, many clients who take anxiolytic drugs for GAD show a considerable reduction in their reliance on medications after receiving CBT (e.g., Barlow et al., 1992; Butler et al., 1991; Öst & Breitholtz, 2000). CBT may also help to reduce the need for excessive visits to medical doctors, which tend to occur more frequently in clients with GAD than in their nonanxious peers. Although CBT has a number of long-term advantages over medication, an exception may involve the treatment of GAD when it occurs comorbidly with depression, in which case medication is increasingly indicated (e.g., Ballenger et al., 2001). However, the benefits of combining psychotherapy with medication for the long-term management of GAD need to be validated in large, carefully controlled studies.

CASE EXAMPLE

In this section, we highlight some of the important issues raised in this chapter by describing the conceptualization and treatment of a female client with GAD.

Case Description

Valerie is a 45-year-old married woman who presented for treatment for chronic worries in a number of areas. She described her worries as being excessive and uncontrollable for many years, and at the time of presentation, Valerie was concerned that she was having a "nervous breakdown" because "her worries were too much to cope with." She reported not being able to fulfill day-to-day responsibilities or make routine decisions. She frequently felt teary, was easily upset, and felt unable to discuss her problems with her husband or friends for fear they would think she was "crazy." She also described feeling chronically tense and on edge and was having difficulty falling asleep.

Valerie reported numerous domains of worry. For example, she worried about her relationship with her husband to whom she had been married for 1 year. In particular, she worried that he would lose interest in her and would want to end their marriage. Despite being financially comfortable (her husband was a company executive and she was employed as a parttime sales assistant), she reported worrying excessively about financial matters. She also worried about her own health as well as the health of her husband, who was 10 years older than her, even though they both had sound physical health. She described worrying about a range of "little things" on a daily basis, such as whether she wore the right clothes for the day's weather, what others were thinking about her, which route she should take to get from one place to another, and whether she would be on time for appointments. She described often "overplanning" for upcoming events due to worry that she would make mistakes or things would go wrong. Thus, although Valerie recognized that her worries were excessive and often unreasonable, she believed that worrying helped her to be better prepared for the worst and to maintain control.

Valerie recognized that her symptoms had become worse about 3 months ago when her father became ill. Valerie described feeling a great deal of pressure to be a "good daughter" and to visit her father every day, regardless of the impact this had on other areas of her life, and despite her father's attempts to reassure her that she did not need to visit him every day.

Valerie described herself as always having been a worrier. She recalled as a child being worried about doing well at school, having friends, and pleasing her parents. She reported being particularly anxious whenever anything "out of the blue" occurred that she was not prepared for and recognized that her tendency to "overplan" for upcoming events dated back into her childhood. She reported feeling as though she was "walking on eggshells" as a child to prevent upsetting her older brother who she described as being hostile and easily angered. She recognized that her anxiety had waxed and waned over the years, but that presently she felt "out of control." Ultimately, she feared that her anxiety would lead to the end of her marriage.

Valerie's assessment using the Anxiety Disorders Interview Schedule-IV (ADIS; Brown, DiNardo, & Barlow, 1994), which is a semistructured diagnostic interview designed specifically for the assessment of anxiety disorders, confirmed that diagnostic criteria were met for GAD. Although recent stressors had exacerbated her worries, Valerie had experienced excessive and uncontrollable worry dating back into her childhood. Criteria also were met for mild depression, but it was conceptualized that Valerie's depressive state was a consequence of the impairment in functioning and distress brought on by her generalized anxiety.

Treatment Conceptualization

Treatment for Valerie was based on a CBT model with the central premise being that worry involves a unique interaction between cognitive, behavioral, and physiological cues of anxiety. Treatment components included psychoeducation, cognitive therapy, worry imagery exposure, relaxation training, and relapse prevention.

Psychoeducation focused on teaching Valerie about the three components of anxiety (i.e., cognitive, behavioral, and physiological) and about the nature of the "flight or fight" response to perceived threat and danger. Particular emphasis was given to socializing Valerie to the concept of metaworries and the positive (e.g., "Worrying helps me to stay in control") and negative beliefs (e.g., "I will go crazy") she held about worry. The contradiction in these beliefs was highlighted and it was emphasized that although it may seem as if worrying gives the illusion of being in control, it actually leads to greater distress and avoidance of feared events, which, in turn, maintains the worry process.

Through self-monitoring, the first goal of treatment was to help Valerie identify the cognitive, behavioral, and physiological signs of anxiety early in the worry process. Valerie was instructed in the use of a self-monitoring form (shown in Figure 3.1) on which she recorded cognitive, behavioral, and physiological cues in anxiety-provoking situations. She responded well to this initial homework task and was competent at identifying cues of anxiety in various situations.

Building on initial self-monitoring, Valerie was instructed to record in an objective manner the thoughts associated with anxiety-provoking situations and the subsequent physical and emotional consequences and behavioral urges that followed. Cognitive distortions (e.g., probability overestimations, catastrophic thinking, and "black and white" thinking) also were introduced and highlighted through examples of these errors reflected in the anxiety-provoking situations Valerie had monitored. Review of Valerie's self-monitoring homework at the commencement of the next session indicated that she was compliant with this procedure and grasped the idea that anxious cognitions play a role in causing and maintaining anxiety.

Valerie was then instructed in the utilization of cognitive techniques to challenge the accuracy of her worrisome thoughts and to generate other alternatives. The concept of challenging worrisome thinking was reinforced by having Valerie review previous episodes of worry and considering objective evidence for other ways of viewing these situations. The idea of generating various alternatives for interpreting situations was introduced by having Valerie use pie charts like the one depicted in Figure 3.2 to generate as many alternatives as possible for interpreting a range of ambiguous scenarios. In addition, her negative metabeliefs about worry (i.e., "worrying will make me go crazy") were challenged through examining the evidence and counterevidence for these appraisals during instances in which Valerie's worrying had been at its peak. Furthermore, through behavioral experiments conducted in session, Valerie focused on images relating to her worst fears coming true (e.g., her husband divorcing her), thereby activating the worry process, and she was encouraged to examine her reactions for objective evidence that she was actually "going crazy." The longer Valerie persisted in focusing on these feared images, she gained evidence that although worrying results in undesirable emotional and somatic sensations, worrying did not cause her to go crazy. Moreover, in light of the new evidence that elevated worrying resulted in negative personal experience, Valerie's positive beliefs, such as "worry helps me keep in control of things," were contrasted with her negative beliefs that worry would "make her go crazy." She was encouraged to explore situations in which she had worried excessively for evidence of whether her worry actually facilitated or hindered coping. Valerie recognized that in many cases, worrying had interfered with her daily activities by causing her to run late for appointments, to forget what she needed to take with her, and to forget important information she had been given because her mind had been "elsewhere."

Although Valerie was competent in identifying the kinds of errors her anxiety-related thoughts reflected and she was able to recognize that her negative and positive beliefs played a role in maintaining her worry, review of her self-monitoring homework indicated that she did not respond well to employing countering techniques out of session. Probing about factors that led to noncompliance revealed that Valerie believed she had so many areas of worry and stress that she was overwhelmed trying to apply cognitive restructuring techniques to all of them. She also felt that at times when she had implemented cognitive techniques, none of the alternatives she had generated felt as believable as her anxiety-related thoughts. At the same time, Valerie was distressed about an argument she had with her husband during the week, stemming from her perception of his behavior as indicating he had "rejected" her.

Further probing about her interpersonal functioning revealed that Valerie often felt that family and friends were critical of her and that she was often hurt by their perceived disregard for her feelings. She recognized that she was particularly fearful of people becoming angry or hostile toward her and traced this fear back to her childhood when she felt she was "walking on eggshells" to avoid triggering anger and hostility from her brother. Consequently, Valerie recognized that she was "sensitive" to how people responded to her and that she avoided certain interpersonal situations through fear of criticism and not being liked. With these background factors in mind, the focus of treatment narrowed to specifically targeting interpersonal aspects of Valerie's functioning, and in particular, her worries concerning her relationship with her husband. It was agreed that all other areas of worry would be "kept on hold" while this interpersonal domain was dealt with. It seemed that setting a clear parameter on the focus of treatment at that point, and in particular focusing on her interpersonal functioning with her husband (her greatest concern), helped Valerie to overcome feelings of being overwhelmed and to comply with the treatment procedures.

Valerie recorded specific situations with her husband in which she expected dangerous or feared outcomes to occur (e.g., her husband becoming angry at her), and situations in which she felt hurt or upset by his actions. She recorded the cognitive, emotional, and physiological cues of anxiety in these situations as well as how she subsequently behaved, how her husband behaved, and how their behavior affected each other. Each situation was worked through in session using countering and challenging techniques to help Valerie explore alternative ways of interpreting these situations. She was encouraged to examine the spiral of events that transpired from her initial threatening interpretation of his actions, to the subsequent emotional and physiological reactions it triggered, and to the impact that her own passive or avoidant behavior had on the situation and her ongoing worry. Using pie charts like the one depicted in Figure 3.2, she generated alternative ways of viewing these situations, and then through mini-experiments discussed in session, Valerie "tried out" new behaviors with her husband (e.g., asking questions if she needed more information, voicing her opinion on things, and taking "the initiative" on certain tasks around the house) in order to test out the validity of alternative perspectives.

To enhance her ability to tolerate negative affect and somatic sensations associated with worry, and to help her habituate to anxiety cues, cognitive strategies were complemented by worry imagery exposure sessions during which Valerie focused on images relating to worries about her marriage. Using the Worry Imagery Form depicted in Figure 3.3, Valerie identified specific instances of anxiety-provoking interpersonal events with her husband (e.g., her husband arriving home late and her husband becoming angry at her) and rank-ordered these situations according to how distressed she was by them. Beginning with the least anxiety-provoking image (i.e., her husband raising his voice), Valerie focused on these images for 15 minutes and, using a Subjective Units of Distress Scale (SUDS) ranging from 0 to 100, Valerie's level of distress was monitored during the exposure period. Initially, Valerie found it difficult to resist the urge to think about other things rather than the worst possible outcomes stemming from these images (e.g., "he will leave me"). As a result, it was necessary to reinforce the purpose of worry imagery exposure and to repeat the exposure exercise until she was able to hold attentional focus on the images and experience reduced levels of anxiety. Worry imagery exposure continued every session until Valerie reported only mild levels of distress, and eventually the imagery exposure exercise was assigned as a homework task and reviewed at the commencement of each session.

Recognizing the importance of relaxation interventions in the treatment of GAD, therapy also included instruction in relaxation. As Valerie reported having had little success in applying progressive muscle relaxation techniques during past treatment attempts as well as a desire to use a form of relaxation that was not time-consuming, she was instructed in the use of a 60-second paced breathing exercise. The primary purpose of this strategy was for Valerie to engage in the breathing exercise at times when she felt acutely anxious and when she recognized a gradual "buildup" of tension and distress. She was instructed to repeat the 60-second breathing cycle as often as required to reduce anxiety symptoms or for as long as time permitted, depending on the situation.

Her first success in applying cognitive and behavioral strategies to interactions with her husband outside of structured hypothesis-testing exercises came when her husband asked her to pick up a new electric drill from a nearby hardware store but then shortly afterward told Valerie not to worry about it. Her initial interpretation was, "He thinks I'll mess this up." However, rather than accepting that her interpretation was the truth and then worrying about this as she usually would, Valerie tested out her hypothesis by asking her husband why he no longer wanted her to pick up the drill, something she would have avoided previously. To Valerie's surprise, her husband did not respond with hostility but stated that he thought it would be easier for them both if he picked up the drill on his way home from work. Through recognizing the triggers of worry (i.e., her husband's change of mind), putting in place cognitive interventions (i.e., "what are other explanations for this?") and positive behavioral strategies (i.e., asking for more information), she was able to obtain disconfirming evidence of her negative thoughts and thereby circumvent her usual spiral of worry. Initial gains achieved in interpersonal functioning with her husband laid the foundation for Valerie to apply cognitive restructuring techniques and positive coping strategies to other domains of worry, such as financial concerns and the health of her family, particularly her father. These other domains of worry were targeted through cognitive restructuring techniques, worry imagery exposure, and behavioral experiments aimed at Valerie taking positive action to deal with anticipated feared outcomes in each of the domains. Problem-solving techniques also were employed to help Valerie establish more realistic expectations concerning the care of her father. Through a cost-benefit analysis, Valerie recognized that it was unrealistic to visit her father every day and that this commitment prevented her from completing daily chores and spending time with her husband, which together, contributed to the tension between them and to her feelings of inadequacy and sense of being overwhelmed. As a result, Valerie decided to visit her father every second day. At times when she worried about this decision, Valerie employed countering techniques to challenge the catastrophic consequences she believed would follow, namely, that people would think she was not "a good daughter" and that her father would deteriorate because she did not visit every day.

Valerie's treatment also included relapse prevention strategies. She was instructed to identify high-risk situations that might trigger worry and anxiety symptoms in the future. Valerie recognized that situations in which she was likely to experience a recurrence of anxiety included interpersonal situations that she perceives as threatening (e.g., discussing certain issues with her husband and receiving perceived criticism from friends), stressful events that come up in her life, and having a busy schedule. She also was instructed to identify early-warning signs of anxiety (e.g., increased muscle tension in her shoulders, difficulty falling asleep, and recognizing that she was "thinking" excessively about certain topics). Valerie kept a record of these potential triggers and early-warning signs of anxiety using various forms and materials accumulated during the course of therapy and she was encouraged to regularly review these materials after treatment was completed.

Valerie's treatment continued for 15 weekly sessions. A posttreatment assessment with the ADIS-IV revealed that diagnostic criteria for GAD and depression were met at subclinical levels. Two follow-up sessions were scheduled with Valerie, each 1 month apart. She was encouraged to make contact if assistance was required thereafter. Of importance in Valerie's treatment was recognizing her early noncompliance with cognitive techniques and examining possible causes of her resistance. Identifying that interpersonal functioning was a primary source of distress, particularly with her husband, and then focusing treatment specifically on this domain was important for reinstating compliance and obtaining initial treatment success. However, initial gains might have been achieved sooner in treatment if the various domains of worry that Valerie reported had been systematically reviewed at the commencement of treatment and an agreement had been reached about which domain to focus on first based on Valerie's perception of the degree of distress and impairment caused by each domain.

CONCLUSION

As outlined in this chapter, CBT is considered the gold standard treatment for GAD and it is the only psychological treatment that is empirically supported. However, CBT leads to clinically significant change in only about half of those clients who receive it, suggesting that there is considerable room for improvement. In this chapter, we reviewed factors associated with the client presenting with GAD and with current treatment approaches that may have an impact on successful treatment of GAD. We also reviewed factors that may increase the likelihood of relapse or recurrence following treatment. In summary, client factors that may impact on initial and long-term treatment outcome of CBT for GAD include being of older age, presenting with co-occurring disorders, experiencing elevated levels of interpersonal difficulty, and having greater difficulty coping with stressful events in daily life. In addition, clients who do not achieve significant cognitive and perceptual change through treatment are less likely to be doing well at posttreatment and at follow-up.

Reflecting that we are yet to develop sufficiently efficacious treatments for GAD (Brown, Barlow, & Liebowitz, 1994), more recent thinking suggests that treatment outcome may be enhanced if cognitive approaches also target underlying metacognitive processes, such as worry about worry itself and the positive and negative beliefs that clients with GAD typically hold about worry (Wells, 1997). Other recent advances in the understanding of the core features of GAD and associated symptoms also may improve treatment outcomes rates for GAD. Some of these advances include the integration of interpersonal strategies with CBT (Borkovec et al., 2002), targeting intolerance of uncertainty in treatment (e.g., Ladouceur et al., 2000), incorporating emotion regulation components into treatment (e.g., Mennin et al., 2002), and integrating mindfulness and acceptance perspectives into existing models and treatment of GAD (e.g., Roemer & Orsillo, 2002).

Perhaps more than any of the other anxiety disorders, the conceptualization and treatment of GAD best reflects the perspectives offered by Antony (2002) and Craske (2003a) in that the challenge for researchers and therapists over the coming years will be to identify which clients with GAD are likely to benefit from which specific interventions, rather than to apply a large number of interventions to all clients with a diagnosis of GAD. Moreover, instead of focusing on distinct diagnostic entities, a more useful approach may be to identify the core dimensions of disorder that are relevant to a particular client and to then select treatment approaches that specifically target those dimensions (Antony, 2002).

REFERENCES

Abel, J. L., & Borkovec, T. D. (1995). Generalizability of DSM-III-R generalized anxiety disorder to proposed DSM-IV criteria and cross-validation of proposed changes. *Journal of Anxiety Disorders, 9,* 303–315.

American Psychiatric Association. (1980). *Diagnostic and statistical manual of mental disorders* (3rd ed.). Washington, DC: Author.

American Psychiatric Association. (1987). *Diagnostic and statistical manual of mental disorders* (3rd ed., rev.). Washington, DC: Author.

American Psychiatric Association. (1994). *Diagnostic and statistical manual of mental disorders* (4th ed.). Washington, DC: Author.

Anderson, D. J., Noyes, R., & Crowe, R. R. (1984). A comparison of panic disorder and generalized anxiety disorder. *American Journal of Psychiatry, 141,* 572–575.

Antony, M. M. (2002). Enhancing current treatments for anxiety disorders. *Clinical Psychology: Science and Practice, 9,* 91–97.

Ballenger, J. C., Davidson, J. R. T., Lecrubier, Y., Nutt, D. J., Borkovec, T. D., Rickels, K., Stein, D. J., & Wittchen, H.-U. (2001). Consensus statement on generalized anxiety disorder from the international consensus group on depression and anxiety. *Journal of Clinical Psychiatry, 62*(Suppl. 11), 53–58.

Barlow, D. H., & Di Nardo, P. A. (1991). The diagnosis of generalized anxiety disorder: Development, current status, and future directions. In R. M. Rapee & D. H. Barlow (Eds.), *Chronic anxiety: Generalized anxiety disorder, and mixed anxiety–depression* (pp. 95–118). New York: Guilford Press.

Barlow, D. H., Raffa, S. D., & Cohen, E. M. (2002). Psychosocial treatments for panic disorder, phobias, and generalized anxiety disorder. In P. E. Nathan & J. M. Gorman (Eds.), *A guide to treatments that work* (2nd ed., pp. 301–335). London: Oxford University Press.

Barlow, D. H., Rapee, R. M., & Brown, T. A. (1992). Behavioral treatment of generalized anxiety disorder. *Behavior Therapy, 23,* 551–570.

Barrett, P. M. (2000). Treatment of childhood anxiety: A developmental perspective. *Clinical Psychology Review, 20,* 479–494.

Barrett, P. M., Dadds, M. R., & Rapee, R. M. (1996). Family treatment of childhood anxiety: A controlled trial. *Journal of Consulting and Clinical Psychology, 64,* 333–342.

Barrett, P. M., Duffy, A. L., Dadds, M. R., & Rapee, R. M. (2001). Cognitive-behavioral treatment of anxiety disorders in children: Long-term (6-year) follow-up. *Journal of Consulting and Clinical Psychology, 69,* 135–141.

Barrett, P. M., Lowry-Webster, H., & Holmes, J. (1998). *The friends program.* Brisbane, Australia: Australian Academic Press.

Beck, A. T., & Emery, G. (1979). *Cognitive therapy of anxiety and phobic disorders.* Philadelphia: Center of Cognitive Therapy.

Beck, A. T., Emery, G., & Greenberg, R. L. (1985). *Anxiety disorders and phobias: A cognitive perspective.* New York: Basic Books.

Bernstein, D. A., Borkovec, T. D., & Hazlett-Stevens, H. (2000). *New editions in progressive relaxation training: A guidebook for helping professionals.* Westport, CT: Praeger.

Bernstein, G. A., & Borchardt, C. M. (1991). Anxiety disorders of childhood and adolescence: A critical review. *Journal of the American Academy of Child and Adolescent Psychiatry, 30,* 519–532.

Biswas, A., & Chattopadhyay, P. K. (2001). Predicting psychotherapeutic outcomes in patients with generalized anxiety disorder. *Journal of Personality and Clinical Studies, 17,* 27–32.

Blazer, D. G., George, L. K., & Hughes, D. (1991). The epidemiology of anxiety disorders: An age comparison. In C. Salzman & B. D. Lebowitz (Eds.), *Anxiety disorders in the elderly* (pp. 180–203). New York: Free Press.

Bond, A. J., Wingrove, J., Curran, H. V., & Lader, M. H. (2002). Treatment of generalized anxiety disorder with a short course of psychological therapy, combined with buspirone or placebo. *Journal of Affective Disorders, 72,* 267–271.

Borison, R. L., Albrecht, J. W., & Diamond, B. I. (1990). Efficacy and safety of a putative anxiolytic agent: Ipsapirone. *Psychopharmacology Bulletin, 26,* 207–210.

Borkovec, T. D. (1994). The nature, functions, and origins of worry. In G. Davey & F. Tallis (Eds.), *Worrying: Perspectives on theory, assessment, and treatment.* (pp. 5–33). New York: Wiley.

Borkovec, T. D. (2002). Training clinic research and the possibility of a National Training Clinics Practice Research Network. *The Behavior Therapist, 25,* 98–103.

Borkovec, T. D., Abel, J. L., & Newman, H. (1995). Effects of psychotherapy on comorbid conditions in generalized anxiety disorder. *Journal of Consulting and Clinical Psychology, 63,* 479–483.

Borkovec, T. D., & Costello, E. (1993). Efficacy of applied relaxation and cognitive-behavioral therapy in the treatment of generalized anxiety disorder. *Journal of Consulting and Clinical Psychology, 61,* 611–619.

Borkovec, T. D., & Hu, S. (1990). The effect of worry on cardiovascular response to phobic imagery. *Behaviour Research and Therapy, 28,* 69–73.

Borkovec, T. D., Lyonfields, J. D., Wiser, S. L., & Diehl, L. (1993). The role of worrisome thinking in the suppression of cardiovascular response to phobic imagery. *Behaviour Research and Therapy, 31,* 321–324.

Borkovec, T. D., Mathews, A. M., Chambers, A., Ebrahimi, S., Lytle, R., & Nelson, R. (1987). The effects of relaxation training with cognitive therapy or nondirective therapy and the role of relaxation induced anxiety in the treatment of generalized anxiety. *Journal of Consulting and Clinical Psychology, 55,* 883–888.

Borkovec, T. D., Newman, M. G., Pincus, A. L., & Lytle, R. (2002). A component analysis of cognitive-behavioral therapy for generalized anxiety disorder and the role of interpersonal problems. *Journal of Consulting and Clinical Psychology, 70,* 288–298.

Borkovec, T. D., & Ruscio, A. M. (2001). Psychotherapy for generalized anxiety disorder. *Journal of Clinical Psychiatry, 62*(Suppl. 11), 37–42.

Borkovec, T. D., Shadick, R., & Hopkins, M. (1991). The nature of normal and pathological worry. In R. M. Rapee & D. H. Barlow (Eds.), *Chronic anxiety: Generalized anxiety disorder, and mixed anxiety–depression* (pp. 29–51). New York: Guilford Press.

Boyer, W. F., & Feighner, J. P. (1993). A placebo-controlled double-blind multicenter trial of two doses of ipsapirone versus diazepam in generalized anxiety disorder. *International Clinical Psychopharmacology, 8,* 173–176.

Brawman-Mintzer, O., Lydiard, R. B., Emmanuel, N., Payeur, R., Johnson, M., Roberts, J., Jarrell, M. P., & Ballenger, J. C. (1993). Psychiatric comorbidity in patients with generalized anxiety disorder. *American Journal of Psychiatry, 150,* 1216–1218.

Brown, T. A., & Barlow, D. H. (1992). Comorbidity among anxiety disorders: Implications for treatment and DSM-IV. *Journal of Consulting and Clinical Psychology, 60,* 835–844.

Brown, T. A., Barlow, D. H., & Liebowitz, M. R. (1994). The empirical basis of generalized anxiety disorder. *American Journal of Psychiatry, 151,* 1272–1280.

Brown, T. A., Campbell, L. A., Lehman, C. L., Grisham, J. R., & Mancill, R. B. (2001). Current and lifetime comorbidity of the DSM-IV anxiety and mood disorders in a large clinical sample. *Journal of Abnormal Psychology, 110,* 585–599.

Brown, T. A., Chorpita, B. F., & Barlow, D. H. (1998). Structural relationships among dimensions of the DSM-IV anxiety and mood disorders and dimensions of negative affect, positive affect, and autonomic arousal. *Journal of Abnormal Psychology, 107,* 179–192.

Brown, T. A., Di Nardo, P. A., & Barlow, D. H. (1994). *Anxiety disorders interview schedule for DSM-IV (ADIS-IV).* Boulder, CO: Graywind.

Brown, T. A., Marten, P. A., & Barlow, D. H. (1995). Discriminant validity of the symptoms constituting the DSM-III-R and DSM-IV associated symptom criterion of generalized anxiety disorder. *Journal of Anxiety Disorders, 9,* 317–328.

Brown, T. A., O'Leary, T. A., & Barlow, D. H. (2001). Generalized anxiety disorder. In D. H. Barlow (Ed.), *Clinical handbook of psychological disorders: A step-by-step treatment manual* (pp. 154–207). New York: Guilford Press.

Butler, G. (1993). Predicting outcome after treatment for generalized anxiety disorder. *Behaviour Research and Therapy, 31,* 211–312.

Butler, G., Fennell, M., Robson, P., & Gelder, M. (1991). Comparison of behavior therapy and cognitive behavior therapy in the treatment of generalized anxiety disorder. *Journal of Consulting and Clinical Psychology, 59,* 167–175.

Chorpita, B. (2001). Control and the development of negative emotion. In M. Vasey & M. R. Dadds (Eds.), *The developmental psychopathology of anxiety* (pp. 112–142). London: Oxford University Press.

Clark, L. A., Watson, D., & Mineka, S. (1994). Temperament, personality, and the mood and anxiety disorders. *Journal of Abnormal Psychology, 103,* 103–116.

Cohen, A. S., Barlow, D. H., & Blanchard, E. B. (1985). The psychophysiology of relaxation-associated panic attacks. *Journal of Abnormal Psychology, 94,* 96–101.

Compton, S. N., Grant, P. J., Chrisman, A. K., Gammon, P. J., Brown, V. L., & March, J. S. (2001). Sertraline in children and adolescents with social anxiety disorder: An open trial. *Journal of the American Academy of Child and Adolescent Psychiatry, 40,* 564–571.

Craske, M. G. (2003a). *Origins of phobias and anxiety disorders: Why more women than men.* Oxford, UK: Elsevier.

Craske, M. G. (2003b). *Integrated treatment manual for anxiety disorders.* Unpublished manuscript, University of California, Los Angeles.

Craske, M. G., Barlow, D. H., & O'Leary, T. A. (1992). *Mastery of your anxiety and worry.* Boulder, CO: Graywind.

Craske, M. G., Rapee, R. M., Jackel, L., & Barlow, D. H. (1989). Qualitative dimensions of worry in DSM-III-R generalized anxiety disorder subjects and nonanxious controls. *Behaviour Research and Therapy, 27,* 397–402.

Craske, M. G., Street, L., & Barlow, D. H. (1989). Instructions to focus upon or distract from internal cues during exposure treatment of agoraphobic avoidance. *Behaviour Research and Therapy, 27,* 663–672.

Davidson, J. R. T., DuPont, R. L., Hedges, D., & Haskins, J. T. (1999). Efficacy, safety, and tolerability of venlafaxine extended release and buspirone in outpatients with generalized anxiety disorder. *Journal of Clinical Psychiatry, 60,* 528–535.

Durham, R. C., & Allan, T. (1993). Psychological treatment of generalized anxiety disorder: A review of the clinical significance of results in outcome studies since 1980. *British Journal of Psychiatry, 163,* 19–26.

Durham, R. C., Allan, T., & Hackett, C. A. (1997). On predicting improvement and relapse in generalized anxiety disorder following psychotherapy. *British Journal of Clinical Psychology, 36,* 101–119.

Feighner, J. P., & Cohn, J. B. (1989). Analysis of individual symptoms in generalized anxiety: A pooled, multistudy, double-blind evaluation of buspirone. *Neuropsychobiology, 21,* 124–130.

Ferreri, M., Hantouche, E. G., & Billardon, M. (1994). Advantages of hydroxyzine in generalized anxiety disorder (GAD): A double-blind placebo-controlled study. *Acta Psychiatrica Scandinavica, 98*(Suppl. 393), 102–108.

Gale, C., & Oakley-Browne, M. (2000). Extracts from "clinical evidence": Anxiety Disorder. *British Medical Journal, 321,* 1204–1207.

Gelenberg, A. J., Lydiard, R. B., Rudolph, R. L., Aguiar, L., Haskins, J. T., & Salinas, E. (2000). Efficacy of venlafaxine extended-release capsules in nondepressed outpatients with generalized anxiety disorder: A 6-month randomized controlled trial. *Journal of the American Medical Association, 283,* 3082–3088.

Gorski, T., & Miller, M. (1982). *Counseling for relapse prevention.* Independence, MO: Independence Press.

124   WATERS *and* CRASKE

Hazlett, R. L., McLeod, D. R., & Hoehn-Saric, R. (1994). Muscle tension in generalized anxiety disorder: Elevated muscle tonus or agitated movement? *Psychophysiology, 31,* 189–195.

Heide, F. J., & Borkovec, T. D. (1983). Relaxation-induced anxiety: Paradoxical anxiety enhancement due to relaxation training. *Journal of Consulting and Clinical Psychology, 51,* 171–182.

Hoehn-Saric, R., & McLeod, D. R. (1988). The peripheral sympathetic nervous system: Its role in normal and pathological anxiety. *Psychiatric Clinics of North America, 11,* 375–386.

Hoehn-Saric, R., McLeod, D. R., & Zimmerli, W. D. (1988). Differential effects of alprazolam and imipramine in generalized anxiety disorder: Somatic versus psychic symptoms. *Journal of Clinical Psychiatry, 49,* 293–301.

Hoehn-Saric, R., McLeod, D. R., & Zimmerli, W. D. (1989). Somatic manifestations in women with generalized anxiety disorder: Psychophysiological responses to psychological stress. *Archives of General Psychiatry, 46,* 1113–1119.

Houck, C. (1998). An open-label pilot study of fluvoxamine for mixed anxiety-depression. *Psychopharmacology Bulletin, 34,* 225–227.

Howard, B. L., & Kendall, P. C. (1996). Cognitive-behavioral family therapy for anxiety-disordered children: A multiple-baseline evaluation. *Cognitive Therapy and Research, 20,* 423–443.

Kabat-Zinn, J. (1994). *Wherever you go there you are.* New York: Hyperion.

Keller, M. B., Lavori, P. W., Wunder, J., Beardslee, W. R., Schwartz, C. E., & Roth, J. (1992). Chronic course of anxiety disorders in children and adolescents. *Journal of the American Academy of Child and Adolescent Psychiatry, 31,* 595–599.

Kendall, P. C. (1994). Treating anxiety disorders in children: Results of a randomized clinical trial. *Journal of Consulting and Clinical Psychology, 62,* 100–110.

Kendall, P. C., Kane, M., Howard, B., & Siqueland, L. (1990). *Cognitive-behavioral treatment of anxious children: Treatment manual.* Temple University: Author.

Kendall, P. C., & Southam-Gerow, M. A. (1996). Long-term follow-up of a cognitive-behavioral therapy for anxiety disordered youth. *Journal of Consulting and Clinical Psychology, 64,* 724–730.

Kessler, R. C., McGonagle, K. A., Zhao S., Nelson, C. B., Hughes, M., Eshleman, S., Wittchen, H.-U., & Kendler, K. (1994). Lifetime and 12-month prevalence of DSM-III-R psychiatric disorders in the United States: Results from the National Comorbidity Survey. *Archives of General Psychiatry, 51,* 8–19.

Klein, E., Colin, V., Stolk, J., & Lenox, R. H. (1994). Alprazolam withdrawal in patients with panic disorder and generalized anxiety disorder: Vulnerability and effect of carbamazepine. *American Journal of Psychiatry, 151,* 1760–1766.

Ladouceur, R., Dugas, M. J., Freeston, M. H., Leger, E., Gagnon, F., & Thibodeau, N. (2000). Efficacy of a new cognitive-behavioral treatment for generalized anxiety disorder: Evaluation in a controlled clinical trial. *Journal of Consulting and Clinical Psychology, 68,* 957–964.

Last, C. G., Perrin, S., Hersen, M., & Kazdin, A. E. (1996). A prospective study of childhood anxiety disorders. *Journal of the American Academy of Child and Adolescent Psychiatry, 35,* 1502–1510.

Leahy, R. L. (2002). Improving homework compliance in the treatment of generalized anxiety disorder. *Journal of Clinical Psychology, 58,* 499–511.

Lucki, I., Rickels, K., & Geller, A. M. (1986). Chronic use of benzodiazepines and psychomotor and cognitive test performance. *Psychopharmacology, 88,* 426–433.

Massion, A. O., Warshaw, M. G., & Keller, M. B. (1993). Quality of life and psychiatric morbidity in panic disorder and generalized anxiety disorder. *American Journal of Psychiatry, 150,* 600–607.

Meichenbaum, D. S., & Jaremko, M. E. (Eds.). (1983). *Stress reduction and prevention.* New York: Plenum Press.

Mennin, D. S., Heimberg, R. G., Turk, C. L., & Fresco, D. M. (2002). Applying an emotion regulation framework to integrative approaches to generalized anxiety disorder. *Clinical Psychology: Science and Practice, 9,* 85–92.

Mohlman, J., Gorenstein, E. E., Kleber, M., de Jesus, M., Gorman, J. M., & Papp, L. A. (2003). Standard and enhanced cognitive-behavior therapy for late-life generalized anxiety disorder: Two pilot investigations. *American Journal of Geriatric Psychiatry, 11,* 24–32.

Newman, M. G. (2000). Generalized anxiety disorder. In M. Hersen & M. Biaggio (Eds.), *Effective brief therapies: A clinician's guide* (pp. 158–178). San Diego: Academic Press.

Öst, L. (1987). Applied relaxation: Description of a copying technique and review of controlled studies. *Behaviour Research and Therapy, 25,* 397–409.

Öst, L., & Breitholtz, E. (2000). Applied relaxation vs. cognitive therapy in the treatment of generalized anxiety disorder, *Behaviour Research and Therapy, 38,* 777–790.

Overholser, J. C., & Nasser, E. H. (2000). Cognitive-behavioral treatment of generalized anxiety disorder. *Journal of Contemporary Psychotherapy, 30,* 149–161.

Pecknold, J. C., Matas, M., Howarth, B. G., Ross, C., Swinson, R., Vezeau, C., & Ungar, W. (1989). Evaluation of buspirone as an antianxiety agent: Buspirone and diazepam versus placebo. *Canadian Journal of Psychiatry, 34,* 766–771.

Power, K. G., Simpson, R. J., Swanson, V., & Wallace, L. A. (1990a). A controlled comparison of cognitive-behaviour therapy, diazepam, and placebo, alone and in combination, for the treatment of generalised anxiety disorder. *Journal of Anxiety Disorders, 4,* 267–292.

Power, K. G., Simpson, R. J., Swanson, V., & Wallace, L. A. (1990b). Controlled comparison of pharmacological and psychological treatment of generalized anxiety disorder in primary care. *British Journal of General Practice, 40,* 289–294.

Rapee, R. M. (1985). The distinction between panic disorder and generalized anxiety disorder: Clinical presentation. *Australian and New Zealand Journal of Psychiatry, 19,* 227–232.

Rapee, R. M. (1991). Generalized anxiety disorder: A review of clinical features and theoretical concepts. *Clinical Psychology Review, 11,* 419–440.

Rickels, K., Case, G., Downing, R. W., & Fridman, R. (1986). One-year follow-up of anxious patients treated with diazepam. *Journal of Clinical Psychopharmacology, 6,* 32–36.

Rickels, K., Schweizer, E., DeMartinis, N., Mandos, L., & Mercer, C. (1997). Gepirone and diazepam in generalized anxiety disorder: A placebo-controlled trial. *Journal of Clinical Psychopharmacology, 17,* 272–277.

Rickels, K., Weisman, K., Norstad, N., Singer, M., Stoltz, D., Brown, A., & Danton, J. (1982). Buspirone and diazepam in anxiety: A controlled study. *Journal of Clinical Psychiatry, 43,* 81–86.

Roemer, L., & Orsillo, S. M. (2002). Expanding our conceptualization of and treatment for generalized anxiety disorder: Integrating mindfulness/Acceptance-based approaches with existing cognitive-behavioral models. *Clinical Psychology: Science and Practice, 9,* 54–75.

Ross, C. A., & Matas, M. (1987). A clinical trial of buspirone and diazepam in the treatment of generalized anxiety disorder. *Canadian Journal of Psychiatry, 32*, 351–355.

Roy-Byrne, P. P., & Cowley, D. S. (2002). Pharmacological treatments for panic disorder, generalized anxiety disorder, specific phobia, and social anxiety disorder. In P. E. Nathan & J. M. Gorman (Eds.), *A guide to treatments that work* (2nd ed., pp. 301–335). London: Oxford University Press.

Roy-Byrne, P. P., & Katon, W. (1997). Generalized anxiety disorder in primary care: The precursor/modifier pathway to increased health care utilization. *Journal of Clinical Psychiatry, 58*(Suppl. 3), 34–40.

Ryan, M. A., Siqueland, L., & Rickels, K. (2001). Placebo-controlled trial of sertraline in the treatment of children with generalized anxiety disorder. *American Journal of Psychiatry, 158*, 2008–2015.

Sanderson, W. C., Beck, A. T., & McGinn, L. K. (1994). Cognitive therapy for generalized anxiety disorder: Significance of comorbid personality disorders. *Journal of Cognitive Psychotherapy, 8*, 13–18.

Schut, A. J., Castonguay, L. G., & Borkovec, T. D. (2001). Compulsive checking behaviors in generalized anxiety disorder. *Journal of Clinical Psychology, 57*, 705–715.

Schweizer, E., & Rickels, K. (1996). The long-term management of generalized anxiety disorder: Issues and dilemmas. *Journal of Clinical Psychiatry, 57*(Suppl. 7), 9–12.

Seivewright, H., Tyrer, P., & Johnson, T. (1998). Prediction of outcome in neurotic disorder: A 5-year prospective study. *Psychological Medicine, 28*, 1149–1157.

Spence, S. H., Donovan, C., & Brechman-Toussaint, M. (2000). The treatment of childhood social phobia: The effectiveness of a social skills training-based, cognitive-behavioural intervention, with and without parental involvement. *Journal of Child Psychology and Psychiatry and Allied Disciplines, 41*, 713–726.

Stanley, M. A., Beck, J. G., & Glassco, J. D. (1996). Treatment of generalized anxiety in older adults: A preliminary comparison of cognitive-behavioral and supportive approaches. *Behavior Therapy, 27*, 565–581.

Thayer, J. F., Friedman, B. H., & Borkovec, T. D. (1996). Autonomic characteristics of generalized anxiety disorder and worry. *Biological Psychiatry, 39*, 255–266.

Velting, O. N., Setzer, N. J., & Albano, A. (2004). Update on and advances in assessment and cognitive-behavioral treatment of anxiety disorders in children and adolescents. *Professional Psychology: Research and Practice, 35*, 42–54.

Versiani, M., Ontiveros, A., Mazzotti, G., Ospina, J., Davila, J., Mata, S., Pacheco, A., Plewes, J., Tamura, R., & Palacios, M. (1999). Fluoxetine versus amitriptyline in the treatment of major depression with associated anxiety (anxious depression): A double-blind comparison. *International Clinical Psychopharmacology, 14*, 321–327.

Weiss, D. D., & Last, C. G. (2001). Developmental variations in the prevalence and manifestations of anxiety disorders. In M. W. Vasey & M. R. Dadds (Eds.), *The developmental psychopathology of anxiety* (pp. 27–42). New York: Oxford University Press.

Wells, A. (1997). *Cognitive therapy of anxiety disorders: A practice manual and conceptual guide.* Chichester, UK: Wiley.

Wells, A. (1999). A cognitive model of generalized anxiety disorder. *Behavior Modification, 23*, 526–555.

Wetherell, J. L., Gatz, M., & Craske, M. G. (2003). Treatment of generalized anxiety disorder in older adults. *Journal of Consulting and Clinical Psychology, 71*, 31–40.

Wittchen, H. U., Zhao, S., Kessler, R. C., & de Boer, A. G. (1994). DSM-III-R generalized anxiety disorder in the National Comorbidity Survey. *Archives of General Psychiatry, 51,* 355–364.

Yonkers, K. A., Dyck, I. R., Warshaw, M., & Keller, M. B. (2000). Factors predicting the clinical course of generalised anxiety disorder. *British Journal of Psychiatry, 176,* 544–549.

Yonkers, K. A., Warshaw, M., Massion, A., & Keller, M. B. (1996). Phenomenology and course of generalized anxiety disorder. *British Journal of Psychiatry, 168,* 308–313.

4

Obsessive–Compulsive Disorder

MARTIN E. FRANKLIN
DAVID S. RIGGS
ANUSHKA PAI

OVERVIEW OF THE DISORDER

DSM-IV Definition

Obsessive–compulsive disorder (OCD) is an anxiety disorder characterized by recurrent obsessions and/or compulsions that interfere substantially with daily functioning (American Psychiatric Association, 1994). Obsessions are "persistent ideas, thoughts, impulses, or images that are experienced as intrusive and inappropriate and cause marked anxiety or distress" (p. 418). Compulsions are "repetitive behaviors . . . or mental acts . . . the goal of which is to prevent or reduce anxiety or distress" (p. 418). Explicit in the fourth edition of the *Diagnostic and Statistical Manual of Mental Disorders* (DSM-IV) definition, obsessions and compulsions are functionally related: Obsessions *cause* marked anxiety or distress, whereas compulsions are overt (behavioral) or covert (mental) actions that are performed in an attempt to *reduce* the distress brought on by obsessions or according to rigid rules. This relationship is supported by findings from the DSM-IV field study on OCD, in which over 90% of participants reported that their compulsions aim to either prevent harm associated with their obsessions or to reduce obsessional distress (Foa et al., 1995). In our view, the absence of any functional link between obsessions and compulsions in adults raises a question about whether or not OCD is the proper diagnosis. This issue is more complicated in young children, who may be unable for developmental reasons to fully articulate their obsessions or describe the functional link between their obsessions and compulsions.

Although the diagnostic criteria for OCD allow for the diagnosis to be made when either obsessions or compulsions are present, data from the DSM-

IV field study indicate that the vast majority (over 90%) of adult obsessive–compulsives manifest both obsessions and behavioral rituals. Many OCD patients also engage in mental rituals (e.g., silently repeating special words or prayers and silently counting). Indeed, when mental rituals are included, only 2% of adults with OCD fail to report both obsessions and compulsions and are classified as "pure" obsessions (Foa et al., 1995). Mental and behavioral rituals (e.g., handwashing) are functionally equivalent in that both serve to reduce obsessional distress, prevent feared harm, or restore safety. Thus, although all obsessions are mental events, compulsions can be either mental or behavioral. Identification of mental rituals is an especially important aspect of cognitive-behavioral treatment planning, as obsessions and compulsions are addressed via different techniques.

DSM-IV also deemphasized the requirement for insight in diagnosing OCD. It has been argued that a continuum of "insight" or "strength of belief" better represents the clinical picture of OCD than the previously prevailing view that *all* patients with OCD recognize the senselessness of their obsessions and compulsions (Kozak & Foa, 1994). The growing consensus about a continuum of insight (Foa et al., 1995; Insel & Akiskal, 1986; Lelliott, Noshirvani, Başoğlu, Marks, & Monteiro, 1988) led to the inclusion of a subtype of OCD "with poor insight" to include individuals who indeed have obsessions and compulsions but do not recognize their senselessness. Clinical impression suggests that this subtype might be especially prevalent in children and adolescents with OCD, perhaps because of their level of cognitive development. A large-scale field trial has not been conducted to confirm the impression that this subtype is more prevalent in children and a fuller understanding of the role of insight in OCD awaits further research.

Classification of Subtypes

In addition to the formal subtype reflecting insight, most OCD classification schemes have focused on the topography of ritualistic activity (i.e., compulsions) rather than on the obsessive content. Although many patients have more than one form of ritual, the predominant one typically determines how the individual's OCD symptoms will be classified. Thus, patients are described as washers, checkers, orderers, and so on. The reliance on compulsions to classify OCD subtypes reflects both the relative ease of observing overt compulsions and the recognition that these rituals are functionally tied to obsessions. Although it can be useful to classify OCD patients based on their rituals, it is important to identify obsessions as well in order to ensure that the function of the ritual is identified.

Ritualistic washing is the most common compulsion and is typically performed to decrease discomfort associated with contamination obsessions. For example, individuals who fear contact with "AIDS germs" clean themselves and their environment excessively in order to prevent either contracting AIDS themselves or spreading it to others. Some washers do not fear that a specific disaster will befall them if they refrain from compulsive washing. Rather, the state of being contaminated itself generates tremendous discomfort. To decrease this distress, they feel compelled to engage in washing rituals.

Another common compulsion is repetitive checking, which is very often performed in order to prevent an anticipated catastrophe. Individuals who fear that a burglar will enter their home, take their valuables, and possibly harm their family will repeatedly check doors and windows to decrease the likelihood of this actually happening. Likewise, individuals who dread that while driving they will run over a pedestrian and fail to notice it will repeatedly retrace their driving route in search of possible victims.

Other rituals such as repeating, ordering, and counting may serve to prevent disasters much as checking does, but often they lack the logical connection to the feared consequence seen in checkers. For example, it is logical (if excessive) to check the front door lock many times if one fears a burglary but illogical to walk up and down the stairs repeatedly to prevent a loved one's death in a motor vehicle accident. Notably, like some washers, many repeaters, orderers and counters perform the ritual just to reduce distress or to ensure that things "feel right" rather than to prevent a feared disaster.

Hoarding is atypical in that many hoarders engage in little compulsive activity but are perhaps better characterized as avoidant. Instead of going to great lengths to collect materials to save, many hoarders simply avoid discarding items they encounter in everyday life (e.g., newspapers and string) for fear of not having them available in the future. Over long periods, consistent avoidance of discarding can result in overwhelming accumulations, even in the absence of active gathering rituals. Hoarded material can also vary from items of some monetary value (e.g., complete sets of *Sports Illustrated* magazines) to those that are worthless (e.g., chicken bones and empty milk containers). A diagnosis of OCD is more complicated when the hoarded material can be viewed as "collectibles." In these cases, the diagnosis relies more heavily on the distress associated with the loss or failure to obtain the collectible object or by the functional impairment resulting directly from the collection and activities associated with collecting (e.g., oven filled with comic books and failure to go to work in order to tend to collection).

In the pediatric population, the most common compulsions are washing and cleaning followed by checking, counting, repeating, touching and straightening (Swedo, Rapoport, Leonard, Lenane, & Cheslow, 1989); corresponding obsessions are fear of contamination, harm to self, harm to a familiar person, and symmetry/exactness urges. As with adult OCD sufferers, most children and adolescents have more than one constellation of OCD symptoms. In almost all cases, these symptoms are driven by one or more dysphoric affects, including anxiety, fear, doubt, disgust, rudimentary urges, and "just so" feelings, which some have labeled sensory incompleteness (Goodman, Rasmussen, Foa, & Price, 1994). For example, washing rituals may be a reaction to contamination fears or a response to feeling "sticky." The developmental stage of the child may influence the child's OCD presentation: For example, because children in general tend to be more magical in their thinking than are adults, our clinical experience has indicated that they are more likely to experience "magical" or superstitious OCD, such as fears that failing to walk up the stairs repeatedly will result in harm befalling a parent during the next morning's commute to work.

OVERVIEW OF EMPIRICALLY SUPPORTED TREATMENTS

Exposure and Ritual Prevention

Exposure and response (ritual) prevention (EX/RP) has proven to be a highly effective form of intervention for OCD (for a comprehensive review, see Franklin & Foa, 2002) and is considered the psychosocial treatment of choice for this disorder (March, Frances, Kahn, & Carpenter, 1997). As implied by the name, EX/RP programs include two major components: exposure to feared stimuli and voluntary abstinence from compulsive rituals. Repeated, prolonged exposure without ritualizing or avoiding is thought to provide information that disconfirms mistaken associations and evaluations held by the patients and to promote habituation to previously feared thoughts and situations (Foa & Kozak, 1986).

Contemporary EX/RP programs typically include two variants of exposure both designed specifically to prompt obsessional distress. The first, *in vivo* exposure, involves the actual confrontation of feared stimuli, such as having the patient who fears contamination from germs touch toilets and sinks. The second form of exposure, typically labeled imaginal exposure, allows for exposure to feared consequences that patients believe will occur if they fail to complete compulsive rituals (e.g., refraining from compulsive praying now will result in demonic possession at some time in the future). Imaginal exposure can help clients to better see the distinction between imagined, unrealistic disasters and reality in which those disasters do not occur.

Exposure, whether *in vivo* or imaginal, is typically conducted in a graduated manner, with situations and thoughts provoking moderate distress confronted before more upsetting ones. The initial order of exposures is usually based on the patient's predicted level of distress prior to initiating any exposure work. However, this order may be changed as treatment progresses should changes in these initial ratings occur. Furthermore, certain exposure exercises may be completed "out of order" for practical reasons. For example, if a patient's car is highly contaminated and yet necessary for transportation to and from session, the therapist might suggest focused exposures to the car even if these exposures are rated as more than moderately distressing on the stimulus hierarchy. When such changes are deemed necessary, of course, they should be fully discussed with the patient. Homework in the form of additional prolonged exposure exercises is assigned during each treatment session and homework completion is considered critical to treatment success.

The second component of EX/RP programs, ritual prevention, is somewhat of a misnomer. Competent therapists do not *prevent* patients from engaging in rituals but, rather, suggest that clients refrain from rituals voluntarily. Therapists may use a variety of strategies to help the patient cease rituals such as providing an explicit rationale and clear instructions for ritual prevention, encouraging attempts at stopping rituals, and verbally reinforcing successful abstinence from rituals. Patients are encouraged to refrain from ritualizing during treatment sessions when exposure exercises are conducted and between sessions while engaging in exposure homework and when the urge to ritualize arises spontaneously. Patients are further asked to record any violations of ritual abstinence that occur between sessions to discuss them with the therapist in the next treatment session. During these discussions, the therapist can provide reinforcement for successful prevention of rituals and develop strategies to help the patient more successfully refrain from rituals in the future.

Empirical support for the efficacy of EX/RP has been garnered from many uncontrolled and controlled studies, most of which have shown that the large majority of patients who complete EX/RP treatment are deemed "treatment responders" (i.e., showing at least a 30–50% reduction in OCD symptoms) at posttreatment and remain so when evaluated months after treatment. Foa and Kozak (1996) reviewed 12 EX/RP outcome studies (total N = 330), and found that an average of 83% of treatment completers were classified as responders (using the individual studies' varied definitions) immediately after treatment. In 16 studies reporting long-term outcome (total N = 376; mean follow-up interval of 29 months), 76% of patients completing treatment were rated as responders. Several meta-analytic studies (e.g., Abramowitz, 1996) have detected large effect sizes for EX/RP with OCD in adults (> 1.0) regardless of the study selection criteria utilized for the various meta-analytic procedures.

Most of the OCD meta-analytic studies did not, however, exclude studies of EX/RP that failed to use some form of control treatment, so their reported effect sizes may overestimate the benefit of EX/RP. More compelling evidence for the efficacy of EX/RP is derived from randomized controlled trials (RCTs) that have demonstrated the superiority of EX/RP in comparison to various control treatments, including relaxation (Fals-Stewart, Marks, & Schafer, 1993), pill placebo (Foa et al., 2005) and anxiety management training (Lindsay, Crino, 7 Andrews, 1997). On the whole, the evidence indicates clearly that EX/RP is superior to these various control treatments, produces substantial and clinically meaningful symptom reductions at posttreatment, and provides durable symptom reduction at long-term follow-up. These findings appear to be particularly robust: They are largely consistent across different sites and procedural variations. However, because there are so many variants of EX/RP treatment, we briefly review the literature of the relative efficacy of the ingredients that comprise EX/RP and comment on their use in clinical practice.

EX/RP Procedural Variations

Exposure versus Ritual Prevention versus EX/RP

Most studies that have examined the efficacy of exposure therapy for OCD also included ritual prevention techniques (Foa & Chambless, 1978; Marks, Stern, Mawson, Cobb, & McDonald, 1980; Marks et al., 1988), thus confounding the effects of these procedures. To separate these effects, Foa, Steketee, Grayson, Turner, and Latimer (1984) randomly assigned patients with washing rituals to either treatment by exposure (EX) only, ritual prevention (RP) only, or their combination (EX/RP). Each treatment was conducted intensively (15 daily 2-hour sessions conducted over 3 weeks) and followed by a home visit. Results indicated that the combined treatment was superior to the single-component treatments on almost every symptom measure at posttreatment and follow-up. Notably, patients who received EX alone reported lower anxiety when confronting feared contaminants than did patients who had received only RP, whereas the RP-alone group reported greater decreases in their urge to ritualize than did the EX-alone group. Thus, it appears that EX and RP affect symptoms differently, and that treatments that do not include *both* EX and RP yield inferior outcome. Clinically, we make ample use of these findings when discussing the rationale for treatment procedures with patients before they commit to a course of EX/RP, and we are not above using dramatic and colorful Powerpoint graphs representing the data from Foa et al. (1984) to drive this critical point home for patients and families alike.

Frequency of Exposure Sessions

EX/RP programs that have achieved excellent results (e.g., Foa et al., 2005; Franklin, Abramowitz, Kozak, Levitt, & Foa, 2000) typically involve daily sessions, but favorable outcomes have also been achieved with more widely spaced sessions (e.g., Abramowitz, Foa, & Franklin, 2003; Warren & Thomas, 2001). Pilot data gathered with a pediatric OCD sample suggest that children and adolescents who received weekly sessions responded very favorably and similarly to those treated intensively (Franklin et al., 1998), but the lack of random assignment to these treatments renders the findings inconclusive. In the absence of a large study that includes random assignment to intensive and less intensive EX/RP regimens, we are forced to rely on our clinical impressions and the relatively weak outcome literature when making decisions about session frequency. We believe that less frequent sessions may suffice for patients whose OCD symptoms are mild or moderate in severity, who readily understand the importance of daily exposure homework, and who adhere strictly to ritual abstinence instructions. Patients with severe symptoms or those who exhibit considerable difficulty complying with exposure homework or ritual prevention are more likely to benefit from a more intensive regimen. Another possible option is to conduct more frequent sessions at the beginning of treatment (e.g., for treatment planning, initial exposures, and initiating ritual prevention) and then taper to less frequent sessions once patients are engaged in the treatment.

Therapist-Assisted versus Self-Exposure

The importance of therapist-aided exposure in EX/RP is unclear. Although one study found that modeling of exposure by the therapists did not enhance overall treatment efficacy (Rachman, Marks, & Hodgson, 1973), patients in this study did prefer treatment that included modeling. Moreover, our clinical experience suggests that patients may be more willing to confront feared situations in the presence of a therapist, and some patients find modeling instructive. Empirical evaluations of the presence of a therapist during exposure have yielded inconsistent results. In one study, patients with OCD who received therapist-aided exposure were more improved immediately posttreatment than those receiving clomipramine and self-exposure, but this difference disappeared by 1-year follow-up (Marks et al., 1988). However, the design of the study introduced various confounds and therefore the results are difficult to interpret. In a second study, no differences between therapist-assisted treatment and self-exposure were detected either at posttreatment or at follow-up (Emmelkamp & van Kraanen, 1977). Unfortunately the number of patients in this study was too small to render these results conclusive. In contrast, meta-analytic findings have suggested that therapist-assisted exposure is more potent than self-exposure (Abramowitz, 1996).

Therapist presence enhanced the efficacy of a single 3-hour exposure session for persons with specific phobia compared to self exposure of equal length (Öst, 1989). Because specific phobias are on the whole less debilitating and easier to treat than OCD, one might surmise that therapist presence could also enhance OCD exposures. The effect of therapist-assisted exposure on treatment outcome awaits a well-controlled study with a sufficiently large sample to afford the necessary power to detect group differences. In our clinical practice, we use both therapist-assisted and self-controlled exposures: We routinely use therapist-assisted exposure during treatment sessions and ask patients to conduct self-directed exposure exercises between sessions. Notably, there are specific cases in which therapist-aided exposure may be detrimental to treatment. In particular, patients who derive reassurance from the presence of another (e.g., checkers who are only anxious when they are the last to leave a room) may fail to experience anxious arousal during exposures in which the therapist is present. In these cases, we typically plan the exercise with the patient but leave the room as they complete the exposure.

Duration of Exposure

Although there is no hard and fast rule for how long exposures should last, prolonged continuous exposure is considered superior to short interrupted exposure (Rabavilas, Boulougouris, & Stefanis, 1977). In general, exposure exercises should continue at least until the patient notices a decrease in obsessional distress. This clinical "rule of thumb" is supported by the empirical finding that improvement following EX/RP was associated with reduced anxiety (habituation) within the exposure session as well as reduced peak anxiety across sessions (Kozak, Foa, & Steketee, 1988). Our therapy sessions for adults are usually scheduled for 90 minutes to allow for homework review, homework assignment, and one imaginal and one *in vivo* exposure exercise to be completed in each therapy session. However, this regimen places practical constraints on patients and therapists with respect to time and billing issues, and no RCT has ever definitively demonstrated that 90-minute sessions are necessary to produce substantial and lasting benefit. Notably, in light of concerns about exceeding the attention span of our younger patients and encouraging pilot data (Franklin et al., 1998; March, Mulle, & Herbel, 1994), our recently completed pediatric OCD treatment outcome study (described in Franklin, Foa, & March, 2003) used 60-minute cognitive-behavioral treatment (CBT) sessions, during which one exposure (either imaginal or *in vivo*) was completed in each session. To reinforce this work, therapists assigned daily exposure homework exercises to be completed between sessions.

Gradual versus Abrupt Exposures

Patients who confront the most distressing situations from the start of therapy have achieved the same gains as patients who confront less distressing situations before confronting the most distressing one (Hodgson, Rachman, & Marks, 1972). However, most patients appear to be more comfortable with a gradual approach. Because patients' willingness to comply with treatment procedures is such a critical aspect of successful EX/RP, situations of moderate difficulty are usually confronted first, followed by several intermediate steps before the most distressing exposures are accomplished. This may be especially important in conducting EX/RP with younger patients, as treatment experts have emphasized the need for hierarchy-driven exposure and a collaborative approach between the therapist and the child in the development of exposure exercises (March & Mulle, 1998).

Use of Imaginal Exposure

The addition of imaginal exposure to a program that includes *in vivo* exposure and ritual prevention appeared to enhance maintenance of treatment gains for OCD patients (Foa, Steketee, & Turner, Fischer, 1980; Steketee, Foa, & Grayson, 1982). However, no such effect was found in a third study (de Arauja, Ito, Marks, & Deale, 1995). This discrepancy may be explained by differences in the treatment program utilized by Foa and colleagues in comparison to that of de Araujo and colleagues (e.g., 90-minute vs. 30-minute imaginal exposures, respectively), and thus the source of the disparate findings cannot be identified.

Clinically, we find imaginal exposure to be very useful, especially for patients whose obsessional fears include disastrous consequences (e.g., killing one's child) and/or for those patients whose fears are not readily translated into *in vivo* exposure exercises (e.g., burning in hell for all eternity due to failure to neutralize blasphemous thoughts). Also, the addition of imagery to *in vivo* exposure may circumvent the cognitive avoidance strategies used by patients who evade thinking about the consequences of exposure while confronting feared situations *in vivo*. Thus, although imaginal exposure may not be essential for successful outcome at posttreatment for *all* OCD patients, it may enhance long-term maintenance and is often a useful adjunct to *in vivo* exercises for patients with fears focusing on disastrous consequences. For patients who do not report any feared disasters consequent to refraining from rituals (other than being extremely distressed), imaginal exposure may not be necessary. Treatment of pediatric patients should include imaginal exposure only if they are developmentally able to complete the task. Imaginal procedures can be adjusted (e.g., written exercises instead of audiotaped scripts listened to with eyes closed) to prevent younger children from confusing fantasy and reality. A detailed account of the presentation of the rationale for imaginal exposure to a young patient is beyond our scope here but can be found elsewhere (Franklin, Abramowitz, Bux, Zoellner, & Feeny, 2002).

Implementation of Ritual Prevention

As noted earlier, exposure appears effective at reducing obsessional distress but is not as effective in reducing compulsions (Foa et al., 1984). To maximize improvement, the patient needs to refrain from ritualizing while engaging in programmatic exposure exercises. In Victor Meyer's (1966) initial EX/RP treatment program, hospital staff actually stopped the patients from performing rituals (e.g., turning off water supply in patient's room). However, physical intervention by others to prevent patients from ritualizing is no longer typical or recommended. In addition to concerns that actual physical prevention is too coercive to be acceptable, it is believed that reliance on this technique may limit generalizability to nontherapy situations in which staff are not present to prevent rituals. Instead of physical prevention, therapists should assist with this difficult task by providing support, encouragement, and suggestions about how to refrain from ritualizing in particular situations. Self-monitoring of rituals may also serve to promote ritual abstinence by increasing patient awareness of rituals and by providing an alternative activity to ritualizing when the urges to do so are high.

Other Treatments Approaches

Pharmacotherapy

A comprehensive review of the OCD pharmacotherapy literature is beyond the scope of this chapter, but such reviews are available elsewhere (see, e.g.,

Dougherty, Rauch, & Jenike, 2002, for adult OCD; March, Franklin, Nelson, & Foa, 2001; Thomsen, 2002, for pediatric OCD). To summarize, it appears that the tricyclic antidepressant clomipramine (e.g., Clomipramine Collaborative Group, 1991; DeVeaugh-Geiss et al., 1992) and the selective serotonin reuptake inhibitors (SSRIs) fluoxetine (e.g., Geller et al., 2001; Tollefson et al., 1994), sertraline (e.g., Greist et al., 1995; March et al., 1998), fluvoxamine (e.g., Riddle et al., 2001), paroxetine (e.g., Wheadon, Bushnell, & Steiner, 1993) and, more recently, citalopram (e.g., Montgomery, Kasper, Stein, Hedegaard, & Bang, 2001) are superior to pill placebo. However, on average the groups treated with medication in these trials still met the criteria for study inclusion, which suggests that even though medications are efficacious, the typical patient treated with SSRI monotherapy still has substantial residual symptoms. In addition to residual symptoms, SSRI treatment for OCD raises other concerns. Some patients experience significant side effects, up to one-third of patients treated with SSRIs do not respond to the medication and, especially with younger patients, concerns are emerging about the long-term implications of remaining on an SSRI. Despite these concerns, there are a number of appealing aspects to SSRI treatment for OCD. Among these are the relative availability of SSRIs (as compared to EX/RP), the ease of administering the treatment (for both the physician and patient), and the fact that it has proven highly effective for at least some OCD patients even if treatment response is neither universal nor complete. For clinically impaired OCD patients who decide that EX/RP is too difficult, too expensive, or unavailable within a reasonable distance from their homes, or who do not believe they are ready to commit to a course of EX/RP, we routinely recommend a course of SSRI monotherapy.

EX/RP plus Pharmacotherapy

The relative efficacy of EX/RP versus EX/RP plus SSRIs has generated much discussion and some empirical study thus far. Marks et al. (1980) compared 4 weeks of initial treatment with clomipramine (CMI) to pill placebo (PBO), followed by an additional 3 weeks of EX/RP or relaxation. In this study, as well as a subsequent study (Marks et al., 1988), the combination of CMI and EX/RP had a small transitory additive effect compared to EX/RP and PBO. Cottraux et al. (1990) found a trend favoring EX/RP plus fluvoxamine (FLV) over EX/RP alone in reducing OCD symptoms at posttreatment, and also that combined treatment yielded slightly greater short-term, but not long-term, improvement in depression than did EX/RP alone. Hohagen et al. (1998) found that EX/RP plus FLV was superior to EX/RP plus PBO in reducing compulsions, while van Balkom et al. (1998) failed to detect any additive effect for FLV over EX/RP alone. Most recently, Foa et al. (2005) did not find any advantage for CMI plus EX/RP over EX/RP alone. Differences in sampling, experimental design, and EX/RP procedures (e.g., number and spacing of sessions) compromise direct comparison of the results of these studies; secondary analyses of data from Foa et al. (2005) and

Cottraux et al. (1990) suggest that procedural variations in EX/RP may have attenuated outcome in the latter study, which may be why the results diverged (Foa, Franklin, & Moser, 2002).

In sum, the data do not support the unequivocal statement that combined treatment is generally superior to EX/RP alone, although clinically there may be circumstances in which combined treatment may be preferable. For example, patients who have significant psychiatric comorbidity such as major depressive disorder might benefit from combined treatment because the medication also ameliorates symptoms of the other disorder that can attenuate CBT compliance (e.g., amotivation). The data do clearly indicate that combined treatment does not interfere with EX/RP alone, and thus patients who are already receiving SSRIs need not discontinue their medication to fully benefit from EX/RP (Franklin et al., 2002).

Cognitive Therapy

Cognitive approaches have been brought to bear in treating OCD, sometimes as formal protocols designed to be alternatives to EX/RP and sometimes less formally, as part of EX/RP programs. As we have discussed elsewhere (e.g., Foa et al., 2002; Franklin et al., 2002), EX/RP therapists are typically interested in changing OCD-related cognitions but tend to use EX/RP procedures and informal cognitive discussions to try to bring about these changes. Thus far studies of cognitive therapy for OCD have yielded some positive findings (e.g., Freeston et al., 1997), and studies comparing cognitive therapies to EX/RP have generally failed to find an advantage of one over the other (e.g., van Balkom et al., 1998), with the exception that group EX/RP may be superior to group CT (McLean et al., 2001). More research is clearly needed to determine whether there is an advantage to using one treatment over the other with certain OCD subtypes (e.g., those with feared consequences vs. those without), and much more to be learned about the mechanisms by which the treatments exert their influence. Clinically we emphasize EX/RP in our work, yet we include informal cognitive interventions in therapy, particularly when they can be used to reinforce the EX/RP interventions. For example, therapists will discuss cognitive risk factors (e.g., thought suppression and thought–action fusion) to explain the maintenance of OCD symptoms and encourage patients to use "positive self-talk" to support themselves when they confront feared situations without ritualizing (e.g., Franklin, Abramowiz, Furr, Kalsy, & Riggs, 2003). We also, conduct informal discussions of the meaning of completed exposures (e.g., "You refrained from checking your stove every day this week and yet the house has not burned down, what do you make of it?") to help patients challenge their beliefs. Our clinical stance is to use such methods to support and enhance EX/RP rather than to replace it. The possibility remains that cognitive therapy is a viable alternative to EX/RP when patients refuse EX/RP, fail to comply with EX/RP procedures, or fail to benefit much even after a complete course.

PREDICTORS OF TREATMENT OUTCOME
AND MAINTENANCE OF GAIN

Identifying divergent outcomes for patient subgroups and identifying change mechanisms are important secondary goals of treatment outcome studies (March & Curry, 1998). Overall group differences in outcome may be (1) *moderated*, wherein predefined subgroups (e.g., groups differing in gender or family characteristics) show differential response to assigned treatment modalities; or (2) *mediated*, whereby postrandomization factors help to explain treatment effects (e.g., attendance at treatment sessions or change in cognitive variables) (Kraemer, 2000; Kraemer, Wilson, Fairburn, & Agras, 2002). Below we summarize the literature on predictors of EX/RP treatment outcome and maintenance of gains. Difficulty in accruing the very large samples needed of patients who have entered and/or completed EX/RP has slowed the scientific study of predictors, and accordingly the literature is replete with inconsistent findings, null results, or studies with clear methodological problems. That said, predictors found thus far empirically and those considered relevant clinically are considered in our subsequent discussions of how best to maximize treatment gains and to promote maintenance over time.

The most studied predictor of response to EX/RP is comorbid depression, which is important clinically because this comorbidity is so common. Studies examining the effects of depression have yielded inconsistent results. Although some studies have found that initial levels of depression were related to less improvement and poorer outcome (Keijsers, Hoogduin, & Schaap, 1994; Steketee, Chambless, & Tran, 2001), others have found little or no effect (Mataix-Cols, Marks, Greist, Kobak, & Baer, 2002; O'Sullivan, Noshirvani, Marks, Monteiro, & Lelliott, 1991; Steketee, Eisen, Dyck, Warshaw, & Rasmussen, 1999). One limitation of the studies conducted thus far is that they assume a linear relationship between depressive and OCD symptoms. When patients were grouped according to their initial levels of depression, Abramowitz, Franklin, Street, Kozak, and Foa (2000) found that only patients who were severely depressed were less likely to respond to EX/RP than patients who were nondepressed or mildly or even moderately depressed. Effects were also found when diagnosis of depression was considered. OCD patients who were nondepressed fared better than those diagnosed with comorbid depression both at posttreatment and follow-up (Abramowitz & Foa, 2000); moreover, highly depressed OCD patients were also at greater risk for relapse following treatment discontinuation (Başoğlu, Lax, Kasvikis, & Marks, 1988). Importantly, although they did not fare as well as the other groups, even the severely depressed patients in Abramowitz et al. (2000) improved significantly with EX/RP.

Personality psychopathology has been thought of as another variable that could hinder improvement from CBT; however, there has been little research examining personality disorders as a predictive factor in EX/RP treatment. The number of comorbid personality disorders with which patients were diagnosed had little predictive value for treatment outcome in several studies (Dreessen, Hoekstra, & Arntz, 1997; de Haan et al., 1997; Franklin, Harap, & Herbert, 2004), but patients with no personality pathology benefited the most from EX/RP in another study (Fals-Stewart & Lucente, 1993). When looking within personality clusters, it appears that different personality traits may affect treatment outcome in various ways. High dependent personality traits were associated with better outcome (Steketee et al., 2001), while passive–aggressive traits were associated with worse outcome (Steketee et al., 2001). Histrionic/borderline traits were associated with successful treatment outcome at posttreatment, but a loss of gains by follow-up (Fals-Stewart & Lucente, 1993). The most studied personality pathology has been the schizotypal trait, but the impact of this characteristic is unclear. Minichiello, Baer, and Jenike (1987) found the schizotypal trait to be associated with poorer outcome, and others have suggested that the schizotypal trait, or a cluster of traits which included the schizotypal trait, were marginally associated with poorer outcome (Dreessen et al., 1997; Fals-Stewart & Lucente, 1993; Steketee et al., 2001).

It has also been suggested that EX/RP may be differentially beneficial depending on the subtype of OCD. Some studies have indicated that washers fare better than checkers, but the results are inconsistent (e.g., Başoğlu et al., 1988; Castle et al., 1994). Patients with primary hoarding symptoms are more likely to drop out of treatment (Mataix-Cols et al., 2002) and less likely to improve (Abramowitz, Franklin, Schwartz, & Furr, 2003). In addition, responders are less likely than non-responders to have any hoarding symptoms (Black et al., 1998). Little research has examined whether certain types of obsessions respond better or worse to EX/RP; however, Mataix-Cols et al. (2002) found that patients with religious/sexual obsessions were the less responsive to treatment. One study also found that obsessions rated as more bizarre or irrational were predictive of poorer outcome (Başoğlu et al., 1988).

Another factor that has been found to be associated with treatment outcome is the patient's insight, or lack of insight, into his or her obsessive–compulsive symptoms (i.e., the degree to which patients are convinced that their feared outcomes will occur if they do not engage in rituals). Foa, Abramowitz, Franklin, and Kozak (1999) found that patients who were convinced or nearly convinced that their feared consequences would come to pass if they refrained from ritualizing (OCD with poor insight) were more severe at posttreatment than those with better insight. Similarly, Başoğlu et al. (1988) found that higher fixity of beliefs, a measure of poor insight, was predictive of poorer outcome in a sample of treated obsessive–compulsives. It is thought that poor insight leads to poorer homework compliance resulting in worse outcome, but an empirical study has yet to examine this (Foa et al., 1999).

There is discrepancy over the predictive power of initial symptom severity. Some studies have found that initial severity has no effect on posttreatment outcome (de Araujo, Ito, & Marks, 1996; Foa et al., 1983), while others have found initial severity to be a predictor of posttreatment outcome

(Başoğlu et al., 1988; Keijsers et al., 1994; Mataix-cols et al., 2002). Studies that included follow-up assessments showed that initial symptom severity had no effects during the follow-up (Başoğlu et al., 1988; O'Sullivan et al., 1991).

Severity at the end of treatment is a strong predictor of severity at follow-up (de Haan et al., 1997; O'Sullivan et al., 1991; Simpson et al., 2004). Simpson et al. (2004) found that patients with more severe OCD at posttreatment were more likely to relapse following EX/RP discontinuation than were patients with less severe OCD. de Haan et al. (1997) found similar results and noted that if a patient was rated as a responder at the end of treatment he or she maintained the gains. In contrast, among patients identified as nonresponders immediately after treatment some were rated as responders at follow-up whereas others were not. Notably, patients who reached responder status after the end of active treatment often had more severe OCD symptoms at the initial assessment (Başoğlu et al., 1988; de Haan et al., 1997). Foa et al. (1983) suggested that patients who were clearly successful during treatment and those who clearly failed to improve at posttreatment maintained their status at follow-up, patients who showed partial improvement were most likely to experience change in their symptoms after the end of active treatment.

Motivation and treatment compliance have also been found to be predictive of outcome. Motivation has been associated with improvement at posttreatment (de Haan et al., 1997; Keijsers et al., 1994), although not at 6-year follow-up (O'Sullivan et al., 1991). Although Lax, Başoğlu, and Marks (1992) found that compliance had no effect on outcome, most patients in their sample were fairly compliant. Another study did find noncompliance to be associated with poor treatment response (Keijsers et al., 1994), and compliance during the first week of treatment was found in one study to be the strongest predictor for treatment outcome, even at 6-month follow-up (de Araujo et al. 1996). Abramowitz, Franklin, Zoellner, and DiBernardo (2002) found that compliance with psychoeducation, in-session exposure, and homework exposure were associated with reductions in OCD severity, although compliance with self-monitoring of rituals was not.

Interpersonal factors might also play a role in treatment outcome of EX/RP. The effects of the quality of the psychotherapeutic relationship on treatment outcome are inconsistent. Keijsers et al. (1994) found that the patient's view of the relationship had an effect on treatment outcome but the therapist's evaluation had no bearing. Arts, Hoogduin, Keijsers, Severeijns, & Schaap (1994) found the opposite to be true. In addition, no further treatment gains were seen when therapists attempted to manipulate the therapeutic relationship. Positive patient ratings of therapist characteristics do not, however, explain away the effects of EX/RP: Lindsay et al. (1997) found that therapists randomly assigned to receive anxiety management training rated their therapists as warm and knowledgeable, yet patients assigned to this treatment did not improve; patients assigned to EX/RP also rated their therapists as warm and knowledgeable, but their OCD symptoms were substantially reduced at posttreatment. On a slightly different note, Renshaw, Chambless, and Steketee

(2003) examined the impact of familial relationships. Their data showed that the degree to which patients felt that their families were critical of them was associated with severity of symptoms at posttreatment.

PRACTICAL STRATEGIES FOR IMPROVING OUTCOME

Therapists using EX/RP to treat patients with OCD are confronted with many, sometimes incompatible, goals. The art of providing effective EX/RP treatment is balancing these various needs. Let us think for a moment about what demands are placed on the clinician when implementing EX/RP. The basic goal of the treatment is to encourage the patient to confront his or her most feared situations and refrain from engaging in the rituals that have provided safety in the past. For some patients, this is the emotional equivalent of asking them to face an armed attacker without fighting back, with only the therapist's word that the attacker will not really hurt them. Achieving this goal is further complicated by the relative brevity of the standard EX/RP treatment (typically no more than 40 hours of therapy over 20 sessions).

To successfully implement EX/RP for OCD, the therapist must design exposure exercises that reflect the functional relationships among the patient's obsessions, compulsions, and avoidance behavior and communicate these interrelationships clearly to the patient. To do this, the therapist must attend to even seemingly minor aspects of the patient's symptoms. The therapist must also work to help the patient develop a sense of trust in the therapist and the therapy as well as instilling a sense of self-confidence that will allow the patient to take the risks involved in the treatment. To do this within the relatively brief course of the standard EX/RP protocol requires the therapist to attend to even seemingly minor matters regarding the therapeutic relationship as well. To examine how the therapist can work to improve the outcome of EX/RP, we proceed step by step through a clinical encounter to identify decisions that may influence the outcome of treatment. We illustrate these decisions using information drawn from many of our clinical experiences.

Initial Meetings

In our standard protocol, the first 4 hours of treatment are allocated to gathering information about the patient's symptoms and developing a treatment plan. These sessions also serve to lay the foundation for the therapeutic relationship and introduce the patient to our model of OCD and philosophy of treatment. This is a lot to accomplish in a rather small amount of time (typically 4 hours over the course of 2 days), so it is important to attend to issues that might facilitate or hinder treatment.

Given that exposure therapy can be quite difficult for the patient, it has the potential to become confrontational with the therapist pushing the client to engage in exposure exercises and the client resisting these attempts. Perhaps the most important mechanism for avoiding this conflict is to develop with the client a sense of mutual effort against the OCD symptoms—in essence, a therapeutic team with the clinician and patient working together to treat the symptoms. Many of our efforts during the first two sessions are designed to foster this sense of teamwork. This collaborative approach may be especially important to convey with younger patients, and the "externalizing" of OCD as a common enemy has been discussed in detail elsewhere (e.g., March & Mulle, 1998).

One of the most important aspects of this process is that we endeavor to keep everything about the treatment as transparent as possible to the patient. This begins even before we meet with the patient for the first treatment session. During the conversation in which the initial appointment is scheduled, we typically inform the patient that the first two sessions will be used to get to know one another and to develop a plan for treatment. If time allows, we provide additional information about what we will be discussing in the initial session and will likely suggest that it is an opportunity for the therapist to learn about the patients specific symptoms and concerns. This provides the patient with a clear expectation of what will occur during the initial session and may help to reduce anticipatory anxiety.

In our experience, the approach that has worked best as a foundation for developing this therapeutic team is to recognize that while we, the clinicians, have a great deal of knowledge as to how best to treat OCD symptoms, each patient represents a new presentation that is shaded with his or her own individual experience with OCD. Thus, we present to the patient a model for the team in which the therapist is the expert in treating OCD, while the patient is the expert in his or her own symptoms and experiences. Working together then, the therapist and client can develop a plan for treating the patient's particular OCD symptoms.

Typically, these initial meetings begin with the therapist introducing the session agenda like this.

> "We have a lot to accomplish today. In particular, we need to figure out how, working together, we can help you to reduce the problems you are having with your OCD symptoms. Mostly this session gives us an opportunity to get to know one another and to exchange some important information. The way I think about it is that I know a great deal about how to treat OCD and you know a lot about your own OCD symptoms and we have to work together to figure out how best to treat your particular symptoms."

Another aspect of developing a team approach with patients is to provide a common language and model of OCD to allow the therapist and patient to communicate accurately about the patient's symptoms and the treatment plan. We typically take a good portion of the first hour of therapy to describe our model of OCD and to carefully define the terms we use during treatment. For example, EX/RP treatment is based on the idea that there is a functional relationship between obsessions (which increase anxiety) and compulsive rituals (which decrease anxiety). However, many of our patients are unaware of these relationships so we take time to explain the model and get the patient to generate examples of his or her own obsessions, rituals and avoidance routines.

For example, a therapist might begin with a discussion of this model and a brief description of the treatment that is being planned as follows.

"You have a set of habits which, as you know, are called obsessive–compulsive symptoms. These are habits of thinking, feeling, and acting which are extremely unpleasant, wasteful, and difficult to get rid of on your own. We are about to begin a treatment that is specifically designed to help you get rid of these symptoms, but before we do, I need to understand as much as I can about your particular symptoms. So most of today's session I am going to ask you to teach me about what you struggle with. To begin, though, I want to talk a little bit about how we understand OCD and make sure that we are on the same page as we talk about your symptoms.

"When we think about obsessions and compulsions, we think about them as two sides of a coin. Obsessions are usually thoughts, images, or impulses that come to your mind even though you don't want them. Most of the time when someone has obsessions they also feel extreme distress or anxiety along with strong urges to do something to reduce the distress. The things people do to make the distress go away are the things we call compulsions or rituals. Most of the time, compulsions are special thoughts or actions, but they could be almost anything that makes the bad feelings related to the obsessions go away. Unfortunately, as you know, the rituals do not work real well, and the distress goes down for a short time only and comes back again. Sometimes, people find that they have to do the ritual over and over again to the point that it seems they are getting in the way of almost everything. What would help me is to get a little sense of some of your obsessions and compulsions.

"What are some of the obsessions that you have? These would be thoughts that make you more upset or anxious?

"What are some of your rituals? What do you do to get a bit of relief from the anxiety and obsessions?"

The team approach that is initiated in this first session colors all of our interactions with the patient. It seems apparent that if we do not work diligently during the initial sessions to form a strong working alliance with the patient we will confront difficulties as treatment progresses. With regard to the therapists, potential obstacles to forming this alliance with the patient typically arise from clinicians neglecting the basic skills for good therapy such as active listening, reflection, and empathy. It is vitally important to remember to use these skills when communicating with patients about their symptoms and distress. Unfortunately, the structure of EX/RP and the fact that it is "manualized" can lead clinicians to neglect the basic therapeutic skills in favor of the treatment techniques. We are often heard to say "good therapy first, manualized therapy second." This is not to say that we drift far from the techniques of EX/RP, only that the techniques work much better in the context of a strong therapeutic alliance.

We make every attempt to ensure that the patient understands the approach to treatment as well as the rationale for the techniques we use. Building on the functional model of OCD we describe the treatment and detail the reasons we prescribe the exposure exercises and proscribe rituals. It is very important to discuss the rationale for treatment and to describe the treatment program in detail. The program requires that the patient abandon his or her OCD habits and, therefore, temporarily experience substantial discomfort. If patients do not understand why they are asked to suffer this short-term distress or are not convinced that treatment will work, they will be unlikely to comply with treatment instructions. A strong link between the model of OCD and the therapeutic techniques also allows the therapist to return to this rationale in later sessions should there be questions about why certain exercises are being included.

An example of how we might present the treatment rationale is presented here for a case of a man with obsessions related to contamination.

> "The treatment we are about to begin is called exposure and response prevention. It is designed to break two types of associations that people with OCD often have. The first one is the association, or connection, between certain objects, situations or thoughts and feelings of anxiety or distress. These are the connections that set off your obsessions. Like when you feel extremely anxious when you have to have to use a public restroom. The second association we want to break is the one between doing your rituals and feeling less anxiety or less distress. You, for example, wash your hands for a long time to reduce your distress. The problem is that you only feel better for a short time and then you begin to feel contaminated and anxious again. It is like you are going around and around on a treadmill, never getting anywhere. You touch something and feel anxious and then wash and feel less anxious for a little while and then back around again. The exposure and ritual prevention treatment works to break the automatic connection between the feelings of anxiety and contamination and your rituals. It will also train you not to ritualize when you are anxious."

As with the formation of the therapeutic alliance, the provision of a clear, understandable rationale for EX/RP is invaluable and may prove critical once treatment starts. Our clinicians often repeat the rationale or parts of it throughout treatment to remind the patient why certain exercises are important or why it is important to refrain from rituals. It is our experience that if this foundation is not in place before beginning exposure exercises, clinicians end up having to take time from later sessions to present the same information again and again.

To help communicate the rationale for EX/RP, particularly in cases in which the patient does not seem to understand the initial description, we have found it useful to spend time educating the patient about aspects of OCD that seem relevant. For example, we discuss the paradox of thought suppression (trying not to think of something almost invariably causes one to think of it), problems of thought–action fusion (believing that thinking something is the same as doing it), and the need to tolerate uncertainty. Each of these issues can be used to illustrate the utility of EX/RP to address problems of OCD. For example, when we describe the endless cycle of obsessions and rituals, we often use the thought suppression paradox to illustrate why we must work to eliminate the rituals.

> "Remember the obsessions increase your anxiety and the rituals decrease it but then it goes up again when your obsession returns. We have to find a way to break that cycle. It would be great if we could just eliminate your obsession, but that is really hard, because it is tough to make yourself not think about something. In fact, the more you try not to think of something, the more it seems to get stuck in your mind. For example, if I ask you not to think of a pink elephant with purple polka dots, what is the first thing you think of? (we have never had a patient deny that they imagine such an elephant). Because that won't work, we have to break the other side of the circle—the rituals. If we can stop the rituals then that will also serve to break the loop that you get in. This will not be easy, because right now the rituals serve to reduce your bad feelings, so when you stop them things will feel bad for a while, but that's part of why I am here—to help you through the rough spots."

Discussions about thought–action fusion and the need to tolerate uncertainty provide useful illustrations for breaking the associations between stimuli and anxious responses. Often persons with OCD make errors in their appraisal of unwanted thoughts. The thoughts are equated with actions such that merely having the thought is just as bad (and therefore distressing) as actually having the event happen. Similarly, the intolerance for uncertainty that is frequently observed among OCD patients reflects a sense of elevated distress in the absence of complete certainty of safety. In both cases, the therapist can impart some basic education about these logical errors while also illustrating how EX/RP is designed to address such associations.

Information gathering is one of the critical aspects of the EX/RP protocol. Without complete and detailed knowledge of a patient's symptoms and the functional relations among them, it is very difficult to develop an effective treatment plan. Importantly, though, information gathering need not stop with the initiation of treatment. The therapist should continue to collect information about obsessions, rituals, and the links between them throughout treatment. This information can be used to update or revise the treatment plan as the program proceeds. We discuss this process of continuous assessment and updating of treatment plans later when we describe ways of optimizing the efficacy of the EX/RP treatment procedures. First, though, we describe some techniques we have developed to maximize the useful information obtained during the initial information gathering stage.

Generally speaking, a therapist wants to maximize the amount of information provided by the patient, as long as it is relevant to the patient's OCD symptoms. Therefore, the first guideline for therapists is to try to open the lines of communication as widely as possible. Providing the patient with a clear goal for this task can be helpful, so we often begin this process with a statement similar to the following.

> "I need to understand, as completely as I can, what your experience of the obsessions and compulsions is like. The more you can teach me about what you struggle with, the better we'll be able to develop a plan to help you. Ultimately, what I need to get is a list of situations that lead you to obsess or to get anxious and a list of the rituals you use to reduce or manage the distress that comes from your obsessions. Why don't you begin by telling me about some of the situations that can lead to obsessions or anxiety."

There is no particular reason to begin with a description of obsessions or of rituals, and therapists generally find themselves working back and forth across the two. In addition to asking about obsessions and rituals, we ask patients to identify situations that they tend to avoid. Typically, these are situations that would raise obsessive concerns were the patient not able to avoid them. Sometimes patients discount these issues because they do not cause problems at the present time. It is important for the therapist to inquire as to whether the obsession would arise should the situation arise in the future. Unless we are completely convinced that the situation would not raise obsessive concerns, it is included on the treatment plan. The primary issues that might arise during this phase of treatment to diminish the effectiveness of EX/RP are those that serve to reduce the amount of useful information the therapist obtains. In most cases this occurs because the therapist fails to ask detailed questions, but some patients are also reticent to talk about some of their symptoms—because they find them either embarrassing or too frightening. To help ensure that therapists ask all the necessary questions, it is important to retain the functional model of OCD as a framework. Obsessions are thoughts (or images) that arise in certain situations (or in the presence of certain stimuli) and produce an increase in anxiety. Compulsive rituals are behaviors or thoughts (or images) that are used to reduce the anxiety associated with obsessions (for practical purposes, we typically group avoidance with rituals as efforts to reduce or manage anxiety). With this model in mind, it matters little where the therapist begins the inquiry as long as he or she understands the following aspects of the patient's symptoms.

1. In what situations do the obsessions arise?
2. What stimuli cue the obsessive concerns?
3. What is the content of the obsession, particularly the ultimate feared consequence?
4. What rituals (including mental rituals) are used to counter the obsession?
5. What is the consequence of not completing a ritual?
6. What situations are avoided because an obsession might occur were they to be encountered?

We have developed a number of approaches to help ensure that therapists ask all the necessary questions to develop a fairly complete idea of the patient's symptoms. First, we provide the therapist with an outline that includes lists of stimuli that cue obsessions, compulsions, and avoided situations to be completed during the information-gathering stage of treatment. Second, we tend to emphasize in training and supervision the need to obtain detailed information about patient symptoms. This is reflected in the instructions we offer the patients and the questions used to obtain this information. For example, we often follow the introduction of the aforementioned information-gathering phase with the following comments.

> "As we go through this, it is really important that I understand every aspect of your obsessions and compulsions, so I want you to try to answer my questions in as much detail as you can. Along the way I will probably ask you a lot of questions to make sure that I understand what it is you are dealing with. Sometimes you may think that certain details are not really important, maybe because these obsessions and rituals have become so much a part of your life they are almost automatic, but they will help me understand your symptoms better. That is important if we are to develop a plan that will really help you."

Then we begin to ask questions about the patient's symptoms.

Another approach that we often use is to ask the patient to describe a typical recent day in detail. Again, we warn them that we will be interrupting frequently to ask questions and get more detail. An example of this might be:

> "What I would like you to do is walk me through a typical day for you from the time you get up to the time you fall asleep at night. I want you to describe each step you take through the day and, most importantly, when and where you run into problems with your OCD. In a way, I want you to pretend that I am riding around on your shoulder and can see everything that you see and hear everything that you hear. But I also need you to tell me when you have obsessions and when the things you are doing are actually rituals. I'll probably stop you here and there to ask you some questions to make sure that I understand what you were doing and thinking at the time. Does that make sense?"

The information obtained throughout the description of a day provides direct evidence or clues as to situations that lead to obsessions and how rituals are used to counter the obsessions. Again, the therapist has to be willing to ask detailed questions to ensure that a full understanding of obsessions and rituals is obtained. This means the therapist must become comfortable asking patients about all activities, including many that are not typically discussed even with a therapist such as grooming, toileting, eating, dressing, sex, and sleeping. Even aspects of the patient's life that seem relatively benign, such as driving, closing doors, using the telephone, or shopping, must be explored in detail. For example, a patient describing his commute to work should be asked if he experienced any obsessions or engaged in any rituals during the trip or upon arriving at work.

In addition to the therapist's failure to ask the necessary questions, patients are sometimes reticent to share information about their OCD symptoms. We find three main reasons for this. First, some patients overlook certain aspects of their OCD because they have become practically automatic or because they have been a part of their lives for so long that they seem "normal." By emphasizing the need to get very detailed information the therapist can counter much of this problem. It is also possible that patients fail to report some aspect of their OCD because they do not define the thought or behavior as an obsession or compulsion. This is another reason why it is important to make sure the patient understands the functional definitions of obsessions and compulsions. There are many instances in which a patient indicates that a particular behavior is not a ritual but, when asked, acknowledges that it serves to reduce anxiety.

In addition to merely overlooking certain obsessions or compulsions, some patients find it difficult to discuss the details of their OCD because they find the content of their obsessions or the specifics of their rituals embarrassing. Again, therapists using EX/RP must remember to use their basic therapeutic skills of empathy, active listening, and normalizing of the patient's feelings to encourage the patient to share necessary information. Also, as the therapist becomes more familiar with the presentation of OCD, he or she may find it useful to offer educated hypotheses of the fears to the patient. This allows the patient to confirm or deny the content of the fears rather than having to express them completely. This also provides an opportunity for the patient to compare his or her actual fears to those proposed by the therapist. If the therapist is accurate, it offers a normalizing experience (i.e., I am not the only person who feels this way). Often, even if the therapist is not correct in the proposed obsession or compulsion, the patient finds it easier to discuss his or her concern because it seems "not so crazy" after hearing what others experience.

Other patients resist discussing some or all of their symptoms because talking about the symptoms serves to increase their anxiety. Sometimes this is simply because the discussion serves to focus their attention on the particular obsession or compulsion. More often, though, the verbalizing of the obsessive fear makes it more likely that the feared consequence will come to pass (e.g., If

I say aloud that I fear my son will die, then it will really happen.). In this case it can be extremely difficult to get them to verbalize the concern to the therapist. Again, good basic clinical skills and offering hypothesized fears to the patient can help, but therapists may also need to be creative to get the necessary information. One strategy that has proven useful is to discuss thought–action fusion as described previously. Alternatively, it may be possible for patients to talk about their fear if they are also given permission to complete a ritual to "undo" the obsession once the discussion is completed. It is also our experience that encouraging patients to discuss some of their fears will make it easier for them to describe their worst fears. Therefore, we often "skip over" particularly difficult aspects of the patient's presentation and return after we have discussed symptoms that they can verbalize. This also offers more opportunities for the therapist to normalize the patient's experience and to develop educated hypotheses as to the nature of the unspoken fears.

Some patients report that they do not have any feared consequences, but rather that they simply feel a great deal of distress if they fail to ritualize or if an obsession is cued. In these cases, it is important for the therapist to inquire, perhaps repeatedly, to confirm that there is not specific feared consequence. In many cases, patients fear not only the presence of the distress but also the persistence of it (e.g., I am afraid I will become upset and it will never go away). In other cases, it is not the persistence of the distress but, rather, the chance that it will interfere with future activities that is feared (e.g., If I get upset, I will not be able to concentrate at work and I'll get fired). The therapist should make sure to evaluate the possibility that there is in fact a feared consequence before developing a treatment plan that does not take any consequences into account.

Treatment Planning

The goal of the treatment planning stage of EX/RP is to lay out a plan for the treatment program that is acceptable to both the therapist and the patient. The concrete manifestation of this treatment plan is a hierarchy of situations that will potentially cue the patient's obsessions or fears and a list of rituals to be eliminated. To develop the hierarchy, the therapist asks the patient to rank the situations identified in the information-gathering stage based on the degree to which each situation will engender feelings of fear or distress. For the purposes of developing this hierarchy, we ask patients to rate each situation on a scale of Subjective Units of Distress (SUDS) ranging from 0 (no distress at all) to 100 (the worst fear I could imagine). Based on these subjective rankings, we develop a hierarchy and, from it, the treatment plan.

The few problems that may arise during the development of the hierarchy do not typically lead to poor outcome or require major adjustments to the EX/RP procedures. The most common problems reflect a conflict between the demands of the task (i.e., generating a complete and accurate hierarchy) and the obsessive concerns of the patient. For example, some patients have a difficult time providing ratings for each situation because their obsessive need to provide precise and accurate answers makes such a subjective task difficult. It is important for therapists to remember that the goal is to develop a working hierarchy that allows for five to six steps from the initiation of exposure exercises and the top of the hierarchy. For this reason, we typically begin exposure exercises with an item rated approximately 50% of the most difficult item and move up the list in steps. For practical purposes, these steps usually approximate a 10-point increase in SUDS ratings. Thus, a distinction of a few points on the SUDS rating is rarely important for clinical purposes. The therapist should remind the patient that the ratings need not be perfectly accurate and that they may be adjusted later if necessary. Also, therapists can encourage patients to use a more limited rating scheme (e.g., rate the situations to the nearest 5 or 10 on the SUDS scale), again reinforcing the idea that the ratings need not be perfect.

Another issue that may arise as the hierarchy develops is the presence of multiple obsessive themes (e.g., a patient who fears both contamination by germs and fire resulting from leaving an electrical appliance turned on). Practically, the structure of EX/RP, particularly the goal of reaching the top of the hierarchy by the sixth session of treatment, encourages a single hierarchy. However, therapists may find it useful for organizational purposes to have the patient rate items on multiple lists first and then combine the lists into a single hierarchy.

Clearly, the biggest potential problem that might arise during the treatment planning stage of EX/RP is the rejection of some aspect of the plan by the patient. Typically, this occurs when the patient identifies one or more potential exposure objects (usually those at the top of the hierarchy) that they do not agree to attempt. Our clinical experience as well as the limited data available suggest that the more completely OCD symptoms remit, the more persistent the gains will be. Therefore, we are reticent to agree to eliminate some objects from the treatment plan. Instead, we try to educate the patient as to why we believe it is important to include the specific exposure exercises in the treatment. Remembering that this must be done within an empathic therapeutic relationship, we do this with three lines of reasoning.

1. We reiterate the rationale for EX/RP.
2. We inform the patient of the data and our experience that indicates that it is important to tackle all the obsessive concerns as completely as possible and that ruling out some exposure exercises is likely to lead to problems returning later.
3. We discuss the concept of overcorrection whereby the patient's natural tendency will be to revert to obsessive–compulsive patterns and we need to push far in the other direction during treatment to overcome this tendency (this last is most useful when the patient relies on the argument that "normal people wouldn't do that").

It is important to remember that the goal of this discussion is not to seize control from the patient (indeed forced exposures tend not to work) but, rather, to explain why we believe that exposure exercises are important. We are attempting to get the patient to *agree* to participate fully in the treatment, not *forcing* the patient into it. If the best attempts to gain agreement fail, the therapist is faced with a difficult decision. One can proceed with treatment while eliminating some proposed exercises or one could suggest that the patient try an alternative treatment for the OCD (or delay EX/RP until he or she is ready to engage in all the exercises).

For a variety of reasons we tend toward the option of initiating treatment even if the patient resists engaging in some exercises. First, even without eliminating all the OCD symptoms, many patients are able to gain significant relief with EX/RP treatment. Second, our clinical experience suggests that if we can help the patient to reduce his or her symptoms, the patient often becomes motivated to attempt the exercises that he or she rejected initially. Third, many of the OCD patients we treat have tried various forms of treatment prior to EX/RP and found little or no relief from their OCD symptoms, so it is unclear to where we would refer them.

When initiating EX/RP without the patient fully agreeing to engage in the exposure exercises, it is important for the therapist to outline the expectations for treatment. We recommend that even should EX/RP be initiated with some limitation on the exposure exercises, therapists should try to reach an agreement with the patient that the question of whether to attempt the exercises will be revisited in the future. The therapist should also explore alternate means for conducting the exposure exercises, including imaginal exposure and exercises that approximate those the patient refuses to complete. Finally, the therapist must make sure that the patient understands that by limiting exposures to be done, he or she may be limiting the effectiveness of the treatment.

Optimizing EX/RP Interventions

In Vivo *Exposure*

The basic intervention of EX/RP is the *in vivo* exposure exercises in which patients are encouraged to systematically confront situations that bring about obsessive fears. Theoretically, the exercises serve to activate the patient's cognitive fear structure and allow new information (e.g., nothing bad happened when I used the public toilet) to be integrated into the system. Ideally, the exercises will last for sufficient time to allow for habituation of the patient's anxiety (typically, 30–45 minutes) and should be done repeatedly.

Obviously, the first challenge for the patient is to actually engage in the exposure. It is important for the therapist to remember how difficult these exercises are for the patient and to empathize with their struggle. Several approaches can help patients to engage in the exposure exercise and are generally appropriate for most patients (for exceptions, see discussion of reassurance later). First, the therapist should remind the patient of the rationale for engaging in these exercises, with particular emphasis on the long-term gains expected with successful completion of the exercise. Second, the therapist should provide concrete instructions for the patient so that the nature of the exercise is very clear. Third, the therapist should be willing to model the exercise for the patient. If the patient is still unable to complete the exposure, the therapist and patient may need to develop a series of small exercises (essentially a brief hierarchy) culminating with the planned exposure. Finally, the therapist should provide substantial reinforcement for patient's attempts at completing exposure exercises. An example illustrating these strategies follows.

In this particular case of a contamination fear, the treatment plan called for an initial exposure exercise of sitting on the floor of the office. The patient initially refused to participate in the exercise stating that it would be too difficult and overwhelming. The therapist empathized with the patient's fears but reminded him of the treatment plan and why it was important to confront these situations. The patient acknowledged that he understood that he needed to "do this" but wondered if they could try something easier first. The therapist asked the patient what he might be willing to try and suggested that perhaps he would be able to touch the floor of the office with his fingers. At the same time the therapist demonstrated this by bending down and touching the floor. The patient agreed and similarly touched the floor. The therapist verbally reinforced and encouraged the patient and suggested that perhaps he could place his hand flat on the floor and leave it there for a few minutes (again demonstrating the task). The patient did and was again reinforced for his efforts. The therapist continued to model a series of additions to the exposure (e.g., touching his arms and then face with contaminated hands, touching the bottom of his shoes) and reinforcing the patient's successful completion of these tasks. Finally, the therapist suggested that they try to complete the exercise that they had initially planned and invited the patient to sit on the floor with him. Both the therapist and the patient then sat on the floor for enough time for the patient to successfully habituate his anxiety.

Another problem that might interfere with effective *in vivo* exercises is the failure of the exercise to elicit the patient's anxiety. There are three possible reasons for this to occur. First, the item may not actually activate the patient's obsessive fears—either because it was misidentified during the information-gathering/treatment-planning phase of therapy or because previous exercises have successfully addressed the same concerns as this particular exercise. Alternatively, the exercise may be designed poorly such that it does not elicit the desired response. For example, a patient with a fear of causing a fire by leaving lights on may not have any such fears if other people are aware that he has left them on. Therefore, if the therapist is aware that the patient has left lights switched on the exercise will not elicit the patient's fear. Finally, it is possible that the exercise fails to elicit the patient's fear because he or she is engaging in rituals that function to reduce the anxiety.

When faced with an exposure exercise that does not produce distress for the patient, the therapist must investigate to see which of these factors is contributing to the lack of arousal. Typically, our first line of inquiry is to explore the possibility that therapist missed an important variable in the exposure or that the exposure was poorly designed. The most common indicator that the exposure is not functioning to activate the patient's anxiety is that the patient reports that his or her SUDS rating during the exposure is substantially below what was estimated during treatment planning. Therefore, the therapist often begins the inquiry as to why the exposure does not elicit anxiety by asking the patient, "Why is this not as difficult as you thought it would be?" Alternatively, the therapist might ask, "Is there something that would make this more anxiety evoking for you?" Patients are often able to describe parameters that if changed might increase their fear and these adjustments can be tried to see if they do indeed result in increased fear. If the patient cannot generate possible variations, the therapist may offer some of his or her own to see if the patient believes that these changes will result in increased arousal. Even if the patient does not believe that altering the exposure will change the feelings it evokes, it may be useful to try a few changes to the exposure to ensure that nothing is missed in the treatment.

If it appears that nothing was missed in the design of the exposure exercise, the therapist must inquire whether the patient is engaging in any rituals (or other behaviors) to help manage his or her arousal. Usually questioning around this issue will begin with a general inquiry such as "I'm wondering if you are doing something or saying something to yourself that seems to be keeping your anxiety down even though you are doing the exercise just like we designed it?" Again, it is important for the therapist to remember the critical nature of the therapeutic relationship and to make this initial question as nonthreatening and noncritical as possible. Should the patient acknowledge that he or she is using rituals (or other behaviors) to reduce anxiety, the therapist can reiterate the rationale for exposure and the importance of confronting anxious feelings in order to overcome them. The therapist should also provide concrete instructions for refraining from the identified behavior as well as any other behaviors that function to reduce (or manage) anxiety during exposure exercises.

Should it appear that the exercise adequately taps the patients anxiety cues and that the patient is not using ritualistic behavior to reduce his or her anxiety, then it is reasonable to conclude that the content of the exposure no longer (perhaps never did) elicit the patient's obsessions. Before eliminating the exercise from the hierarchy altogether, though, the therapist should ask the patient to engage in a similar exposure outside the office to see if more anxiety is elicited in different settings. If the patient is able to complete the exercise on his or her own without significant anxiety, it can be removed from the list (though the therapist may wish to keep it in reserve for later exposure trials to make sure that the anxiety is no longer a problem).

Imaginal Exposure

In general, the problems that arise during imaginal exposure exercises mirror those that occur during *in vivo* exercises—patients may refuse to participate or the exercise may fail to elicit anxiety. In addition, patients may find it diffi-cult to complete the imaginal tasks because they have a difficult time generat-ing an image of their feared consequence. Sometimes this reflects a difficulty using their imagination, but more often this problem arises because the thera-pist has misidentified some aspect of the patient's feared consequences. Similar to the *in vivo* situation, then, it is important for the therapist to work with the patient to identify what aspects of the image need to be changed, omitted, or added. A similar line of inquiry should be followed if the patient reports that he or she is able to imagine the scene sufficiently well but it still fails to elicit anxiety.

Similar to *in vivo* exposures, the first assumption when an imaginal expo-sure fails to elicit the expected anxiety is that some aspect of the feared stimu-lus or consequence has not been included in the imagery. If, however, the patient reports that the imagery is accurate, then the most likely explanation for the lack of anxious arousal is that the patient is using rituals or other be-havior to reduce the negative emotions. As in the case of *in vivo* exposures, it falls to the therapist to ask patients if they are doing or saying or thinking any-thing that might be serving to reduce the expected anxious feelings. Some likely candidates include "self-reassurance" in which patients offer themselves assurance that the consequences will not actually happen. Other self-statements, such as reminding oneself that the exercise is imaginary, can be used to man-age anxiety as well. Should such strategies be identified, the therapist must remind the patient of the goals of the exercise and the reasons for engaging in it. Therapists should also ask patients whether they are doing anything while listening to their imaginal exposure tapes. Sometimes patients report that they were driving to work or cooking dinner as the tape was playing, decreasing their ability to vividly picture the images that the exposure evokes. In such cases, patients should be reminded that they should set aside some time for imaginal exposures when no other distractions will interfere.

Imaginal exposure is commonly used when some aspect of the patients fear cannot be activated through *in vivo* exercises (e.g., when faced with the fear of burning down one's house we would not recommend that the patient actually do this). Typically, the aspect of the fear that is not available to *in vivo* exercises in-volves the feared consequences of certain actions or refraining from rituals. In some cases though patients lack specific consequences to their obsessions. In these cases, imaginal exposure is not likely to provide benefits beyond those ob-tained from *in vivo* exposure. However, imaginal exposures may be useful as ini-tial steps toward eventual *in vivo* exposure. For example, the therapist might conduct an imaginal exposure to using a public restroom for the session prior to the one in which an *in vivo* exposure to the restroom is planned.

Ritual Prevention

Ritual prevention, the second component of EX/RP is perhaps a more difficult issue that the exposure exercises. Exposures are typically conducted as planned time-limited exercises first with the therapist and later by the patient alone as part of specific homework assignments. In contrast, ritual prevention is a goal that represents a shift in behavior across many, perhaps all, aspects of a patient's life. In short, the patient is instructed to refrain from all compulsive or ritualistic behaviors regardless of the situation. In the ideal case, this restriction is complete from the initial day of treatment. However, there are bound to be occasions when the patient cannot or does not follow these instructions. In practice, therefore, we have developed several approaches designed to maximize the prevention of rituals and to address potential problems that arise when patients do engage in rituals.

Strategies for encouraging ritual prevention begin early in the information-gathering and treatment-planning phases. Several aspects of these early treatment stages are designed, wholly or in part, to set the groundwork for ritual prevention. First, when describing the treatment, we describe the goal of ritual prevention and share the expectation that the patient will be able to inhibit many of his or her rituals once treatment begins. Second, we get the patient used to attending to his or her rituals by having the patient monitor the rituals during the treatment-planning phase of treatment (some patients report that simply monitoring their compulsions results in decreased frequency and duration of rituals). Self-monitoring of rituals continues throughout treatment, though we expect few rituals to be reported after ritual prevention is initiated. Third, during the session the therapist identifies links between specific obsessional cues (to be use for exposure exercises) and compulsive rituals. This information can be used to make the ritual prevention task easier by eliminating exposure to some obsessional cues early in treatment in order to reduce the strength of the patient's urges to ritualize. For example, if it becomes clear that using a public restroom will almost invariably lead to strong urges for the patient to wash his hands, it is better to limit the patient's contact with public restrooms than to allow the ritual washing to occur. In general, when faced with a choice between avoidance of an obsessional cue and contact with that cue followed by ritualistic behavior, we choose avoidance. Importantly, the treatment plan should include exposure exercises to the obsessional cues at an appropriate point in treatment. After that, avoidance should be discouraged.

Several problems may arise with regard to patients following the ritual prevention instructions. The most common of these is simply that they give in to the urge to ritualize. In fact, these "slips" are so common that when we initiate the ritual prevention, we typically tell patients that we expect to see some slips recorded on their self-monitoring sheets. To strengthen this message, therapists may also point out that we do not expect perfection, in fact we tend to discourage it because most obsessive–compulsive patients tend toward perfectionism in some or all aspects of their lives. When slips are reported, therapists must remember how difficult this task is for the patient. The basic instructions should be reiterated and some time spent helping the patient develop strategies for resisting the urges in the future, but the therapist must be careful not to be punitive in his or her corrections. Also, it is important to reinforce the patient's attempts, particularly when successful, at preventing rituals.

A second problem arises when patients refuse to resist their urges to ritualize. If the refusal to follow the instructions to prevent the rituals is general (e.g., the patient refuses to give up any rituals, or will refrain from only a few of the many rituals he or she has), then EX/RP is probably not the most appropriate approach to treating the OCD symptoms and the patient should be referred for an alternate form of treatment. More likely, though, the patient will agree to eliminate most compulsions but will want to hold on to one or two "really important" ones. This problem is parallel to the patient who does not immediately agree to complete all of the planned exposure exercises. The therapist is again faced with a decision, whether to require the patient to try and resist all rituals or agree that some ritual may be retained during the initial portion of treatment and addressed at a later point.

Our experience suggests that attempting to initiate EX/RP treatment without working to eliminate all rituals is extremely difficult. The retention of some rituals negates many of the exposure exercises and prevents patients from habituating their fear. Essentially, by continuing to ritualize, patients retain the belief that their feared situations and/or thoughts are dangerous. This is not to say that we will not treat patients who continue to ritualize, only that it makes the treatment more difficult and potentially less effective. When agreeing to begin treatment without prohibiting all rituals, the therapist must be extremely clear that the ultimate goal is to eliminate all the rituals. Also, it is important to minimize the need for rituals. Thus, the therapist may instruct the patient to avoid situations that were not previously avoided in order to reduce the frequency with which rituals are used to manage feelings of anxiety.

A third potential problem with prescribed ritual prevention arises when the RP instructions conflict with demands of life. In this case, patients do not steadfastly refuse to follow ritual prevention instructions, but rather there are reasons that it is not possible to completely refrain from behaviors that have become ritualized. For example, common RP instructions for a compulsive washer would be to refrain from washing (i.e., handwashing, showering, perhaps even brushing of teeth) for 3 days. However, this may create problems when the patient goes to work or school. Here again, the therapist must remember that the goal of the RP instructions is to "break" the association between the ritualistic behavior and the sense of safety resulting from the removal of the feared object. Thus, washing itself is not a problem, but washing to decontaminate or protect oneself from all potential illness is. Therefore, one way to modify RP instructions when it is unrealistic for patients to refrain from rituals entirely is to find a way to "undo" them (this strategy can also be used to counter "slips" when they occur). To undo a ritual, the therapist and patient must find a behavior that reverses the anxiety reducing function of the compulsive behavior. For example, after washing one's hands a patient could "recontaminate" them by touching something that was previously contaminated. Thus, after showering in the morning, a patient could touch the side of the toilet. The result is that the patient is clean but contaminated and the shower did not serve to protect him from germs.

One other issue that must be attended to if EX/RP is to be successful is the problem of mental rituals. As the label implies, these are rituals that the patient completes mentally; typically these are words, sayings, prayers, or images that are repeated silently to oneself. In the past, patients who used only mental rituals were identified as "pure obsessionals" because they had no observable rituals. However, with rituals defined functionally, it has become clear that mental activities can serve as both obsessions (increasing anxiety) and compulsions (decreasing anxiety). The difficulty in working with mental rituals arises because they are observable only to the patient. Thus, therapists are completely dependent on the patient to monitor and control these mental rituals. In addition, these rituals tend to be briefer and more automatic than many of the observable rituals such as handwashing and checking. Therefore, the patient may have some difficulty resisting the urge to engage in the mental ritual ("it just happens" or "it was easier to give in" are common complaints from patients trying to prevent mental rituals).

When treating a patient with mental rituals, it is vitally important for the therapist to identify which mental activities function as obsessions and which as compulsions because the instructions to the patient for how to handle each of these mental events are exactly opposite. A patient should not try to prevent obsessions; in fact, he or she should probably enhance them to encourage habituation. In contrast, the patient should resist or prevent the mental events that function as rituals (i.e., to reduce anxiety). As with other rituals, strategies such as avoiding cues for specific obsessions may be necessary to allow patients to reduce the urges to ritualize initially. Similarly, therapists may want to help the patient develop strategies for "undoing" the mental rituals as they are often difficult to resist.

Homework

Homework assignments are a vital part of the EX/RP treatment program (for a more detailed discussion, see Franklin, Huppert, & Roth, in press). Homework usually requires 1–3 hours daily in addition to the treatment sessions and consists of additional exposure exercises to be done between treatment sessions at the patient's home or elsewhere (e.g., shopping malls or a relative's home). We suggest that the patient monitor his or her SUDs level every 10 minutes during the homework exposures. In some cases, it will be impossible for the patient to maintain an exposure for 45–60 minutes. In these cases, the therapist should work with the patient to develop a plan that will allow the exposure to be prolonged. For example, instead of asking the patient to spend 45 minutes sitting in the restroom of a local restaurant, one might suggest that he or she contaminate a handkerchief on the toilet seat and carry this "contamination rag" in a pocket.

Obviously the primary problem that can arise with regard to homework is lack of compliance. Without the support and encouragement of the therapist, the patient may find it very difficult to engage in the exposure exercises. One thing that a therapist can do to facilitate homework compliance is offer substantial reinforcement for the actual completion of the assignments. Also, carefully planning the assignments to maximize the chances of success can aid compliance. Practically, this translates into designing homework assignments to include exercises that have already been successfully completed in session. Also, therapists should consider ways to incorporate exposure homework into activities in which the patient engages naturally. For example, if a patient walks his dog every evening but avoids walking on the grass (or cleans ritualistically if he must walk on the grass) then planning an exposure to the grass that coincides with walking the dog may encourage compliance with the homework assignment.

A support person (e.g., parent, spouse, or close friend) identified by the patient can also be useful in ensuring compliance with homework. The patient is instructed to rely on this person for support during exposures and the support person is asked to help monitor compliance with response-prevention instructions. If the patient experiences difficulty resisting the urge to ritualize, the support person should be contacted to offer support. Because the support person will be involved in the therapy, the therapist should allocate time during the information-gathering phase to describe the treatment and discuss its rationale with the support person.

The therapist should make an effort to ensure that the support person and the patient find a mutually agreed-on way for the support person to offer constructive criticism and observations. In making these suggestions, one should be sensitive to any difficulties that have arisen in the past. For example, Mr. B, who served as his wife's primary source of reassurance, also criticized her severely when he "caught" her performing her handwashing ritual. To prevent these responses from hampering treatment, the therapist spent time with the couple negotiating appropriate responses to requests for reassurance and a means for the husband to help supervise his wife's response prevention without being critical.

STRATEGIES FOR PREVENTING
RELAPSE AND RECURRENCE

The empirical literature on prediction of acute and long-term treatment outcome can be informative with respect to helping patients maintain their gains, as can our collective clinical experience. Next we discuss a number of points that we try to underscore in order to promote maintenance of gains, and later we provide clinical examples of how to manage common difficulties that patients encounter after acute EX/RP treatment has been completed. Because good posttreatment status may be predictive of long-term maintenance of gains, many of the clinical strategies we use to maximize benefit during acute treatment are also thought to help patients *remain* well. However, there are also several strategies that we employ specifically to address maintenance, although many of these strategies are introduced toward the end of acute treatment rather than after treatment is completed.

Emphasize How Progress Was Made in the First Place

Patients who have made substantial progress in EX/RP often become alarmed at the prospect of having to fight OCD "on their own" once the treatment course has been completed. Throughout treatment, patients are aware that they can have booster sessions with their therapist once acute treatment is over (e.g., bimonthly sessions, monthly sessions, followed by check-ins as needed) and that more generally, their therapists will be available to provide assistance down the road should it be needed. Also, we spend a good deal of time in later EX/RP sessions emphasizing to patients that their significant progress is largely a result of their own hard work. Through this work they have become more knowledgeable about OCD, the theoretical foundation of EX/RP, and the implementation of treatment procedures. We remind our patients that, now that they have completed a course of EX/RP, they are more knowledgeable about these key issues than are many if not most mental health professionals. We ask them to recount how they were able to make progress on reducing their fear of items that were confronted early on in treatment, and quiz them on what to do if a new obsession were to occur. Patients are often able to answer such questions without difficulty at this stage of treatment and can develop EX/RP treatment plans that flow logically from CBT theory, and we take every opportunity we can to reinforce their newfound knowledge in order to allay concerns that the therapist, clinic, and so on, was primarily responsible for the change and that relapse must necessarily follow if the contact is decreased. With younger patients we formalize this process by holding a graduation ceremony in the last session (see March & Mulle, 1998) in which we present a certificate of achievement, invite relatives, and provide refreshments. The similarity between completing an EX/RP program successfully and graduating from school is emphasized in order to reinforce the patient's achievement of mastery over the subject matter and the need for further "self-study" to retain the knowledge can also be underscored simultaneously.

Normalize Posttreatment Obsessions

By the time the latter stages of acute EX/RP treatment have been reached, the patient should already be quite familiar with the fact that most if not all people have occasional unwanted ideas, thoughts, or images that promote at least some distress (Rachman & deSilva, 1978). Accordingly, patients who are still experiencing obsessions toward the end of treatment should be told that not only is this to be expected because the patient has a biological vulnerability to obsessions but it should be expected because obsessions are ubiquitous. It is very important to highlight this point, because the patient who is soon to leave treatment may be frightened by the fact that obsessions are still present or, in the case in which the patient has made very substantial progress, could recur. We emphasize that the presence of an obsession should no longer be a cause for alarm, as the treatment focused specifically on developing effective methods to deal with obsessions successfully. Instead, the patient should be instructed to openly acknowledge the presence of obsessions when they occur, allow them to be fully present, refrain from any intentional efforts to neutralize or avoid them, and simply allow them to pass of their own accord and in their own good time. When obsessional themes persist or when a particularly strong obsession occurs, patients should consider whether more formal imaginal or *in vivo* exposure will be needed, and they should continue to resist the urge to try to make the obsession itself or the resulting distress go away, because this is the very process that maintains the OCD. We have been accused of pessimism by emphasizing the likely persistence of obsessions even after a very successful treatment course, but we believe strongly that it is more therapeutic to prepare the patient for this likely possibility than to turn a blind eye to data about the persistence of subclinical obsessions in treated and untreated OCD patients (e.g., Skoog & Skoog, 1999).

Discuss Lapses and Relapses

As noted previously, we underscore the ubiquity of obsessions and thus their likely occurrence even after treatment has been completed successfully. In keeping with this same spirit of preparing patients for a long-term battle against OCD, a plan should be put in place toward the end of treatment for managing significant lapses or a relapse. This plan should include psychoeducation about what to expect in the long run with respect to obsessions and compulsions, define lapses (temporary slip-ups in refraining from rituals and/ or other avoidance behaviors) and relapses (a return to the old ways of managing obsessional distress), and provide tailored instructions about what to do when the OCD is especially troublesome. We are careful at this stage to emphasize that an occasional obsession does not even constitute a "lapse" but is better viewed as a natural occurrence that then involves a set of choices, some of which are likely to further weaken the OCD and some of which can strengthen it. The *response* to a given obsession is thus emphasized over its mere occurrence, and patients should be instructed that responding by simply recognizing the obsession and letting it come and go without making efforts to hasten its departure is associated with good long-term outcome.

When the patient's response to an obsession involves rituals and/or other avoidance behaviors, this constitutes a lapse and should be addressed. Sometimes the rituals are less intentional (i.e., they occur almost automatically because of the long history of responding in this manner). If this is indeed the case, the patient should be instructed to make a note of the lapse and, if feasible, to engage in immediate reexposure, which means essentially spoiling the ritual. For example, if a patient with past washing compulsions notices that he has wiped his hands quickly on his pants immediately prior to eating finger food, the best strategy to prevent OCD from slowly creeping back into the picture more prominently would be to reexpose by immediately contaminating the wiped hands with something in the immediate environment that still prompts at least some obsessional distress (e.g., lunchroom table and patient's own shoes), then proceeding with the meal. Sometimes lapses are more intentional (i.e., the patient clearly recognized the obsession and chose intentionally to avoid or to ritualize). Again, in this circumstance immediate reexposure would be helpful: The patient could spoil the ritual and get back on track quickly. When reexposure is not feasible (e.g., patient checked her luggage repeatedly immediately before placing the bags on a conveyor belt in an airport) or when the patient is unwilling to engage in reexposure, the instructions change somewhat. In that circumstance the patient should be told that ignoring the lapse or catastrophizing it are both likely to be unhelpful, and that instead the patient should examine what happened, consider what could be done in future similar circumstances, and create a specific exposure and response prevention plan to be followed the next time a similar opportunity arises. Patients who are experiencing frequent intentional lapses over the course of several days and find themselves thinking about feared stimuli as things to be avoided at all costs may be in the midst of a relapse and should be encouraged to contact the therapist and inform their designated support person that they are experiencing significant difficulty. We emphasize that one or even an occasional lapse does not constitute a relapse, because OCD patients often become hypervigilant about this issue after treatment has been completed.

Encourage Lifestyle Adjustments

For many untreated OCD patients, trying to cope with their OCD is a full-time job. Underemployment and other forms of functional impairment are quite common, and the functional impact of the symptoms can sometimes result in "derailing" from expected developmental trajectories to the point where even when the OCD is under much better control, the consequences of having had OCD for decades sometimes remain. For patients such as these, there are other posttreatment tasks that warrant clinical attention, such as reestablishing professional and personal contacts, developing greater confidence in their ability to cope with life's other challenges, determining what to do with the time now regained from engaging in hours of OCD-related activities, mending fences with loved ones caught in OCD's crossfire, and building a life without OCD that is meaningful and sufficiently challenging. Often patients who have been unemployed for years because of OCD-related disability fear that the return to gainful employment will trigger recurrence of symptoms and are thus reluctant to take on these challenges, yet they also fear that failing to do so will leave them with too much idle time than is likely to be healthy. It is important to carefully assess the challenges that face the OCD patient who is completing a successful course of EX/RP, because problems in reintegrating into their social roles can threaten the stability of the treatment gains by increasing stress. We encourage our patients at this stage of treatment to consider returning to or developing new hobbies (e.g., exercise regimen) that can help fill in the idle time and increase their sense of accomplishment and worth, both of which are often compromised by the effects of OCD.

We once encountered a patient whose OCD checking and perfectionism began at age 8 and persisted essentially untreated for over 40 years. He completed a full course of EX/RP, learned to confront feared thoughts and situations without engaging in rituals, and became very adept at spotting the vestiges of his OCD wherever it occurred, conducting exposures on the spot to keep the OCD at bay. His posttreatment OCD symptoms were quite minimal and it was clear to him and to the therapist that he had benefited greatly from the treatment, yet nevertheless the patient was sad at the last treatment visit. When the therapist asked about this affect, the patient responded by telling the therapist that even though the treatment worked wonders and left him essentially symptom-free, he was preoccupied by the many things he felt he could have accomplished in his life (e.g., graduating from college and pursuing a career in law as he had always imagined) had he received the treatment years earlier. It was important clinically to allow the patient to grieve for these significant losses, which were discussed to an extent in subsequent booster sessions, yet at the same time it was also important to make sure that the patient did not focus on what could no longer be accomplished but instead consider what could be done still. Accordingly, the therapist and patient constructed an extensive list of things that the patient could work on now that would be fulfilling and meaningful (e.g., spending more time with his children) that could provide a more balanced focus against what was no longer deemed feasible.

CASE EXAMPLE

We present here a composite case example to help summarize the material presented previously in a clinically coherent manner; the use of a composite is preferable to protect the confidentiality of specific patients and to allow us to illustrate a greater variety of clinical issues than would ordinarily arise in any single case. Our composite adult patient, who we will call Hope, presented for EX/RP after having already tried an SSRI for approximately 6 months. The SSRI was apparently helpful for Hope's depression but did not change her or have much impact on her OCD symptoms. Like most OCD patients, Hope presented with several different obsessions and compulsions, with the primary fears currently focused on intrusive thoughts and images of harming her children intentionally and associated reassurance seeking and mental rituals (e.g., repeating "God forgive me" many times over in response to the images), as well as fears of harm befalling her family because of her carelessness and associated checking rituals (e.g., checking locks at night and checking stove). Hope and her husband shared responsibility for taking care of their three children, who ranged in age from 8 months to 8 years. Hope's obsessive fears of harming the children intentionally were more pronounced when she was alone with the children, especially the infant, whereas her fears of accidentally harming the family were more prominent when she was leaving for work (she had just started back to working some night shifts as a nurse at a local hospital) with her children and husband still at home or when she was locking up for the night with everyone home.

Psychoeducation began in the very first treatment session, when Hope asked the therapist repeatedly whether he thought she was "like Andrea Yates," and whether she was likely to harm her children. The therapist explained that the symptoms she reported at intake were consistent with the OCD diagnosis, that she was unlikely to harm anyone given her lack of history of violence and her obvious love of her family, but that her OCD (note that the externalizing of OCD begins early on in treatment) would probably not be satisfied with any answer other than an unequivocal guarantee of safety. The trouble with the attempts to get such guarantees, the therapist continued, is that these rituals serve to maintain the OCD without reducing the actual risk to her family, which was extremely low anyway given her history. Although not providing guarantees, the therapist provided support and encouragement, acknowledged that the patient's obvious goal was to reduce these intrusive thoughts and images, but noted that the neutralizing process had to be reversed in order to help her to ultimately achieve the goal of a reduction in these kinds of thoughts and the accompanying distress. The therapist then began to explain how he would try to help by pointing out when he noticed when she was seeking reassurance in session, and he would try to help her develop alternative strategies for handling obsessional distress.

With this important exchange completed, treatment planning continued in accordance with the EX/RP protocol. The therapist was intentionally specific when asking about the nature of the harm-related thoughts and would often precede these questions by remarking about other patients with similar obsessional fears (e.g., "I saw someone a few months ago who would get more intense intrusive thoughts about harming their kids in the kitchen because of the big butcher block of knives, does it work that way for you, too?"). This approach must be taken artfully but is advocated because it serves to model directness about the content of obsessions, increases the chance that essential pieces of information are obtained from patients who are ordinarily reticent to discuss the thoughts in this much detail (e.g., presence of mental rituals to neutralize the most distressing elements of the obsessions), and provides a subtle opportunity for exposure early on in treatment. Separate hierarchies were created for intentional and accidental harm-related thoughts and for the situations that evoked those thoughts, and a list was made of the patient's typical rituals and passive avoidances. Therapist and patient agreed that the intentional harm was more distressing and omnipresent and that imaginal and *in vivo* exposures designed to combat these symptoms would be initiated on this theme. Patients who are about to embark on exercises that will put them face to face with the thoughts of harming their children must be fully versed in the theoretical rationale for doing so, perhaps most so for imaginal exposures. Imaginal exposure for such patients can be titrated by beginning with less graphic material or by asking patients to engage in writing exercises before committing to the creation of image scripts that will be presented, audiotaped, and listened to in the present tense. Accordingly, the therapist began with more benign harm-related stimuli: He asked Hope to write, "I might hit my children," repeatedly on a piece of paper and then, when she habituated to that, he asked her to "up the anty," which she did by writing, "I want to hit my children," and then later "I will hit my youngest son in the head," "I want to chop up my entire family and place them in plastic bags for disposal at sea," and so on. The therapist discussed the purpose of the exercise before, during, and after and helped Hope process the meaning of having engaged in this exercise and, perhaps more importantly, the meaning of having gotten used to writing increasingly specific and violent thoughts on paper.

In vivo exposures for such cases often involve increasing direct contact between the patient and the person he or she is afraid of harming, then gradually incorporating the specific thoughts into the exercise to allow the patient to learn that having the thought and the opportunity does not necessarily lead to engaging in the feared action. *In vivo* exposure in this case began with the therapist in the office. In accordance with the prespecified symptom hierarchy, a large carving knife was placed on the therapist's desk during the second exposure session, and the therapist asked the patient first to pick up the knife, then to make stabbing motions in the air with the knife, next to make the stabbing motions in the therapist's direction. These practices raised her anxiety only a little bit, which in turn made the therapist consider what factors were preventing it from increasing further. When queried about this, Hope noted that if she were to actually lose control and attempt to stab the therapist that she would be unlikely to be successful in harming him because of their considerable difference in size and strength. The exposure was modified by having the therapist turn his back to the patient and work on his computer while she stood behind him—accordingly, Hope's anxiety rose significantly. Nevertheless she habituated within only a few minutes, and then the therapist encouraged Hope to incorporate violent images into the *in vivo* exposure to test her hypothesis that having the thoughts while having the opportunity would greatly increase the risk, and she imagined herself stabbing the unsuspecting therapist between the shoulder blades while he worked. With this exposure under her belt, she was asked to create something similar for homework that would allow her the same opportunity to test her hypothesis and yet still would not be too overwhelming to complete without avoiding or ritualizing. Hope chose to cut vegetables for dinner with a sharp knife while her youngest child sat close by in his high chair, and gradually faded in thoughts of harming him with the knife just as she had practiced with the therapist in session. Together these exercises helped to disconfirm her belief that the thoughts would lead to the actions—the therapist discussed this change in thinking, encouraged Hope to "push the envelope" in subsequent sessions, and to continue to confront OCD rather than feed it by ritualizing and avoiding. Hope did imaginal and *in vivo* exposures to more and more graphic images, learned to take advantage of opportunities to confront OCD rather than to avoid (e.g., making sure that she bathed the infant rather than her husband), gradually did that exposure when her husband and older children were not home, and became more and more consistent in allowing obsessions to come and go of their own accord without neutralizing or avoiding.

Hope continued in this same way for 15 sessions, and toward the end of treatment we began to incorporate many of the suggestions made earlier in order to promote maintenance of gains: Hope was given the clear expectation that these harm-related and perhaps even new obsessions would likely occur from time to time at the very least, but that she was now better equipped to combat her obsessional fears via exposure and response prevention. Like many OCD patients, Hope had also noticed that stress increased the frequency and intensity of her obsessions, and she was instructed to increase her attention to OCD during such times and to conduct exposures when the going got tough rather than rationalizing avoidance during difficult times. With patients who have fears of harming vulnerable others, interpersonal difficulties and anger in particular can trigger or exacerbate these obsessions. Accordingly, Hope had developed the tendency to allow her husband to manage negative interactions with the older children for fear that negative exchanges would prompt obsessions about harming her children; Hope was instructed to shift back to staying in these situations rather than avoiding them so that she could participate more actively in this important parenting task and take advantage of the opportunity to push back against OCD by refusing to give any ground. Lifestyle changes were also incorporated: Hope was encouraged to go out more frequently with her husband and with friends, which served both as an exposure opportunity to confront fears of harm befalling the family while she was away from home but also to reduce her overall stress level and growing sense that, "my time is not my own." Hope made significant progress and maintained that progress even through a few lapses, and reported that she remained confident that she would be able to manage any future difficulties successfully. She remained on her medication for 9 months after EX/RP had finished and decided to continue this regimen because her side effects were minimal, her depressive symptoms were under good control, and she felt she was not yet ready to "rock the boat" by discontinuing them.

CONCLUSION

"The more you do the better you will do" is one of the summary statements that can be derived both from the empirical literature and from our collective clinical experience with OCD. Accordingly, the clinical approaches to psycho-education, treatment planning, and using the EX/RP techniques described in detail earlier are recommended as strategies for helping patient not only make but also maintain clinically significant improvement and should be discussed as such from the beginning. We also emphasize early on that treatment is best thought of from a teaching perspective, in that patients will learn from their therapists specific strategies and ways to cope more effectively with obsessions and urges to ritualize and passively avoid. By emphasizing the transfer of control and responsibility for treatment over the course of the therapy, we seek to empower patients and help them "own" the progress that is made during EX/RP. It is especially important to do this because EX/RP is typically a short-term treatment that comes with an explicit expectation that the patient's symptoms will not be completely eradicated by the end of the acute phase, nor will the vulnerability to obsessions be expunged forever. Patients should be encouraged that their newfound knowledge of how to deal with the same old obsessions when they inevitably arise and their improved ability to quickly recognize new obsessions and their knowledge of what to do when confronted with new obsessional themes leave them in a better position to battle OCD successfully in the long run. Therapists should also schedule booster sessions in accordance with their patients' needs and should generally leave the door open for contact in the future should the need arise.

REFERENCES

Abramowitz, J. S. (1996). Variants of exposure and response prevention in the treatment of obsessive–compulsive disorder: A meta-analysis. *Behavior Therapy, 27*, 583–600.

Abramowitz, J. S., & Foa, E. B. (2000). Does major depressive disorder influence outcome of exposure and response prevention for OCD? *Behavior Therapy, 31*, 795–800.

Abramowitz, J. S., Foa, E. B., & Franklin, M. E. (2003). Exposure and ritual prevention for obsessive–compulsive disorder: Effects of intensive versus twice-weekly sessions. *Journal of Consulting and Clinical Psychology, 71*, 394–398.

Abramowitz, J. S., Franklin, M. E., Schwartz, S. A., & Furr, J. M. (2003). Symptom presentation and outcome of cognitive-behavior therapy for obsessive–compulsive disorder. *Journal of Consulting and Clinical Psychology, 71*, 1049–1057.

Abramowitz, J. S., Franklin, M. E., Street, G. P., Kozak, M. J., & Foa, E. B. (2000). Effects of comorbid depression on response to treatment for obsessive–compulsive disorder. *Behavior Therapy, 31*, 517–528.

Abramowitz, J. S., Franklin, M. E., Zoellner, L. A., & DiBernardo, C. (2002). Treatment compliance and outcome of cognitive-behavioral therapy for obsessive–compulsive disorder. *Behavior Modification, 26*, 447–463.

American Psychiatric Association. (1994). *Diagnostic and statistical manual of mental disorders* (4th ed.). Washington, DC: Author.

Arts, W., Hoogduin, K., Keijsers, G., Severeijns, R., & Schaap, G. (1994). A quasi-experimental study into the effect of enhancing the quality of the patient–therapist relationship in the outpatient treatment of obsessive–compulsive neurosis. In S. Borgo

& L. Sibilia (Eds.), *The patient–therapist relationship: Its many dimensions* (pp. 25–31). Roma: Consiglio Nazionale delle Ricerche.

Başoğlu, M., Lax, T., Kasvikis, Y., & Marks, I. M. (1988). Predictors of improvement in obsessive–compulsive disorder. *Journal of Anxiety Disorders, 2,* 299–317.

Black, D. W., Monahan, P., Gable, J., Blum, N., Clancy, G., & Baker, P. (1998). Hoarding and treatment response in 38 nondepressed subjects with obsessive–compulsive disorder. *Journal of Clinical Psychiatry, 59*(8), 420–425.

Castle, D. J., Deale, A., Marks, I. M., Cutts, F., Chaudory, Y., Stewart, A., et al. (1994). Obsessive–compulsive disorder: Prediction of outcome from behavioural psychotherapy. *Acta Psychiatrica Scandinavica, 89*(6), 393–398.

Clomipramine Collaborative Group. (1991). Clomipramine in the treatment of patients with obsessive–compulsive disorder. *Archives of General Psychiatry, 48,* 730–738.

Cottraux, J., Mollard, E., Bouvard, M., Marks, I., Sluys, M., Nury, A. M., Douge, R., & Ciadella, P. (1990). A controlled study of fluvoxamine and exposure in obsessive–compulsive disorder. *International Clinical Psychopharmacology, 5,* 17–30.

de Araujo, L. A., Ito, L. M., & Marks, I. M. (1996). Early compliance and other factors predicting outcome of exposure for obsessive–compulsive disorder. *British Journal of Psychiatry, 169,* 747–752.

de Araujo, L. A., Ito, L. M., Marks, I. M., & Deale, A. (1995). Does imagined exposure to the consequences of not ritualising enhance live exposure for OCD? A controlled study. I. Main outcome. *British Journal of Psychiatry, 167,* 65–70.

de Haan, E., van Oppen, P., van Balkom, A. J., Spinhoven, P., Hoogduin, K. A., & Van Dyck, R. (1997). Prediction of outcome and early vs. late improvement in OCD patients treated with cognitive behaviour therapy and pharmacotherapy. *Acta Psychiatrica Scandinavica, 96*(5), 354–361.

DeVeaugh-Geiss, J., Moroz, G., Biederman, J., Cantwell, D., Fontaine, R., Greist, J. H., Reichler, R., Katz, R., & Landau, P. (1992). Clomipramine hydrochloride in childhood and adolescent obsessive–compulsive disorder—A multicenter trial. *Journal of the American Academy of Child and Adolescent Psychiatry, 31*(1), 45–49.

Dougherty, D. D., Rauch, S. L., & Jenike, M. A. (2002). Pharmacological treatments for obsessive compulsive disorder. In P. Nathan & J. Gorman (Eds.), *A guide to treatments that work* (2nd ed., pp. 387–410). Oxford, UK: Oxford University Press.

Dreessen, L., Hoekstra, R., & Arntz, A. (1997). Personality disorders do not influence the results of cognitive and behavior therapy for obsessive compulsive disorder. *Journal of Anxiety Disorders, 11*(5), 503–521.

Emmelkamp, P. M. G., & van Kraanen, J. (1977). Therapist-controlled exposure *in vivo*: A comparison with obsessive–compulsive patients. *Behaviour Research and Therapy, 15,* 491–495.

Fals-Stewart, W., & Lucente, S. (1993). An MCMI cluster typology of obsessive–compulsives: A measure of personality characteristics and its relationship to treatment participation, compliance and outcome in behavior therapy. *Journal of Psychiatric Research, 27,* 139–154.

Fals-Stewart, W., Marks, A. P., & Schafer, J. (1993). A comparison of behavioral group therapy and individual behavior therapy in treating obsessive–compulsive disorder. *Journal of Nervous and Mental Disease, 181,* 189–193.

Foa, E. B., Abramowitz, J. S., Franklin, M. E., & Kozak, M. J. (1999). Feared consequences, fixity of belief, and treatment outcome in OCD. *Behavior Therapy, 30,* 717–724.

Foa, E. B., & Chambless, D. L. (1978). Habituation of subjective anxiety during flooding in imagery. *Behaviour Research and Therapy, 16*(6), 391–399.

Foa, E. B., Franklin, M. E., & Moser, J. (2002). Context in the clinic: How well do CBT and medications work in combination? *Biological Psychiatry, 51*, 989–997.

Foa, E. B., Grayson, J. B., Steketee, G. S., Doppelt, H. G., Turner, R. M., & Latimer, P. R. (1983). Success and failure in the behavioral treatment of obsessive–compulsives. *Journal of Consulting and Clinical Psychology, 51*, 287–297.

Foa, E. B., & Kozak, M. J. (1986). Emotional processing of fear: Exposure to corrective information. *Psychological Bulletin, 99*, 20–35.

Foa, E. B., & Kozak, M. J. (1996). Psychological treatment for obsessive–compulsive disorder. In M. R. Mavissakalian & R. F. Prien (Eds.), *Long-term treatments of anxiety disorders* (pp. 285–309). Washington, DC: American Psychiatric Press.

Foa, E. B., Kozak, M. J., Goodman, W. K., Hollander, E., Jenike, M., & Rasmussen, S. (1995). DSM-IV field trial: Obsessive–compulsive disorder. *American Journal of Psychiatry, 15*, 90–94.

Foa, E. B., Liebowitz, M. R., Kozak, M. J., Davies, S. O., Campeas, R., Franklin, M. E., Huppert, J. D., Kjernisted, K., Rowan, V., Schmidt, A. B., Simpson, H. B., & Tu, X. (2005). Treatment of obsessive–compulsive disorder by exposure and ritual prevention, clomipramine, and their combination: A randomized, placebo-controlled trial. *American Journal of Psychiatry, 162*, 151–161.

Foa, E. B., Steketee, G., Grayson, J. B., Turner, R. M., & Latimer, P. (1984). Deliberate exposure and blocking of obsessive–compulsive rituals: Immediate and long-term effects. *Behavior Therapy, 15*, 450–472.

Foa, E. B., Steketee, G. S., & Milby, J. B. (1980). Differential effects of exposure and response prevention in obsessive–compulsive washers. *Journal of Consulting and Clinical Psychology, 48*, 71–79.

Foa, E. B., Steketee, G., Turner, R. M., & Fischer, S. C. (1980). Effects of imaginal exposure to feared disasters in obsessive–compulsive checkers. *Behaviour Research and Therapy, 18*, 449–455.

Franklin, M. E., Abramowitz, J. S., Bux, D. A., Zoellner, L. A., & Feeny, N. C. (2002). Cognitive-behavioral therapy with and without medication in the treatment of obsessive–compulsive disorder. *Professional Psychology: Research and Practice, 33*, 162–168.

Franklin, M. E., Abramowitz, J. S., Furr, J., Kalsy, S., & Riggs, D. S. (2003). A naturalistic examination of therapist experience and outcome of exposure and ritual prevention for OCD. *Psychotherapy Research, 13*, 153–167.

Franklin, M. E., Abramowitz, J. S., Kozak, M. J., Levitt, J., & Foa, E. B. (2000). Effectiveness of exposure and ritual prevention for obsessive–compulsive disorder: Randomized compared with non-randomized samples. *Journal of Consulting and Clinical Psychology, 68*, 594–602.

Franklin, M. E., & Foa, E. B. (2002). Cognitive-behavioral treatment of obsessive compulsive disorder. In P. Nathan & J. Gorman (Eds.), *A guide to treatments that work* (2nd ed., pp. 367–386). Oxford, UK: Oxford University Press.

Franklin, M. E., Foa, E. B., & March, J. S. (2003). The Pediatric OCD Treatment Study (POTS): Rationale, design and methods. *Journal of Child and Adolescent Psychopharmacology, 13*(Suppl. 1), 39–52.

Franklin, M. E., Harap, S., & Herbert, J. D. (2004). *Effects of Axis II personality disorders on exposure and ritual prevention treatment outcome for OCD.* Manuscript in preparation.

Franklin, M. E., Huppert, J. D., & Roth, D. A. (in press). Obsessions and compulsions. In N. Kazantzis, F. P. Deane, K. R. Ronan, & L. L'Abate (Eds.), *Using homework assignments in cognitive-behavior therapy.* New York: Brunner-Routledge.

Franklin, M. E., Kozak, M. J., Cashman, L., Coles, M., Rheingold, A., & Foa, E. B. (1998). Cognitive behavioral treatment of pediatric obsessive–compulsive disorder: An open clinical trial. *Journal of the American Academy of Child and Adolescent Psychiatry, 37,* 412–419.

Freeston, M. H., Ladouceur, R., Gagnon, F., Thibodeau, N., Rheaume, J., LeTarte, L., & Bujold, A. (1997). Cognitive-behavioral treatment of obsessive thoughts: A controlled study. *Journal of Consulting and Clinical Psychology, 65,* 405–413.

Geller, D. A., Hoog, S. L., Heiligenstein, J. H., Ricardi, R. K., Tamura, R., Kluszynski, S., & Jacobson, J. G. (2001). Fluoxetine treatment for obsessive–compulsive disorder in children and adolescents: A placebo-controlled clinical trial. *Journal of the American Academy of Child and Adolescent Psychiatry, 40,* 773–779.

Goodman, W., Rasmussen, S., Foa, E., & Price, L. (1994). Obsessive–compulsive disorder. In R. Prien & D. Robinson (Eds.), *Clinical evaluation of psychotropic drugs: Principles and guidelines* (pp. 431–466). New York: Raven Press.

Greist, J., Chouinard, G., DuBoff, E., Halaris, A., Kim, S. W., Koran, L., et al. (1995). Double-blind parallel comparison of three dosages of sertraline and placebo in outpatients with obsessive–compulsive disorder. *Archives of General Psychiatry, 52,* 289–295.

Hiss, H., Foa, E. B., & Kozak, M. J. (1994). Relapse prevention program for treatment of obsessive–compulsive disorder. *Journal of Consulting and Clinical Psychology, 62,* 801–808.

Hodgson, R., Rachman, S., & Marks, I. M. (1972). The treatment of chronic obsessive–compulsive neurosis: Follow-up and further findings. *Behaviour Research and Therapy, 10*(2), 181–189.

Hohagen, F., Winkelmann, G., Rasche-Räuschle, H., Hand, I., König, A., Münchau, N., Hiss, H., Geiger-Kabisch, C., Käppler, C., Schramm, P., Rey, E., Aldenhoff, J., & Berger, M. (1998). Combination of behaviour therapy with fluvoxamine in comparison with behaviour therapy and placebo. *British Journal of Psychiatry, 173*(Suppl. 35), 71–78.

Insel, T. R., & Akiskal, H. S. (1986). Obsessive–compulsive disorder with psychotic features: A phenomenologic analysis. *American Journal of Psychiatry, 143*(12), 1527–1533.

Keijsers, G. P. J., Hoogduin, C. A. L., & Schaap, C. P. D. R. (1994). Predictors of treatment outcome in the behavioural treatment of obsessive–compulsive disorder. *British Journal of Psychiatry, 165,* 781–786.

Kozak, M. J., & Foa, E. B. (1994). Obsessions, overvalued ideas, and delusions in obsessive–compulsive disorder. *Behaviour Research and Therapy, 32,* 343–353.

Kozak, M. J., Foa, E. B., & Steketee, G. (1988). Process and outcome of exposure treatment with obsessive–compulsives: Psychophysiological indicators of emotional processing. *Behavior Therapy, 19*(2), 157–169.

Kraemer, H. C. (2000). Pitfalls of multisite randomized clinical trials of efficacy and effectiveness. *Schizophrenic Bulletin, 26,* 533–541.

Kraemer, H. C., Wilson, G. T., Fairburn, C. G., & Agras, W. S. (2002). Mediators and moderators of treatment effects in randomized clinical trials. *Archives of General Psychiatry, 59,* 877–883.

Lax, T., Başoğlu, M., & Marks, I. M. (1992). Expectancy and compliance as predictors of outcome in obsessive–compulsive disorder. *Behavioural Psychotherapy, 20,* 257–266.

Lelliott, P. T., Noshirvani, H. F., Başoğlu, M., Marks, I. M., & Monteiro, W. O. (1988). Obsessive–compulsive beliefs and treatment outcome. *Psychological Medicine, 18,* 697–702.

Lindsay, M., Crino, R., & Andrews, G. (1997). Controlled trial of exposure and response prevention in obsessive–compulsive disorder. *British Journal of Psychiatry, 171,* 135–139.

March, J. S., Biederman, J., Wolkow, R., Safferman, A., Mardekian, J., Cook, E. H., Cutler, N. R., Dominguez, R., Ferguson, J., Muller, B., Riesenberg, R., Rosenthal, M., Sallee, F. R., & Wagner, K. D. (1998). Sertraline in children and adolescents with obsessive–compulsive disorder: A multicenter randomized controlled trial. *Journal of the American Medical Association, 280,* 1752–1756.

March, J. S., & Curry, J. F. (1998). Predicting the outcome of treatment. *Journal of Abnormal Child Psychology, 26,* 39–51.

March, J. S., Franklin, M. E., Nelson, A. H., & Foa, E. B. (2001). Cognitive-behavioral psychotherapy for pediatric obsessive–compulsive disorder. *Journal of Clinical Child Psychology, 30,* 8–18.

March, J., Frances, A., Kahn, D., & Carpenter, D. (1997). Expert consensus guidelines: Treatment of obsessive–compulsive disorder. *Journal of Clinical Psychiatry, 58*(Suppl. 4), 1–72.

March, J., & Mulle, K. (1998). *OCD in children and adolescents: A cognitive-behavioral treatment manual.* New York: Guilford Press.

March, J. S., Mulle, K., & Herbel, B. (1994). Behavioral psychotherapy for children and adolescents with obsessive–compulsive disorder: an open trial of a new protocol-driven treatment package. *Journal of the American Academy of Child and Adolescent Psychiatry, 33,* 333–341.

Marks, I. M., Lelliott, P. T., Başoğlu, M., Noshirvani, H., Monteiro, W., Cohen, D., & Kasvikis, Y. (1988). Clomipramine, self-exposure and therapist-aided exposure for obsessive–compulsive rituals. *British Journal of Psychiatry, 152,* 522–534.

Marks, I. M., Stern, R. S., Mawson, D., Cobb, J., & McDonald, R. (1980). Clomipramine and exposure for obsessive–compulsive rituals—I. *British Journal of Psychiatry, 136,* 1–25.

Mataix-Cols, D., Marks, I. M., Greist, J. H., Kobak, K. A., & Baer, L. (2002). Obsessive–compulsive symptom dimensions as predictors of compliance with and response to behaviour therapy: Results from a controlled trial. *Psychotherapy and Psychosomatics, 71*(5), 255–262.

McLean, P. D., Whittal, M. L., Thordarson, D. S., Taylor, S., Soechting, I., Koch, W. J., Paterson, R., & Anderson, K. S. (2001). Cognitive versus behavior therapy in the group treatment of obsessive–compulsive disorder. *Journal of Consulting and Clinical Psychology, 69,* 205–214.

Meyer, V. (1966). Modification of expectations in cases with obsessional rituals. *Behaviour Research and Therapy, 4,* 273–280.

Minichiello, W. E., Baer, L., & Jenike, M. A. (1987). Schizotypal personality disorder: A poor prognostic indicator for behavior therapy in the treatment of obsessive–compulsive disorder. *Journal of Anxiety Disorders, 1*(3), 273–276.

Montgomery, S. A., Kasper, S., Stein, D. J., Hedegaard, K., & Bang, L. O. M. (2001). Citalopram 20 mg, 40 mg and 60 mg are all effective and well tolerated compared with placebo in obsessive–compulsive disorder. *International Clinical Psychopharmacology, 16,* 75–86.

O'Sullivan, G., Noshirvani, H., Marks, I., Monteiro, W., & Lelliott, P. (1991). Six-year follow-up after exposure and clomipramine therapy for obsessive–compulsive disorder. *Journal of Clinical Psychiatry, 52,* 150–155.

Öst, L. G. (1989). One-session treatment for specific phobias. *Behaviour Research and Therapy, 27,* 1–7.

Rabavilas, A. D., Boulougouris, J. C., & Stefanis, C. (1976). Duration of flooding sessions in the treatment of obsessive–compulsive patients. *Behaviour Research and Therapy, 14,* 349–355.

Rachman, S., & DeSilva, P. (1978). Abnormal and normal obsessions. *Behaviour Research and Therapy, 16,* 233–248.

Rachman, S., Marks, I. M., & Hodgson, R. (1973). The treatment of obsessive–compulsive neurotics by modeling. *Behaviour Research and Therapy, 8,* 383–392.

Renshaw, K. D., Chambless, D. L., & Steketee, G. (2003). Perceived criticism predicts severity of anxiety symptoms after behavioral treatment in patients with obsessive–compulsive disorder and panic disorder with agoraphobia. *Journal of Clinical Psychology, 59*(4), 411–421.

Riddle, M. A., Reeve, E. A., Yaryura-Tobias, J. A., Yang, H. M., Claghorn, J. L., Gaffney, G., Greist, J. H., Holland, D., McConville, B. J., Pigott, T., & Walkup, J. T. (2001). Fluvoxamine for children and adolescents with obsessive–compulsive disorder: A randomized, controlled, multicenter trial. *Journal of the American Academy of Child and Adolescent Psychiatry, 40,* 222–229.

Simpson, H. B., Liebowitz, M. R., Foa, E. B., Kozak, M. J., Schmidt, A. B., Rowan, V., Petkova, E., Kjernisted, K., Huppert, J. D., Franklin, M. E., Davies, S. O., & Campeas, R. (2004). Post-treatment effects of exposure therapy versus clomipramine in OCD. *Depression and Anxiety, 19,* 225–233.

Skoog, G., & Skoog, I. (1999). A 40-year follow-up of patients with obsessive–compulsive disorder. *Archives of General Psychiatry, 56*(2), 121–127.

Steketee, G., Chambless, D. L., & Tran, G. Q. (2001). Effects of axis I and II comorbidity on behavior therapy outcome for obsessive–compulsive disorder and agoraphobia. *Comprehensive Psychiatry, 42*(1), 76–86.

Steketee, G., Eisen, J., Dyck, I., Warshaw, M., & Rasmussen, S. (1999). Predictors of course in obsessive–compulsive disorder. *Psychiatry Research, 89*(3), 229–238.

Steketee, G. S., Foa, E. B., & Grayson, J. B. (1982). Recent advances in the treatment of obsessive–compulsives. *Archives of General Psychiatry, 39,* 1365–1371.

Swedo, S. E., Rapoport, J. L., Leonard, H. L., Lenane, M., & Cheslow, D. (1989). Obsessive–compulsive disorder in children and adolescents: Clinical phenomenology of 70 consecutive cases. *Archives of General Psychiatry, 46,* 335–341.

Thomsen, P. H. (2002). Pharmacological treatment of pediatric obsessive compulsive disorder. *Expert Review in Neurotherapeutics, 2,* 549–554.

Tollefson, G. D., Rampey, A. H., Potvin, J. H., Jenike, M. A., Rush, A. J., Dominguez, R. A., et al. (1994). A multicenter investigation of fixed-dose fluoxetine in the treatment of obsessive–compulsive disorders. *Archives of General Psychiatry, 51,* 559–567.

van Balkom, A. J. L. M., de Haan, E., van Oppen, P., Spinhoven, P., Hoogduin, K. A. L., Vermeulen, A. W. A., & van Dyck, R. (1998). Cognitive and behavioral therapies alone and in combination with fluvoxamine in the treatment of obsessive–compulsive disorder. *Journal of Nervous and Mental Disease, 186,* 492–499.

Warren, R., & Thomas, J. C. (2001). Cognitive-behavior therapy of obsessive–compulsive disorder in private practice: An effectiveness study. *Journal of Anxiety Disorders, 15,* 277–285.

Wheadon, D. E., Bushnell, W. D., & Steiner, M. (1993, December). *A fixed dose comparison of 20, 40 or 60 mg paroxetine to placebo in the treatment of OCD.* Paper presented at the annual meeting of the American College of Neuropsychopharmaclogy, Honolulu.

5

Posttraumatic Stress Disorder

NORAH C. FEENY
EDNA B. FOA

To date, much evidence has been accumulated regarding the effectiveness of psychosocial treatments for anxiety disorders. There now exist controlled studies illustrating the efficacy of these treatments (in particular, cognitive-behavioral therapy [CBT]) across the anxiety disorders (e.g., Brown & Barlow, 1992; Foa, Franklin, & Moser, 2002). In the case of posttraumatic stress disorder (PTSD), a series of randomized controlled trials evaluating cognitive-behavioral interventions have demonstrated both short- and longer-term improvements following such treatments (e.g., Foa, Dancu, et al., 1999; Foa, Rothbaum, Riggs, & Murdock, 1991; Marks, Lovell, Noshirvani, Livanou, & Thrasher, 1998; Resick, Nishith, Weaver, Astin, & Feuer, 2002). Indeed, long-term follow-up results suggest that approximately 60–70% of patients are PTSD diagnosis-free (see Foa & Rothbaum, 1998, for a review).

Despite the fact that efficacious treatments have been developed for PTSD and other anxiety disorders, clients vary in their likelihood to complete and benefit from such treatments; outcome depends on both specific client characteristics and specific treatment characteristics (e.g., Feeny, Zoellner, & Foa, 2000b; Taylor et al., 2001). Unfortunately, we know relatively little about factors that influence an individual's response to treatment and propensity for relapse. In this chapter we focus on these important issues: improving cognitive-behavioral treatment outcome for PTSD and reducing relapse for both pharmacological and cognitive-behavioral interventions. First, we provide an overview of trauma and PTSD, describe theoretical conceptualizations of the disorder, and review treatment outcome data. We then discuss predictors of treatment improvement and relapse and practical strategies for improving outcome and reducing relapse rates following treatment for PTSD.

We end the chapter with a case example highlighting issues related to maximizing outcome during CBT and preventing relapse following CBT.

OVERVIEW OF THE DISORDER

Prevalence of Trauma

According to the fourth edition of the *Diagnostic and Statistical Manual of Mental Disorders* (DSM-IV; American Psychiatric Association, 1994) a trauma is defined as an event that involves a perceived or actual threat and elicits an extreme emotional response (i.e., helplessness, horror, or terror). Whereas trauma used to be conceptualized as uncommon and "outside the realm of human experience" (American Psychiatric Association, 1987), large epidemiological studies have established extremely high rates of trauma exposure among adults. For example, Kessler, Sonnega, Bromet, Hughes, and Nelson (1995) examined a nationally representative sample of 6,000 people ages 15–54 and found that 60% of men and 51% of women reported experiencing at least one traumatic event in their lifetime. Similar findings emerged from Norris's (1992) study using a large, racially diverse sample; 73.6% of men and 64.8% of women reported experiencing at least one traumatic event. Somewhat lower prevalence was found in a sample of young members of a health maintenance organization: 43% of men and 38.5% of women experienced a trauma in their lifetime (Breslau, Davis, Andreski, & Peterson, 1991). Consistent with Norris's results, in a representative sample of 4,000 women, almost 70% reported having experienced a traumatic event at one point in their lives (Resnick, Kilpatrick, Dansky, Saunders, & Best, 1993). In addition to high rates of single trauma exposure, women are at high risk for experiencing multiple episodes of violence throughout their lives, including sexual assault (e.g., Resnick et al., 1993). Taken together, studies suggest that trauma is quite common among adults in the United States and that women in particular are at risk for interpersonal violence.

Diagnostic Criteria and Prevalence

It is important to note that most people are resilient in the aftermath of trauma and do not develop long-lasting psychopathology. However, the constellation of psychological difficulties that is observed most often following a trauma is called PTSD. The symptoms of PTSD fall into three clusters: reexperiencing the trauma (e.g., intrusive and distressing thoughts, flashbacks, and nightmares), avoidance of trauma-related reminders (e.g., avoidance of trauma-related thoughts, feelings, and reminders; emotional numbing; and sense of foreshortened future), and hyperarousal symptoms (e.g., sleep disturbance, irritability, and hypervigilance). While most people experience symptoms of PTSD shortly after a traumatic event, the majority also experience a natural reduction in these difficulties over the following several months (e.g.,

Riggs, Rothbaum, & Foa, 1995; Rothbaum, Foa, Riggs, Murdock, & Walsh, 1992). Some trauma survivors, however, continue to experience significant PTSD symptoms for months (Riggs et al., 1995; Rothbaum et al., 1992) and years after exposure to the traumatic event (Kessler et al., 1995).

In the general population, the lifetime prevalence of PTSD is estimated to be 9% (Breslau et al., 1991). It is of note that women appear to be about two times as likely to develop PTSD than men (e.g., 10.4% of women vs. 5% of men in the general population; Kessler et al., 1995). Overall, rates of PTSD among those who are exposed to trauma are higher of course, with lifetime prevalence estimated at 24%. However, among trauma survivors, prevalence of current PTSD varies quite widely; for example, 15% of Vietnam combat veterans (Kulka et al., 1990), 12–65% of female assault survivors (Resnick et al., 1993; Rothbaum et al., 1992), and up to 40% of survivors of serious motor vehicle accidents (Taylor & Koch, 1995) have been reported to meet diagnostic criteria.

Patterns of Natural Recovery Following Assault

As described previously, most people recover naturally in the aftermath of trauma, but some traumatic experiences (e.g., rape) are more likely to lead to PTSD than others (e.g., natural disasters). Two studies have examined patterns of recovery and PTSD following assault: one in a sample of female rape survivors (Rothbaum et al., 1992) and the other in a sample of mixed-gender non-sexual assault survivors (Riggs et al., 1995). In both studies, participants were assessed weekly for at least 12 weeks, beginning shortly after the assault. The results of the studies paralleled one another, both showing high levels of PTSD in the immediate aftermath of the assaults and then a gradual reduction of these symptoms with time for many. Rothbaum et al. (1992) found, for example, that within 2 weeks of a sexual assault, 94% of the women met symptom criteria (but not duration) for PTSD. By 12 weeks after the sexual assault, rates of PTSD had declined significantly among these women; however, 47% continued to experience symptoms meeting PTSD criteria. Those women for whom PTSD criteria were not met 3 months after the assault showed a pattern of consistent improvement over the 3 months of the study. Women who had PTSD 3 months after the assault showed little symptom reduction after the 1-month assessment. Assessments conducted 6 and 9 months after the assault revealed that 41.7% of women experienced symptoms meeting criteria for PTSD at each time point. In the Riggs et al. (1995) study, within 2 weeks of an assault, 90% of rape survivors and 62% of non-sexual assault survivors had symptoms meeting criteria for PTSD. One month after the assaults, rates of PTSD dropped to 60% for rape, and 44% for non-sexual assault survivors. The rate of PTSD had further dropped to 51% and 21% for rape and non-sexual assault survivors, respectively, by 3 months after the assaults.

These studies further underscore that even following severe traumas, PTSD is not the norm, and of those who develop PTSD, not all go on develop chronic PTSD. Thus, it is important for us to begin to understand what differentiates those who will develop chronic PTSD from those who will not. At this point, a range of variables have been suggested as playing a role in the development of PTSD, including severity of initial PTSD symptoms (e.g., Rothbaum et al., 1992), numbing (Feeny, Zoellner, Fitzgibbons, & Foa, 2000), assault type (e.g., Weaver, Kilpatrick, Resnick, Best, & Saunders, 1997), anger (e.g., Feeny, Zoellner, & Foa, 2000a; Riggs, Dancu, Gershuny, Greenberg, & Foa, 1992), and dissociation (e.g., Bremner & Brett, 1997). Theories regarding the development and maintenance of PTSD are presented here.

CONCEPTUALIZATIONS OF POSTTRAUMATIC STRESS DISORDER

Learning and cognitive theories have influenced current cognitive-behavioral conceptualizations of the development and maintenance of PTSD. Learning theories of PTSD include both classical and operant conditioning principles. Cognitive theories emphasize the role of thoughts in mediating the development and maintenance of pathological anxiety. To lay the theoretical groundwork for cognitive-behavioral interventions for PTSD, we next briefly review cognitive-behavioral conceptualizations of the disorder.

Learning Theory: Two-Factor Theory of Fear

Mowrer's (1960) two-factor conditioning theory provided the framework for early behavioral theories of PTSD. In this theory, classical (factor one) and operant (factor two) conditioning are understood as the mechanisms facilitating the development and maintenance of fear. As such, anxiety is acquired through classical conditioning, in which a neutral stimulus (conditioned stimulus [CS]) is paired with an aversive stimulus (unconditioned stimulus [UCS]), so that the CS develops the ability to cause a conditioned fear response. Specific to PTSD, previously neutral stimuli that are connected with the traumatic event are hypothesized to come to provoke anxiety themselves (e.g., Foa, Steketee, & Rothbaum, 1989).

Operant conditioning, the second factor in Mowrer's theory, explains the maintenance of avoidance behavior. Individuals learn to eliminate or reduce trauma-related fear by avoiding, or escaping from, the CSs. Avoidance behaviors are established through negative reinforcement—that is, through their ability to stop the anxiety. In turn, avoidance prevents learning that the CS is not in itself dangerous, and as a result, fear and avoidance are maintained. Learning theories led to the development of exposure techniques, which have become the treatment of choice for phobias (cf. Barlow, 2002) and obsessive–compulsive disorder (see Franklin & Foa, 2002). Exposure therapies have also been found to be very effective in the treatment of PTSD and we review this evidence later in the chapter.

Cognitive Theories

In contrast to behavioral accounts of anxiety, cognitive approaches focus on interpretations of events rather than on the events themselves. It is postulated that these interpretations mediate the particular emotional and behavioral reactions to a given event. Pathological emotions (e.g., extreme, prolonged, and disruptive) are thought to be the result of inaccurate or distorted interpretations; for example, the overestimation of danger leads to unrealistic fear. Cognitive theory was first developed to explain depression (Beck, Rush, Shaw & Emery, 1979) and was later expanded to explain anxiety disorders as well (e.g., Beck, Emery & Greenberg, 1985; Clark, 1986).

Some have suggested that traumatic events cause shifts in an individual's thoughts and beliefs, and that these changes determine one's response to trauma (e.g., Ehlers & Clark, 2000; Epstein, 1991; Foa & Rothbaum, 1998; Foa et al., 1989; Horowitz, 1986; Janoff-Bulman, 1992; Resick & Schnicke, 1992). These theories all emphasize the importance of thoughts and interpretations in determining reactions to trauma, but each focuses on different sets of cognitions. For example, Janoff-Bulman (1992) hypothesized that there are three categories of basic assumptions held by people in general: benevolence of the world, meaningfulness of the world, and worthiness of the self. Further, she hypothesized that traumatic experiences violate these basic assumptions (Janoff-Bulman, 1992).

Emotional Processing Theory

Foa and Kozak (1986) integrated learning and cognitive theories of anxiety disorders within an information-processing framework. Underlying this theory is the notion that fear or anxiety reflects the activation of a cognitive structure that serves as a program for escaping danger. This cognitive structure includes three kinds of information: information about the feared stimulus; information about verbal, physiological, and behavioral responses; and information about the meaning of the stimulus and response elements of the structure. According to Foa and Kozak (1986), fear becomes pathological when the structure includes (1) excessive response representations, such that the fear becomes disruptively intense; (2) unrealistic elements, such as associations that do not accurately represent reality; and (3) erroneous interpretations such as "my anxiety will never go away."

Later, Foa and her colleagues (Foa & Riggs, 1993; Foa et al., 1989; Foa & Rothbaum, 1998) expanded emotional processing theory to explain why natural recovery is arrested in individuals with PTSD. Foa and colleagues (e.g., Foa & Riggs, 1993; Foa & Rothbaum, 1998) have hypothesized that elevated perceptions of world dangerousness and self-incompetence, including the perception that PTSD symptoms signify weakness, underlie PTSD. In support of this theory, Foa, Ehlers, Clark, Tolin, and Orsillo (1999) found that exaggerated perceptions about the dangerousness of the world and negative thoughts about the self distinguished individuals with PTSD from both trauma victims without PTSD and from nontraumatized individuals. Thus, from the perspective of emotional processing theory, treatment for PTSD should facilitate emotional engagement with traumatic memories, promote trauma-related fear reduction, and modify the distorted cognitions that contribute to the maintenance of PTSD.

Ehlers and her colleagues (e.g., Ehlers & Clark, 2000) have focused on dysfunctional meanings attributed to PTSD symptoms themselves (i.e., intrusive thoughts) and have suggested that these interpretations play an important role in the maintenance of the disorder. They hypothesize that the negative meanings (e.g., "these thoughts mean I'm crazy") increase the level of distress associated with the intrusions and they determine the extent of cognitive and behavioral avoidance. Support for this notion was obtained by Steil and Ehlers (2000), who found that dysfunctional meanings of intrusions predicted PTSD severity beyond intrusion frequency and the use of avoidance strategies. As with emotional processing theory, these results suggest that cognitive interventions for PTSD focus on trauma-related negative or distorted perceptions of across a variety of domains (e.g., symptoms, self, others, and the world).

OVERVIEW OF EMPIRICALLY SUPPORTED TREATMENTS

Cognitive-Behavioral Therapies

Informed by the aforementioned conceptualizations, several cognitive-behavioral therapies have been developed and tested in prospective, randomized studies for PTSD (for reviews see Foa & Meadows, 1997; Foa & Rothbaum, 1998). Among them are prolonged exposure (PE), stress inoculation training (SIT), cognitive restructuring (CR), cognitive processing therapy (CPT), and eye movement desensitization and reprocessing (EMDR). In this section, we review selected outcome studies that evaluate the efficacy of these treatments.

In the treatment of PTSD, many programs include some form of exposure. Such exposure typically includes imaginally reliving the traumatic event repeatedly and *in vivo* confrontation with avoided trauma-related situations that are not objectively dangerous. PE consists of a variety of therapeutic components, including psychoeducation, breathing retraining, repeated recounting of the traumatic event (i.e., imaginal exposure), and encouragement to systematically confront trauma-related reminders (i.e., in vivo exposure). Overall, four prospective, large-scale randomized clinical trials to date demonstrate the efficacy of PE for sexual and nonsexual assault victims (Foa et al., 1991; Foa, Dancu, et al., 1999; Foa et al., 2001; Resick et al., 2002). In the first randomized clinical trial, the efficacy of PE, SIT, supportive counseling (SC), and a wait-list control were compared for female sexual assault survivors with chronic PTSD (Foa et al., 1991). PE and SIT showed significant pre- to posttreatment reductions on symptoms from the reexperiencing and avoidance clusters of PTSD while SC and wait list did not. Also, at the end of treatment, 50% of patients in SIT and 40% of PE no longer met criteria for PTSD; in contrast, only 10% of SC patients and none in the wait list lost their diagnosis. At follow-up, there was a tendency for patients in the PE group to show further improvement in PTSD symptoms whereas patients in SIT and SC did not show such further improvements.

In a second study, the efficacy of PE and SIT were compared to a combination of both treatments (PE/SIT), and a wait-list condition (Foa, Dancu, et al., 1999). All three active treatments resulted in considerable symptom reduction and were more effective than a wait-list condition. However, PE seemed somewhat superior to the other treatments: It led to greater reductions of anxiety and depression and resulted in fewer dropouts than did SIT and PE/SIT. In addition, at the end of treatment, 70% of patients in PE, 58% in SIT and 54% in PE/SIT lost their PTSD diagnosis, in comparison to none in the wait-list condition. Moreover, the percentage of women achieving good end-state functioning tended to be higher for PE than for SIT or PE/SIT (52%, 42%, and 36% respectively). Also, at follow-up, women who received PE exhibited better social functioning than did those who received SIT or PE/SIT.

In a recently completed randomized trial (Foa et al., 2001), PE was compared with a program that includes PE and CR (PE/CR) in female victims of sexual and nonsexual assault. Preliminary results continue to suggest that PE produces improvement on multiple outcome indices: independent evaluator and self-ratings of PTSD severity, depression, general anxiety, and social functioning. Similar to the PE/SIT findings, combining PE with CR did not improve the efficacy and efficiency of PE.

Exposure therapy has also been found effective for PTSD resulting from various traumas in men and women (Marks et al., 1998; Tarrier et al., 1999; Taylor et al., 2003). In an examination of PE in a sample of mixed trauma victims with chronic PTSD, Marks et al. (1998) compared PE to CR, PE/CR, and a relaxation control condition (R). The results parallel those of the Foa, Dancu, et al. (1999) study. PE, CR, and PE/CR were all quite effective and superior to the relaxation control. At posttreatment, good end-state functioning was found for 53% of clients in PE, 32% in CR and PE/CR, and 15% in relaxation. Thus, both PE and CR were effective, and combining them did not improve efficacy.

Tarrier et al. (1999) compared imaginal exposure only to cognitive therapy in a group of patients with PTSD resulting mostly from criminal victimization and automobile accidents. Imaginal exposure and cognitive therapy were equally effective in ameliorating PTSD symptoms. However, the effects of both treatments were considerably more modest than those reported in previous studies.

Overall, then, exposure therapy that includes both *in vivo* and imaginal exposure has emerged across well-controlled trials as a clearly efficacious and efficient treatment. In the recent treatment guidelines developed by experts in the field in conjunction with International Society for Traumatic Stress Studies

(ISTSS), exposure therapy emerged as the most empirically supported intervention for PTSD. It is also important to note that while concerns have been raised by some clinicians and researchers that exposure therapy is too difficult to tolerate, and thus leads to symptom worsening and treatment dropout, there is recent evidence that exposure therapy is indeed tolerable. For example, Foa, Zoellner, Feeny, Hembree, and Alvarez-Conrad (2002) examined self-reported symptom exacerbation in a sample of women with chronic assault-related PTSD receiving PE. Results indicated that only a minority of participants exhibited reliable symptom exacerbation during treatment: 10.5% reported an increase in PTSD symptoms, 21.1%, in anxiety, and 9.2%, in depression. Importantly, patients who reported such symptom exacerbation benefited from PE as much as those who did not report such exacerbation and were not more likely to drop out of treatment. Thus, although some patients experienced a brief exacerbation of symptoms during PE, this exacerbation was unrelated to eventual symptom reduction or outcome or treatment completion. With respect to the completion of treatment, further evidence exists that exposure therapy is tolerable. An examination of dropout rates from various CBT treatments for PTSD across 17 controlled studies indicated no significant difference in dropout rates among exposure therapy, cognitive therapy, SIT, combined treatments, and EMDR (Hembree et al., 2003). Thus, exposure therapy did not produce a higher rate of treatment dropouts than other PTSD treatments.

Several cognitive therapy programs have also been validated for use with PTSD (CR; Marks et al., 1998; CPT; Resick & Schnicke, 1992; Resick et al., 2002; Tarrier et al., 1999). As reviewed earlier, two RCTs support the efficacy of cognitive therapy alone in the treatment of PTSD (Marks et al., 1998; Tarrier et al., 1999). CPT was developed specifically for use with rape victims and includes CR and written exposure (i.e., writing the traumatic memories and reading the account aloud to the therapist). In a quasi-experimental design, CPT was compared to a naturally occurring wait-list control group. Overall, women who received CPT improved significantly from pre- to posttreatment (about 50% reduction in PTSD symptoms) whereas the wait-list group did not show significant improvement. In a second study, Resick et al. (2002) compared the efficacy of a 12-session CPT, a 9-session PE, and a wait-list control in rape victims with chronic PTSD. Results of the RCT indicated that after 9 weeks of PE and 12 of CPT, both treatments were highly effective in reducing PTSD: at posttreatment, in only 19.5% of completers in CPT and 17.5% in PE were criteria for PTSD still met. Among completers, 76% of the CPT and 58% of the PE clients met criteria for good end-state functioning (i.e., low PTSD and depression). Gains were maintained over time as well. At 3-month follow-up, 16.2% of those who received CPT and 29.7% who received PE were PTSD positive. Finally, at 9-month follow-up, 19.2% of CPT and 15.4% of PE clients were PTSD positive and 64% of the CPT and 68% of the PE participants experienced improvements meeting criteria for

good end-state functioning. In sum, CPT appears to be an efficacious intervention for the short- and long-term treatment of PTSD. This study also provides
further evidence for the efficacy of PE.

EMDR (Shapiro, 1995) is a form of exposure accompanied by saccadic
eye movements that has been the focus of considerable controversy due to initial claims regarding remarkable success in only a single session (Shapiro,
1989). Of the studies evaluating the efficacy of EMDR, only some used well-
controlled designs and thus yielded clearly interpretable results. One well-
controlled study evaluated the efficacy of EMDR relative to a wait-list control
condition for PTSD in female rape victims (Rothbaum, 1997). Three sessions
of EMDR resulted in greater improvement for PTSD symptoms (57% reduction in independently evaluated PTSD at posttreatment and 71% in self-
reported PTSD at follow-up), relative to the wait-list condition (10% reduction
at posttreatment). However, in contrast to other controlled studies, one therapist conducted all treatments and therefore the contribution of therapist and
treatment effects are confounded. A direct comparison between EMDR and a
combined treatment of PE plus SIT (called trauma treatment protocol, TTP)
was conducted by Devilly and Spence (1999). Both TTP and EMDR reduced
PTSD severity (63% and 46%, respectively), but TTP clients maintained their
gains at follow-up whereas EMDR clients showed higher rates of relapse
(symptom reduction at follow-up of 61% vs. 12%, respectively): At follow-
up, the effect size of TTP was 1.13 vs. 0.31 for EMDR.

Rothbaum and Astin (2001) compared PE, EMDR, and wait list among
female sexual assault victims. Compared to wait list, both treatments resulted
in significant improvement in PTSD severity and related psychopathology.
Immediately after treatment, 70% of participants receiving PE and 50% receiving EMDR achieved good end-state functioning (> 50% reduction of
PTSD severity, Beck Depression Inventory (BDI) score < 10, State–Trait Anxiety Inventory-State (STAI-S) score < 40), compared to 0% in wait list. The
active treatments were significantly different from wait list, but did not differ
from one another. At follow-up, however, significantly more participants receiving PE (78%) achieved good end-state functioning than did participants
receiving EMDR (35%).

The most recently published well-designed RCT examined EMDR in
comparison to exposure therapy and relaxation training (Taylor et al., 2003).
The three treatments were on average efficacious in reducing PTSD and did
not differ in attrition rates, in rates of symptoms worsening, or in their effects
on numbing and hyperarousal symptoms. However, exposure was more effective than EMDR and relaxation in reducing avoidance and reexperiencing
symptoms, tended to be faster in reducing avoidance, and tended to yield a
greater proportion of participants who no longer had symptoms meeting criteria for PTSD after treatment. EMDR did not differ from the control condition, relaxation.

Overall then, there is evidence for the efficacy of EMDR. Importantly, however, a recent meta-analysis found EMDR no more effective than exposure therapy programs (Davidson & Parker, 2001). Moreover, the meta-analysis suggested that the eye movements integral to the treatment are unnecessary (Davidson & Parker, 2001).

In summary, several CBT programs have received empirical support in controlled studies: PE, SIT, cognitive therapy, CPT, and EMDR.

Pharmacotherapy

Research in the area of pharmacotherapy for PTSD has expanded dramatically in the last 5 years. At this point, at least seven well-controlled trials have been conducted for the treatment of PTSD (Yehuda, Marshall, Penkower, & Wong, 2002). Based on current knowledge, several early trials were probably too short to fully assess treatment response. However, the existing research shows treatment of PTSD with pharmacotherapy to be promising. Both tricyclic antidepressants (TCAs) and phenelzine, a monoamine oxidase inhibitor (MAOI), have been shown to reduce intrusive and avoidant symptoms among war veterans with PTSD (Davidson et al., 1990; Helzer, Robins, & McEvoy, 1987; Kosten, Frank, Dan, McDougle, & Giller, 1991).

Evidence has also begun to accumulate regarding the efficacy of selective serotonin reuptake inhibitors (SSRIs) in the treatment of PTSD. Three open-label studies with the fluoxetine have shown benefits in both combat veterans (McDougle, Southwick, Charney, & St. James, 1991; Shay, 1992) and sexually traumatized women with PTSD (Davidson, Roth, & Newman, 1991). In a double-blind controlled trial, van der Kolk et al. (1994) showed benefits of fluoxetine over placebo in patients with PTSD. In a placebo-controlled study of fluoxetine conducted with 53 civilians, an early and robust effect of fluoxetine was seen on all measures of PTSD symptoms (Davidson et al., 1990). In addition, on a measure of end-state functioning, over 40% of those on fluoxetine were classified as responders, in comparison to 3% on placebo (Connor, Sutherland, Tupler, Malik, & Davidson, 1999). In a recently presented multicenter, randomized, placebo-controlled trial, Martenyi, Brown, Zhang, Prakash, and Koke (2001) also reported the efficacy of fluoxetine in the treatment of civilian and combat related PTSD.

Empirical support also exists for the use of paroxetine in the treatment of chronic PTSD (Marshall et al., 1998; Tucker et al., 2001). An open trial showed that 65% of those with PTSD had Clinical Global Impression-Improvement (CGI-I) ratings of "much improved" or "very much improved" after 12 weeks of treatment (Marshall et al., 1998). A recently completed multicenter, randomized controlled trial also showed paroxetine (20 and 40 mg) to be superior to placebo on primary outcome measures at study endpoint (Marshall, Beebe, Oldham, & Zaninelli, 2001). Moreover, paroxetine resulted in significant reductions compared to placebo on all symptom clusters of PTSD, as well as impairment and depression. Importantly, paroxetine has been approved by the Food and Drug Administration for the treatment of PTSD.

Sertraline has also been shown in open trials to be a viable treatment option (e.g., Kline, Dow, Brown, & Matloff, 1994), specifically with female victims of sexual assault (Rothbaum, Ninan, & Thomas, 1996). In a 12-week open trial of sertraline with rape victims, PTSD scores were decreased on average by 53% (Rothbaum et al., 1996). In addition, 80% of the sample was classified as treatment responders. To date, two large multicenter, 12-week randomized, placebo-controlled trials have been published (Brady et al., 2000; Davidson et al., 2001). Both studies support the efficacy of sertraline in the treatment of chronic PTSD. In the Davidson et al. (2001) study, sertraline produced a higher response rate (60%) than placebo (38%), with a 44.6% reduction in symptoms. Most responders met criteria for response by week 4, with an overall 11% discontinuation rate from sertraline due to adverse events. In the Brady et al. (2000) study, sertraline produced larger symptom reductions than placebo on 75% of the main outcome measures. When utilizing conservative last observation carried forward analyses, treatment with sertraline resulted in a responder rate of 53%, compared with 32% for placebo. Interestingly, the majority of symptom reduction took place within 10 weeks of onset of treatment. Indeed, the benefit of sertraline treatment was evident early on, with an average 25% improvement in PTSD in the first 2 weeks. These results are particularly impressive given that the mean duration of PTSD was more than 10 years. In addition, in this sample, sertraline was well tolerated. Furthermore, recent data from a large randomized trial suggest that sertraline not only reduces PTSD symptoms but increases quality of life (Rapaport, Endicott, & Clary, 2002). Sertraline was the first SSRI to be approved by the Food and Drug Administration for the short- and long-term treatment of PTSD.

Some work has also begun to explore the efficacy of dual-action medications in the treatment of PTSD. Mirtazapine, for example, a medication with both serotonergic and noradrenergic effects, has been tested in open and randomized trials with encouraging results (Connor, Davidson, Weisler, & Ahearn, 1999; Davidson et al., 2003). In a small, randomized trial comparing mirtazapine to placebo, mirtazapine showed a higher rate of overall response that placebo (64.7% vs. 20%) and was more effective than placebo on some measures of PTSD and anxiety. Notably, mirtazapine was well tolerated in this study and may prove to be a useful medication for PTSD, though more study is needed.

In summary, evidence has accumulated in the last 5 to 10 years regarding the efficacy and safety of a variety of pharmacological interventions for PTSD. Currently, however, sertraline and paroxetine are the only medications approved by the Food and Drug Administration for use with PTSD. It is of note that no studies to date have directly investigated the relative efficacy of medications and CBT. This is one of the remaining important questions to be addressed in the treatment outcome literature for PTSD.

PREDICTORS OF COGNITIVE-BEHAVIORAL THERAPY COMPLETION AND TREATMENT OUTCOME

While we know a great deal at this point about effective treatments for PTSD, we know less about who will benefit from *which* treatment. As reviewed earlier, efficacious treatments for PTSD do exist, but clients vary in their likelihood to complete and benefit from such treatments; outcome depends on both specific client characteristics and specific treatment characteristics (e.g., Feeny et al., 2000b; Taylor et al., 2001). Recently, a few studies have investigated predictors of treatment outcome. Taylor et al. (2001) investigated patterns of treatment completion and outcome among 58 motor vehicle accident victims with PTSD. Participants received a cognitive-behavioral treatment that included education, relaxation, CR, and imaginal and *in vivo* exposure. Fourteen percent of the sample (N = 8) did not complete treatment; when completers were compared to dropouts on baseline characteristics, very few differences emerged. With regard to treatment outcome, cluster analysis revealed two patterns, one for responders and one for partial responders. In comparison to responders, partial responders to treatment showed more severe pretreatment numbing symptoms, as well as greater depression, pain, and accident-related anger, as well as lower levels of global functioning. It is of note that responders and partial responders did not differ in number of sessions attended, homework compliance, stressors occurring during therapy, or the presence or absence of accident-related litigation.

Tarrier, Sommerfield, Pilgrim, and Faragher (2000) explored factors associated with outcomes of imaginal exposure and cognitive therapy for PTSD. Characteristics of the trauma, patient, treatment, and pretreatment symptom measures were all investigated as predictors of PTSD outcome. Of 11 variables associated with pre- to posttreatment change in PTSD, stepwise regression selected three to explain 36.5 % of the outcome: duration of therapy (shorter treatment predictive of better outcome), gender (females had better outcomes), and suicide risk (higher risk predicted worse outcome). Of nine variables associated with pre- to follow-up change in PTSD, stepwise regression again selected three to explain 36.9% of the outcome: number of missed therapy sessions (fewer sessions missed leads to better outcome), residential status (living alone predicted worse outcome), and the presence of generalized anxiety disorder (related to worse outcome). Interestingly, the best predictor of outcome was inconsistent attendance at therapy sessions.

Another recent study explored pretreatment beliefs about mistrust, helplessness, meaninglessness, and unjustness of the world and their relation to short- and long-term PTSD treatment outcome among patients randomized to exposure, CR, their combination, or relaxation (Livanou et al., 2002). These baseline beliefs were related to PTSD severity before treatment but were not predictive of treatment outcome. At posttreatment, however, sense of control over symptoms and attribution of gains to personal efforts predicted maintenance of gains at follow-up.

In a final study exploring predictors of treatment dropout and outcome among two samples of patients receiving PE for PTSD, van Minnen, Arntz, and Keijsers (2002) found only one consistent predictor across the two groups: Patients with more severe PTSD prior to treatment showed more PTSD at posttreatment and follow-up. Indications were found that benzodiazepine use was related to less dropout but also less positive treatment outcome, and alcohol use was related to increased dropout. The authors concluded that pretreatment variables were not powerful or reliable predictors of PTSD treatment outcome or dropout and that clients should not routinely be excluded from receiving PE based on pretreatment characteristics.

PRACTICAL STRATEGIES FOR IMPROVING OUTCOME

Dealing with Common Treatment Obstacles

As the recent ISTSS treatment guidelines concluded that exposure therapy was the most empirically supported intervention for PTSD, we focus on this treatment in our discussion of treatment obstacles. Theoretically, from the perspective of emotional processing theory, in order to modify fear structures perpetuating pathological anxiety, treatment for PTSD should facilitate emotional engagement with traumatic memories. In the treatment of PTSD, several factors have been identified as obstacles to effective emotional engagement: emotional numbing, extreme anxiety, and anger (e.g., Hembree, Marshall, Fitzgibbons, & Foa, 2002; Jaycox & Foa, 1996). We discuss these obstacles and how to deal with them in exposure treatment later. In addition, we also discuss dealing with comorbidity in treatment.

Emotional Numbing

Some researchers consider emotional numbing a cardinal feature of PTSD. Empirical support for the pivotal position of emotional numbing in PTSD comes from a prospective study looking at the symptomatology of female rape and assault survivors 12 weeks posttrauma. The presence of numbing symptoms best identified individuals with PTSD as indicated by their high specificity and predictive power of PTSD diagnosis compared to the other DSM-III-R (American Psychiatric Association, 1987) PTSD symptoms (Foa, Riggs, & Gershuny, 1995). Similarly, Feeny, Zoelner, Fitzgibbons, et al. (2000) found that among assault survivors, even after depression and dissociation were accounted for, early numbing contributed to the prediction of later PTSD. Foa, Zinbarg, and Rothbaum (1992) proposed that avoidance and numbing involve two separate mechanisms. Avoidance, they posited, involves strategic, effortful processes aimed at avoiding trauma-related stimuli. Numbing, on the other hand, involves automatic processes that are the result of continuous hyperarousal (Barlow, 2002; Foa & Riggs, 1993). Expanding on this hypothesis, Foa, Riggs, and Gershuny (1995) suggested that when effortful strategies aimed at reducing distress associated with memories of the trauma fail, a "shutting down" of the affective system takes place and this process is expressed as numbing symptoms. Numbing then, impedes emotional processing and treatment outcome by blocking effective emotional engagement.

Any time during exposure therapy when emotional engagement is not optimal, as with emotional numbing (or emotional underengagement with the traumatic memory), the rationale for processing traumatic events via exposure is reiterated, and the importance of emotional engagement with the trauma memories is emphasized. Clients who are not engaged during imaginal exposure to the trauma memory can be prompted for additional details in order to facilitate engagement. This prompting can include questions about details of what happened, as well as what the client was thinking, feeling, seeing or hearing at the time.

Extreme Anxiety/Overengagement

In some cases, clients experience extreme anxiety during imaginal exposure, which may elicit fear of losing control. As we have described, it is important that clients with PTSD engage with the memory in order to process it. However, clinical observations suggest that overengagement can impede treatment efficacy. It is important that clients maintain the sense that they are safe and "grounded" in the present while recounting the trauma memory with their therapist. This can be particularly challenging when working with clients who have very severe PTSD or who have severe flashbacks. In these cases, exposure procedures often need to be slightly modified to modulate clients' distress to tolerable levels. Such procedural modifications include instructing the patient to keep her eyes open, using the past tense, making eye contact with and conversing with the patient about the story she is relating, and providing frequent, "grounding" comments (e.g., "You are safe here. . . . The memory can not hurt you. . . . I'm here to help you").

Anger

Anger, although a common reaction following trauma, has been conceptualized to reflect emotional disengagement from trauma memories, which has been thought to hinder recovery (Foa & Rothbaum, 1998; Horowitz, 1986; Putnam, 1989). Studies have found a positive relationship between anger and PTSD in combat veterans (Chemtob, Hamada, Roitblat, & Muraoka, 1994; Woolfolk & Grady, 1988) and women victims of various traumas (Koenen, Hearst-Ikeda, Caulfied, & Muldar, 1997). Results consistent with the hypothesis that elevated anger is positively related to the development of PTSD were reported by Riggs et al. (1992). In a prospective study of PTSD, they found that 1 week after an assault, victims were angrier than nonvictims, and that anger elevation at 1 week was predictive of PTSD severity 1 month later. Similarly, Feeny et al. (2000a) demonstrated at 4 weeks after an assault that anger expression was predictive of later PTSD severity.

These findings, that early anger is related to later PTSD severity, are consistent with results demonstrating that fear activation (emotional engagement) during imaginal exposure, as measured by facial expression, promoted successful outcome and that pretreatment anger hindered activation and outcome (Foa, Riggs, Massie, & Yarczower, 1995). In contrast to these findings, however, Cahill, Rauch, Hembree, and Foa (2003) found that among female assault survivors, CBT for PTSD reduced anger, and that pretreatment anger did not reduce the efficacy of CBT for PTSD and associated psychopathology. In light of these conflicting results, it is important that additional research explore the impact of anger on treatment outcome for PTSD.

The view that repeated engagement with the trauma memory is necessary in order to successfully resolve the traumatic experience has been shared by many theorists (e.g., Foa & Rothbaum, 1998; Horowitz, 1986). Thus, if as has been suggested, PTSD reflects a failure to emotionally process the event, then anger may be one factor that impedes mechanisms underlying both "natural" emotional processing and emotional processing during treatment.

So, with this hypothesis in mind, anger that is frequent or intense enough such that it impedes emotional engagement with the trauma memory may need to be dealt with in order to maximize treatment outcome. In the delivery of PE, our first responses include validating clients' anger and empathizing with them. However, we also teach patients that while anger is reasonable and often quite justified in response to trauma, it is also one of the symptoms of PTSD. We discuss with those clients who are experiencing high levels of anger that while understandable and valid, anger can be an obstacle to engaging with the fear and distress, which is also an important part of their ongoing difficulties in the aftermath of the traumatic event. The rationale is reviewed, and the suggestion made to the patient that she try to put the anger aside so that she can fully engage in the exposure procedures and maximize the benefit of the treatment.

Comorbidity

Comorbidity is quite common among those with PTSD (e.g., Breslau et al., 1991; Kessler et al., 1995). Often then, those who seek treatment for PTSD will also be experiencing other mood, anxiety, and substance use disorders. While space constraints limit our ability to address dealing with the range of possible comorbidity in detail here, we would like to offer some general guidelines for treatment delivery. A thorough assessment should always precede treatment and will help guide treatment decisions. Exposure therapy is appropriate and efficacious for those with a primary diagnosis of chronic PTSD and a range of comorbidity. However, clients with PTSD who are acutely suicidal or actively self-mutilating should receive treatment aimed at stabilization of these symptoms prior to starting exposure therapy. Similarly, if such symptoms emerge or worsen during exposure therapy, exposure should stop until safety has been reestablished.

The utilization of exposure therapy with clients who have comorbid substance use disorders has generated some controversy, and these clients may need treatment aimed at their substance abuse first as well. Unfortunately, despite the fact that PTSD and substance dependence are commonly co-occurring, concurrent treatment of these disorders using exposure therapy has received limited empirical study (Back, Dansky, Carroll, Foa, & Brady, 2001). However, some interventions developed to treat comorbid substance use disorders and PTSD have incorporated imaginal exposure (Back et al., 2001) and open-trial pilot data have indicated efficacy in reducing PTSD severity in patient with substance use disorders and PTSD patients (Brady, Dansky, Back, Foa, & Carroll, 2001; Triffleman, Carroll, & Kellogg, 1999).

Overall, it is important to note that studies published to date supporting the efficacy of exposure therapy have included participants with comorbidity. For example, in Foa, Dancu, et al.'s (1999) study of PE and SIT for assault-related chronic PTSD, exclusion criteria were limited (high suicide risk, current psychosis, severe dissociation, current substance abuse) and designed only to ensure clinically appropriate care. Thus, a substantial number of participants met criteria for current comorbid Axis I diagnoses (46%) and many had experienced prior assaults in childhood or adulthood (about 48% in each). Yet, the treatment was effective for most of the participants. Similarly, Resick et al.'s (2002) study comparing PE and CPT utilized limited exclusion criteria (e.g., current psychosis, current substance dependence, and suicidal intent) in an attempt to enroll a clinically representative sample. As a result, the majority of patients had experienced multiple violent events, had moderate to severe levels of depression, and had struggled with PTSD for many years (an average of 8½ years). Yet, again both treatments were quite successful. Moreover, exposure therapy has been shown to reduce levels of depression and general anxiety in addition to improving PTSD (e.g., Foa, Dancu, et al., 1999).

So, comorbidity *per se* should not typically be a reason to abandon the utilization of exposure therapy. Instead, flexible delivery of exposure therapy with a clear focus on PTSD will often have a substantial impact on comorbid conditions. Thus, we often inform clients who present with comorbidity that maintaining a clear focus on their PTSD symptoms is one of the best ways we know to help them with their PTSD and co-occurring diagnoses.

Combining Treatments to Improve Outcome?

Some have assumed that in the treatment of PTSD, the more treatment procedures employed, the better the outcome for clients. Several studies have examined the hypothesis that treatment programs combining several procedures will be more efficacious than programs using fewer procedures (for a review and discussion see Foa, Rothbaum, & Furr, 2003). In one such study that was described earlier, Marks et al. (1998) compared the relative efficacy of PE and CR together to the efficacy of either alone for ameliorating chronic PTSD and associated symptoms. Their results demonstrated that while both PE and CR were effective in their own right, combining them did not enhance outcome.

Similarly, Foa, Dancu, et al. (1999) found that the combination of PE and SIT was not superior to PE alone or SIT alone in reducing PTSD severity. Finally, results from a recently completed treatment study failed to detect superiority for the combination of PE and CR over PE alone in reducing overall PTSD severity (Foa et al., 2001). Taken together, these three studies do not provide evidence that adding procedures increases the therapeutic efficacy of exposure therapy. In fact, programs containing too many procedures may even increase dropout rates or reduce efficiency.

Additional evidence that more is not necessarily better comes from a small sample randomized comparison of exposure therapy versus CBT (i.e., exposure plus cognitive therapy) conducted with severely traumatized refugees with PTSD (Paunovic & Öst, 2001). Both treatments were equally effective: No differences were seen on any measures of psychopathology after treatment. Both therapies resulted in reduction of PTSD, anxiety, and depression symptoms. These results underscore the efficacy of exposure therapy across multiple symptom domains with a difficult-to-treat sample.

Some studies suggest the efficacy of multiple component treatment packages (e.g., efficacy of SIT, Foa et al., 1991; Foa, Dancu, et al., 1999; cognitive processing therapy, Resick & Schnicke, 1992; Resick et al., 2002; and panic control treatment, Falsetti & Resnick, 2000), but there have been no studies conducted to date that have shown exposure therapy with additional components to be more effective than exposure alone in treating PTSD and associated symptoms. In a recent review of the treatment outcome studies, Foa, Rothbaum, and Furr (2003) concluded that the addition of cognitive therapy does not improve outcome of exposure treatment that includes both *in vivo* and imaginal exposure; in contrast, the addition of procedures that enable patients to confront traumatic memories improves cognitive therapy.

To date, no randomized studies have been conducted examining the comparative efficacy of CBT and medication to their combination. However, one trial is currently examining the augmentation of sertraline with prolonged exposure in the treatment of men and women with PTSD (Cahill, Foa, et al., 2003). After 10 weeks of open-label treatment with sertraline, participants who evidence at least 20% symptom reduction are then randomized to 5 weeks of continued sertraline with or without 10 sessions (2 per week for 5 weeks) of prolonged exposure. Preliminary results show a strong effect of medication during the first 10 weeks of treatment. In addition, augmented treatment with PE produced lower relapse rates 6 months after treatment than did sertraline alone.

PREDICTING AND PREVENTING RELAPSE

What Factors Influence Relapse?

The literature related to relapse after cognitive-behavioral treatment for PTSD is virtually nonexistent. Across CBT studies, on average, gains are maintained following treatment (e.g., Foa et al., 1991; Foa, Dancu, et al., 1999; Marks et al., 1998; Resick et al., 2002). Of course, some individuals do lapse, or relapse, following successful CBT, and we discuss how to minimize the likelihood for relapse later.

In contrast to the paucity of empirical investigation of relapse following CBT, a few studies have examined relapse following medication treatment for PTSD. In an investigation of relapse with fluoxetine versus placebo, Martenyi, Brown, Zhang, Koke, and Prakash (2002) found that with continued fluoxetine treatment, the risk of relapse was substantially less (5.8% relapsed) than for those who did not receive continued treatment (16.1%).

Londborg et al. (2001) examined relapse among patients who received 24 weeks of open-label treatment with sertraline after completing a 12-week placebo-controlled, double-blind study. Only those who initially received sertraline were examined. The vast majority of those who responded to acute sertraline treatment maintained their response over the 6 months of continuation treatment. In the same patient population, Davidson et al. (2001) examined the ability of sertraline compared to placebo to prevent relapse over 28 weeks in patients with PTSD (following both the 12-week acute trial and subsequent 24 weeks of open-label treatment with sertraline described earlier). Patients were randomly assigned to 28 weeks of maintenance treatment with sertraline or placebo. The investigators found that continued treatment with sertraline yielded lower PTSD relapse rates than placebo (5 % vs. 26%). In addition, participants who received placebo were 6.4 times more likely to relapse than those who receive sertraline.

As described previously, Cahill, Foa, et al. (2003) showed that augmented treatment with PE produced lower relapse rates 6 months after treatment than did treatment with sertraline alone. Thirty-one percent of those who received 15 weeks of sertraline alone and benefited substantially later relapsed, while 0% of those who received PE relapsed.

Together, these results highlight the importance of maintenance treatment in the long-term medication management of disorders like PTSD.

Maintenance of Gains and Relapse Prevention Following Cognitive-Behavioral Therapy

Although most people who receive and benefit from CBT for PTSD maintain their gains over time, symptom worsening or relapse may occur among some individuals. Several strategies are often used to maximize the likelihood maintenance of gains, among them are normalizing and anticipating brief symptom exacerbations, using treatment tools to manage symptom worsening (e.g., imaginal exposure tapes, *in vivo* assignments, and breathing), and planning for booster visits.

Normalizing and Anticipating Brief Symptom Exacerbations

In the delivery of cognitive-behavioral interventions, in particular PE, the last session is an opportunity to discuss with a client the fact that while he or she may be doing quite well now, it is likely that PTSD symptoms or general anxiety will get worse in the future, due to normal life stressors. This is not framed as "relapse" but as "lapse" and is normalized as a common reaction to life stress, and as an opportunity to practice skills that were previously helpful. This can also be a time to identify with the client particular skills he or she would like to practice on his or her own.

Using Treatment Tools to Manage Symptom Worsening

In the event that PTSD symptoms do get worse with time, clients are informed in advance to use the tools that they found effective over the course of treatment to manage symptom worsening following treatment. For example, clients are instructed to reinitiate *in vivo* exercises they found helpful in the past, to begin again to practice their breathing retraining nightly, or to return to listening to imaginal exposure tapes daily until symptoms abate. At the end of treatment, questions such as "What will you do if in two or three months you start to have nightmares and intrusive thoughts again?" can help clients to mentally prepare for these situations. Clients can also be told that with continued practice of skills and techniques that they have learned, they may continue to feel even better with time.

Planning for Booster Visits

Planning for booster visits is another practical strategy that can be used to prevent relapse and facilitate the maintenance of gains. Particularly for clients who have poor social support networks or severe ongoing life stressors, one or two booster sessions can be scheduled preemptively at the end of treatment. For other clients, they can be informed how to reach their therapist in the event of symptom worsening that they feel unable to manage effectively on their own. The content of booster sessions should be within a PE framework and should include an assessment of current PTSD, a review of the treatment rationale, and a plan for how to manage the current symptom worsening. Such plans can range from encouragement to actively reengage in treatment strategies such as listening to exposure tapes and doing *in vivo* exposure on their own to providing referrals for other mental health professionals (e.g., in the case of severe depression) to reinitiating PTSD-related treatment to restore and consolidate earlier gains.

CASE EXAMPLE

In this section we describe the case of a woman who received PE in order to highlight practical strategies useful for optimizing PTSD treatment outcome and preventing relapse. PE, as we described earlier, consists of a variety of therapeutic components, including psychoeducation about PTSD and common reactions to trauma, breathing retraining, repeated recounting of the traumatic event (i.e., imaginal exposure), and encouragement to systematically confront trauma-related reminders (i.e., *in vivo* exposure). The client received 10 weekly sessions of treatment lasting 1½ to 2 hours in duration. Pre-, post- and follow-up assessments were conducted by an evaluator who was blind to treatment assignment. For a detailed description of the treatment program see Foa and Rothbaum (1998).

Background

Sherry was a 36-year-old African American woman who was married and a full-time mother to her 6-year-old son when she sought treatment. Immediately after high school, she had attended 2 years of college but dropped out after her sophomore year because she could not manage the academic demands. Sherry sought treatment for PTSD symptoms related to repeated physical and sexual abuse perpetrated by her older brother between the ages of 9 and 17. Sherry's brother had repeatedly fondled her after sneaking into her bedroom until she was 12, and as she got older, he turned to physically assaulting her instead. During her teen years, her brother flew into a rage and beat her very badly on several occasions. When she was 17, he beat and then strangled Sherry until she blacked out. This was the last time he ever attacked her and she identified this assault as the worst. Sherry never informed her parents of the sexual or physical abuse (though she suspected they knew) and never pressed legal charges against her brother. When treatment was initiated, she had intermittent contact with her brother. While Sherry was very uncomfortable around him, she was not realistically concerned that he would attack her again.

Pretreatment Assessment

At her initial assessment, the Structured Clinical Interview for DSM-IV (First, Spitzer, Gibbon, & Williams, 1996) was administered along with a variety of self-report scales including the Posttraumatic Stress Scale—Interview Version (PSS-I; Foa, Riggs, Dancu, & Rothbaum, 1993). Current DSM-IV criteria were met for PTSD, recurrent major depressive disorder, and social phobia. Sherry's PTSD was very severe (PSS-I = 47) and was determined to be the primary disorder. Sherry's depression was also quite severe, and she had struggled with ongoing suicidal thoughts for years. Although she had never made a suicide attempt, in the past year she reported "almost overdosing" twice using a bottle of aspirin. Sherry was unable to work outside the home but was, with much effort, successfully raising her son. Her relationship with her husband was close, but strained, due to her high level of irritability, poor functioning, and avoidance of emotional and sexual intimacy. Her relationships with her mother and father were distant but very conflictual, in part because they maintained close contact with her brother.

Treatment Course

Sherry received 10 sessions of manualized PE therapy aimed at reducing her PTSD and associated psychopathology. Her treatment was provided in the context of a PTSD treatment trial in which she had the choice to receive either an SSRI or PE. Sherry chose to receive PE saying, "I have to talk about what happened—it just won't go away." Sherry called about treatment after seeing this study advertised in a newspaper and had never sought mental health treatment previously. Imaginal exposure was focused on the physical assault described earlier in which Sherry was strangled by her brother. This memory was considerably more distressing and vivid than any of her other memories of her brother's abuse. Sherry explained that this was the only time she truly believed that she was going to die.

Optimizing Outcome

Earlier, we described three factors that can impair effective emotional engagement: numbing, extreme anxiety, and extreme anger. For Sherry, numbing/underengagement with the trauma memory was evident from the start of treatment and threatened to impede her progress. As imaginal exposure was initiated, Sherry retold the story of the beating and strangling in a "police report" fashion, with little emotion and seemingly little connection to the story. She had great difficulty visualizing what had happened to her, particularly from the point in the memory when her brother put his hands on her neck. Sherry's self-reported distress during the first several sessions of imaginal exposure was quite low, and she said several times she "couldn't feel much of anything."

The therapist used several standard strategies to more effectively engage her with the trauma memory. First, the therapist reiterated the rationale for exposure and highlighted to Sherry how important it was to emotionally engage with the memory even though it was very distressing. Second, the therapist tried to explore with Sherry what was preventing her from connecting with the memory. It became clear that Sherry was very afraid that she would lose control and "not be able to put herself back together" if she really let herself feel how terrified she was that day. Her therapist empathized with her and validated these feelings but also discussed with her that although very distressing, the memory itself could not hurt her, and that with time, her distress would lessen. In addition, the therapist asked about specific ways to be supportive and help Sherry feel safe during exposure. Third, during exposure, the therapist interacted with Sherry in ways to increase her emotional connection to the memory. For example, using the present tense, the therapist asked brief questions and probed for details (e.g., "Describe what your brother's face looks like". . . . "Describe the room you are in" . . . "What are you wearing?"). The therapist's use of the present tense in asking questions was quite effective in helping Sherry to use the present tense herself and to engage more fully. The therapist also probed for feelings and thoughts (e.g., "What are you feeling?" . . . "What are you thinking as your brother swings at you?") to help Sherry engage with the memory and her feelings. As therapy progressed, the therapist also began to probe for more sensory information, especially related to the strangling (e.g., "How hard is he choking you—what does it feel like?" . . . "Can you breathe?" . . . "What is the pain like?").

These strategies enabled Sherry to connect with the trauma memory much more effectively during imaginal exposure (both in session and when she listened to her exposure tapes for homework). In the short run, this improved engagement led to increased anxiety during exposure. However, by session 8, Sherry reported significant reductions in distress as she recounted the story, and also in her PTSD and depressive symptoms.

Posttreatment Evaluation

At the end of treatment, Sherry was substantially improved. Criteria for PTSD were no longer met, and she had very few residual symptoms (PSS-I = 2, self-report version [PSS-SR] = 0). Criteria for depression were no longer met either, and for the first time in years, her suicidal thoughts remitted. Her functioning also improved and she began to look for a job.

Relapse Prevention

As a standard part of PE, the last session of treatment is devoted in part to relapse prevention. Thus, in Sherry's last session, she and her therapist had an interactive discussion about all the hard work she had done, the excellent progress she had made, what skills she found to be most useful, and when to use them in the future. Even though she found it difficult, Sherry clearly identified imaginal exposure as the most helpful tool for her over the course of treatment. She knew that if her PTSD symptoms were to return, one of the first things she would do would be to begin to listen to her imaginal exposure tapes again. Though Sherry was doing very well at the end of treatment, the objectives of this discussion were to ensure that she felt that she could handle increases in PTSD symptoms with the tools she had learned in treatment, and to normalize for her brief periods of symptom worsening. She and her therapist also talked about the possibility of booster sessions in the event that her symptoms worsened to the degree that she felt unable to manage them on her own.

Approximately 6 months after treatment ended, Sherry's husband lost his job, and they were forced to move out of the home they rented, as they could no longer afford it. They decided that their only option was to live with Sherry's mother temporarily while they saved money for a new place to live. However, this meant substantially more frequent contact with her brother as he visited the house frequently, often without notice. After several weeks of this new living arrangement, Sherry called her therapist for advice, as she was experiencing an increase in intrusive trauma-related thoughts, nightmares, and avoidance. Unfortunately, since the move, Sherry had many of her belongings in storage and had no access to her old exposure tapes. She and the therapist scheduled a booster session, and in this session assessed Sherry's level of PTSD (PSS-I = 19) and reviewed treatment tools that would be useful in light of this symptom increase. They also evaluated Sherry's safety, and Sherry reported that neither she nor her husband were concerned that she was in any danger due to this increased contact with her brother (he had not physically attacked her in over 15 years). In light of this, the therapist reviewed the treatment rationale and made a plan with Sherry for how to manage the current symptom worsening. The therapist provided Sherry with a copy of her final imaginal exposure tape and instructed to her to begin to listen to it again daily as well as to reinitiate her breathing practice and confrontation of avoided situations. At a 2-week follow-up booster session, Sherry reported she had "done all of her homework" and according to interview and self-report, her PTSD symptoms were reduced by 50%. She planned to continue to listen to her exposure tape daily for at least the next week, or until she felt her symptoms were under control and manageable.

12-Month Follow-Up Evaluation

Twelve months after completing treatment, Sherry was doing quite well. Her symptoms did not meet criteria for either PTSD or depression and once again she had very few residual symptoms (PSS-I = 3,[PSS-SR] = 0). She had a full-time job at a library and she and her husband and son were once again living in their own house. After the follow-up assessment, Sherry wrote a note to her therapist in which she conveyed optimism about the future and reported that she felt "more able to handle things" and wrote, "I know now that burying pain doesn't work—I've learned to face it . . . ."

CONCLUSION

Although most people are resilient in the aftermath of trauma, a minority of trauma survivors continues to experience impairing PTSD symptoms for months and even years. Fortunately, we have cognitive-behavioral and pharmacological treatments that have been shown to effectively reduce PTSD and associated psychopathology. Among cognitive-behavioral interventions, to date, PE has received the most empirical support with the widest range of trauma populations. Treatment programs that combine PE with other therapies (e.g., SIT and CT) have not been found to be more effective than PE alone, but more research is needed in this area. Among pharmacological interventions, sertraline and paroxetine have been approved by the Food and Drug Administration for the treatment of adults with PTSD. Though no studies have directly investigated the relative efficacy of medications and CBT, there is preliminary evidence that medication outcomes can be enhanced and relapse reduced by augmenting medication with PE.

In contrast to how much we know about effective treatments for PTSD, we know little about how to predict who will complete and benefit from which treatment for PTSD. Recently, some studies have investigated predictors of treatment outcome, but findings have been somewhat mixed. Overall, pretreatment symptom severity, low levels of functioning, noncompliance with treatment demands, and inconsistent treatment attendance appear to be factors that impede treatment response. Most people who receive and benefit from CBT for PTSD do maintain their gains over time, though symptom worsening or relapse may occur among some individuals. Studies that have examined relapse following medication treatment have clearly indicated the need for maintenance treatment in the long-term medication management of PTSD. Continued systematic study of factors related to treatment non-response, dropout, and maintenance of gains will inform methods for enhancing short- and long-term treatment efficacy and reducing treatment dropout.

REFERENCES

American Psychiatric Association. (1987). *Diagnostic and statistical manual of mental disorders* (3rd ed., revised). Washington, DC: American Psychiatric Press.

American Psychiatric Association. (1994). *Diagnostic and statistical manual of mental disorders* (4th ed.). Washington, DC: American Psychiatric Press.

Back, S. E., Dansky, B. S., Carroll, K. M., Foa, E. B., & Brady, K. T. (2001). Exposure therapy in the treatment of PTSD among cocaine-dependent individuals: Description of procedures. *Journal of Substance Abuse Treatment, 21,* 35–45.

Barlow, D. H. (2002). *Anxiety and its disorders: The nature and treatment of anxiety and panic* (2nd ed.). New York: Guilford Press.

Beck, A. T., Emery, G., & Greenberg, R. L. (1985). *Anxiety disorders and phobias.* New York: Basic Books.

Beck, A. T., Rush, A. J., Shaw, B. F., & Emery, G. (1979). *Cognitive therapy of depression.* New York: Guilford Press.

Brady, K. T., Dansky, B. S., Back, S. E., Foa, E. B., & Carroll, K. M. (2001). Exposure therapy in the treatment of PTSD among cocaine-dependent individuals: Preliminary findings. *Journal of Substance Abuse Treatment, 21,* 47–54.

Brady, K., Pearlstein, T., Asnis, G. M., Baker, D., Rothbaum, B., Sikes, C. R., & Farfel, G. M. (2000). Efficacy and safety of Zoloft treatment of posttraumatic stress disorder: A randomized controlled trial. *Journal of the American Medical Association, 283,* 1837–1844.

Bremner, J. D., & Brett, E. (1997). Trauma-related dissociative states and long-term psychopathology in posttraumatic stress disorder. *Journal of Traumatic Stress, 10,* 37–49.

Breslau, N., Davis, G. C., Andreski, P., & Peterson, E. (1991). Traumatic events and posttraumatic stress disorder in an urban population of young adults. *Archives General Psychiatry, 48,* 218–228.

Brown, T. A., & Barlow, D. H. (1992). Comorbidity among anxiety disorders: Implications for treatment and DSM-IV. *Journal of Consulting and Clinical Psychology, 60,* 835–844.

Cahill, S. P., Foa, E. B., Rothbaum, B., Connor, K., Smith, R., & Davidson, J. R. T. (2003, March). *Augmentation of sertraline with prolonged exposure (PE) in the treatment of PTSD: Does PE protect against relapse?* Poster presented at annual convention of the Anxiety Disorders Association of America, Toronto, Ontario, Canada.

Cahill, S. P., Rauch, S. A., Hembree, E. A., & Foa, E. B. (2003). Effect of cognitive-behavioral treatments for PTSD on anger. *Journal of Cognitive Psychotherapy, 17*(2), 113–131.

Chemtob, C. M., Hamada, R. S., Roitblat, H. L., & Muraoka, M. Y. (1994). Anger, impulsivity, and anger control in combat-related posttraumatic stress disorder. *Journal of Consulting and Clinical Psychology, 62,* 827–832.

Clark, D. M. (1986). A cognitive approach to panic. *Behaviour Research and Therapy, 24,* 461–470.

Connor, K. M., Davidson, J.R.T., Weisler, R. H., & Ahearn, E. (1999). A pilot study of mirtazapine in post-traumatic stress disorder. *International Clinical Pharamacology, 13,* 111–113.

Connor, K. M., Sutherland, S. M., Tupler, L. A., Malik, M. L., & Davidson, J. R. T. (1999). Fluoxetine in post-traumatic stress disorder: Randomised, double-blind study. *British Journal of Psychiatry, 175,* 17–22.

Davidson, J., Kudler, H., Smith, R., Mahorney, S. L., Lipper, S., Hammett, E., Saunders, W. B., & Cavenar, J. O., Jr. (1990). Treatment of posttraumatic stress disorder with amitriptyline and placebo. *Archives of General Psychiatry, 47,* 259–266.

Davidson, J., Pearlstein, T., Londborg, P., Brady, K. T., Rothbaum, B., Bell, J., Maddock, R., Hegel, M. T., & Farfel, G. (2001). Efficacy of sertraline in preventing relapse of posttraumatic stress disorder: Results of a 28-week double-blind, placebo-controlled study. *American Journal Psychiatry, 158,* 1974–1981.

Davidson, J., Roth, S., & Newman, E. (1991). Fluoxetine in post-traumatic stress disorder. *Journal of Traumatic Stress, 4,* 419–423.

Davidson, J. R. T., Weisler, R. H., Butterfield, M. I., Casat, C. D., Connor, K. M., Barnett, S., & van Meter, S. (2003). Mirtazapine vs. placebo in posttraumatic stress disorder: A pilot trial. *Biological Psychiatry, 53,* 188–191.

Davidson P. R., & Parker, K. C. H. (2001). Eye movement desensitization and reprocessing (EMDR): A meta-analysis. *Journal of Consulting and Clinical Psychology, 69,* 305–316.

Devilly, G. J., & Spence, S. H. (1999). The relative efficacy and treatment distress of EMDR and a cognitive-behavior trauma treatment protocol in the amelioration of posttraumatic stress disorder. *Journal of Anxiety Disorders, 13,* 131–157.

Ehlers, A., & Clark, D. M. (2000). A cognitive model of persistent posttraumatic stress disorder. *Behaviour Research and Therapy, 38,* 319–345.

Epstein, S. (1991). The self-concept, traumatic neurosis, and the structure of personality. In D. Ozer, J. M. Healy, Jr., & A. J. Stewart (Eds.), *Perspectives on personality* (Vol. 3, pp. 63–98). London: Jessica Kingsley.

Falsetti, S. A., & Resnick, H. S. (2000). Cognitive behavioral treatment for PTSD with comorbid panic attacks. *Journal of Contemporary Psychotherapy, 30,* 163–179.

Feeny, N. C., Zoellner, L. A., Fitzgibbons, L. A., & Foa, E. B. (2000). Exploring the roles of emotional numbing, depression, and dissociation in PTSD. *Journal of Traumatic Stress, 13,* 489–498.

Feeny, N. C., Zoellner, L. A., & Foa, E. B. (2000a). Anger, dissociation, and posttraumatic stress disorder among female assault victims. *Journal of Traumatic Stress*, *13*, 89–100.

Feeny, N. C., Zoellner, L. A., & Foa, E. B. (2000b, November). *Patterns of recovery women with chronic PTSD.* Paper presented at annual meeting of the Association for Advancement of Behavior Therapy, New Orleans, LA.

First, M. B., Spitzer, R. L., Gibbon, M., & Williams, J. B. W. (1996). *Structured Clinical Interview for Axis I DSM-IV Disorders Research Version—Patient Edition (SCID-I/P, ver. 2.0).* New York: New York State Psychiatric Institute, Biometrics Research Department.

Foa, E. B., Dancu, C. V., Hembree, E. A., Jaycox, L. H., Meadows, E. A., & Street, G. P. (1999). A comparison of exposure therapy, stress inoculation training, and their combination for reducing posttraumatic stress disorder in female assault victims. *Journal of Consulting and Clinical Psychology, 67*, 194–200.

Foa, E. B., Ehlers, A., Clark, D., Tolin, D. F., & Orsillo, S. (1999). Posttraumatic cognitions inventory (PTCI): Development and comparison with other measures. *Psychological Assessment, 11*, 303–314.

Foa, E. B., Franklin, M. E., & Moser, J. (2002). Context in the clinic: How well to cognitive-behavioral therapies and medications work in combination? *Biological Psychiatry, 52*, 989–997.

Foa, E. B., Hembree, E. A., Cahill, S., Feeny, N. C., Zoellner, L. A., & Jaycox, L. (2001, November). *Treatment of PTSD with PE, PE/CR, and waitlist.* Paper presented at annual International Society for Traumatic Stress Studies (ISTSS) conference, New Orleans, LA.

Foa, E. B., & Kozak, M. J. (1986). Emotional processing of fear: Exposure to corrective information. *Psychological Bulletin, 99*, 20–35.

Foa, E. B., & Meadows, E. A. (1997). Psychosocial treatments for post-traumatic stress disorder: A critical review. In J. Spence, J. M. Darley, & D. J. Foss (Eds.), *Annual review of psychology* (Vol. 48, pp. 449–480). Palo Alto, CA: Annual Reviews.

Foa, E. B., & Riggs, D. S. (1993). Post-traumatic stress disorder in rape victims. In J. Oldham, M. B. Riba, & A. Tasman (Eds.), *American psychiatric press review of psychiatry* (Vol. 12, pp. 273–303). Washington, DC: American Psychiatric Press.

Foa, E. B., Riggs, D. S., Dancu, C. V., & Rothbaum, B. O. (1993). Reliability and validity of a brief instrument for assessing posttraumatic stress disorder. *Journal of Traumatic Stress, 6*, 459–473.

Foa, E. B., Riggs, D. S., & Gershuny, B. S. (1995). Arousal, numbing, and intrusion: Symptom structure of PTSD following assault. *American Journal of Psychiatry, 152*, 116–120.

Foa, E. B., Riggs, D. S., Massie, E. D., & Yarczower, M. (1995). The impact of fear activation and anger on the efficacy of exposure treatment for posttraumatic stress disorder. *Behavior Therapy, 26*, 487–499.

Foa, E. B., & Rothbaum, B. O. (1998). *Treating the trauma of rape.* New York: Guilford Press.

Foa, E. B., Rothbaum, B. O., & Furr, J. M. (2003). Augmenting exposure therapy with other CBT procedures. *Psychiatric Annals, 33*, 47–53.

Foa, E. B., Rothbaum, B. O., Riggs, D. S., & Murdock, T. (1991). Treatment of post-traumatic stress disorder in rape victims: A comparison between cognitive-behavioral procedures and counseling. *Journal of Consulting and Clinical Psychology, 59*, 715–723.

Foa, E. B., Steketee, G., & Rothbaum, B. (1989). Behavioral/cognitive conceptualizations of post-traumatic stress disorder. *Behavior Therapy, 20,* 155–176.

Foa, E. B., Zinbarg, R., & Rothbaum, B. O. (1992). Uncontrollability and unpredictability in post-traumatic stress disorder: An animal model. *Psychological Bulletin, 112,* 218–238.

Foa, E. B., Zoellner, L. A., Feeny, N. C., Hembree, E. A., & Alvarez-Conrad, J. (2002). Is imaginal exposure related to an exacerbation of symptoms? *Journal of Consulting and Clinical Psychology, 70,* 1022–1028.

Franklin, M. E., & Foa, E. B. (2002). Cognitive behavioral treatments for obsessive compulsive disorder. In P. E. Nathan & J. M. Gorman (Eds.), *A guide to treatments that work* (pp. 367–386). New York: Oxford University Press.

Helzer, J. E., Robins, L. N., & McEvoy, L. (1987). Post-traumatic stress disorder in the general population: Findings of the Epidemiologic Catchment Area Survey. *New England Journal of Medicine, 317,* 1630–1634.

Hembree, E. A., Foa, E. B., Dorfan, N. M., Street, G., Kowalski, A., & Tu, X. (2003). Do patients drop out prematurely from exposure therapy for PTSD? *Journal of Traumatic Stress, 16,* 555–562.

Hembree, E. A., Marshall, R. D., Fitzgibbons, L. A., & Foa, E. B. (2002). The difficult-to-treat patient with posttraumatic stress disorder. In M. J. Dewan & R. W. Pies (Eds.), *The difficult-to-treat psychiatric patient* (pp. 149–178). Washington, DC: American Psychiatric Press.

Horowitz, M. J. (1986). *Stress response syndromes* (2nd ed.). Northvale, NJ: Jason Aronson.

Janoff-Bulman, R. (1992). *Shattered assumptions: Towards a new psychology of trauma.* New York: Free Press.

Jaycox, L., & Foa, E. B. (1996). Obstacles in implementing exposure therapy for PTSD: Case discussions and practical solutions. *Clinical Psychology and Psychotherapy, 3,* 176–184.

Kessler, R. C., Sonnega, A., Bromet, E., Hughes, M., & Nelson, C. B. (1995). Posttraumatic stress disorder in the National Comorbidity Survey. *Archives of General Psychiatry, 52,* 1048–1060.

Kline, N. A., Dow, B. M., Brown, S. A., & Matloff, J. L. (1994). Zoloft efficacy in depressed combat veterans with posttraumatic stress disorder. *American Journal of Psychiatry, 151,* 621.

Koenen, K., Hearst-Ikeda, D., Caulfield, M. B., & Muldar, R. (1997, November). *The relationship of anger and coping to PTSD symptoms in traumatized women.* Poster presented at the 31st annual meeting of the Association for Advancement of Behavior Therapy, Miami, FL.

Kosten, T. R., Frank, J. B., Dan, E., McDougle, C. J., & Giller, E. L. (1991). Pharmacotherapy for posttraumatic stress disorder using phenelzine or imipramine. *Journal of Nervous and Mental Disease, 179,* 336–370.

Kulka, R. A., Schlenger, W. E., Fairbank, J. A., Hough, R. L., Jordan, B. K., Marmar, C. R., & Weiss, D. S. (1990). *Trauma and the Vietnam war generation.* New York: Brunner/Mazel.

Livanou, M., Başoğlu, M., Marks, I. M., De Silva, P., Noshirvani, H., Lovell, K., & Thrasher, S. (2002). Beliefs, sense of control and treatment outcome in post-traumatic stress disorder. *Psychological Medicine, 32,* 157–165.

Londborg, P. D., Hegel, M. T., Goldstein, S., Goldstein, D., Himmelhoch, J. M., Maddock, R., Patterson, W. M., Rausch, J., & Farfel, G. M. (2001). Sertraline treatment of posttraumatic stress disorder: Results of 24 weeks of open-label continuation treatment. *Journal of Clinical Psychiatry, 62,* 325–331.

Marks, I., Lovell, K., Noshirvani, H., Livanou, M., & Thrasher, S. (1998). Treatment of posttraumatic stress disorder by exposure and/or cognitive restructuring. *Archives of General Psychiatry, 55,* 317–325.

Marshall, R. D., Beebe, K. L., Oldham, M., & Zaninelli, R. (2001). Efficacy and safety of paroxetine treatment of chronic PTSD: A fixed dosage, multicenter placebo controlled study. *American Journal of Psychiatry, 158,* 1982–1988.

Marshall, R. D., Schneier, F. R., Knight, B. A., Charles, B. G., Abbate, L. A., Goetz, D., Campeas, R., & Liebowitz, M. R. (1998). An open trial of paroxetine in patients with noncombat-related, chronic posttraumatic stress disorder. *Journal of Clinical Psychopharmacology, 18,* 10–18.

Martenyi, F., Brown, E., Zhang, H., Koke, S., & Prakash, A. (2002). Fluoxetine v. placebo in prevention of relapse in post-traumatic stress disorder. *British Journal of Psychiatry, 181,* 315–320.

Martenyi, F., Brown, E., Zhang, H., Prakash, A., & Koke, S. (2001, May). *Fluoxetine vs. placebo in posttraumatic stress disorder.* Poster presented at the meeting of the American Psychiatric Association, New Orleans, LA.

McDougle, C. J., Southwick, S. M., Charney, D. S., & St. James, R. L. (1991). An open trial of fluoxetine in the treatment of posttraumatic stress disorder. *Journal of Clinical Psychopharmacology, 11,* 325–327.

Mowrer, O. A. (1960). *Learning theory and behavior.* New York: Wiley.

Norris, F. H. (1992). Epidemiology of trauma: Frequency and impact of different potentially traumatic events on different demographic groups. *Journal of Consulting and Clinical Psychology, 60,* 409–418.

Paunovic, N., & Öst, L.-G. (2001). Cognitive behavioral therapy vs. exposure therapy in treatment of PTSD in refugees. *Behaviour Research and Therapy, 39,* 1183–1197.

Putnam, F. W. (1989). Pierre Janet and modern views of dissociation. *Journal of Traumatic Stress, 2,* 413–429.

Rapaport, M. H., Endicott J., & Clary, C. M. (2002). Posttraumatic stress disorder and quality of life: Results across 64 weeks of sertraline treatment. *Journal of Clinical Psychiatry, 63,* 59–65.

Resick, P. A., Nishith, P., & Weaver, T., Astin, M. C., & Feuer, C. A. (2002). A comparison of cognitive processing therapy, prolonged exposure, and a waiting condition for the treatment of posttraumatic stress disorder in female rape victims. *Journal of Consulting and Clinical Psychology, 70,* 867–879.

Resick, P. A., & Schnicke, M. K. (1992). Cognitive processing therapy for sexual assault victims. *Journal of Consulting and Clinical Psychology, 60,* 748–756.

Resnick, H. S., Kilpatrick, D. G., Dansky, B. S., Saunders, B. E., & Best, C. L. (1993). Prevalence of civilian trauma and posttraumatic stress disorder in a representative national sample of women. *Journal of Consulting and Clinical Psychology, 61,* 984–991.

Riggs, D. S., Dancu, C. V., Gershuny, B. S., Greenberg, D., & Foa, E. B. (1992). Anger and post-traumatic stress disorder in female crime victims. *Journal of Traumatic Stress, 5,* 613–625.

Riggs, D. S., Rothbaum, B. O., & Foa, E. B. (1995). A prospective examination of symptoms of posttraumatic stress disorder in victims of non-assault. *Journal of Interpersonal Violence, 2,* 201–214.

Rothbaum, B. O. (1997). A controlled study of eye movement desensitization and reprocessing in the treatment of posttraumatic stress disordered sexual assault victims. *Bulletin of the Menninger Clinic, 61,* 317–334.

Rothbaum, B. O., & Astin, M. (2001, December). *Prolonged Exposure vs. EMDR For PTSD Rape Victims.* Paper presented at the annual meeting of the International Society for Traumatic Stress Studies, New Orleans, LA.

Rothbaum, B. O., Foa, E. B., Riggs, D. S., Murdock, T., & Walsh, W. (1992). A prospective examination of post-traumatic stress disorder in rape victims. *Journal of Traumatic Stress, 5,* 455–475.

Rothbaum, B. O., Ninan, P. T., & Thomas, L. (1996). Sertraline in the treatment of rape victims with posttraumatic stress disorder. *Journal of Traumatic Stress, 9,* 865–871.

Shapiro, F. (1989). Eye movement desensitization: A new treatment for post-traumatic stress disorder. *Journal of Behavior Therapy and Experimental Psychiatry, 20,* 211–217.

Shapiro, F. (1995). *Eye movement desensitization and reprocessing: Basic principles, protocols, and procedures.* New York: Guilford Press.

Shay, J. (1992). Fluoxetine reduces explosiveness and elevates mood of Vietnam combat vets with PTSD. *Journal of Traumatic Stress, 5,* 97–101.

Steil, R., & Ehlers, A. (2000). Dysfunctional meaning of posttraumatic intrusions in chronic PTSD. *Behaviour Research and Therapy, 38,* 537–558.

Tarrier, N., Pilgrim, H., Sommerfield, C., Faragher, B., Reynolds, M., Graham, E., & Barrowclough, C. (1999). A randomized trial of cognitive therapy and imaginal exposure in the treatment of chronic posttraumatic stress disorder. *Journal of Consulting and Clinical Psychology, 67,* 13–18.

Tarrier, N., Sommerfield, C., Pilgrim, H., & Faragher, B. (2000). Factors associated with outcome of cognitive-behavioral treatment of chronic post-traumatic stress disorder. *Behaviour Research and Therapy, 38,* 191–202.

Taylor, S., & Koch, W. J. (1995). Anxiety disorders due to motor vehicle accidents: Nature and treatment. *Clinical Psychology Review, 15,* 721–738.

Taylor, S., Koch, W. J., Fecteau, G., Fedoroff, I. C., Thordarson, D. S., & Nicki, R. M. (2001). Posttraumatic stress disorder arising after road traffic collisions: Patterns of response to cognitive-behavioral therapy. *Journal of Consulting and Clinical Psychology, 63,* 541–551.

Taylor, S., Thordarson, D. S., Maxfield, L., Fedoroff, I. C., Lovell, K., & Ogrodniczuk, J. (2003). Comparative efficacy, speed, and adverse effects of three PTSD treatments: Exposure therapy, EMDR, and relaxation training. *Journal of Consulting and Clinical Psychology, 71,* 330–338.

Triffleman, E., Carroll, K., & Kellogg, S. (1999). Substance dependence posttraumatic stress disorder therapy. *Journal of Substance Abuse Treatment, 17,* 3–14.

Tucker, P., Zaninelli, R., Yehuda, R., Ruggerio, L., Dillingham, K., & Pitts, C. D. (2001). Paroxetine in the treatment of chronic posttraumatic stress disorder: Results of a placebo-controlled, flexible-dosage trial. *Journal of Clinical Psychiatry, 62,* 860–868.

van der Kolk, B. A., Dreyfuss, D., Michaels, M., Shera, D., Berkowitz, R., Fisler, R. E., & Saxe, G. N. (1994). Fluoxetine in posttraumatic stress disorder. *Journal of Clinical Psychiatry, 55,* 517–522.

van Minnen, A., Arntz, A., & Keijsers, G. P. J. (2002). Prolonged exposure in patients with chronic PTSD: Predictors of treatment outcome and dropout. *Behaviour Research and Therapy, 40,* 439–457.

Weaver, T., Kilpatrick, D. G., Resnick, H. S., Best, C. L., & Saunders, B. E. (1997). An examination of physical assault and childhood victimization histories within a national probability sample of women. In G. K. Kantor & J. L. Jasinski (Eds.), *Out of darkness: Contemporary perspectives on family violence* (pp. 34–46). Thousand Oaks, CA: Sage.

Woolfolk, R. L., & Grady, D. A. (1988). Combat-related posttraumatic stress disorder: Patterns of symptomatology in help-seeking Vietnam veterans. *Journal of Nervous and Mental Disorders, 176,* 107–111.

Yehuda, R., Marshall, R., Penkower, A., & Wong, C. (2002). Pharmacological treatments for posttraumatic stress disorder. In P. E. Nathan & J. M. Gorman (Eds.), *A guide to treatments that work* (pp. 411–445). New York: Oxford University Press.

6

Depression

KAREN ROWA
PETER J. BIELING
ZINDEL V. SEGAL

In recent years there has been increasing attention paid not only to achieving full treatment response among depressed clients but also to the prevention of relapse or recurrence once symptoms have remitted. A wealth of data suggests that when depression is "partially" as opposed to "fully" treated, risk for relapse remains very high (e.g., see Keller, 2003). These findings highlight the need to optimize treatment to help people achieve a full response. On the other hand, even after people are treated to full remission, risk for relapse or recurrence remains a substantial problem, especially for those who have experienced multiple previous episodes of depression. Acute treatments that include relapse prevention strategies as well as stand-alone relapse prevention programs are sorely needed.

In this chapter, we aim to address both issues by offering suggestions for improving outcome of cognitive-behavioral therapy (CBT) for depression as well as strategies for keeping treated people well. This chapter begins with an overview of empirically supported treatments for depression and an examination of predictors of outcome in CBT for depression. We then describe strategies to improve or optimize CBT to achieve a more robust response as well as situations in which modification to standard CBT are necessary. We conclude with an analysis of the predictors of relapse and recurrence and a variety of emerging strategies to prevent relapse.

OVERVIEW OF THE DISORDER

Major depressive disorder (MDD) is characterized by the presence of at least one major depressive episode, which involves at least 2 weeks of depressed mood or loss of interest accompanied by four or more other symptoms (American Psychiatric Association, 2000a). These other symptoms include changes in weight or appetite, dysregulated sleep, physical agitation or retardation, loss of energy, feelings of worthlessness or excessive guilt, difficulty concentrating or making decisions, and suicidal ideation, plan, or attempt. Depressive episodes can be categorized as mild, moderate, severe, or severe with psychotic features (i.e., the presence of delusions or hallucinations).

Symptoms of depression may also manifest themselves in a less severe but more long-standing constellation of symptoms than seen in MDD. Dysthymic disorder is characterized by at least 2 years of chronically depressed mood accompanied by at minimum two other symptoms of depression, including poor appetite or overeating, sleep disturbance, low energy, low self-esteem, poor concentration or difficulty making decisions, and feelings of hopelessness (American Psychiatric Association, 2000a).

Although the minimum length of illness necessary to receive a diagnosis of dysthymia is 2 years, the average duration of illness may be much longer (e.g., median duration of 5 years; Rounsaville, Shokomskas, & Prusoff, 1988). Due to the chronic and long-standing nature of dysthymia and its substantial comorbidity with Axis II disorders (Pepper, Klein, Anderson, Ouimette, & Lizardi, 1995), some have argued that this constellation of symptoms is better understood as a personality disorder than an Axis I disorder. The recognition of dsythymia as an Axis I or II disorder likely depends on whether one focuses on the similarity of symptoms to major depression or the early onset and chronic nature of the disorder.

Although MDD and dysthymia are separate diagnostic categories, they can coexist within an individual. This phenomenon is most commonly known as "double depression" and involves one or more major depressive episodes superimposed on a preexisting dysthymia. Double depression is distinct from chronic major depression, wherein an individual experiences the symptoms of a major depressive episode continuously for at least 2 years. The value of this diagnostic convention is unclear as some studies suggest better prognosis for the major depressive episode in double depression than for chronic MDD (Keller & Shapiro, 1982), while other studies have found no difference in response to treatment for double depression versus chronic major depression (Thase et al., 1994).

In recent years, there has been a growing recognition of another "subtype" of depression, subsyndromal or minor depression, which has implications for relapse rates. This phenomenon occurs when a person has clinically significant symptoms of depression but experiences fewer symptoms than are required for full diagnosis. The recognition of subsyndromal depression is important for several reasons. First, studies suggest that individuals with subsyndromal depression may be at higher risk for the development of major depression (e.g., Horwath, Johnson, Klerman, & Weissman, 1992). Further, individuals with subsyndromal depression often experience significant functional impairment, making this an important clinical phenomenon in its own right (Brent, Birmaher, Kolko, Baugher, & Bridge, 2001; Broadhead, Blazer, George, & Tse, 1990). Finally, residual depressive symptoms after treatment may leave people vulnerable to quicker and more frequent relapse (Judd et al., 1998), suggesting that treating most but not all the symptoms of depression may not be as useful as treating to complete remission.

OVERVIEW OF EMPIRICALLY SUPPORTED TREATMENTS

There are a number of empirically supported treatments for depression, including pharmacotherapy, stimulant treatments, and different forms of psychotherapy. Although results for individuals vary, pharmacotherapy and psychotherapy seem to yield similar rates of remission in MDD (e.g., Casacalenda, Perry, & Looper, 2002). Because a comprehensive review of all known efficacious treatment options for depression is beyond the scope of this chapter, interested readers are referred to Lambert and Davis (2002) as well as recent treatment guidelines from the Canadian Psychiatric Association (2001) and the American Psychiatric Association (2000b).

Medications

A number of medications have been shown to be effective in treating depression, with little evidence for the superiority of any one class of antidepressant over another (Mulrow et al., 1998). An extensive review of randomized controlled trials of antidepressant medication for MDD found that response rates were between 50 and 55% while response rates to placebo were 25–30% (Depression Guideline Panel, 1993). More recently, these results were replicated with studies involving newer antidepressants (Mulrow et al., 1998), though other reviews using different methodologies suggest there are actually negligible differences between antidepressant and placebo effects (Kirsch, Moore, Scoboria, & Nicholls, 2002). The Kirsch et al. (2002) study included all data submitted to the U.S. Food and Drug Administration for approval of particular antidepressants, ostensibly eliminating a potential publication bias inherent in other reviews and meta-analyses.

The first class of medications widely used in the treatment of depression was the tricyclic antidepressants. Though these medications are still in use for the treatment of depression, they are not as widely prescribed as newer forms of antidepressants due to less tolerable side effect profiles and lethality in overdose. Some of the newer empirically supported antidepressant medications include the selective serotonin reuptake inhibitors (SSRIs; e.g., fluoxetine), norepinephrine dopamine reuptake inhibitors (NDRIs; e.g., bupropion), selective serotonin norepinephrine reuptake inhibitors (SNRIs; e.g., venlafaxine), serotonin-$_2$ antagonists–reuptake inhibitors (SARIs; e.g., trazodone), and noradrenergic–specific serotonergic antidepressants (NaSSAs; e.g., mirtazapine). Studies have also supported the use of monoamine oxidase inhibitors (MAOIs) though this class of drugs is often used as a last option in treating depression. MAOIs can have potentially dangerous effects when combined with other prescription and nonprescription medications and foods containing tyramine. Thus, dietary restrictions are essential when taking MAOIs, and this has limited their use.

There is less research on the efficacy of antidepressants for dysthymia or subsyndromal depression. There seems to be growing evidence for the efficacy of medications for dysthymia, but there is little difference in response to medication and placebo for subsyndromal depression (Simon, 2002).

Although the antidepressant medications are generally useful in the treatment of depression, they are not universally effective and often require additional strategies to enhance response. One strategy is to combine two antidepressants if the first yields only a partial response. Antidepressants may also be augmented with other types of medications including lithium, thyroid hormone, buspirone, or atypical antipsychotics (e.g., olanzepine or risperidone) to boost their effectiveness (Bezchlibnyk-Butler & Jeffries, 2002). Pharmacotherapy can also be combined with psychotherapy in the treatment of depression. However, it is not clear that combination treatment is superior to either treatment alone (for a review, see Segal, Vincent, & Levitt, 2002). Some studies suggest that combining pharmacotherapy with CBT is more useful than either treatment alone (e.g., Keller et al., 2000; Thase et al., 1997) while other studies have found no difference between combined therapies and monotherapies (Depression Guideline Panel, 1993).

Stimulant Treatments

Before the advent of effective antidepressant medications, electroconvulsive therapy (ECT) was frequently used in the treatment of depression. Although its use remains somewhat controversial, research has shown ECT to be an effective treatment for depression, and some have argued that it deserves better status than a "last resort" treatment (Fink, 2001). ECT works by inducing a grand mal seizure, which is often followed by a reduction in depressive symptoms. Through a full course of ECT (i.e., 6–20 treatments), clients may experience a significant reduction or full remission of symptoms. Most clients typically take antidepressants after ECT to maintain gains, though continuation ECT after acute treatment is currently being investigated (see Andrade & Kurinji, 2002).

Another stimulant treatment for depression is transcranial magnetic stimulation (TMS), which has been studied only since the mid-1990s (George et al., 2001). TMS involves placing a magnet over a person's scalp to modify electrical signals in the brain, though the exact mechanism of action is unknown. Evidence for its efficacy has been equivocal. Some studies have found no difference between TMS and placebo groups (Manes et al., 2001), while other studies have found TMS to be superior in its antidepressant effects to placebo (Berman et al., 2000; George et al., 1997, 2000). Some authors have argued that the interpretation of results may be hampered by the variation of parameters across studies (e.g., intensity and location of stimulation) (Padberg et al., 2002). Thus, future studies that control for these variables will be helpful in assessing the utility of TMS as a treatment for depression.

Psychological Treatments

Cognitive therapy of depression, pioneered by Aaron T. Beck in the 1960s and 1970s, is a short-term, goal-oriented therapy that focuses on the relationship between thoughts, emotions, and behaviors. Individuals vulnerable to depression are thought to hold negative beliefs about themselves, others, the world, and the future, through which incoming information is filtered (Clark, Beck, & Alford, 1999). These negative core beliefs affect the content of situationally bound automatic thoughts, which have an impact on a person's affective and behavioral responses in a variety of situations.

There is a great deal of empirical evidence supporting the efficacy of cognitive therapy for depression. Several meta-analyses and qualitative reviews suggest that CBT is similar to or even slightly more efficacious than antidepressant medications in the treatment of depression (e.g., DeRubeis, Gelfand, Tang, & Simons, 1999). The National Institute of Mental Health (NIMH) Treatment of Depression Collaborative Research Program (TDCRP) found that CBT was similar in treatment outcome to interpersonal therapy or imipramine (Elkin et al., 1989). Much less research has evaluated the efficacy of CBT for dysthymic disorder, with initial findings suggesting a combination of CBT (or a variant of CBT termed "cognitive-behavioral analysis system of psychotherapy") and antidepressant medication is more effective than placebo (Keller et al., 2000; Ravindran et al., 1999).

Interpersonal therapy (IPT) was developed specifically for the treatment of depression and focuses on improving a variety of relational factors in a person's life. The content of sessions in IPT involves examination of one of four main interpersonal domains: unresolved grief, role disputes, role transition, or social isolation. There are a much smaller number of empirical studies evaluating the efficacy of IPT, but studies are very encouraging. For example, studies have suggested that IPT is equivalent to amitriptyline (Reynolds et al., 1996) and CBT (Elkin et al., 1989) in treating depression, though the combination of IPT and medication has been found to be superior to monotherapies (Reynolds et al., 1996). Similar to results of CBT for dysthymia, the combination of IPT and antidepressants seems to be more effective than either treatment alone for this disorder (Browne et al., 2002).

Behavior therapy (BT) for depression, often combined with cognitive strategies in a CBT protocol, focuses on increasing a person's activity level, especially activities that provide a source of positive reinforcement (e.g., mastery and pleasure activities). BT also focuses on identifying and modifying sources of punishment or lack of positive reinforcement in a person's life (e.g., social skills training to reduce the number of unsatisfying social exchanges).

Studies have supported the utility of BT for depression, finding it to be equivalent to amitriptyline and better than dynamic therapy and relaxation in one study (McLean & Hakstian, 1979) and equivalent to CBT in another (Jacobson et al., 1996). In the latter study, both BT and CBT showed symptom improvement at the end of treatment, and between 50 and 65% of participants maintained gains across a 24-month follow-up (Gortner, Gollan, Dobson, & Jacobson, 1998).

PREDICTORS OF TREATMENT OUTCOME

How Do We Know Who Will Benefit from Cognitive-Behavioral Therapy?

Although the volume of studies on the outcome of CBT and other treatments for depression is large, there is much less information on the predictors of successful outcome using CBT or other psychotherapeutic approaches. This question is of practical and theoretical importance, allowing better informed decisions about the provision of particular services in specific form for particular clients (Paul, 1967).

Severity and Chronicity of Depression

One of the most well-studied set of predictors of outcome are variables related to the characteristics and history of the individual's depression. For example, several studies suggest that more severe pretreatment depression predicts poorer response to CBT (see Hamilton & Dobson, 2002, for a review). Another predictor of poor outcome in CBT is the chronicity of a person's depression. Evidence is fairly consistent that chronically depressed individuals show poorer response to treatment than do more acutely depressed individuals (Hamilton & Dobson, 2002; Thase et al., 1994). Results for recurrent major depression are less consistent, with some studies finding that recurrent depression is associated with poorer outcome (Thase, 1992), while other studies have found no relationship (e.g., Jarrett, Eaves, Brannemann, & Rush, 1991) or a tendency for individuals with recurrent depression to respond favorably to CBT (Sotsky et al., 1991).

Comorbidity

Patterns of comorbidity may also contribute to treatment outcome. Depression is highly comorbid with anxiety disorders, eating disorders, substance use disorders, and personality disorders (Enns et al., 2001). Despite high rates of comorbidity, there is little research that can meaningfully address the degree to which comorbid conditions affect treatment outcome as comorbid disorders are often exclusion criteria in controlled trials. From the existing studies, results suggest either no differences in outcome (Gelhart & King, 2001;

Woody, McLean, Taylor, & Koch, 1999) or that individuals with double depression and comorbid anxiety may do less well than those with just major depression or dysthymia (Gelhart & King, 2001).

Depression is also associated with high rates of personality disorders. A review by Hirschfeld (1999) suggested that the rates of Axis II comorbidity may be between 41% and 81% for samples of depressed individuals. The presence of personality disorders or features has a negative impact on outcome for psychotherapy (including CBT) (Ball, Kearney, Wilhelm, Dewhurst-Savellis, & Barton, 2000; Hardy et al., 1995; Merrill, Tolbert, & Wade, 2003; Pilkonis & Frank, 1988; Shea et al., 1990). For example, in the NIMH TDCRP, individuals with personality disorders were more likely to have residual depressive symptoms at the end of treatment (Shea et al., 1990). Kuyken, Kurzer, DeRubeis, Beck, and Brown (2001) found that stronger avoidant and paranoid beliefs were associated with poorer CBT outcome.

Further research has examined the impact of individual differences in universal personality traits such as neuroticism (i.e., the disposition to experience emotional instability and negative emotions) on treatment outcome. Clients with higher neuroticism scores do less well in a variety of treatments (Duggan, Lee, & Murray, 1990) and take longer to achieve remission (O'Leary & Costello, 2001).

Few studies have examined the impact of comorbid substance use disorders or eating disorders on treatment for depression in adults. However, one study of CBT for depressed adolescents found that comorbid substance use disorders were associated with a longer time to recovery (72 weeks vs. 10 weeks for adolescents with just depression) and lower global assessment of functioning scores at the end of treatment (Rohde, Clarke, Lewinsohn, Seeley, & Kaufman, 2001), once again suggesting the interfering role of comorbid conditions on the treatment of depression.

Characteristics of the Affected Individual

A number of demographic variables have been examined to understand their impact on outcome in treatment of depression. Although many studies suggest that younger people do better in CBT (e.g., Sotsky et al., 1991) and other structured therapies (Ezquiaga, Garcia, Pallares, & Bravo, 1999), other studies have found that age has no predictive validity (Jarrett et al., 1991). Moreover, some studies suggest that older adults (i.e., 65 and older) benefit from CBT in a comparable way to younger individuals (Hamilton & Dobson, 2002). It is also important to distinguish age at treatment from age at onset of depression, as younger age at onset may be more predictive of negative outcome than age at time of treatment (Belsher & Costello, 1988).

One demographic variable that is clearly linked with outcome in CBT is marital status. With little exception, individuals who are married do better in CBT (Jarrett et al., 1991) and are less likely to relapse after treatment (Thase, 1992) than unmarried, separated, or divorced individuals. However, it may not be marriage per se that has such powerful effects but degree of satisfaction with one's marriage (Whisman, 2001). In related observations, more severe depressive symptoms were related to lower levels of social support and less satisfaction with that support (Ezquiaga et al., 1999). Thus, being married, and, more important, being satisfied with that relationship, is associated with better outcomes in therapy.

Marital status may also be associated with another predictor of outcome, interpersonal style. Individuals who demonstrate fewer interpersonal problems (e.g., avoidance or interpersonal distress) may have both a higher rate of satisfactory marriages as well as better outcomes in CBT and other therapies. Indeed, distal variables such as strong friendships in adolescence are predictive of recovery from chronic major depression (Coryell, Endicott, & Keller, 1990), indicating a role of social support that may be mediated by interpersonal style. Some studies have found that high levels of interpersonal distress as measured by the Inventory of Interpersonal Problems (IIP) were characteristic of both positive responders and negative responders (Mohr et al., 1990) and others have found no impact of interpersonal problems on treatment outcome (Horowitz, Rosenberg, Baer, Ureno, & Villaseñor, 1988). A more recent study found that an underinvolved, avoidant style may be related to posttreatment severity of depression through the therapeutic alliance. Underinvolved clients were less able to form a strong alliance with their therapist, which in turn predicted outcome (Hardy et al., 2001).

Cognitive Vulnerability

There is a growing interest in the role of cognitive vulnerability in predicting treatment outcome. The most frequently studied construct has been dysfunctional attitudes. According to the cognitive model of depression, dysfunctional attitudes, typically assessed by the Dysfunctional Attitudes Scale (DAS; Weissman, 1979), play a central role in contributing to and maintaining depressive affect.

Blatt, Quinlan, Pilkonis, and Shea (1995) found that higher pretreatment perfectionism scores on the DAS predicted more impairment across multiple measures of posttreatment adjustment and were linked to higher dropout rates. More generally, higher pretreatment levels of dysfunctional attitudes have been associated with poorer outcome and greater chance of relapse following successful treatment (see Hamilton & Dobson, 2002, for a review). This finding has been replicated both for individual and group CBT as well as for response to medication and placebo (Peselow, Robins, Block, Barouche, & Fieve, 1990). Relatedly, reductions in DAS scores later in treatment predict better outcomes in CBT (Furlong & Oei, 2002), and the DAS predicts outcome over and above the variance accounted for by nonspecific therapy factors (Oei & Shuttlewood, 1997).

Some authors have suggested that it is not the presence of dysfunctional attitudes that will most strongly affect treatment outcome but the interaction of dysfunctional attitudes and stressful life events. Although there have been some inconsistent results on this topic, several studies have found support for the interaction of preexisting dysfunctional attitudes with a negative life event in predicting a worsening of depressive symptoms (e.g., Joiner, Metalsky, Lew, & Klocek, 1999). Following from these ideas, some authors have argued that individuals showing evidence of a negative life event and elevated dysfunctional attitudes should preferentially respond to CBT because CBT is designed to target these issues. Research on this hypothesis has produced mixed results. In one study, individuals with high levels of dysfunctional attitudes and co-occurring negative life events responded most successfully to CBT, along with individuals with low levels of dysfunctional attitudes and no negative life events (Simons, Gordon, Monroe, & Thase, 1995). However, Spangler, Simons, Monroe, and Thase (1997) did not replicate this result, finding that CBT was effective regardless of participants' pretreatment DAS scores or the presence of life events.

In sum, few demographic characteristics of clients reliably predict outcome of CBT. There is good evidence that being married and having a later age at onset of depression may be associated with more successful outcomes. In addition, the presence of strong dysfunctional beliefs may be a negative prognostic indicator for CBT, while change in dysfunctional beliefs during therapy is associated with a more robust and lasting response to intervention.

Characteristics of Cognitive-Behavioral Treatment That Affect Outcome

In addition to features that all psychotherapies share, CBT has a number of unique characteristics. A hallmark of CBT is the expectation that clients will complete homework assignments between therapy sessions. CBT is offered in both group and individual formats, a trend that is increasingly popular and distinct from some schools of psychotherapy that only offer therapy in an individual format. Like most other therapies, CBT also relies on a strong working alliance, a rationale for understanding one's problems, a framework for change, and interpersonal factors such as empathy and support.

Early studies have clearly emphasized the importance of homework completion and the therapist's reactions to homework tasks in CBT. Using retrospective therapist ratings of homework compliance, Persons, Burns, and Perloff (1988) demonstrated that homework completers did significantly better in therapy than did those who did not complete homework, and this was especially true for severely depressed individuals who completed homework. Similarly, Neimeyer and Feixas (1990) showed that CBT that included homework assignments was more effective than CBT without homework. Although most studies on homework compliance in CBT are correlational in nature, Burns and Spangler (2000) used structural equation modeling and demonstrated a potential causal relation between homework completion and a reduction in depressive symptoms. Thus, homework compliance, as rated by retrospective reports (Persons et al., 1988), therapists (Addis & Jacobson, 2000), or independent raters (Bryant, Simons, & Thase, 1999), is associated with better outcomes in CBT for depression.

In addition to homework compliance, researchers have been interested in the client's acceptance of the treatment rationale as a predictor of outcome. A greater acceptance of the treatment rationale may encourage greater investment in homework assignments or it may have unique effects on outcome. In an early study, Fennell and Teasdale (1987) found that clients' positive reactions to homework assignments predicted a faster response to CBT. Reactions to homework likely reflect an understanding of and investment in the treatment rationale. Addis and Jacobson (2000) found that early acceptance of the rationale made a unique and independent contribution to change in treatment and ultimate outcome, even when homework compliance ratings were included in the analyses.

The Therapeutic Alliance

It is an accepted maxim that the therapeutic alliance has a significant effect on the progress and outcome of treatment. Research on both CBT (e.g., Castonguay, Goldfried, Wiser, Raue, & Hayes, 1996; Gaston, Thompson, Gallagher, Cournoyer, & Gagnon, 1998; Krupnick et al., 1996; Persons & Burns, 1985; Safran & Waller, 1991; Stiles, Agnew-Davies, Hardy, Barkham, & Shapiro, 1998) and other forms of psychotherapy (Horvath & Symonds, 1991) have suggested that a positive alliance is correlated with positive outcomes. However, these studies have been criticized for failing to control for symptom change that occurred before the alliance was assessed, thus confounding the temporal relationship between these constructs. When this confound has been addressed, results have suggested that positive changes in symptoms may contribute to a better therapeutic alliance, rather than vice versa (Feeley, DeRubeis, & Gelfand, 1999). In another study, the perceived agreement between client and therapist on the goals and tasks of therapy predicted change in dysfunctional beliefs in CBT, but the bond between client and therapist did not (Rector, Zuroff, & Segal, 1999). On the other hand, a strong therapeutic bond seemed to provide the context in which changes in dysfunctional beliefs resulted in significant symptom reduction. Taken together, results from these studies suggest that both the connection between client and therapist and their agreement on the "work" of therapy may be important in facilitating change, while symptom change helps to foster a strong bond between client and therapist.

Studies have examined the relative efficacy of CBT for depression when offered in group or individual formats. Group CBT is often used as it is assumed to be cost-effective with the additional benefit of providing a support network for participants. Studies generally suggest that group and individual CBT for depression are similarly effective, and both are more effective than no treatment (Robinson, Berman, & Neimeyer, 1990).

Factors That Do Not Affect Outcome

There are a number of variables that do not show any relationship to outcome despite "clinical lore" and anecdotal evidence. For example, practitioners have long questioned whether the gender of the therapist and/or the gender match between therapist and client is of importance. Research from other models of therapy is equivocal, with most studies suggesting that there may be an impact of therapist gender on client satisfaction but little impact on outcome (e.g., Jones, Krupnick, & Kerig, 1987). In a study on gender issues in CBT, IPT, medication, or placebo, Zlotnick, Elkin, and Shea (1998) found no impact of gender of therapist or match between therapist and client on outcome, attrition, or the client's perception of therapist empathy across all therapeutic conditions. Thus, preliminary studies on this issue within a CBT framework have provided no evidence for the effects of therapist gender on outcome.

Gender itself does not consistently predict outcome of CBT. Scant research has examined this question despite the clear gender bias in prevalence of depression and research suggesting that being female is a predictor of recurrence of depression (Lee & Murray, 1988; Mueller et al., 1999). Research on other therapy modalities has demonstrated gender differences in response to type of therapy (Ogrondniczuk, Piper, Joyce, & McCallum, 2001) as well as across various therapies (Frank et al., 2002; Katon et al., 2002). However, in CBT, men and women seem to respond similarly (Thase et al., 1994).

Intelligence also does not predict outcome in CBT (Haaga, DeRubeis, Stewart, & Beck, 1991). In fact, a study of fluid intelligence (i.e., the ability to reason through or solve novel problems) in older adults with anxiety disorders found no relation between scores on a test of fluid intelligence and outcome in CBT (Doubleday, King, & Papageorgiou, 2002). These results require replication in a population of depressed individuals but suggest that intelligence likely does not predict outcome.

PRACTICAL STRATEGIES FOR IMPROVING OUTCOME

Our review of predictors has several implications for future research and current practice. First, there are many contradictory findings across studies when investigating predictors of outcome, and in some areas of interest there is little empirical research (e.g., the impact of all types of comorbidity on outcome; gender differences in outcome). More research is needed to discern whether these factors are reliably associated with outcome.

Second, there are a number of predictors of poor outcome in CBT that clinicians can do little about at the time of assessment or treatment initiation (e.g., age of onset and chronicity of depression). Although these variables may lower the probability of a robust or sustained response to CBT, we have inadequate data to determine any individual's likelihood of benefiting from treatment. In addition, these same factors may also predict poor response to other known efficacious treatments, including medication and combination treatments. Thus, the clinician is faced with difficult choices when individuals have a number of "negative" demographic predictors. The most reasonable strategy may be to provide a time-limited course of CBT with a view of creating as much improvement as possible and understanding that it may be unreasonable to expect full remission. However, because full remission is the most optimal outcome to protect against relapse, an initial, time-limited course of treatment may need to be followed by additional treatment or booster sessions for this subgroup of clients. Of course, expectations are important not only for therapists but also for the client. Even when there are a number of negative indicators of outcome, it will still be important to instill hope for improvement and motivate the client to try strategies to reduce impairment and severity of symptoms, tempered by the reality that therapy may not always be a "magic bullet."

For the purposes of this chapter, the most relevant set of predictors of CBT outcome is one that can be modified to some extent before or during therapy. Next, we describe these modifiable factors and some practical suggestions for improving outcome in CBT.

Diagnostic Assessment and Suitability Screening

Although a thorough description of diagnostic and assessment issues is beyond the scope of this chapter, a complete diagnostic screening is crucial prior to CBT. A thorough workup on Axes I and II can facilitate the selection of the most appropriate treatment methods and allow the clinician to ascertain whether comorbid conditions are present that might affect outcome.

In addition to these basic diagnostic screens, a suitability interview is an important tool to ascertain a number of predictors of outcome prior to commencing treatment. With this tool, the "fit" between client and the treatment modality can be assessed. Suitability interviewing may also have the added benefit of enhancing a client's readiness for a brief, focused treatment such as CBT. In the process of completing a suitability assessment for CBT, clients may make significant progress in understanding their depression simply by answering questions about their compatibility with the cognitive model. For example, clients might compare their own thinking process to the model described by the therapist and thereby come to a new understanding about how their thoughts "drive" their depressive affect and behavior.

In their book on interpersonal factors in depression, Safran and Segal (1990) provide a suitability interview for CBT that rates suitability across 10 dimensions. These include (1) the client's ability to notice automatic thoughts, (2) the client's awareness of emotions and ability to discriminate between various emotional states, (3) the degree to which clients accept responsibility for change, (4) the compatibility between clients' understanding of their problem and the cognitive model, (5) the ability of client and therapist to form an initial therapeutic alliance, (6) the ability of clients to have trusting relationships in their lives, (7) the duration of difficulties with depression, (8) the degree to which various disruptive processes (e.g., intellectualization, overinclusiveness) may interfere with therapy, (9) the ability of the client to maintain focus on a particular problem, and (10) the client's optimism that change is possible. Scores on this instrument have shown moderate correlations with both client and therapist ratings of success in treatment (Safran & Segal, 1990).

Some authors also advocate a self-screening device before therapy is initiated, especially in outpatient clinics that may offer a host of treatment choices. This process may increase the likelihood of identifying motivated clients who are interested in being involved in CBT, while screening out clients who are not yet ready or who prefer a different model of intervention. For example, Westra, Boardman, and Moran-Tynski (2000) describe a process in an anxiety disorders clinic in which clients were asked to complete a decisional balance exercise about attending a CBT group and then contact the clinic if they were interested in moving forward with therapy. By using these two simple steps, the authors reported a drop in their first appointment no-show rate from 35% to 0% and found that 96% of candidates who were interviewed for CBT were suitable for the program, compared to 73% before these procedures were implemented.

Overall, suitability screening can be seen to involve two steps: (1) a client-centered step in which the client selects CBT as his or her preferred treatment and (2) a clinician-centered step in which the clinician attempts to determine whether the client is ready for CBT and is, in fact, likely to benefit. The first of the suitability steps is to ascertain the client's interest in and desire to pursue CBT. This is clearly less relevant when treatment is offered in a "CBT only" setting to which clients have self-referred because they have learned about CBT and believe it would be useful for them. However, when referrals come from other sources (e.g., a family physician recommends CBT), or when clients present to clinics that offer multiple treatment modalities, educating the client about the unique benefits of CBT will be a very useful first step. The work of Westra et al. (2000) suggests that going a step further and having the client take some responsibility for initiating treatment may increase attendance and compliance rates. Self-selection to CBT, which likely involves a host of factors such as the client's level of motivation and beliefs about the value of "talking therapy," should be bolstered by more concerted screening involving the treating clinician.

Finally, it should be recognized that, even in randomized controlled trials with carefully screened and selected participants who presumably are reasonably suitable for CBT, response is not universal (i.e., 51% of participants treated with CBT achieved remission in the NIMH TDCRP; Elkin et al., 1989), and a significant minority of clients will still have quite troubling symptoms at the end of the trial. Thus, the approaches we describe next could be useful for clinicians in two ways: as methods to improve response in those less suitable for CBT or as enhancements for suitable clients in order to help them achieve full remission.

Motivational Issues in Treatment

A number of the modifiable predictors of negative outcome outlined previously may be related to the client's struggles to commit to therapy and maintain motivation to complete the tasks of therapy. In their seminal work on change processes, Prochaska and DiClemente (1984) outlined the stages of readiness for change in substance-abusing populations. This work has subsequently been expanded for use with other populations and has spawned a body of literature that is useful to consider when dealing with motivational issues both before and during therapy. According to Prochaska (2000), there are six stages of change. In *precontemplation*, people do not recognize that they have a problem, have little interest in changing their behavior, and are unlikely to seek treatment. At the *contemplation* stage, people realize they have a problem, may seek advice about it, but are not ready to act and do not know how to go about making changes. In *preparation*, people are ready to make changes, and in *action*, people are making the desired changes. After making these changes, people work at sustaining changes and not relapsing in the *maintenance* stage, and finally, if changes are maintained with no further effort, people have reached the *termination* stage. There are numerous instruments designed to assess stages of change that are widely available and applicable to different problems and settings. One excellent source of these measures is the University of Rhode Island's Cancer Prevention Research Center (1991). These measures provide information about the client's current stage of change.

Knowing a client's current stage of change can be used to enhance motivation for CBT prior to the commencement of treatment. Westra and Phoenix (2003) have developed a protocol for motivational enhancement therapy for anxiety based on work by Miller and Rollnick (1991), and many of these ideas could be useful when working with a depressed client. The goal of their five-session protocol is to facilitate readiness for change in CBT by helping the client to examine and become aware of the problem, its impact on one's life, its impact on important others, and its consistency with valued goals. To do this, therapists are encouraged to maintain a neutral stance about the necessity of change, resisting the urge to embrace the "pro-change" role. Wherever possible, the client is encouraged to voice the arguments for change.

Borrowing from Westra and Phoenix's protocol as well as the work of Prochaska and colleagues, motivational enhancement sessions could include (1) education about the stages of change and identification of the client's current stage; (2) listing the pros and cons of both the *status quo* and changing it (i.e., accomplishing some valued goals); (3) brainstorming other problems for which the client was able to make important changes and borrowing ideas and inspiration from those experiences; (4) having the therapist and client switch roles (i.e., have the client take a pro-change stance with the therapist playing the devil's advocate, forcing the client to think of strong arguments for change); and (5) having the client elaborate on the most important personal costs of depression. For the latter strategy, it would be important to ensure that clients know that if they wish, many of these consequences may be averted with successful treatment.

Not only do motivational issues manifest themselves at the outset of therapy, but they may also emerge over the course of CBT. For example, clients may make initial gains but then fail to complete homework or use newly acquired coping skills when encountering a difficult problem they are ambivalent about changing. At this point, it may be useful to call on some of the aforementioned strategies in reference to the particular problem at hand.

Enhancing Cognitive-Behavioral Techniques

Studies have suggested that the provision of CBT-specific tools and techniques early in therapy predicts a greater reduction in depression (Feeley et al., 1999). Thus, on a practical note, therapists can ensure that early therapy sessions include both information gathering for their conceptualization of the problem as well as instruction on how to identify, evaluate, and modify dysfunctional cognitions, schedule mastery and pleasure activities, set goals, and so on. Clearly, CBT includes sharing a set of tools, or a technology, for modifying one's mood or behavior, and these tools should be emphasized early and often.

Length of treatment may also affect outcome. Studies suggest that longer courses of CBT for depression are associated with improvements even for severely depressed clients (e.g., Thase, Simons, Cahalane, McGeary, & Harden, 1991). Following from this, outcome may be enhanced simply by providing a longer course of treatment, depending on pretreatment severity. Thus, although studies suggest that it is the provision of tools early in therapy that enhances outcome, increasing the length of treatment in severe depression may provide the opportunity for repetition and rehearsal of strategies for this more difficult population.

Compliance with Treatment

Homework

As discussed earlier, a clear predictor of outcome in CBT for depression is homework completion but, more substantially, the integration and discussion of homework in the session. Clearly, homework needs to play a central role in CBT. In fact, one study found that the beneficial effects of homework completion were more pronounced for those with more severe depression (Persons et al., 1988), suggesting that improving homework completion may even help clients with refractory depression. However, getting clients to complete homework can be a challenge. There are a number of strategies to enhance the probability that a client will complete homework tasks (e.g., J. Beck, 1995; Greenberger & Padesky, 1995). When homework is assigned, it is useful to provide a clear rationale for why the particular task is being assigned. Early in therapy, this rationale may be more didactic, but later in therapy, the task would ideally be suggested by the client or determined collaboratively by client and therapist. It is often useful to actually begin the homework assignment during the therapy session. Once again, this is especially useful early in therapy or if the assignment involves a new form or a newly developed skill. Clearly, homework that is "disembodied" from the session (e.g., a therapist handing out a homework sheet as the client leaves the session without explaining what to do or why) has the potential to be confusing or misunderstood. Even worse, the tie between the session and the assigned homework can become so tenuous that the intent of the exercise may be lost on the client.

It may also be useful to anticipate any obstacles that may arise as the client attempts to complete the assigned homework. Clients may become concerned that they do not understand how to complete the assignment, they will not have the time or opportunity to complete the task, or it will make them feel worse to focus on their symptoms (J. Beck, 1995). Once potential obstacles are identified, therapist and client can troubleshoot these difficulties. For example, the therapist can clarify any confusing instructions, normalize the intensification of symptoms at the start of therapy, provide further rationale for why the assignment might be useful, and help the client rearrange his or her schedule to better accommodate homework tasks. If homework involves another person, the therapist can help the client come up with a backup plan if that person is not available.

Once clients have completed homework, it is important that it be reviewed in the very next session. In a study of homework compliance, Bryant et al. (1999) found that therapist review of previous homework was associated with greater compliance on subsequent homework assignments. By reviewing the homework, the therapist communicates its importance to the therapy.

Treatment Rationale

Clients may have misgivings about the rationale for CBT, including how this model of illness fits their experience. It is clear that acceptance of the rationale enhances outcome (Addis & Jacobson, 2000), and thus it is an important area on which to focus. In addition to using a suitability interview to assess and enhance the rationale for CBT at the outset of treatment, difficulties with the rationale can be elucidated by asking for feedback from the client. Difficulties with comprehension of the model can be addressed by using visual aids (e.g., drawing diagrams of the interaction between thoughts, feelings, and behaviors and writing out a basic conceptualization diagram), assigning reading materials (e.g., chapters from a workbook such as *Mind Over Mood*; Greenberger & Padesky, 1995), or using analogies. One analogy that we have found useful is to liken the examination of automatic thoughts to listening to both sides of an argument. Most clients will readily say it is not that useful to hear only one side of an argument when making a decision, so listening to both sides (i.e., evidence for and against the "hot" cognition) is the most reasonable course of action.

At times, a client's model of his or her illness may interfere with acceptance of the rationale for CBT. Clients may have a variety of explanations for why they are depressed, and they are likely to get a variety of messages from many sources about the causes of depression. A particular obstacle is in place when the client believes in an exclusively biological or genetic model of his or her illness (e.g., depression is the result of a chemical imbalance). A mistaken corollary of such a view is that only a biological manipulation can therefore result in change. In situations such as this, the provision of psychoeducation about the biopsychosocial model of depression may be useful. Critically, the biopsychosocial model has the advantage of being broadly inclusive, so it is unlikely to make the client's view "wrong" and the therapist's view "right." Thus, therapists are not likely to find themselves in unproductive, and alliance-threatening, debates about the causes of depression. Instead, CBT simply becomes one useful route into a complex and interconnected system. In addition, research findings on regional changes in brain functioning after CBT may be useful for the client to consider (e.g., Goldapple et al., 2004). Comparing depression to a chronic medical illness (e.g., diabetes) that requires both medication and other, more behavioral management strategies might also offer a useful analogy. Clients may be hesitant to try a psychological treatment for what they consider a biological problem because the mechanism of change does not make sense to them. However, there are many treatments we readily use that work but for which the mechanism is unclear or counterintuitive. For example, aspirin relieves headaches, but the mechanism of its action on pain sensations remains elusive. Similarly, behavioral interventions make a difference in many problems that clearly have biological underpinnings. For example, for that same headache, reducing stimulation by lying in a darkened room may work as well as aspirin. Again, the mechanism of action is unclear, but the intervention is no less effective. The metaphor could be extended to rehabilitation exercises for a broken bone. Full recovery would not be possible if the bone was not properly set, but it also would not be possible if there was no rehabilitation effort to gradually and planfully regain the ability to use that part of the body. By explaining that CBT can be effective for symptoms of depression, even if the cause is multidetermined, the therapist may place the client in a better position to suspend disbelief and use the techniques with an open mind. To some extent, the entire process of CBT becomes an experiment to collect relevant data.

Cognitive-Behavioral Therapy for Comorbid Conditions

Because comorbidity is almost normative in depression and is often associated with reduced treatment response, it is important to address the issue of common co-occurring disorders. Comorbid depression and anxiety disorders are the most likely combination, and these can be addressed in two main ways: (1) sequential treatment of each disorder and (2) combined treatment for both disorders. Sequential treatment involves treating one problem in isolation and then addressing the next problem, once the primary problem has successfully remitted. In sequential treatment, it is essential to determine which problem needs to be addressed first. Some useful questions to address include the following: Which problem does the client want to deal with first? Which problem is most impairing and distressing? Does one problem need to be dealt with first before the other can even be addressed? Which problem would result in the most benefit if it were treated successfully? Are the two disorders functionally related, so that treatment of one might influence the course of the other? For example, a client presenting with comorbid depression and panic disorder may want to work on his or her depression but cannot reliably attend appointments due to interference from panic attacks. In this case, it may be most useful to treat the panic attacks first and then proceed to treat the depression. Some studies suggest that sequential treatment of comorbid panic and depression yields similar outcomes to treatment of panic (McLean, Woody, Taylor, & Koch, 1998), and there is no carryover effect of the treatment of panic on symptoms of depression (Woody et al., 1999). Thus, sequential treatment may simply be like treating each problem in isolation, with no drawbacks *or* benefits from addressing the other condition. On the other hand, preliminary research suggests that the order of sequential treatment may be important, at least in treating depression and comorbid panic. In a case series, Chudzik, McCabe, Bieling, Antony, and Swinson (2003) found evidence for the value of treating panic symptoms before depression. They noted clinical examples in which participants could not complete behavioral activation exercises because of interference from panic attacks.

Treatment of depression with comorbid anxiety can also involve some amalgamation of treatment protocols and strategies within a single treatment. For example, if avoidance is getting in the way of behavioral activation exercises, the concept of exposure may be introduced to help the client systematically expose him- or herself to the feared situations. The client may also begin scheduling mastery and pleasure activities, addressing inactivation due to depression and avoidance due to anxiety. Cognitive strategies, common to CBT for both anxiety and depression, can be used to address both the client's fearful and depressogenic cognitions.

Realistic Depression

It is not uncommon in CBT to find that there is truth in a client's automatic thoughts or interpretations. Further, many clients who present for treatment are immersed in difficult and stressful life situations (e.g., health problems, marital difficulties, and financial problems). When faced with these circumstances in therapy, a therapist's first job is to help the client disentangle truth from distortion, even in the context of terrible life conditions. Indeed, people under duress are prone to cognitive distortions. For example, Moorey (1996) points out that a common or natural reaction to the death of a loved one is to feel sad and think about how we will miss the loved one. On the other hand, thoughts such as "I'll never be happy again" may be overgeneralizations that are characteristic of a depressed state. By encouraging clients to consider evidence and alternatives for all their automatic thoughts, they will be better able to challenge distortions and identify "realistic" thoughts that need further attention.

In the case of thoughts and circumstances that are truly difficult, the therapist can help by providing support, exploring ways of coping, facilitating adjustment to difficult events, and helping the client bring meaning to difficulties. For example, Moorey (1996) suggests that it can sometimes be useful to help a client learn to distract himself from thoughts that are not adaptive. Further, if a client has undergone an acute stressor (loss of a job, death of a loved one, diagnosis of an illness, etc.), it may be useful to examine beliefs and assumptions that hinder the process of adjustment. Moorey (1996) described a client who had recently been diagnosed with cancer who believed that she should not burden others with her problems. By withholding her feelings and difficulties from others, she only increased her own feelings of depression, isolation, and hopelessness. The focus of CBT could be to examine the utility of this belief and conduct behavioral experiments about the effect of increased self-disclosure.

Cognitive-Behavioral Therapy for Persons with Cognitive or Language Difficulties

CBT can be an effective therapy for people with mild cognitive deficits, with some practical modifications. Expectations for material to be covered in sessions and homework may need to be tempered. Similarly, concepts can be simplified. For example, if the person has difficulty providing numerical ratings of moods, they can instead use labels such as "low," "medium," and "high." If the process of evidence gathering is too challenging for a client to complete outside the therapist's presence, the therapist and client can come up with coping statements or balanced thoughts that can be written down for the client to review on his own. Clients with cognitive deficits will also benefit from the repetition of ideas and concepts, in language that is as simple as possible.

If the client and therapist have different first languages and language matching is not possible, visual aids (e.g., pictures of faces with different expressions to assess mood) can be extremely helpful. When assessing any obstacles to homework, it may be important to consider whether language difficulties may interfere with written assignments (i.e., if verbal skills in a particular language are stronger than written skills). If this is the case, clients can be invited to complete assignments in their first language, then explain their work to the therapist in the therapist's language. Explanations of CBT strategies can likewise be translated into the language of the client. It is often possible, with careful and slow explanations, to have a client come up with a term in his or her first language that expresses a CBT principle. This will make it easier for the client to remember and experience the technique. Many CBT resources are now available in a number of languages, and such materials are readily available using the Internet. It is especially useful for therapists if a manual they have used has been translated to another language.

Ways to Improve the Alliance in Cognitive-Behavioral Therapy

A solid therapeutic alliance is fundamental in CBT. Although practical ways to improve the alliance have not received a great deal of empirical attention in the CBT literature, they have been a source of interest in other forms of psychotherapy. A recent review of this topic by Ackerman and Hilsenroth (2003) highlighted (1) personal attributes of the therapist and (2) therapy techniques that positively influence the therapeutic alliance. Personal variables include attributes that convey a sense that the client is important (e.g., warmth, interest, and alertness), that the therapist knows what he or she is doing (e.g., experience and confidence), and that the therapy session is a safe place to discuss and process the client's problems (e.g., honesty and respect). One study suggested that therapist experience is associated with a stronger alliance because more experienced therapists are better at establishing the goals of treatment and making progress toward these goals (Mallinckrodt & Nelson, 1991). This result suggests that a focus on setting clear goals, a crucial component of CBT for depression, should have the added benefit of strengthening the alliance. Further, therapist flexibility is associated with a stronger alliance, suggesting that the ability of a therapist to shift plans and set a flexible agenda will be important.

Many of the therapy techniques associated with a strong alliance are encouraged within a CBT model. For example, being active and attending to a client's experience is a fundamental part of CBT and has been shown to foster the alliance. The collaborative efforts of therapists have been useful in building an alliance, including behaviors such as communicating hope, developing therapy goals, noting progress toward goals, being open-minded, and working with clients (Ackerman, Hilsenroth, Baity, & Blagys, 2000; Luborsky, Crits-Christoph, Alexander, Margolis, & Cohen, 1983). Although these studies involved a therapy other than CBT, these techniques can also be emphasized in CBT. In a study that focused on CBT for cocaine dependence, useful techniques for alliance building included guided discovery, focusing on important thoughts, and homework (Crits-Christoph et al., 1998). Thus, therapist activities that suggest support facilitate a sense of collaboration, and a focus on setting and working toward goals can help provide a solid working relationship in which change can occur.

There are some interpersonal styles that have been documented to be detrimental to the therapeutic alliance. As noted previously, an underinvolved, avoidant interpersonal style on the part of the client may challenge the therapist's ability to easily foster a connection (Hardy et al., 2001). From this perspective, there will be some clients with whom a positive therapeutic relationship will be difficult to establish. Being aware of one's own emotional and physical reactions to clients is important in understanding and then dealing with any negative response. It is also important to adjust expectations about clients' ability to form a trusting, collaborative relationship and to look for any beliefs, assumptions, or experiences that may hinder this process. For example, if mistrust and paranoia are part of the clinical presentation, these will undoubtedly have an impact on the formation of the therapeutic relationship, often resulting in impasses and slowing the process of therapy. Interpersonal beliefs of all kinds are likely to extend into the therapy relationship, making it difficult to establish a positive alliance until the client is made aware of the belief and its impact in therapy and other aspects of life. There is tremendous potential for the therapeutic relationship to help disconfirm dysfunctional interpersonal beliefs. This is similar in many ways to the concept of the corrective emotional experience described in other forms of therapy (Strupp, 1984). However, in CBT the emphasis would be on the implications of the therapeutic experience for the client's beliefs as well as the affective features of this experience.

Summary

Although there are some predictors of outcome that cannot be modified, there are a number of practical strategies therapists can use to maximize CBT outcome. These strategies include modifications of and additions to a standard CBT protocol. In addition, therapists can consider ways to enhance the alliance between therapist and client in ways that provide an environment in which change can occur.

PREDICTORS OF RELAPSE AND RECURRENCE

It is commonly understood that depression is a disorder with a high risk of relapse (i.e., the reemergence of symptoms of depression after a depression-free period of 2 weeks or longer) and recurrence (i.e., the emergence of a new depressive episode after full recovery from the original episode) (Frank et al., 1991). Numerous studies have reported on the high incidence of relapse or recurrence in depression, even after remission of a particular episode or successful treatment. Although recommendations have been made about the precise definitions of relapse and recurrence, few authors have followed these definitions in practice. For this reason, the terms "relapse" and "recurrence" are used somewhat interchangeably through the following section. In a 5-year study of the naturalistic course of depression, the odds of a person remaining well for the full 5 years of the study was only one in five (Keller, 1994). Further, 70% of clients in the NIMH TDCRP had significant symptoms of depression within 18 months of achieving remission of symptoms (Shea et al., 1992). These findings have spurred the development of a number of research programs and an evolving clinical focus on "wellness" that goes beyond treatment of an acute episode. Both stand-alone prevention programs and CBT enhancements (e.g., maintenance sessions) have been investigated, and self-help resources for clients are becoming available (e.g., Bieling & Antony, 2003).

Demographic Predictors, Illness Factors, and Treatment Factors

Given the high rate of relapse and recurrence, understanding their predictors and developing treatments that prevent relapse and recurrence have become imperative for researchers and clinicians. What factors can help us understand if, and why, symptoms will return? One set of very important variables is related to the course of the person's past illness. Just as a history of more depressive episodes predicts worse outcome in CBT, a larger number and longer duration of previous episodes is linked with a greater chance of recurrence of symptoms (Kessing, Anderson, Mortensen, & Bolwig, 1998; Lewinsohn, Clarke, Seeley, & Rohde, 1994; Mueller et al., 1999). Further, the severity of a depressive episode predicts relapse, with more severe episodes linked to greater chance of relapse (O'Leary, Costello, Gormley, & Webb, 2000).

Demographic characteristics may also predict recurrence. In a large-scale case register study of hospitalizations for depression, Kessing, Anderson, and Mortensen (1998) found a number of sociodemographic predictors of recurrence of depression (as defined by rehospitalization). For example, females were more likely to experience a recurrence of symptoms than males, as were unmarried individuals, results which were replicated in a long-term observational follow-up of recovered clients (Mueller et al., 1999). Further, recurrence seemed to be less likely for older individuals.

Few studies have examined factors regarding treatment and relapse. One such study found that slower symptom reduction in the first 10 sessions of CBT predicted quicker relapse at 3- and 6-month follow-up (Santor & Segal, 2001).

Stressful Life Events

A considerable body of evidence demonstrates a link between stressors and the onset of major depression, and more recent evidence suggests that those stressors that precipitate relapse may often come as a result of the individual's own behavior, a phenomenon termed "stress generation" (Hammen, 1991). For example, Hammen found that the stressors experienced by women were related to specific self-defeating behaviors and environments constructed by these women, an assertion that has been supported by recent and compelling evidence from Kendler, Karkowski, and Prescott (1999). Using a large population-based twin registry, Kendler et al. assessed the level of dependence of 15 classes of life events (i.e., the degree to which the stressful life event could have resulted from the participant's behavior). The association with depression onset was significantly stronger for dependent life events. Kendler et al. interpreted these findings to suggest that *individuals predisposed to major depres-*

sion select themselves into high-risk environments. This would affect not only onset of depression but also risk of relapse due to ongoing stress generation.

On the other hand, Post (1992) has argued that stressful life events are important triggers only of initial depressive episodes, and their influence on recurrence becomes increasingly less as individuals experience further episodes of depression. In other words, this theory suggests that a person's neural circuitry becomes "sensitized" by stressful life events or that negative schema are made increasingly accessible by such events so that the individual begins to respond to lower and lower levels of stress in maladaptive ways (Segal, Williams, Teasdale, & Gemar, 1996). A study by Daley, Hammen, and Rao (2000) in which 128 young women were followed for 5 years provides some support for this assertion. In this study, the presence of current, episodic life stress predicted depressive relapse and recurrence, while chronic stress levels were only predictive of initial episodes.

Cognitive Vulnerability

It may not simply be the presence of stressful life events that predicts relapse but the interaction of life events and cognitive vulnerability. Studies have suggested that people at risk for relapse or recurrence display information-processing biases during periods of low mood. Segal, Shaw, Vella, and Katz (1992) found that the occurrence of an achievement-related stressor increased risk of relapse for self-critical individuals, suggesting that it may be the congruence of a negative life event with one's personality style or self-concept that increases risk of relapse. Studies also suggest that nondepressed individuals show biases in memory after experiencing a mood induction, being less able to recall positive events and more likely to recall negative events (Segal & Ingram, 1994; Teasdale, 1988). In one of the only studies that examined the association of these biases with actual rates of relapse, Segal, Gemar, and Williams (1999) found that ratings of dysfunctional attitudes after a mood challenge predicted relapse in a 30-month follow-up after successful pharmacotherapy or cognitive therapy. In this study, it was not dysfunctional attitudes in general that predicted relapse but, rather, those that were primed by a sad mood.

Research also supports the notion that a depressive attributional style may increase the risk of depressive relapse (Abramson, Metalsky, & Alloy, 1989). This style involves making negative inferences about the cause, consequences, and meaning of a negative life event, which is thought to contribute to feelings of hopelessness that, in turn, contribute to depressed mood. In a test of this hypothesis, Abramson et al. (1999) identified nondepressed individuals who were high or low on a measure of depressive attributional style and found that high-scoring individuals with a history of depressive episodes were more likely to experience recurrences in their depression than low scoring individuals.

Residual Depressive Symptoms

As mentioned earlier, the presence of residual symptoms of depression after treatment is over has been linked with a higher chance of relapse (Clark et al., 1999) and a faster rate of recurrence (Kanai et al., 2003). For example, a study by Judd et al. (1998) followed an asymptomatic recovered group and a residual symptom recovered group to see whether one would relapse quicker than the other. Participants with residual depressive symptoms relapsed over three times faster than the asymptomatic group, and this variable was more predictive of relapse than a past history of major depressive episodes.

Comorbid Pathology

Not only do comorbid personality disorders and certain personality dimensions interfere with outcome in CBT for depression, but the presence of these features predicts a higher rate of recurrence. In a study following young adults with remitted depression, Hart, Craighead, and Craighead (2001) found that higher scores on Cluster B personality traits predicted recurrence of depression. Further, elevated neuroticism scores are linked with recurrence (Berlanga, Heinze, Torres, Apiquian, & Caballero, 1999). Other forms of comorbidity (e.g., bipolar disorder, substance abuse disorders, and anxiety disorders) are also predictive of risk of relapse (Coryell, Endicott, & Keller, 1991; Daley et al., 2000; Giles, Jarrett, Biggs, Guzick, & Rush, 1989).

PRACTICAL STRATEGIES FOR PREVENTING RELAPSE

Relapse Prevention in Cognitive-Behavioral Therapy

The concept of relapse prevention, an idea common to many types of therapy, is especially relevant in CBT. According to Judith Beck (1995), relapse prevention is an ongoing process in CBT. Indeed, there are things a therapist can do beginning in the first session to help a client prevent relapse once gains have been made. It is in this spirit that clients are taught and encouraged to "be their own therapists" in CBT; this allows the client to identify lapses and use cognitive and behavioral strategies to prevent lapses from becoming relapses. Judith Beck (1995) outlines a number of specific strategies to facilitate this process. For example, when educating the client about the course of depression, the therapist can normalize fluctuations in mood, both during therapy and after therapy has ended. Thus, if the client later experiences depressed mood, a bad day, and so on, he or she will have realistic expectations regarding the meaning of these events. Further, the therapist can help the client make a plan for how to handle these events, using the therapy session early on in CBT, and having a self-therapy plan for after treatment has ended. As therapy draws to a close, one strategy to help inoculate a client against relapse is to taper sessions. If sessions have been held on a weekly basis, the therapist and client might try to hold biweekly sessions, then monthly sessions, and so forth. Tapering sessions provides the opportunity for the client to become accustomed to functioning with increasing independence, that is, without the structure of weekly therapy sessions. At times, a client may seem prepared for termination but may quickly encounter difficulties that require attention. At other times, a client may not feel ready for termination but may surprise himself with his ability to function independently.

Follow-Up Sessions

Another way to be alert for signs of relapse is to schedule follow-up sessions after the termination of regular therapy sessions. The spacing of these sessions is arbitrary (e.g., J. Beck, 1995, recommends 3-, 6-, and 9-month follow-up sessions), but they can be very useful. They provide the client with a goal to work toward and may enhance motivation to continue working on valued goals (i.e., they will have to "check in" with their therapist at some point and may not want to turn up "empty handed"). During these sessions the therapist can reinforce previously acquired learning and skills, review progress, highlight successfully handled problems, and troubleshoot problem-solving difficulties. Time may also be spent setting new goals for the client to work on. Follow-up sessions also provide the therapist an opportunity to look for signs of relapse or recurrence before the client reenters a full depressive episode.

Maintenance Cognitive-Behavioral Therapy

Another idea to prevent relapse once acute CBT has been discontinued is to provide maintenance therapy sessions. Maintenance therapy is more consistent than follow-up sessions but also less frequent than acute therapy sessions. Although this strategy has not been the focus of a great deal of research, two studies provide initial support for the efficacy of maintenance sessions. One study examined the combination of maintenance IPT and medication across a 7-year follow-up (Reynolds et al., 1999). During this period, 80% of depressed participants remained well. In contrast to naturalistic relapse rates, this is an impressive statistic. Another study specifically examined maintenance CBT, provided monthly for 8 months (Jarrett et al., 2001). In this study, previously depressed clients were randomly assigned to receive either maintenance CBT or monthly clinical evaluations and then followed for 2 years. At the end of the follow-up period, the group that received monthly evaluations had three times greater chance of relapsing than the maintenance CBT group (31% vs. 10% chance of relapse). Thus, maintenance CBT seems like a promising strategy to attenuate the likelihood of relapse for depressed individuals.

How often and for how long should maintenance therapy be scheduled? The answer to this question is unclear. Studies described earlier have used monthly sessions and have achieved significant benefit with as few as eight monthly sessions. Until further research clarifies these parameters, it seems that therapist and client can be flexible about scheduling sessions without spacing sessions too close (i.e., too similar to active therapy) or too far apart to be of benefit to clients.

Structure of maintenance therapy sessions can parallel that of a regular CBT session. The content of sessions can highlight a number of important topics including reviewing skills and progress, problem solving around current difficulties, devising behavioral experiments to test assumptions, and core belief work. Sessions should also address the important distinction between "lapses" in progress and a "relapse." A lapse is a temporary fluctuation in progress that is normal and expected. A relapse is a return to previous symptom levels. It is critically important for clients to distinguish between these two phenomena. Lapses may be best helped by a self-therapy session, completing a thought record, brief telephone contact with one's therapist, or simply "riding it out." Relapses are more serious and may necessitate a return to treatment (even if this is time-limited), introduction of a new mode of treatment (e.g., antidepressant medications, augmentation of a medication, and a different type of psychotherapy), or a more intrusive intervention (e.g., hospitalization for serious suicidality). Clients may benefit from listing the signs of a lapse (e.g., transient fluctuations in mood and fluctuations tied to a time-limited trigger) and signs of relapse (prolonged worsening of mood that does not respond to self-therapy, links to long-term stressors, active suicidality, prolonged decrease in functioning, etc.) to clarify the difference between these two phenomena.

When discussing maintenance therapy, clients may disclose feelings of ambivalence about being involved in further sessions. Once acute symptoms of depression have remitted and clients feel like their "normal" selves, they may be less motivated to schedule regular sessions. Further, if clients feel well, they may not want to pay attention to periods of sadness or depression or "look for" these types of difficulties (i.e., emotional avoidance; Bieling & Antony, 2003). Clients may interpret the suggestion of maintenance CBT as a sign that they are still not well or are at risk for becoming depressed again. In any of these situations, it can be useful to examine costs and benefits of being involved in maintenance therapy. Costs may include time, expense, or fears of dwelling on negative feelings. Benefits may include continued work on staying well, reinforcing skills or ideas learned in therapy, or preventing a lapse from becoming a relapse. Bieling and Antony (2003) provide an analogy of visiting the dentist on a regular basis, whether one has a toothache or not. Such regular visits have a maintenance and prevention function, and this preventive strategy can be emphasized for clients contemplating maintenance CBT.

Lifestyle Changes

Considerable evidence supports the utility of exercise in improving symptoms of depression (for a review, see Tkachuk & Martin, 1999). Most studies have examined low to moderate intensity of either aerobic or nonaerobic exercise, occurring approximately three times per week. Beneficial effects have also been found for a short duration of exercise, spaced more closely together (i.e., walking on a treadmill 30 minutes a day for 10 days; Dimeo, Bauer, Varahram, Proest, & Halter, 2000). The mechanism by which exercise affects mood is unclear, but its beneficial effects are evident. Thus, it may be useful to encourage depressed clients to adopt a regular exercise program that can be maintained after regular therapy sessions cease.

Combination Therapies

There are a number of instances in which clients may best benefit from a combination of CBT and pharmacotherapy. Although the superiority of combination therapy to either type of therapy in isolation is unclear across groups (Segal, Vincent, & Leavitt, 2002), it may prove immensely useful for specific clients. Situations in which combination treatment may be considered include a lack of response to an adequate dose of either therapy on its own, clients who present with a long and chronic history of depression, or the presence of endogenous symptoms of depression. In other words, if depressive symptoms appear to be minimally linked to life stressors or environmental triggers, it may be useful to augment CBT with a medication. Further, it may also be reasonable to consider combination therapy for "realistic" depression, discussed earlier. Studies generally support the use of a sequential strategy in treating depression, in addition to using CBT or medications as monotherapies, in which acute symptoms are targeted by an antidepressant medication and residual symptoms are addressed by CBT. This strategy is useful in decreasing rates of relapse (Fava, Fabbri, & Sonino, 2002).

Other Therapies

There may also be clients who are not interested in CBT, for whom adequate trials of CBT have not been helpful, and whose problems might be better served by a different modality of therapy. One randomized controlled trial has found IPT to be as effective as CBT (Elkin et al., 1989), and it should be considered, particularly when the client's presenting problems are interpersonal in nature. As reviewed earlier, IPT focuses on problems that fall into one of four categories of interpersonal issues: unresolved grief, role disputes, role transition, or social isolation. If, for example, the client has just lost his job and is experiencing depression related to this loss, either IPT or CBT would be appropriate referrals.

Mindfulness-Based Cognitive Therapy

In response to the high rates of relapse in depression, a group of researchers has designed an intervention targeted specifically at the prevention of relapse

(Segal, Williams, & Teasdale, 2002). Mindfulness-based cognitive therapy (MBCT) integrates aspects of mindfulness meditation with traditional cognitive therapy. This intervention, usually offered in group format, aims to help people with depression to detach and decenter from their thoughts, allowing them to observe their thought processes rather than getting caught up in them. Through this process, it is hoped that participants will gain perspective on their thought processes, have more control over their focus of attention, and be better able to notice any shifts in their thought processes that might signal the return of depression. Thus, the goal of MBCT is not to achieve happiness but to achieve freedom from depression (Segal, Williams, & Teasdale, 2002). Although study of this intervention is relatively new, the results of the first comprehensive study comparing MBCT to treatment as usual (TAU) for recovered clients were very promising. For clients with three or more previous episodes of depression, risk of relapse over 60 weeks was 66% in the TAU group as compared to 37% in the MBCT group (Teasdale et al., 2000).

Mindfulness involves "paying attention in a particular way—on purpose, in the present moment, and nonjudgementally" (Kabat-Zinn, 1990, p. 4). Participants in this treatment are encouraged to adopt the attitudes of nonjudging, patience, nonstriving, acceptance, and letting go. Nonjudging involves witnessing but not evaluating, one's own experience. Patience and nonstriving involve being with an experience instead of working toward an experience (e.g., not even striving to be mindful during a mindfulness practice). Acceptance involves letting an experience be what it may. For example, in relation to depression, acceptance would mean being understanding about the presence of unwanted or negative thoughts. Finally, letting go involves having an experience rather than thinking about having an experience. For example, the more a person thinks about how she is interacting with others, the more stilted and awkward the encounter may be. If the individual is able to focus less on what he or she is doing and more on the experience of the conversation itself, the more likely it is that the conversation will flow.

Although a full description of MBCT is beyond the scope of this chapter, we briefly review the components of an initial MBCT session to provide readers with an idea of how these concepts appear in practice. After initial introductions, group members are introduced to the experiential nature of MBCT by completing the "raisin exercise." Each participant is given a raisin and then encouraged to feel, smell, taste, and eat the raisin mindfully, noticing and experiencing what happens when they eat it. Naturally, participants will have numerous thoughts and feelings while doing this exercise, and this feedback can be used to illustrate how people do not often bring awareness to simple tasks like eating. In fact, the mind's tendency to be thinking of past or future events during the raisin exercise can be related to how automatically one's mind can "pull away" from the present and begin to ruminate or worry about other issues. The next exercise in an initial MBCT session is the "body scan." Participants are encouraged to pay attention to various parts of their bodies, with an emphasis on curiosity rather than judgment. Noticing bodily changes is useful not only in coming to understand the physical components of depressed mood (e.g., muscle tightness) but also in helping participants approach emotion in a different, more physical, way than they are used to. Sessions in MBCT end with the assignment of homework, which may include formal practice in meditation as well as encouragement to generalize a mindful state to everyday activities. For more details on MBCT, please see Segal, Williams, and Teasdale (2002).

CASE EXAMPLE

Jim, a 44 year-old never-married man, presented to a specialty CBT clinic for treatment of long-standing depressed mood. He reported numerous depressive episodes starting in his teens, most of which were triggered by some difficult life event (the end of a relationship, job loss, etc.). His most recent depressive episode, which had been ongoing for a number of months by the time he presented for treatment, was triggered by the loss of his most recent job when his company downsized.

Upon initial presentation, Jim received a thorough diagnostic assessment. Results suggested that he met criteria for major depressive disorder, recurrent, severe. Jim also met criteria for an anxiety disorder not otherwise specified. He described some social anxiety, but did not meet full DSM-IV (American Psychiatric Association, 1994) criteria for this disorder. His anxiety symptoms included discomfort being around others, including writing or talking in front of others.

Prior to commencing treatment, the therapist completed a suitability interview with Jim, as outlined by Safran and Segal (1990). This interview indicated that Jim was a reasonably suitable candidate for CBT, but it also highlighted some issues that may have presented problems for CBT. Jim demonstrated some difficulty identifying and discussing his emotional experience, instead using vague terms like being "upset" in specific situations. His avoidance of discussing emotions was paralleled by his use of avoidance as a general coping strategy. Also, his depression was chronic, and his level of premorbid functioning did not appear to be very high.

These areas of concern, particularly the identification of emotions and thoughts, were noted by the therapist and became the initial focus in therapy. Early therapy sessions focused on identifying and rating emotions, using two aids in this process. First, Jim was provided a copy of the mood list from *Mind Over Mood* (Greenberger & Padesky, 1995) and was asked to use this list when completing the mood column of a thought record. By providing this resource for Jim, he considered his moods in more specific terms than he originally used, and he was also forced to focus on his emotional experience when choosing a mood. Jim was also asked to rate his mood both within sessions and between sessions using pictures that represented various mood states.

Although this initial intervention helped Jim consider and identify his emotional experience, his use of avoidance as a coping strategy became apparent in other ways. For example, Jim had significant problems completing homework and often arrived at sessions without having completed any assignments. Jim's avoidance also interfered with initial efforts at behavioral activation, leaving him doing very little in his day-to-day life. The therapist initially checked out Jim's understanding of the assignments and the reason for doing them. Once it became clear that Jim's comprehension of the rationale was not the problem, the therapist began to explore the emotions and thoughts associated with Jim's avoidance. Jim identified a number of automatic thoughts about completing assignments, including "I won't do them [the forms] right," "I hate my writing," and "Doing this [activity] won't help and I might feel worse." The primary emotions Jim experienced included anxiety and hopelessness. Evidence gathering and cognitive restructuring were somewhat helpful for Jim's mood, but they were not enough to convince him to try the assignments. At this point, the therapist decided to step back from trying to convince Jim to try exercises and instead work with Jim to figure out if it was worth it to him to take the risk of trying homework. The therapist and Jim completed an advantages and disadvantages list for completing homework, with the therapist doing the writing in session. Jim's list of advantages far outnumbered his list of disadvantages, and when he was asked to rate the importance of each item to his life, Jim realized that the advantages of trying homework also reflected valued aspects of his life (e.g., he might not feel so depressed all the time and he would not feel like a failure if he gave this therapy a good effort). At this point, he indicated slightly more willingness to try homework, though he continued to be reticent.

Once Jim's specific fears were identified and he expressed more willingness to broach the subject of his avoidance, the therapist suggested that she and Jim approach his fears as possibilities and design experiments within session to test them out. For example, they agreed to have Jim complete a monitoring sheet in session and to rate his anxiety and depression throughout the process. Jim was fearful that his anxiety and depression would skyrocket as he monitored his thoughts and feelings, but he agreed that it was worth it to him to put this idea to the test. Session four was devoted to testing this assumption, with the added benefit of helping Jim learn how to use some of the forms used in CBT. During this exercise, the therapist continued to do most of the writing for Jim as he was still anxious about writing in front of others. Jim was pleased to realize that his levels of anxiety and depression did not dramatically increase with monitoring, and he reported feeling slightly better about making such an accomplishment within the session.

Next, the therapist and Jim agreed to focus on his fears of writing in front of others, noting that Jim's avoidance of writing things down could be a potential barrier to progress. The therapist described the process of repeatedly exposing oneself to a feared situation until the situation no longer elicited the same amount of fear. Jim and the therapist decided to use session five to complete an exposure in which Jim would repeatedly write in front of the therapist until his anxiety about doing so declined. At the start of the session, Jim rated his anxiety about writing in front of the therapist as 60 (on a 0–100 scale), but after 25 minutes, it had dropped to 30, and he reported feeling more comfortable about writing in session and about bringing written work into session. These exercises allowed Jim to more fully engage in the therapy process over the next several sessions. Further, these experiments provided Jim with enough confidence to generalize his gains to some initial behavioral activation exercises. Over the next several weeks, Jim began to wake up earlier and schedule some small activities into his day.

Although therapy proceeded fairly smoothly for the next several sessions, a roadblock occurred at session eight. Jim informed the therapist that his unemployment insurance had been terminated, and he had not been able to bring himself to check his bank account balance to see if he had enough money for this month's rent. He reported that his anxiety level had shot up, and he had reverted back to old habits of isolating himself from others and sleeping most of the day. Jim absolutely refused to check his balance, and therefore he did not know the actual state of his finances. In light of these difficult circumstances, the therapist tried to help Jim differentiate his realistic concerns from catastrophic or distorted concerns:

THERAPIST: Jim, what do you think will happen if you look at your bank balance?

JIM: I'm afraid it will be bad news—that I don't have enough to get through the month.

THERAPIST: Are there any other possible outcomes?

JIM: Well, it's possible that I could make it through this month, but I'm not sure. I haven't looked at things for a long time.

THERAPIST: Are you afraid of anything else to do with looking at your finances?

JIM: I just don't know if I can handle it. What if I freak out? I feel like such a loser.

THERAPIST: Those sound like important thoughts to look at a little closer. Should we spend some time on thoughts of being a loser and your fears of not being able to handle the news, no matter what the outcome is?

The therapist proceeded to help Jim with thought records about being a "loser," which tied into his core beliefs of worthlessness. Although anyone might feel frustrated at himself for being in a difficult financial situation, it seemed as though Jim equated his money problems with a general sense of worthlessness. The therapist also spent time with Jim brainstorming other difficult situations that he had successfully navigated in the past. It turned out that Jim had been in financial trouble before, and he had always been able to do what it took to pay his bills, even if it meant temporarily borrowing money from his family or going on public assistance. Although Jim was able to see that some of his thoughts were distorted, even in this difficult situation, he was unable to bypass his anxiety about facing this stressful situation, and he was not able to look into his financial situation for several weeks. This avoidance had a deleterious effect on Jim's treatment, as it became the primary focus, but he could not make any progress on solving the problem. After a number of weeks, the therapist decided to return to the advantages and disadvantages list that had proved useful earlier in therapy. Once again, the therapist disengaged from trying to convince Jim to face his concerns and instead helped Jim examine the reasons for avoiding and the reasons for approaching his fears. Although Jim began to feel it would be useful to face his financial fears, he indicated extreme discomfort about doing this on his own. Thus, Jim and his therapist decided to treat his fears as the targets of exposure therapy. They broke Jim's fears down into small steps and then had Jim systematically expose himself to each step until he was able to tackle his most feared situation—dealing with his current money problems. For example, the initial exposure involved the therapist and Jim looking at old bank statements together, then visiting the waiting areas of local banks. Through this process, Jim worked up to the point where he could bring his most recent bank statement to session and review it in the therapist's presence. Upon reviewing his statement, Jim found that he was indeed in serious financial trouble, and the therapist and Jim spent the rest of the session brainstorming ways Jim could deal with this problem. Jim also began a thought record in session about being "pathetic" and completed this thought record for homework.

At the conclusion of therapy, Jim had achieved significant reduction in symptoms of depression. He did not have another job, but he had successfully arranged for public assistance to support himself while he looked for a job. He also began a volunteer position with a local charity to increase his level of activity. This position helped Jim with his feelings of worthlessness.

Upon reflection, if motivational strategies had not been helpful for Jim, it may have been useful to investigate other treatment options when he became paralyzed in the current therapy. He was not taking any medications and had indicated a preference to remain medication free. However, given his state of distress when his unemployment insurance was cut off, the addition of an antidepressant medication may have been useful.

CONCLUSION

Paul's (1967) question "What therapy works for whom … " has been partially answered in the last three decades. It is clear that CBT is an effective treatment for depression. But it is also clear that not everyone derives the maximum possible benefit from CBT and that relapse and recurrence are significant problems in the treatment of depression. In this chapter, we provided suggestions for ways to maximize treatment outcome and relapse prevention by drawing on our understanding of the factors that influence outcome. In the coming years, we are hopeful that more and more data will be available to guide CBT clinicians working in everyday settings with "real" client populations.

REFERENCES

Abramson, L. Y., Alloy, L. B., Hogan, M. E., Whitehouse, W. G., Donovan, P., Rose, D. T., Panzarella, C., & Raniere, D. (1999). Cognitive vulnerability to depression: Theory and evidence. *Journal of Cognitive Psychotherapy, 13*, 5–20.

Abramson, L. Y., Metalsky, G. I., & Alloy, L. B. (1989). Hopelessness depression: A theory-based subtype of depression. *Psychological Review, 96*, 358–372.

Ackerman, S. J., & Hilsenroth, M. J. (2003). A review of therapist characteristics and techniques positively impacting he therapeutic alliance. *Clinical Psychology Review, 23*, 1–33.

Ackerman, S. J., Hilsenroth, M. J., Baity, M. R., & Blagys, M. D. (2000). Interaction of therapeutic process and alliance during psychological assessment. *Journal of Personality Assessment, 75*, 82–109.

Addis, M. E., & Jacobson, N. S. (2000). A closer look at the treatment rationale and homework compliance in the cognitive-behavioral treatment of depression. *Cognitive Therapy and Research, 24*, 313–326.

American Psychiatric Association. (1994). *Diagnostic and statistical manual of mental disorders* (4th ed.). Washington, DC: Author.

American Psychiatric Association. (2000a). *Diagnostic and statistical manual of mental disorders* (4th ed., text rev.). Washington, DC: Author.

American Psychiatric Association. (2000b). *Practice guideline for the treatment of clients with major depression.* Retrieved September 3, 2002, from the American Psychiatric Association web site: www.psych.org/clin_res/Depression2e.book.cfm.

Andrade, C., & Kurinji, S. (2002). Continuation and maintenance ECT: A review of recent research. *Journal of ECT, 18*, 149–158.

Ball, J., Kearney, B., Wilhelm, K., Dewhurst-Savellis, J., & Barton, B. (2000). Cognitive behaviour therapy and assertion training groups for patients with depression and comorbid personality disorders. *Behavioural and Cognitive Psychotherapy, 28*, 71–85.

Beck, J. S. (1995). *Cognitive therapy: Basics and beyond.* New York: Guilford Press.

Belsher, G., & Costello, C. G. (1988). Relapse after recover from unipolar depression: A critical review. *Psychological Bulletin, 104*, 84–96.

Berlanga, C., Heinze, G., Torres, M., Apiquian, R., & Caballero, A. (1999). Personality and clinical predictors of recurrence of depression. *Psychiatric Services, 50*, 376–380.

Berman, R. M., Narasinham, M., Sanacora, G., Miano, A. P., Hoffman, R. E., Hu, X. S., Charney, D. S., & Boutros, N. N. (2000). A randomized clinical trial of repetitive transcranial magnetic stimulation in the treatment of major depression. *Biological Psychiatry, 47*, 332–337.

Bezchlibnyk-Butler, K. Z., & Jeffries, J. J. (2002). *Clinical handbook of psychotropic drugs* (12th ed.). Seattle, WA: Hogrefe & Huber.

Bieling, P. J., & Antony, M. M. (2003). *Ending the depression cycle: A step-by-step guide for preventing relapse.* Oakland, CA: New Harbinger.

Blatt, S. J., Quinlan, D. M., Pilkonis, P. A., & Shea, M. T. (1995). Impact of perfectionism and need for approval on the brief treatment of depression: The National Institute of Mental Health Treatment of Depression Collaborative Research Program revisited. *Journal of Consulting and Clinical Psychology, 63*, 125–132.

Brent, D. A., Birmaher, B., Kolko, D., Baugher, M., & Bridge, J. (2001). Subsyndromal depression in adolescents after a brief psychotherapy trial: Course and outcome. *Journal of Affective Disorders, 63*, 51–58.

Broadhead, W. E., Blazer, D. G., George, L. K., & Tse, C. K. (1990). Depression, disability days, and days lost from work in a prospective epidemiologic survey. *Journal of the American Medical Association, 264*, 2524–2528.

Browne, G., Steiner, M., Roberts, J., Gafni, A., Byrne, C., Dunn, E., Bell, B., Mills, M., Chalklin, L., Wallik, D., & Kraemer, J. (2002). Sertraline and/or interpersonal psychotherapy for clients with dysthymic disorder in primary care: 6-month comparison with longitudinal 2-year follow-up of effectiveness and costs. *Journal of Affective Disorders, 68*, 317–330.

Bryant, M. J., Simons, A. D., & Thase, M. E. (1999). Therapist skill and client variables in homework compliance: Controlling and uncontrolled variable in cognitive therapy outcome research. *Cognitive Therapy and Research, 23*, 381–399.

Burns, D. D., & Spangler, D. L. (2000). Does psychotherapy homework lead to improvements in depression in cognitive-behavioral therapy or does improvement lead to increased homework compliance? *Journal of Consulting and Clinical Psychology, 68*, 46–56.

Canadian Psychiatric Association. (2001). *Clinical practice guidelines for the treatment of depressive disorders.* Retrieved August 12, 2003, from the Canadian Psychiatric Association web site: www.cpa-apc.org/Publications/Clinical_Guidelines/depression/clinicalGuidelinesDepression.asp.

Cancer Prevention Research Center. (1991). *Measures.* Retrieved July 30, 2003, from the University of Rhode Island, Cancer Prevention Research Center web site: www.uri.edu/research/cprc/measures.htm.

Casacalenda, N., Perry, J. C., & Looper, K. (2002). Remission in major depressive disorder: A comparison of pharmacotherapy, psychotherapy, and control conditions. *American Journal of Psychiatry, 159*, 1354–1360.

Castonguay, L. G., Goldfried, M. R., Wiser, S., Raue, P. J., & Hayes, A. M. (1996). Predicting the effect of cognitive therapy for depression: A study of unique and common factors. *Journal of Consulting and Clinical Psychology, 64*, 497–504.

Chudzik, S. M., McCabe, R. E., Bieling, P. J., Antony, M. M., & Swinson, R. P. (2003, June). *Treatment of comorbid panic disorder and depression: A preliminary case series examination.* Poster presented at the Canadian Psychological Association Conference, Hamilton, Ontario.

Clark, D. A., Beck, A. T., & Alford, B. A. (1999). *Scientific foundations of cognitive theory and therapy of depression.* New York: Wiley.

Coryell, W., Endicott, J., & Keller, M. (1990). Outcome of patients with chronic affective disorder: A five-year follow-up. *American Journal of Psychiatry, 147*, 1627–1633.

Coryell, W., Endicott, J., & Keller, M. B. (1991). Predictors of relapse into major depressive disorder in a nonclinical population. *American Journal of Psychiatry, 148*, 1353–1358.

Crits-Christoph, P., Siqueland, J., Chittams, J., Barber, P., Beck, A. T., Liese, B., Onken, L. S., Thase, M. E., Frank, A., Luborsky, L., Mark, D., Mercer, D., Najavits, L. M., & Woody, G. (1998). Training in cognitive, supportive-expressive, and drug counseling therapies for cocaine dependence. *Journal of Consulting and Clinical Psychology, 66,* 484–492.

Daley, S. E., Hammen, C., & Rao, U. (2000). Predictors of first onset and recurrence of major depression in young women during the 5 years following high school graduation. *Journal of Abnormal Psychology, 109,* 525–533.

Depression Guideline Panel. (1993). *Clinical Practice Guideline Number 5. Depression in primary care: 2. Treatment of major depression* (AHCPR Publication No. 93-0551). Rockville, MD: U.S. Department of Health and Human Services, Agency for Health Care Policy and Research.

DeRubeis, R. J., Gelfand, L. A., Tang, T. Z., & Simons, A. D. (1999). Medications versus cognitive behavior therapy for severely depressed outpatients: Mega-analysis of four randomized comparisons. *American Journal of Psychiatry, 156,* 1007–1013.

Dimeo, F., Bauer, M., Varahram, I., Proest, G., & Halter, U. (2000). Benefits from aerobic exercise in clients with major depression: A pilot study. *Psychosomatic Medicine, 62,* 633–638.

Doubleday, E. K., King, P., & Papageorgiou, C. (2002). Relationship between fluid intelligence and ability to benefit from cognitive-behavioural therapy in older adults: A preliminary investigation. *British Journal of Clinical Psychology, 41,* 423–428.

Duggan, C. F., Lee, A. S., & Murray, R. M. (1990). Does personality predict long-term outcome in depression? *British Journal of Psychiatry, 157,* 19–24.

Elkin, I., Shea, T., Watkins, J. T., Imber, S. D., Sotsky, S. M., Collins, J. F., Glass, D. R., Pilkonis, P. A., Leber, W. R., Docherty, J. P., Fiester, S. J., & Parloff, M. B. (1989). National Institute of Mental Health Treatment of Depression Collaborative Research Program: General effectiveness of treatments. *Archives of General Psychiatry, 46,* 971–982.

Enns, M. W., Swenson, J. R., McIntyre, R. S., Swinson, R. P., Kennedy, S. H., & the CANMAT Depression Working Group. (2001). Clinical guidelines for the treatment of depressive disorders: Comorbidity. *Canadian Journal of Psychiatry, 46*(Suppl. 1), 77S–90S.

Ezquiaga, E., Garcia, A., Pallares, T., & Bravo, M. F. (1999). Psychosocial predictors of outcome in major depression: A prospective 12-month study. *Journal of Affective Disorders, 52,* 209–216.

Fava, G. A., Fabbri, S., & Sonino, N. (2002). Residual symptoms in depression: An emerging therapeutic target. *Progress in Neuro-Psychopharmacology and Biological Psychiatry, 26,* 1019–1027.

Feely, M., DeRubeis, R. J., & Gelfand, L. A. (1999). The temporal relation of adherence and alliance to symptom change in cognitive therapy for depression. *Journal of Consulting and Clinical Psychology, 67,* 578–582.

Fennell, M. J., & Teasdale, J. D. (1987). Cognitive therapy for depression: Individual differences and the process of change. *Cognitive Therapy and Research, 11,* 253–271.

Fink, M. (2001). Convulsive therapy: A review of the first 55 years. *Journal of Affective Disorders, 63,* 1–15.

Frank, E., Prien, R. F., Jarrett, R. B., Keller, M. B., Kupfer, D. J., Lavori, P. W., Rush, A. J., & Weissman, M. M. (1991). Conceptualization and rationale for consensus definitions of terms in major depressive disorder: Remission, recovery, relapse, and recurrence. *Archives of General Psychiatry, 48,* 851–855.

Frank, E., Rucci, P., Katon, W., Barrett, J., Williams, J. W., Jr., Oxman, T., Sullivan, M., & Cornell, J. (2002). Correlates of remission in primary care clients treated for minor depression. *General Hospital Psychiatry, 24,* 12–19.

Furlong, M., & Oei, T. P. S. (2002). Changes to automatic thoughts and dysfuntional attitudes in group CBT for depression. *Behavioural and Cognitive Psychotherapy, 30,* 351–360.

Gaston, L., Thompson, L., Gallagher, D., Cournoyer, L. G., & Gagnon, R. (1998). Alliance, technique, and their interactions in predicting outcome of behavioral, cognitive, and brief dynamic therapy. *Psychotherapy Research, 8,* 190–209.

Gelhart, R. P., & King, H. L. (2001). The influence of comorbid risk factors on the effectiveness of cognitive-behavioral treatment of depression. *Cognitive and Behavioral Practice, 8,* 18–28.

George, M. S., Nahas, Z., Li, X. B., Chae, J. H., Oliver, N., Najib, A., & Anderson, B. (2001). New depression treatment strategies: What does the future hold for therapeutic uses of minimally invasive brain stimulation? In J. Greden (Ed.), *Treatment of recurrent depression* (pp. 103–133). Washington, DC: American Psychiatric Press.

George, M. S., Nahas, Z., Molloy, M., Speer, A. M., Oliver, N. C., Li, X. B., Arana, G. W., Risch, S. C., & Ballenger, J. C. (2000). A controlled trial of daily left prefrontal cortex TMS for treating depression. *Biological Psychiatry, 48,* 962–970.

George, M. S., Wassermann, E. M., Kimbrell, T. A., Little, J. T., Williams, W. E., Danielson, A. L., Greenberg, B. D., Hallett, M., & Post, R. M. (1997). Mood improvement following daily left pre-frontal repetitive transcranial magnetic stimulation in patients with depression: A placebo-controlled crossover trial. *American Journal of Psychiatry, 154,* 1752–1756.

Giles, D. E., Jarrett, R. B., Biggs, M. M., Guzick, D. S., & Rush, A. J. (1989). Clinical predictors of recurrence in depression. *American Journal of Psychiatry, 146,* 764–767.

Goldapple, K., Segal, Z., Garson, C., Lau, M., Bieling, P., Kennedy, S., & Mayburg, H. (2004). Modulation of cortical-limbic pathways in major depression. *Archives of General Psychiatry, 61,* 34–41.

Gortner, E. T., Gollan, J. K., Dobson, K. S., & Jacobson, N. S. (1998). Cognitive-behavioral treatment for depression: Relapse prevention. *Journal of Consulting and Clinical Psychology, 66,* 377–384.

Greenberger, D., & Padesky, C. A. (1995). *Mind over mood (client manual).* New York: Guilford Press.

Haaga, D. A., DeRubeis, R. J., Stewart, B. L., & Beck, A. T. (1991). Relationship of intelligence with cognitive therapy outcome. *Behaviour Research and Therapy, 29,* 277–281.

Hamilton, K. E., & Dobson, K. S. (2002). Cognitive therapy of depression: Pretreatment client predictors of outcome. *Clinical Psychology Review, 22,* 875–893.

Hammen, C. (1991). Generation of stress in the course of unipolar depression. *Journal of Abnormal Psychology, 100,* 555–561.

Hardy, G. E., Barkham, M. Shapiro, D. A., Stiles, W. B., Rees, A., & Reynolds, S. (1995). Impact of cluster C personality disorders on outcomes of contrasting brief psychotherapies for depression. *Journal of Consulting and Clinical Psychology, 63,* 997–1004.

Hardy, G. E., Cahill, J., Shapiro, D. A., Barkham, M., Rees, A., & Macaskill, N. (2001). Client interpersonal and cognitive styles as predictors of response to time-limited cognitive therapy for depression. *Journal of Consulting and Clinical Psychology, 69,* 841–845.

Hart, A. B., Craighead, W. E., & Craighead, L. W. (2001). Predicting recurrence of major depressive disorder in young adults: A prospective study. *Journal of Abnormal Psychology, 110,* 633–643.

Hirschfeld, R. M. A. (1999). Personality disorders and depression: Comorbidity. *Depression and Anxiety, 10,* 142–146.

Horowitz, L. M., Rosenberg, S. E., Baer, B. A., Ureno, G., & Villaseñor, V. S. (1988). Inventory of Interpersonal Problems: Psychometric properties and clinical applications. *Journal of Consulting and Clinical Psychology, 56,* 885–892.

Horvath, A. O., & Symonds, B. D. (1991). Relation between working alliance and outcome in psychotherapy: A meta-analysis. *Journal of Counseling Psychology, 38,* 139–149.

Horwath, E., Johnson, J., Klerman, G. L., & Weissman, M. M. (1992). Depressive symptoms as relative and attributable risk factors for first-onset major depression. *Archives of General Psychiatry, 49,* 817–823.

Jacobson, N. S., Dobson, K. S., Truax, P. A., Addis, M. E., Koerner, K., Gollan, J. K., Gortner, E., & Prince, S. E. (1996). A component analysis of cognitive-behavioral treatment for depression. *Journal of Consulting and Clinical Psychology, 64,* 295–304.

Jarrett, R. B., Eaves, G. G., Brannemann, B. D., & Rush, A. J. (1991). Clinical, cognitive, and demographic predictors of response to cognitive therapy for depression: A preliminary report. *Psychiatry Research, 37,* 245–260.

Jarrett, R. B., Kraft, D., Doyle, J., Foster, B. M., Eaves, G. G., & Silver, P. C. (2001). Preventing recurrent depression using cognitive therapy with and without a continuation phase. *Archives of General Psychiatry, 58,* 381–388.

Joiner, T. E., Metalsky, G. I., Lew, A., & Klocek, J. (1999). Testing the causal mediation component of Beck's theory of depression: Evidence for specific mediation. *Cognitive Therapy and Research, 23,* 401–412.

Jones, E. E., Krupnick, J. L., & Kerig, P. K. (1987). Some gender effects in a brief psychotherapy. *Psychotherapy: Theory, Research, Practice, and Training, 24,* 336–352.

Judd, L. L., Akiskal, H. S., Maser, J. D., Zeller, P. J., Endicott, J., Coryell, W., Paulus, M. P., Kunovac, J. L., Leon, A. C., Mueller, T. I., Rice, J. A., & Keller, M. B. (1998). Major depressive disorder: A prospective study of residual subthreshold depressive symptoms as predictor of rapid relapse. *Journal of Affective Disorders, 50,* 97–108.

Kabat-Zinn, J. (1990). *Full catastophe living: The program of the Stress Reduction Clinic at the University of Massachusetts Medical Center.* New York: Delta.

Kanai, T., Takeuchi, H., Furukawa, T. A., Yoshimura, R., Imaizumi, T., Kitamura, T., & Takahashi, K. (2003). Time to recurrence after recovery from major depressive episodes and its predictors. *Psychological Medicine, 33,* 839–845.

Katon, W., Russo, J., Frank, E., Barrett, J., Williams, J. W., Jr., Oxman, T., Sullivan, M., & Cornell, J. (2002). Predictors of nonresponse to treatment in primary care patients with dysthymia. *General Hospital Psychiatry, 24,* 20–27.

Keller, M. B. (1994). Depression: A long term illness. *British Journal of Psychiatry, 165*(Suppl. 26), 9–15.

Keller, M. B. (2003). Past, present, and future directions for defining optimal treatment outcome in depression. *Journal of the American Medical Association, 289,* 3152–3160.

Keller, M. B., McCullough, J. P., Klein, D. N., Arnow, B., Dunner, D. L., Gelenberg, A. J., Markowitz, J. C., Nemeroff, C. B., Russell, J. M., Thase, M. E., Trivedi, M. H., & Zajecka, J. (2000). A comparison of nefazodone, the cognitive behavioral-analysis system of psychotherapy, and their combination for the treatment of chronic depression. *New England Journal of Medicine, 342,* 1462–1470.

Keller, M. B., & Shapiro, R. W. (1982). Double depression: Super-imposition of acute depressive episodes on chronic depressive disorders. *American Journal of Psychiatry, 139,* 438–442.

Kendler, K. S., Karkowski, L. M., & Prescott, C. A. (1999). Causal relationship between stressful life events and the onset of major depression. *American Journal of Psychiatry, 156,* 837–848.

Kessing, L. V., Anderson, P. K., & Mortensen, P. B. (1998). Predictors of recurrence in affective disorder: A case register study. *Journal of Affective Disorders, 49,* 101–108.

Kessing, L. V., Anderson, P. K., Mortensen, P. B., & Bolwig, T. G. (1998). Recurrence in affective disorder: A case register study. *British Journal of Psychiatry, 172,* 73–78.

Kirsch, I., Moore, T. J., Scoboria, A., Nicholls, S. S. (2002, July 15). The emperor's new drugs: An analysis of antidepressant medication data submitted to the U.S. Food and Drug Administration. *Prevention and Treatment, 5,* Article 23. Retrieved July 27, 2003, from www.journals.apa.org/prevention/volume5/pre0050023a.html.

Krupnick, J. L., Sotsky, S. M., Simmens, S., Moyer, J., Elkin, I., Watkins, J., & Pilkonis, P. A. (1996). The role of the therapeutic alliance in psychotherapy and pharmacotherapy outcome: Findings in the National Institute of Mental Health Treatment of Depression Collaborative Research Program. *Journal of Consulting and Clinical Psychology, 64,* 532–539.

Kuyken, W., Kurzer, N., DeRubeis, R. J., Beck, A. T., & Brown, G. K. (2001). Response to cognitive therapy in depression: The role of maladaptive beliefs and personality disorders. *Journal of Consulting and Clinical Psychology, 69,* 560–566.

Lambert, M. J., & Davis, M. J. (2002). Treatment for depression: What the research says. In M. A. Reinecke & M. R. Davison (Eds.), *Comparative treatments of depression* (pp. 21–46). New York: Springer.

Lee, A. S., & Murray, R. M. (1988). The long-term outcome of Maudsley depressives. *British Journal of Psychiatry, 153,* 741–751.

Lewinsohn, P. M., Clarke, G. N., Seeley, J. R., & Rohde, P. (1994). Major depression in community adolescents: Age at onset, episode duration, and time to recurrence. *Journal of the American Academy of Child and Adolescent Psychiatry, 33,* 809–818.

Luborsky, L., Crits-Christoph, P., Alexander, L., Margolis, M., & Cohen, M. (1983). Two helping alliance methods for predicting outcomes of psychotherapy, a counting signs vs. a global rating method. *Journal of Nervous and Mental Disorder, 171,* 480–491.

Mallinckrodt, B., & Nelson, M. L. (1991). Counselor training level and the formation of the psychotherapeutic working alliance. *Journal of Counseling Psychology, 38,* 133–138.

Manes, F., Jorge, R., Morcuende, M., Yamada, T., Paradiso, S., & Robinson, R. G. (2001). A controlled study of repetitive transcranial magnetic stimulation as a treatment of depression in the elderly. *International Psychogeriatrics, 13,* 225–231.

McLean, P. D., & Hakstian, A. R. (1979). Clinical depression: Comparative efficacy of outpatient treatments. *Journal of Consulting and Clinical Psychology, 47,* 818–836.

McLean, P. D., Woody, S., Taylor, S., & Koch, W. J. (1998). Comorbid panic disorder and major depression: Implications for cognitive-behavioral treatment. *Journal of Consulting and Clinical Psychology, 66,* 240–247.

Merrill, K. A., Tolbert, V. E., & Wade, W. A. (2003). Effectiveness of cognitive therapy for depression in a community mental health center: A benchmarking study. *Journal of Consulting and Clinical Psychology, 71,* 404–409.

Miller, W. R., & Rollnick, S. (1991). *Motivational interviewing: Preparing people to change addictive behavior.* New York: Guilford Press.

Mohr, D. C., Beutler, L. E., Engle, D., Shoham-Salomon, V., Bergan, J., Kaszniak, A. W., & Yost, E. B. (1990). Identification of patients at risk for nonresponse and negative outcome in psychotherapy. *Journal of Consulting and Clinical Psychology, 58,* 622–628.

Moorey, S. (1996). When bad things happen to rational people: Cognitive therapy in adverse life circumstances. In P. M. Salkovskis (Ed.), *Frontiers of cognitive therapy* (pp. 450–469). New York: Guilford Press.

Mueller, T. I., Leon, A. C., Keller, M. B., Soloman, D. A., Endicott, J., Coryell, W., Warshaw, M., & Maser, J. D. (1999). Recurrence after recovery from major depressive disorder during 15 years of observational follow-up. *American Journal of Psychiatry, 156,* 1000–1006.

Mulrow, C. D., Williams, J. W., Trivedi, M., Chiquette, E., Aguilar, C., Cornell, J. E., Badgett, R., Noel, P. H., Lawrence, V., Lee, S., Luther, M., Ramirez, G., Richardon, W. S., & Stamm, K. (1998). Treatment of major depression: Newer pharmacotherapies. *Psychopharmacologial Bulletin, 34,* 409–795.

Neimeyer, R. A., & Feixas, G. (1990). The role of homework and skill acquisition in the outcome of group cognitive therapy for depression. *Behavior Therapy, 21,* 281–292.

Oei, T. P. S., & Shuttlewood, G. J. (1997). Comparison of specific and nonspecific factors in group cognitive therapy for depression. *Journal of Behavior Therapy and Experimental Psychiatry, 28,* 221–231.

Ogrodniczuk, J. S., Piper, W. E., Joyce, A. S., & McCallum, M. (2001). Effect of patient gender on outcome in two forms of short-term individual psychotherapy. *Journal of Psychotherapy Practice and Research, 10,* 69–78.

O'Leary, D., & Costello F. (2001). Personality and outcome in depression: An 18-month prospective follow-up study. *Journal of Affective Disorders, 63,* 67–78.

O'Leary, D., Costello, F., Gormley, N., & Webb, M. (2000). Remission onset and relapse in depression: An 18-month prospective study of course for 100 first admission clients. *Journal of Affective Disorders, 57,* 159–171.

Padberg, F., Zwanzger, P., Keck, M. E., Kathmann, N., Mikhaiel, P., Ella, R., Rupprecht, P., Thoma, H., Hampel, H., Toschi, N., & Muller, H. (2002). Repetitive transcranial magnetic stimulation (rTMS) in major depression: Relation between efficacy and stimulation intensity. *Neuropsychopharmacology, 27,* 638–645.

Paul, G. L. (1967). Strategy of outcome research in psychotherapy. *Journal of Consulting Psychology, 31,* 109–118.

Pepper, C. M., Klein, D. N., Anderson, L. P., Ouimette, P. C., & Lizardi, H. (1995). DSM-III-R Axis II comorbidity in dysthymia and major depression. *American Journal of Psychiatry, 152,* 239–247.

Persons, J. B., & Burns, D. D. (1985). Mechanisms of action of cognitive therapy: The relative contributions of technical and interpersonal interventions. *Cognitive Therapy and Research, 9,* 539–551.

Persons, J. B., Burns, D. D., & Perloff, J. M. (1988). Predictors of dropout and outcome in cognitive therapy for depression in a private practice setting. *Cognitive Therapy and Research, 12,* 557–575.

Peselow, E. D., Robins, C., Block, P., Barouche, F., & Fieve, R. R. (1990). Dysfunctional attitudes in depressed patients before and after clinical treatment and in normal control subjects. *American Journal of Psychiatry, 147,* 439–444.

Pilkonis, P. A., & Frank, E. (1988). Personality pathology in recurrent depression: Naure, prevalence, and relationship to treatment response. *American Journal of Psychiatry, 145,* 435–441.

Post, R. M. (1992). Transduction of psychosocial stress into the neurobiology of recurrent affective disorder. *American Journal of Psychiatry, 149,* 999–1010.

Prochaska, J. O. (2000). Change at differing stages. In R. E. Ingram & C. R. Snyder (Eds.), *Handbook of psychological change: Psychotherapy processes and practices for the 21st century* (pp. 109–127). New York: Wiley.

Prochaska, J. O., & DiClemente, C. C. (1984). *The transtheoretical approach: Crossing traditional boundaries of therapy.* Homewood, IL: Dow Jones / Irwin.

Ravindran, A. V., Anisman, H., Merali, Z., Charbonneau, Y., Telner, J., Bialik, R. J., Wiens, A., Ellis, J., & Griffiths, J. (1999). Treatment of primary dysthymia with group cognitive therapy and pharmacotherapy: Clinical symptoms and functional impairments. *American Journal of Psychiatry, 156,* 1608–1617.

Rector, N. A., Zuroff, D. C., & Segal, Z. V. (1999). Cognitive change and the therapeutic alliance: The role of technical and nontechnical factors in cognitive therapy. *Psychotherapy, 36,* 320–328.

Reynolds, C. F., III., Frank, E., Perel, J. M., Imber, S. D., Cornes, C., Miller, M. D., Mazumdar, S., Houck, P. R., Dew, M. A., Stack, J. A., Pollock, B. G., & Kupfer, D. J. (1999). Nortriptyline and interpersonal psychotherapy as maintenance therapies for recurrent major depression: A randomized controlled trial in patients older than 59 years. *Journal of the American Medical Association, 281,* 39–45.

Reynolds, C. F., III., Frank, E., Perel, J. M., Mazumdar, S., Dew, M. A., Begley, A., Houck, P. R., Hall, M., Mulsant, B., Shear, M. K., Miller, M. D., Cornes, C., & Kupfer, D. J. (1996). High relapse rate after discontinuation of adjunctive medication for elderly clients with recurrent major depression. *American Journal of Psychiatry, 153,* 1418–1422.

Robinson, L. A., Berman, J. S., & Neimeyer, R. A. (1990). Psychotherapy for the treatment of depression: A comprehensive review of controlled outcome research. *Psychological Bulletin, 108,* 30–49.

Rohde, P., Clarke, G. N., Lewinsohn, P. M., Seeley, J. R., & Kaufman, N. K. (2001). Impact of comorbidity on a cognitive-behavioral group treatment for adolescent depression. *Journal of the American Academy of Child and Adolescent Psychiatry, 40,* 795–802.

Rounsaville, B. J., Shokomskas, D., & Prusoff, B. A. (1988). Chronic mood disorders in depressed outpatients: Diagnosis and response to pharmacotherapy. *Journal of Affective Disorders, 2,* 72–78.

Safran, J. D., & Segal, Z. V. (1990). *Interpersonal process in cognitive therapy.* New York: Basic Books.

Safran, J. D., & Wallner, L. K. (1991). The relative predictive validity of two therapeutic alliance measures in cognitive therapy. *Psychological Assessment, 3,* 188–195.

Santor, D. A., & Segal, Z. V. (2001). Predicting symptom return from rate of symptom reduction in cognitive-behavior therapy for depression. *Cognitive Therapy and Research, 25,* 117–135.

Segal, Z. V., Gemar, M., & Williams, S. (1999). Differential cognitive response to a mood challenge following successful cognitive therapy or pharmacotherapy for unipolar depression. *Journal of Abnormal Psychology, 108,* 3–10.

Segal, Z. V., & Ingram, R. E. (1994). Mood priming and construct activation in tests of cognitive vulnerability to unipolar depression. *Clinical Psychology Review, 14,* 663–695.

Segal, Z. V., Shaw, B. F., Vella, D. D., & Katz, R. (1992). Cognitive and life stress predictors of relapse in remitted unipolar depressed patients: Test of the congruency hypothesis. *Journal of Abnormal Psychology, 101,* 26–36.

Segal, Z. V., Vincent, P., & Levitt, A. (2002). Efficacy of combined, sequential and crossover psychotherapy and pharmacotherapy in improving outcomes in depression. *Journal of Psychiatry and Neurosciences, 27,* 281–290.

Segal, Z. V., Williams, J. M., & Teasdale, J. D. (2002). *Preventing depression: Mindfulness-based cognitive therapy.* New York: Guilford Press.

Segal, Z. V., Williams, J. M., Teasdale, J. D., & Gemar, M. (1996). A cognitive science perspective on kindling and episode sensitization in recurrent affective disorder. *Psychological Medicine, 26,* 371–380.

Shea, M. T., Elkin, I., Imber, S. D., Sotsky, S. M., Watkins, J. T., Collins, J. F., Pilkonis, P. A., Beckham, E., Glass, D. R., Dolan, R. T., & Parloff, M. B. (1992). Course of depressive symptoms over follow up: Findings from the NIMH Treatment of Depression Collaborative Research Program. *Archives of General Psychiatry, 49,* 782–787.

Shea, M. T., Pilkonis, P. A., Beckham, E., Collins, J. F., Elkin, I., Sotsky, S. M., & Docherty, J. P. (1990). Personality disorders and treatment outcome in the NIMH Treatment of Depression Collaborative Research Program. *American Journal of Psychiatry, 147,* 711–718.

Simon, G. E. (2002). Evidence review: Efficacy and effectiveness of antidepressant treatment in primary care. *General Hospital Psychiatry, 24,* 213–224.

Simons, A. D., Gordon, J. S., Monroe, S. M., & Thase, M. E. (1995). Toward an integration of psychologic, social, and biological factors in depression: Effects on outcome and course of cognitive therapy. *Journal of Consulting and Clinical Psychology, 63,* 369–377.

Sotsky, S. M., Glass, D. R., Shea, M. T., Pilkonis, P. A., Collins, J. F., Elkin, I., Watkins, J. T., Imber, S. D., Leber, W. R., Moyer, J., & Oliveri, M. E. (1991). Patient predictors of response to psychotherapy and pharmocotherapy: Findings in the NIMH Treatment of Depression Collaborative Research Program. *American Journal of Psychiatry, 148,* 997–1008.

Spangler, D. L., Simons, A. D., Monroe, S. M., & Thase, M. E. (1997). Response to cognitive-behavioral therapy in depression: Effects of pretreatment cognitive dysfunction and life stress. *Journal of Consulting and Clinical Psychology, 65,* 568–575.

Stiles, W. B., Agnew-Davies, R., Hardy, G. E., Barkham, M., & Shapiro, D. A. (1998). Relations of the alliance with psychotherapy outcome findings in the second Sheffield Psychotherapy Project. *Journal of Consulting and Clinical Psychology, 66,* 791–802.

Strupp, H. H. (1984). *Psychotherapy in a new key: A guide to time-limited dynamic psychotherapy.* New York: Basic Books.

Teasdale, J. D. (1988). Cognitive vulnerability to persistent depression. *Cognitive and Emotion, 2,* 247–274.

Teasdale, J. D., Segal, Z. V., Williams, J. M. G., Ridgeway, V. A., Soulsby, J. M., & Lau, M. A. (2000). Prevention of relapse/recurrence in major depression by mindfulness-based cognitive therapy. *Journal of Consulting and Clinical Psychology, 68,* 615–623.

Thase, M. E. (1992). Long-term treatments of recurrent depressive disorders. *Journal of Clinical Psychiatry, 53*(Suppl.), 32–44.

Thase, M. E., Greenhouse, J. B., Frank, E., Reynolds, C. F., Pilkonis, P. A., Hurley, K.,

Grochocinski, V., & Kupfer, D. J. (1997). Treatment of major depression with psychotherapy or psychotherapy-pharmacotherapy combinations. *Archives of General Psychiatry, 54*, 989–991.

Thase, M. E., Reynolds, C. F., Frank, E., Simons, A. D., Garamoni, G. .D., McGeary, J., Harden, T., Fasiczka, A. L., & Cahalane, J. F. (1994). Response to cognitive-behavioral therapy in chronic depression. *Journal of Psychotherapy Practice and Research, 3*, 204–214.

Thase, M. E., Simons, A. D., Cahalane, J., McGeary, J., & Harden, T. (1991). Severity of depression and response to cognitive behavior therapy. *American Journal of Psychiatry, 148*, 784–789.

Tkachuk, G. A., & Martin, G. L. (1999). Exercise therapy for patients with psychiatric disorders: Research and clinical implications. *Professional Psychology: Research and Practice, 30*, 275–282.

Weissman, A. (1979). The Dysfunctional Attitudes Scale: A validation study. *Dissertation Abstracts International, 40*, 1389B–1390B.

Westra, H. A., Boardman, C., & Moran-Tynski, S. (2000). The impact of providing preassessment informaiton on no-show rates. *Canadian Journal of Psychiatry, 45*, 572.

Westra, H. A., & Phoenix, E. (2003). *Motivational enhancement therapy in two cases of anxiety disorder: New responses to treatment refractoriness.* Unpublished manuscript, University of Western Ontario.

Whisman, M. A. (2001). Marital adjustment and outcome following treatments for depression. *Journal of Consulting and Clinical Psychology, 69*, 125–129.

Woody, S., McLean, P. D., Taylor, S., & Koch, W. J. (1999). Treatment of depression in the context of panic disorder. *Journal of Affective Disorders, 531*, 163–174.

Zlotnick, C., Elkin, I., & Shea, M. T. (1998). Does the gender of a patient or the gender of a therapist affect the treatment of patients with major depression? *Journal of Consulting and Clinical Psychology, 66*, 655–659.

7

Bipolar Disorder

DOMINIC LAM
WARREN MANSELL

OVERVIEW OF THE DISORDER

Bipolar disorder is a common illness. About 1% of the U.S. population is afflicted with it (Weissman, Leaf, Tischler, & Blazer, 1988). It affects approximately equal numbers of men and women and the median age of onset is 19 years (Burke, Burke, Regier, & Rae, 1990). There is strong evidence of a genetic component. The concordance rate for monozygotic twins raised together is about 80% (Bertelsen, Harvald, & Hauge 1977) and the concordance rate for monozygotic twins raised apart is about 67% (Price, 1968). In a recent twin study examining the overlap between unipolar depression and bipolar disorder, McGuffin et al. (2003) showed that although there are substantial genetic and nonshared environmental correlations between mania and depression, most of the genetic liability to mania is specific to the manic syndrome.

Bipolar disorder runs a natural course of high relapse and recurrences, as suggested by naturalistic studies (Gitlin, Swendsen, Heller, & Hammen, 1995; Winokur, Coryell, Keller, Endicott, & Akiskal, 1993). For bipolar patients who have had one episode of mania, between 85 and 95% will have further multiple recurrences (Keller, 1985), with patients typically averaging 0.6 episodes per year (Winokur et al., 1993). Even with maintenance medication, the 5-year risk of relapse for bipolar disorder is over 70% (Gitlin et al., 1995). With such high rates of relapse and recurrence, it is not surprising that bipolar disorder is very costly to both patients with the disorder and to society at large. In a 1979 report, the U.S. Department of Health concluded that, without adequate treatment, an average woman with an onset of bipolar disorder in her mid-20s effectively loses 9 years of life, 12 years of normal health, and

14 years of working life (U.S. Department of Health Education and Welfare Medical Practice Report, 1979). According to the World Health Organization (2002), bipolar disorder ranked fourth in the leading causes of years of life lived with disability and ninth in the leading causes of disability-adjusted years in adults in the year 2000. Consequently, the illness imposes a high economic burden on societal resources. Rice and Miller (1995), for example, estimated that bipolar disorder posed a total burden of $30.4 billion in 1990, representing 21% of the costs of all mental illnesses in the United States. In the United Kingdom, Guptar and Guest (2002) estimated that the annual National Health Service cost of managing bipolar disorder was £199 million.

According to the fourth edition (text revision) of the *Diagnostic and Statistical Manual of Mental Disorders* (DSM-IV-TR; American Psychiatric Association, 2000), bipolar depression is characterized by the presence of both major depressive episodes (MDEs) and either manic, mixed, or hypomanic episodes. To meet diagnostic criteria for an MDE, the patient must have five (or more) characteristic symptoms of depression during the same 2-week period and these symptoms must represent a change from previous functioning. At least one of the symptoms must be either depressed mood or marked diminished interest or pleasure in activities that were previously enjoyed. Other criteria include significant weight loss when not dieting (or weight gain) or decrease (or increase) in appetite, insomnia or hypersomnia; psychomotor agitation or retardation, loss of energy, feelings of worthlessness or excessive guilt, impaired concentration or indecisiveness and recurrent thoughts of death or recurrent suicidal ideation. These symptoms have to be present most of the day and nearly every day.

The criteria for DSM-IV-TR (American Psychiatric Association, 2000) criteria for mania are a distinct period of abnormally and persistently elevated, expansive, or irritable mood lasting for 1 week. During the period of mood disturbance, at least three of the following symptoms have to be present to a significant degree: inflated self-esteem or grandiosity; decreased need for sleep (e.g., feeling rested after only 3 hours of sleep); more talkative than usual or pressure of speech; flight of ideas or subjective experience that thoughts are racing; distractibility; increase in goal-directed activity or psychomotor agitation; and excessive involvement in pleasurable activities that have a high potential for painful consequences. One of the symptoms has to be either inflated self-esteem or irritability. If irritability is the persistent mood, then four other symptoms have to be present.

For a hypomanic episode, the criteria are similar to a manic episode with the exception that the duration is at least 4 days. If it is the same duration as mania, the episode cannot be severe enough to cause marked impairment in social or occupational functioning. If there are psychotic features, or the episode leads to hospitalization, a diagnosis of mania rather than hypomania is made.

Mixed bipolar episodes, as defined by DSM criteria, are rare. For mixed episodes, the criteria for both a manic episode and for an MDE have to be fulfilled nearly every day for at least a 2-week period. Furthermore, the mood disturbance has to be sufficiently severe to cause marked social or occupational impairment or psychotic features must be present. Clinicians are asked to specify that the patient's symptoms are rapid cycling if he or she has had at least four episodes of a mood disturbance in the previous 12 months that met criteria for a major depression, manic, mixed, or hypomanic episode.

There are two subtypes for bipolar illness. For patients to suffer from bipolar I disorder, there has to be at least one manic episode or mixed episode and one MDE. For patients to suffer from bipolar II disorder, there has to be at least one hypomanic episode and one MDE but no manic or mixed episodes.

OVERVIEW OF EMPIRICALLY SUPPORTED TREATMENTS

Pharmacotherapy

Until recently, the treatment of choice for bipolar disorder has been pharmacotherapy. For the acute phase of severe manic or mixed episodes, oral administration of an antipsychotic or valproate is usually the treatment of choice for their rapid antimanic effect (American Psychiatric Association, 2002). Atypical antipsychotics are also used because of their generally more favorable short-term adverse effects. Adjunctive treatment with a benzodiazepine such as clonazepam or lorazepam may be used to promote sleep for agitated or overactive patients in the short term. In terms of treatment for bipolar depression, the prescribing psychiatrist usually ensures an adequate serum level of the mood stabilizers if the patient is already on long-term prophylactic treatment. If the depression is severe, an antidepressant such as a selective serotonin reuptake inhibitor (SSRI) is usually prescribed (Grunze et al., 2002). There is a risk of switch to mania or mood instability during treatment for depression. Antidepressants appear less likely to induce mania when added to lithium, valproate or an antipsychotic. Tricyclic antidepressants carry a greater risk of precipitating a switch to mania than other antidepressants.

To prevent relapses, bipolar disorder has typically been treated by mood stabilizers. Although lithium has a known effectiveness in reducing relapse rates, the National Institute on Mental Health (NIMH) workshop on the Treatment of Bipolar Disorders (Prien & Potter, 1990) found that lithium is ineffective for between 20 and 40% of patients, often because of side effects and poor compliance. Some studies indicated a 2-year relapse rate of around 50% in patients on lithium (Solomon Keitner, Miller, Shea, & Keller, 1995). In a more recent review, it was again concluded that lithium provides a prophylactic response for only about two-thirds of patients with bipolar disorder (Goodwin, 2002).

Newer mood stabilizers are generally of equivalent efficacy to lithium (Moncrieff, 1995; Solomon et al., 1995). Carbamazepine and valproate appeared to prevent relapse as monotherapy even though there is still a paucity of data from randomized placebo-controlled trials (Keck & McElroy,

2002). Lamotrigine has been found to have a long-term role in delaying or preventing the recurrence of depressive episodes, but lithium and divalproex sodium remains the first-line treatment (Calabrese, Shelton, Rapport, Kimmel, & Elhaj, 2002). Other antipsychotics such as clozapine and olanzapine are also used clinically, but more research is needed as the adverse side effects associated with these antipsychotics may outweigh the benefits (Kusumakar, 2002).

Psychotherapy

There was a paucity of psychotherapy specific to bipolar disorder until the late 1990s. Partly owing to the limited effects of drug treatment for bipolar disorder, psychological therapy in conjunction with pharmacotherapy has become a growing area of development. The psychoanalytic/psychodynamic schools demonstrate a long history of speculation about the etiology of bipolar disorder in early parent–child interactions, later relationships, and intrapsychic mechanisms (Abraham, 1911/1953; Klein, 1950). No controlled studies using psychodynamic psychotherapy have been reported.

To date, all evidence-based psychological therapies specific to bipolar disorder use a diathesis-stress model, emphasizing the importance of both the biological and psychological aspect of the disorder. It is thought that while medication targets the biological vulnerability to the illness, psychotherapy can help patients and their families cope better with the illness. Several kinds of psychological interventions have been studied using randomized controlled designs:

Interpersonal and Social Rhythm Therapy

Research indicates that manic episodes are more likely to be preceded by disruptions in the sleep–wake cycle than episodes of depression or episode-free periods (Malkoff-Schwartz et al., 1998). Interpersonal and social rhythm therapy (IPSRT) encourages patients to develop regular routines of eating, sleeping, exercise, and social interaction and to reduce interpersonal stress. Current evidence suggests that IPSRT helps prevent depressive but not manic symptoms (Frank, 1999). However, the final results of this study are not yet published.

Early Symptom Identification

Several studies suggest that people with bipolar disorder can learn to identify the early warning signs of a relapse and adopt suitable coping strategies (Lam & Wong, 1997; Lam, Wong, & Sham, 2001). A controlled trial compared early symptom identification to treatment as usual (TAU) (Perry, Tarrier, Morriss, McCarthy, & Limb, 1998). The study found that treatment adopting the approach of helping patients to detect their idiosyncratic early warnings of relapse and seek prompt medical help reduced the number of relapses of manic episodes, but not episodes of depression, relative to TAU.

Family-Focused Treatment

Research indicates that higher levels of criticism and emotional involvement by the parents or spouses of patients leads to a worse clinical outcome (Priebe, Wildgrube, & Moller-Oerlinghausen, 1989). To target these factors, family-focused treatment (FFT) involves psychoeducation, problem solving, and training in communication skills. A study has shown that FFT is superior to a brief family psychoeducation and crisis management in reducing relapse rates (Miklowitz et al., 2000).

Medication Compliance Therapy

Medication compliance therapy involves the use of cognitive behavioral principles, such as motivational interviewing, pros and cons tables, and downward arrow techniques, to help enhance patients' drug compliance. A controlled study (Cochran, 1984) found that relative to standard clinical care, the treatment group had fewer affective episodes triggered by lithium noncompliance at 6-month follow-up. There were no significant group differences in medication compliance according to patients' and relatives' reports. According to the prescribing psychiatrists, patients in the treatment group had significantly better compliance than the control group. However, the psychiatrists were not blind to patients' group status. The investigators also failed to obtain serum lithium levels in a significant proportion of patients. These findings suggest tentatively that patients may have benefited from the general effects of the cognitive-behavioral principles learned in therapy.

Group Education

In a study by Colom et al. (2003), 120 bipolar patients were randomized to receive group psychoeducation or a nonstructured group intervention. Both groups were receiving medication and were matched for age and gender. The psychoeducation groups consisted of 8 to 12 euthymic patients who received 20, 1½-hour sessions of psychoeducation. The content of these sessions focused on a medical model of the illness. It covered four major areas: illness awareness, treatment compliance, early detection of prodromal symptoms and recurrences, and lifestyle regularity. In the control group, there was nonspecific interaction with no psychoeducational feedback given. At the 24-month follow-up, significantly fewer patients in the intervention group relapsed than in the control group.

Cognitive-Behavioral Therapy

Different teams of researchers have found support for cognitive-behavioral therapy (CBT) as a treatment for bipolar disorder. It typically involves some elements of the aforementioned approaches such as psychoeducation, medication compliance therapy, adopting regular sleep–wake routines, learning to monitor early warning signs of mania and depression, and developing effective coping strategies for mood swings (Lam, Jones, Bright, & Hayward, 1999). Coming to terms with the illness itself is of major importance to patients with bipolar disorder, and cognitive therapy can help patients to grieve over their losses while challenging more dysfunctional beliefs such as "I have no control over my illness." Early on in therapy, patients are encouraged to produce a life-review chart that illustrates the development of episodes over time and the life events and changes in medication or life stresses that may have contributed to them. The life chart allows patients to see their illness in perspective and to identify vulnerabilities and the factors that may have contributed to their past episodes. Patients with bipolar disorder are often currently depressed or have residual depressive symptoms. Therefore, CBT for bipolar disorder also incorporates standard elements of cognitive therapy for unipolar depression such as negative automatic thought diaries and the identification, restructuring, and testing of dysfunctional assumptions. Attempts are made to link mood to behavior and cognition. Certain assumptions appear to be more specific to bipolar disorder and specifically relate to beliefs in high personal goal attainment and independence from others (Lam, Wright, & Smith, 2004). Some people with bipolar disorder also report rigid beliefs about the positive value of their hypomanic symptoms, which are often addressed through a collaborative discussion of the pros and cons that are discussed later in this chapter. Activity schedules are used to monitor and structure the wake–sleep routine.

Several pilot studies of CBT for bipolar disorder have shown encouraging results. Zaretsky, Segal, and Gemar (1999) conducted a study to treat depression in patients with bipolar disorder. They showed equivalent reductions in depression symptoms in unipolar and bipolar patients over 20 sessions of therapy but smaller nonsignificant changes in dysfunctional assumptions in the bipolar group. Lam et al. (2000) compared 12 to 20 sessions of CBT to treatment as usual of mood stabilizers and outpatient appointments and demonstrated fewer bipolar episodes, less mood fluctuations, and higher social functioning over 6 months. Scott, Garland, and Moorhead (2001) showed that 25 sessions of cognitive therapy led to greater reductions in symptoms of mania and depression and greater improvement in global functioning over 6 months relative to a waiting-list control group. A large-scale randomized controlled trial of CBT for bipolar disorder has now been conducted (Lam et al., 2003). At 12 months, cognitive therapy led to fewer bipolar episodes, fewer days in a bipolar episode and fewer bipolar admissions relative to TAU. The cognitive therapy group also had a high social functioning and lower levels of depression at 6 months; these gains were maintained over 12 months but not to a statistically significant degree.

Taken together, there is empirical support for both pharmacological and combined psychological and pharmacological therapy. The research studies to date indicate that a variety of psychological interventions can be effective, with CBT receiving the most empirical support. There are few large-scale randomized controlled trials at present.

PREDICTORS OF TREATMENT OUTCOME

Only two studies have reported on factors that predict treatment outcome in bipolar disorder. The literature on FFT (Miklowitz et al., 2000) has illuminated the importance of criticism and emotional involvement in the family members of patients with bipolar disorder. Patients whose families are highly critical and have a high level of emotional overinvolvement tend to have significantly more frequent relapses and poorer outcome. Patients from high expressed emotion (EE) families tend to benefit more from FFT than do patients from low EE families.

In a study of cognitive therapy for bipolar disorder, Lam, Wright, and Sham (2005) developed a measure called Sense of Hyper-positive Self Scale (SHPSS), which predicted patients' response to therapy. The authors observed clinically that some bipolar patients like being in a state of constant "high" (i.e., positive mood and being behaviorally active). This state of constant high may not even reach clinical hypomania. They value the perceived attributes associated with this state of mild hypomania such as being "dynamic, persuasive and productive." The authors hypothesized that patients with high scores on the SHPSS would not respond well to short-term focused cognitive therapy which emphasizes the monitoring and regulating of mood, thoughts, and behavior in order to prevent further episodes. Furthermore, it was hypothesized that high goal-attainment dysfunctional attitudes (Lam et al., 2005) would contribute to the "SHPSS" scores when mood levels were controlled for. In Lam et al.'s (2003) relapse prevention study, SHPSS scores were found to moderate the effect of therapy. In the cognitive therapy group, significantly more patients who scored high on the SHPSS relapsed during the 6 months compared to patients who scored low on the SHPSS. No such effect was found in the control group. As hypothesized, high scores on the subscale of goal attainment of the Dysfunctional Attitudes Scale (DAS) predicted the SHPSS score when mood scores were controlled for. Furthermore, the individual DAS goal-attainment items that predicted SHPSS significantly were "I ought to be able to solve my problems quickly and without a great deal of effort" and "I should be happy all the time." It is also interesting to note that patients who dropped out of therapy prematurely during the study had higher DAS goal-attainment beliefs at baseline (Lam, Wright, & Sham, 2004). Hence both the SHPSS and the DAS goal attainment predicted how patients fared in cognitive therapy.

PRACTICAL STRATEGIES FOR IMPROVING OUTCOME

Tackling High Goal-Attainment Beliefs and Disorganization

In the Lam et al. (2003) study, patients who dropped out of therapy prematurely did not fare well. Compared to those who stayed to finish a course of therapy, the inadequate treatment group had more previous hospitalizations for bipolar episodes and higher DAS goal-attainment beliefs at baseline. This translated into highly driven behavior and disorganization, leading to sleeplessness, poor daily routine, and eventually a bipolar episode. After a bipolar episode, these patients often believe that they need to "catching up for lost time." This can lead to a vicious cycle of more driven behavior, disorganization, and further relapses. Figure 7.1 summarizes the vicious cycle of high goal attainment.

Often these patients are very driven but too distracted to accomplish any tasks. Patients who are disorganized in their routine may find it difficult to organize themselves to attend therapy sessions regularly. They often miss sessions or come to sessions late and can get upset if the therapist is unwilling to extend the session over the hour. Traditional cognitive techniques are useful to helping to retain this group of patients in therapy. Useful techniques that can be used at an early stage of therapy include drawing up "pros and cons" of highly driven beliefs and behavior as well as activity scheduling in a collaborative way. With patients who are irritable and disorganized, it is often necessary to balance being understanding with working patiently within the therapeutic boundary. Similar to tackling disorganization, activity scheduling in a collaborative way may be useful to help this group of patients to get back to normal functioning in a gradual way. Ultimately, if the therapist can maintain a collaborative empirical stance toward the patient at this difficult stage, the potential for an improved outcome is greater.

Tackling Valuing the Time of Being "High"

Some bipolar patients like the experience of being behaviorally activated and in a state of high arousal. They feel more productive, eloquent, creative, and attractive as people. These patients even come with evidence that they were being highly productive at work when they were high. Unfortunately, when they get into a clinical state of mania or hypomania, they become distractible,

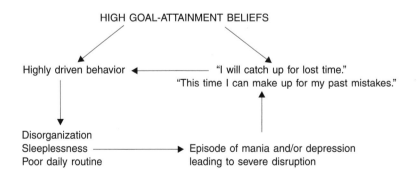

FIGURE 7.1. Example of a vicious cycle for patients with high goal-attainment beliefs.

irritable, destructive, and unproductive. A helpful strategy is to respect the patient's view, particularly as it may be true that there were periods in the patient's life he or she achieved a lot while in such a "high" state. Therapists then can help the patient to examine the evidence and look for pros and cons of being in a permanently high state. Most patients come to therapy because their life is not working out the way they want it to be. It may be they found it hard to stay a bit high and keep functioning without switching into a manic state, which in turn may lead to depressive episodes. In a collaborative way, patients can be helped to tread a fine line of being in a desirable state of slightly high and functioning well without flipping into a clinical state. Often it may be helpful to examine the other neglected domains such as family life, marriages, physical well-being, and psychological well-being. Therapists can then help patients to redress their balance in life more, leading to more contentment.

Involving the Family

It is often useful to involve family members as help at hand when patients need them. However, some bipolar patients have a very strong sense of autonomy. Care must be taken to get patients' explicit consent about the details of family involvement. If this does not happen, patients' sense of autonomy can easily be offended, leading to possible future conflicts in the family.

As has been reported in the expressed emotion literature (e.g., Miklowitz et al., 2000), some family members can be very worried about patients and become too protective or overinvolved. This is most likely to occur when the onset of the disorder was during early adolescence, about the time patients have just left home to go to college. Our experience is that most bipolar patients manage to leave their parents and set up their own home. However, this does not necessarily mean that patients have become truly autonomous. Even well into adulthood, they may still be in daily contact with their parents and consult them excessively about every decision. Some parents have confessed during joint sessions with patients that they have found it difficult to "let go" because patients had such severe breakdowns just when they left home. Therapists ought to be sensitive to these issues. Excessive concerns and worries should be tackled by scheduling some family meetings specifically for these purposes. The family members' concerns and worries can be explicitly explored. Therapists can help the family and the patient to agree on a more appropriate level of independence.

However, family members can be very good help at hand. For example, it is often helpful to get family members' help in eliciting idiosyncratic early signs of relapse, particularly for patients who are not very aware of these signs. In any case, it is helpful for patients and their family members to discuss explicitly what may be helpful and unhelpful involvement. A clear and explicit agreement of what family members can offer as help has to be negotiated. For some patients, this may not be an issue and they may already have good contingency plans for their family members (e.g., taking control of finances in order to minimize any financial loss during a manic episode). Some patients express that being manic and psychotic or being depressed can be very lonely. It then opens doors for family members to provide support that patients value. Patients without family support may be helped to access support through other means such as a trusted friend. To minimize the adverse effects of undetected episodes, extra care should be taken to ensure early detection and treatment for those without a supportive network.

Medication Compliance

Some patients want to discontinue medication, particularly when they have been doing well in therapy. Taking medication has the connotation of being ill and drugs do have unwanted side effects. However, to date, there is no evidence that psychotherapy *on its own* is effective in preventing further episodes. While it is understandable that patients wish to discontinue medication, they should be helped to carefully examine past experiences. Often a life chart detailing onsets and length of episodes, medication, life events, job, education achievement, and relationships can be very informative. Patients can then examine whether mood stabilizers truly prevent or delay relapses. It is also informative to examine the extent of patients' attainment of other life goals when they have fewer episodes. Armed with such information, patients can then be persuaded to consult their prescribing psychiatrists who, like patients, often find such systemic information very helpful. Our experience is that with some coaching, most bipolar patients are able to discuss various treatment options with their psychiatrist. It can be very therapeutic for them to feel they are taking an active role in their treatment.

Alcohol Problems

Alcohol is a common problem in bipolar disorder. When depressed, some patients use alcohol to treat their depression. When they are manic, they use alcohol as fuel. Therapists should be on the lookout for these problems and work with patients to use other strategies to deal with their mood. For example, some patients find it useful to engage in a pleasurable behavior that does not lead to overactivity, such as going for a walk or reading. Specialty alcohol services should be consulted however if the problem is severe.

Social Anxiety and Stigma

It is not uncommon for patients to feel shame and embarrassment, particularly after a psychotic or manic breakdown, which could be very public. Some shame may be realistic and based on indiscretion or embarrassing mistakes when their judgment was affected. However, others may be negatively distorted and based on misinterpretations of other people's reactions. Therapists should also be sensitive that social stigma may be greater in certain cultures. For example, in some cultures, seeking psychiatric help is seen as "loss of face" or loss of dignity. Patients may not articulate their sense of being stigmatized or socially anxious. However, behaviorally they may avoid contact with certain people or situations (Perlick et al., 2001) and hence can never reality-test their worst fears. As a result, this avoidance may result in further social loss unnecessarily. The traditional cognitive-behavioral techniques of articulating their worst fears, formulating a collaborative model, testing out predictions, and evaluating evidence can be helpful (e.g., Clark & Wells, 1995). We would predict that such techniques would improve outcome for socially anxious patients by broadening their social support network and reducing counterproductive avoidance behaviors.

Comorbid Anxiety Disorders

Bipolar disorder, just like unipolar depression, may occur in the context of an anxiety disorder (Cassano, Pini, Saettoni, & Dell'Osso, 1999; Cosoff & Hafner, 1998; Perugi et al., 1999). At present, there is no evidence of a causal relationship between anxiety disorders and mania. However, anxiety is known to lead to reduced sleep, greater fluctuations in mood, and increased physiological activation, all of which are problematic for patients with bipolar disorder. One case study has indicated that it can be fruitful to use a cognitive approach to treat comorbid anxiety disorders in a patient with bipolar disorder (Mansell & Lam, 2004). However, the therapist should be aware of the effects of any increase in stress that may be experienced by patients carrying out exposure therapy or behavioral experiments, especially in patients deemed at high imminent risk of bipolar relapse. Ultimately, however, we would expect treatment for comorbid anxiety disorders to have a beneficial effect for these patients through decreasing stress and hyperarousal.

Interpersonal Processes during Therapy

We have already noted that many bipolar patients have very high personal standards. They may have strong personal opinions, have high qualifications, and be actively engaged in creative pursuits. Furthermore, many patients are already knowledgeable about their condition and may have read self-help guides and autobiographies. These factors can sometimes work to the advantage of the therapy. For example, some patients may be very willing to conscientiously complete mood scales and diaries and discuss them in therapy. However, the same factors may also lead the patient to take on more "homework" than they can actually manage. This is likely to reflect the patient's dysfunctional beliefs that he or she has to excel or be perfect in order to be respected. It could also reflect patients' belief of "having to catch up for lost time." Typically, they are just recovering form a bipolar episode and already taking on a lot in order to get back to their ideal self of being competent and productive. They become overwhelmed with goal-orientated tasks. Within CBT the patient and therapist can tackle the pros and cons of such beliefs and treat the choice of how much homework to do as collaborative experiment. This not only helps assess how much work is feasible but also makes it explicit to the patient that it was best to be realistic about what can be achieved without being too stressed. They do not need to take on large amounts of homework to prove themselves and to gain the approval of the therapist. The patient may begin by suggesting what they believe to be a manageable amount of homework. In the following sessions, they can report on whether the assignments did indeed turn out to be manageable. Such skills gradually generalize to everyday situations, thereby reducing the amount of pressure they create for themselves.

Regarding the process of therapy, these factors may also lead patients to evaluate the therapist by their own high standards, leading the therapist to feel under pressure to provide unambiguous advice or interpretations. The therapist may be able to preempt this situation by adopting a respectful stance to the patient's abilities and being explicit about the patient's rights to autonomy from an early stage in therapy. When put under pressure, the therapist may have to acknowledge the genuine lack of information on some of the complexities of bipolar disorder and therefore explain that therapy will be a collaborative and empirical process for both of them.

Children and Adolescents

Little research has been conducted on psychological therapy for children and adolescents with bipolar disorder. One recent study has indicated that families can learn about mood fluctuations and coping strategies within "multifamily psychoeducation groups" (Fristad, Goldberg-Arnold, & Gavazzi, 2002).

Older Adults

Many older adults will have lived with bipolar disorder throughout their adult life. As a consequence, they may have experienced a long series of losses associated with their illness. It might be necessary to adapt therapy to allow patients to grieve and develop a coherent story of the impact their illness has had on their lives. A life chart can provide a useful aid for this purpose. Other older adults may have experienced their first episode of mania after the age of 50, and there is emerging evidence that this patient group does not have a family history of the illness (Moorhead & Young, 2003). These patients may have difficult questions to ask about why their disorder appeared so late in life and may want to understand the onset of their mania in the context of the life events leading up to the episode. The therapist may therefore need to work with the patient on these issues while also pay-

ing close attention to the patient's current functioning and risk of future relapse.

PREDICTORS OF RELAPSE AND
RECURRENCE AFTER THERAPY

Because research evidence for the efficacy on psychotherapy specific to bipolar
disorder is still emerging, there is not much evidence to suggest what may predict outcome after psychological treatment. However, several areas of research
may shed some light in this area: EE, coping with bipolar prodromes, the disruption of social rhythms and high goal-attainment dysfunctional attitudes.
These findings have guided the recent development of psychotherapies specific
to bipolar affective disorder.

Similar to research in schizophrenia, studies have found that high levels
of criticism or emotional overinvolvement in parents or spouses led to poor
outcomes in terms of relapses or poor symptomatic outcome in bipolar disorder (Hornig, Hoffman, Rozendaal, & Dingemans, 1977; Miklowitz, Goldstein, Nuechterlein, Snyder, & Mintz 1998; Priebe et al., 1989). Psychological
treatments that do not target EE may leave patients in a more vulnerable position for relapse. However, this issue is not always clear. There is evidence that
EE levels do subside after an acute episode (Lam, 1991). Hence the relationship is not strictly causal. High EE responses may exacerbate the episode
rather than cause it.

In terms of prodromes, bipolar patients were found to be able to report
prodromes (Altman et al., 1992; Lam & Wong, 1997; Molnar, Feeney, &
Fava, 1988; Smith & Tarrier, 1992). One study found that bipolar patients
were able to report common prodromes reliably over 18 months (Lam et al.,
2001). Furthermore, patients' ability to cope with manic prodromes predicted
their level of social functioning and relapses 18 months later. There is evidence
that social functioning, particularly functioning at work, could predict shorter
times to relapse (Gitlin et al., 1995). Hence, levels of social functioning may
predict how patients fare even after therapy. Patients' ability to detect and
cope well with bipolar symptoms and mood fluctuations may be an important
factor, which could affect the course of their illness after therapy.

In terms of life events, there is evidence that life events that disrupt sleep–
wake routines play an important role prior to the onset of a manic episode.
Bipolar patients are also known to relapse after long distance traveling or jet
lag (Jauhar & Weller, 1982; Lam et al., 2001). Malkoff-Schwartz et al. (1998)
found that in the 8 weeks prior to manic episodes, a significantly greater
proportion of patients had social rhythm disruption events compared with the
8-week episode-free control period.

Some bipolar patients have extreme goal-attainment attitudes, such as "If
I try hard enough I should be able to excel in anything I attempt" (Lam,
Wright, & Smith, 2004). It was found that bipolar patients with these beliefs

had more frequent previous relapses. As a result of these attitudes they are often behaviorally engaged in achievement activities at the expense of a good routine of regular meals, adequate sleep and exercise. Hence it is possible that highly driven behaviors and disorganized routine could lead to future relapses.

PRACTICAL STRATEGIES FOR
PREVENTING RELAPSE AND RECURRENCE

Based on the aforementioned risk factors, the practical strategies for preventing relapses and recurrences include tackling residual symptoms, monitoring and coping with prodromes or relapse early warning, promoting routine and sleep, and tackling high goal-attainment dysfunctional beliefs. Furthermore, medication taken lifelong is always an issue for bipolar patients. There is evidence that significantly more patients who had rapid discontinuation of lithium experienced relapses compared to gradual discontinuation (Faedda, Tondo, Baldessarini, Suppes, & Tohen, 1993). Hence counseling and advising about medication discontinuation are always warranted.

It is known that clinically stable bipolar patients still display mood swings or subclinical fluctuations that are unrelated to prodromes of a relapse (Molnar, Fava, Zielezny, Spinks, & Loretan, 1987). Patients with significant residual symptoms are likely to relapse into depression by going from residual symptoms to prodromal stages and full-blown episodes, the so called rollback phenomenon. Hence it is important to tackle any significant residual symptoms with cognitive-behavioral techniques such as activity scheduling and negative automatic thought diaries.

Prodromes are defined as the interval from the time that the first symptoms are recognized to the time when the symptoms reach maximum severity (Molnar et al., 1988). In several relapse prevention studies, patients are helped to systematically map out their relapse signature and are taught strategies to cope with the prodromal stage in an adaptive way (Lam et al., 2000; Lam et al., 2003; Perry et al., 1998; Scott et al., 2001). The goal is to "nip it in the bud" at an earliest stage of an episode. Lam et al. (1999) gives a full description of how to work with patients to map out their idiosyncratic relapse signature and to develop good coping strategies. Briefly, an open-ended question approach is advocated in which patients are asked what types of behavioral, cognitive, and affective warnings may lead them to think that they are relapsing into a mania or a depressive episode, respectively. Each warning is written on a piece of paper. Care is taken to make sure that these warnings are described in the patients' own words. The sheets of paper are then sorted into warnings that typically happen in the very early stages and those that happen in the late stages of the prodromal period. Anything that does not belong to the early or late stages is placed into a pile of the middle stage. Affect, such as irritability or depression, is subjective and hard to gauge and hence is always anchored in patients' social environment. Patients are always asked, for example, how the depression or irritability shows itself. Preferably they should be able to name the people with whom they are normally irritated at different stages of the prodromal period. Patients and therapists then work on good coping strategies at the different stages of the prodromal phase. Good coping strategies include seeking medical help early. There is a lot of variability with regard to the length of the prodromal phases. Some patients can have a full-blown manic attack within days of recognizing the first signs of relapse. For them, an agreement can be made with the prescribing psychiatrists to have some tranquillizers at hand so that they can start taking some early while awaiting an outpatient appointment. A mutually respectful and trusting relationship between patients and psychiatrists can be extremely useful.

As there is evidence that good sleep and daily routine are important in preventing relapses, patients should also be advised to restart their activity schedules when they feel life is getting too hectic. This is particularly important at the early stages of either a manic or a depressed episode. When patients are just getting into a manic episode, the temptation to overengage in goal-directed behavior can be very strong. On the contrary, when patients are beginning to sink into a depression, the temptation is to curl up and ruminate. Activity scheduling in order to prioritize and do the minimum can be very important in helping patients to cope with entering either a depressive or a manic episode. As stated earlier, patients with very highly driven beliefs sometimes overcompensate when they are out of an episode in order to "catch up for lost time" due to previous illness. Therapists should use cognitive-behavioral skills to work with patients collaboratively to tackle these highly driven beliefs and behavior. These include a historical review of onset of past episodes, pros and cons of these extreme beliefs, and setting realistic goals while convalescing.

As patients get more stable, the issue of whether to continue with mood-stabilizing medication forever is often raised. This is particularly the case for female patients in the reproductive period of their lives. As stated previously, there is evidence from a randomized controlled study that significantly more patients relapse quickly in rapid discontinuation than medically guided gradual discontinuation of mood stabilizers (Faedda et al., 1993). While patients may want to discontinue their medication abruptly when trying to conceive or if they find out that they are pregnant, rapid discontinuation of medication may leave them particularly vulnerable to relapses. It is at this time that they particularly need frequent and careful professional support. It is often necessary to go through the pros and cons of conceiving urgently because "time is running out." After giving birth, patients are particularly vulnerable to postnatal depression or mania. A frank discussion about making sure they have been stable for a while and have enough support around them prior to trying to conceive is important. Generating pros and cons for the choice to breast-feed or to stay stable so that they can bond with and look after their babies is often helpful. Discussing these issues with a trusted therapist who remains impartial and helpful can be a very positive experience that may enable patients to have a fruitful discussion with their prescribing psychiatrist at some stage.

CASE EXAMPLE

Michael was a 25-year-old trainee accountant with an investment bank. He had received a diagnosis of bipolar disorder following one episode of depression and one episode of mania. There was a family history of bipolar disorder. Both his sister and his maternal aunt were very disabled by their bipolar illness. His 25-year-old twin sister was still living at home. She lost her job and friends years ago and was attending a day center. Michael had been scared that he may develop the illness as well. He had reported being well until the year prior to therapy, when he experienced an episode of generalized anxiety and depression that was treated with antidepressant medication. The hypomanic symptoms emerged while he was in hospital for a medical procedure, but they were initially labeled an anxiety reaction. The next day a diagnosis of a manic episode entailed a transfer to a psychiatric hospital. Michael was eventually stabilized on a low dose of antipsychotic medication.

Cognitive therapy began 5 months after the onset of the manic episode. At the time of assessment, he reported no significant signs of depression (BDI = 3; Beck Depression Inventory; Beck & Steer, 1993), manic symptoms (ISS–Activation = 0; Internal State Scale; Bauer et al., 1991), or anxiety (BAI = 4; Beck Anxiety Inventory; Beck, Epstein, Brown, & Steer, 1988). He reported no other present symptoms. However, he identified several aims of therapy: (1) to understand what may have triggered the depression and mania, in order to help prevent future relapses; (2) to address his difficulties with making decisions, unrelenting standards, and self-criticism; and (3) to learn how to deal with the stigma of the diagnosis.

Michael attended 17 sessions of cognitive therapy. The initial sessions involved producing a life chart of his illness and the particular events that led up to the episodes of depression and mania. Michael reported that he had always been an extremely conscientious individual and had high standards for his own performance. He also wanted to be able to control every aspect of his life. This led him to worry about whether he had performed well enough and made the correct decision in all areas of his life. Often he would work extremely hard to achieve these perfectionist standards. There were examples of his performing well academically all through his life. It was hypothesized that this high goal-attainment cognitive style had combined with a range of stressors to lead up to the recent bipolar episodes with marked anxiety symptoms. The stressors included pressure at work partly owing to his taking on too many responsibilities, isolating himself from his peers because he felt that they would think he could not cope, medical illness, sleep disruption due to work, and rejection by a prospective partner.

Following the identification of these factors, the early, middle, and late warning signs for depression and mania were identified and written down, along with the generation of suitable coping strategies. The middle sessions of therapy were focused mainly on addressing the dysfunctional assumptions that were hypothesized as putting him at risk of future episodes. He was taught how to use problem-solving techniques and pros and cons tables to help make decisions and diaries to identify and challenge negative automatic thoughts. Michael's dysfunctional assumptions included "I am going to fail as a person if I do not make the right decision," "My superiors will think I am incompetent unless I perform perfectly," and "If I do not take (full) control, things would go horribly wrong." Michael carried out behavioral experiments to challenge his assumptions, such as making decisions without covering for every possible negative outcome and delegating and postponing work. The middle–end sessions of therapy were focused mainly on dealing with the issues concerning the diagnosis, in particular whether and how to disclose to friends, possible partners, colleagues, and employers. The final sessions involved a review of the strategies covered and when would be appropriate to use them in the absence of a therapist.

There were several obstacles to effective therapy. First, Michael reported few current psychiatric symptoms. Therefore, current depression or anxiety was unlikely to decrease as a consequence of therapy; but it was certainly possible that they could increase as Michael began to examine his beliefs and try out new behaviors. To prepare for this, the therapist discussed the possibility that the patient might experience an increase in symptoms during therapy, but that the symptoms would be closely monitored. Indeed this would provide an opportunity for the patient to try out the techniques he was learning to prevent a future relapse. Second, and related to the foregoing, Michael, reported negative automatic thoughts in the absence of an intense emotional response, possibly due to his effort to control his emotions. Therefore, the therapist spent more time using downward arrow techniques to try to identify the "hot cognitions."

Third, Michael's interaction in therapy was sometimes a mix of mistrusting the therapist and making demands on him. He sometimes asked for information but repeated the same questions in subsequent sessions in order to check that the information was correct. Mixed with this mistrust, he sometimes made unreasonable demands on the psychiatrist and the therapist. These could include frequent demands in writing to his superior at work, prescribing certain medications, and finding out about his prospects at work. It sometimes proved difficult to maintain a collaborative therapeutic stance owing to the patient's interpersonal pattern of mistrust and demands. As part of taking control, Michael would expect as much information as possible from the therapist and yet pertinent personal issues were often discussed in a very academic way. He took notes in therapy diligently, but the process was so detached that the therapist felt it was like giving a lecture to Michael about the facts of bipolar disorder. Therefore, at several points during the treatment, the therapist chose to reiterate the collaborative nature of cognitive therapy and redirect the aims of the therapy as a joint empirical process.

Fourth, the patient occasionally displayed an ambivalence concerning whether he did qualify for a diagnosis of bipolar affective disorder for several reasons including the fact that he had been taking antidepressant medication at the time of onset and that the symptoms had emerged so rapidly. His worst fear was that, like his sister who was diagnosed with the illness, he would also lose his job and his friends. The patient was encouraged to discuss his diagnosis with his psychiatrist, and the therapist and patient discussed the pros and cons of taking or not taking relevant precautions. The patient eventually committed himself to the diagnosis and to maintaining both the psychological and pharmacological prophylactic measures. Michael and his psychiatrist agreed that the mood prophylactic medication would be reviewed at a later date after a lengthy period of stability.

At the end of therapy, Michael reported that he had gained a better understanding of bipolar affective disorder, his personal risk factors, and how to prevent a relapse. He maintained the same levels of anxiety and hypomanic symptoms throughout therapy, although his symptoms of depression rose slightly (BDI = 9). However Michael plunged himself back to work as soon as possible despite the therapist's advice against the behavior of "catching for lost time." He was experiencing depression and anxiety symptoms again due to returning to work prematurely and taking on too much work. His general practitioner asked him to take a week off from work. Michael saw it as evidence of him losing control of his intellect. He catastrophized and made suicide threats. His condition alarmed his parents. They contacted the emergency psychiatrist who admitted Michael. The admission was only a brief one. Michael was given further sessions to discuss the nature of emotions and exploring the meaning of experiencing and displaying emotions to himself. He was also persuaded to take the brief lapse as an opportunity to take stock, and he was helped to see that a slight relapse can be a learning experience. Michael became more accepting of the importance of making emotional connections to issues being discussed in sessions and used this episode to learn how to manage his illness. Therapy became more connected to his emotions. He no longer took notes diligently in therapy sessions to accumulate knowledge in an intellectual and controlled way. Michael has been well for over 18 months.

CONCLUSION

Evidence for the efficacy of psychotherapy specific for bipolar disorder has only emerged in the last 5 years. These psychotherapies include group psychoeducation, family therapy, and individual therapies including cognitive therapy and interpersonal therapy. So far the evidence is encouraging.

As with other mood disorders, cognitive therapy has produced by far the most evidence of efficacy for patients suffering from bipolar disorder. Several pilot studies and one randomized controlled study have all produced good results. Bipolar disorder is a difficult condition to treat. It is pleasing to see evidence of treatment efficacy for cognitive therapy in patients suffering from bipolar disorder. However, more important, it is necessary to identify individuals who do not respond to the current cognitive therapy treatment manuals and examine their characteristics in order to improve treatment further. We have evidence that patients with a high sense of hyper-positive self may not respond as well to cognitive therapy. These patients typically are disorganized and behaviorally activated. They also have beliefs of high goal attainment and are difficult to engage. Development of specific techniques to engage these patients and to tackle disorganization and high goal-attainment beliefs are necessary if we are to improve the treatment outcome

Another urgent objective for the cognitive therapy treatment of bipolar disorder is to understand the cognitive processes in manic patients. The cognitive model for depression is well developed. Many facets of the cognitive model for unipolar depression seem to be equally applicable to bipolar depression. However, very little is known about the information processing of manic patients. Cognitive-behavioral models of the maintenance of psychological disorders has resulted in important advances in treatment (Beck, Rush, Shaw, & Emery, 1979; Clark 1986; Fairburn, Shafran, & Cooper, 1999). A maintenance model for mania would be very helpful to guide treatment further.

REFERENCES

Abraham, K. (1953). Notes on the psycho-analytical investigation and treatment of manic–depressive insanity and allied conditions. In *Selected papers on psychoanalysis*. New York: Basic Books. (Original work published 1911)

Altman, E. S., Rea, M. M., Mintz, J., Miklowitz, D. J., Goldstein, M. J., & Hwang, S. (1992). Prodromal symptoms and signs of bipolar relapse: A report based on prospectively collected data. *Psychiatry Research, 41*, 1–8.

American Psychiatric Association. (2000). *Diagnostic and statistical manual of mental disorders* (4th ed., text rev.). Washington, DC: Author.

American Psychiatric Association. (2002). Practice guideline for the treatment of patients with bipolar disorder (revision). *American Journal of Psychiatry, 159*(Suppl. 4), 1–50.

Bauer, M. S., Crits-Christoph, P., Ball, W. A., Dewees, E., McAllister, T., Alahi, P., Cacciola, J., & Whybrow, P. C. (1991). Independent assessment of manic and depressive symptoms by self-rating: Scale characteristics and implications for the study of mania. *Archives of General Psychiatry, 48*, 807–812.

Beck, A. T., Epstein, N., Brown, G., & Steer, R. A. (1988). An inventory for measuring clinical anxiety: Psychometric properties. *Journal of Consulting and Clinical Psychology, 56*, 893–897.

Beck, A. T., Rush, A. J., Shaw B. F., & Emery, G. (1979). *Cognitive theory of depression*. New York: Guilford Press.

Beck, A. T., & Steer R. A. (1993). *Beck Depression Inventory Manual*. San Antonio, TX: Psychological Corporation.

Bertelsen, A., Harvald, B., & Hauge, M. (1977). A Danish twin study of manic depressive disorders. *British Journal of Psychiatry, 130*, 330–351.

Burke, K. C., Burke, J. D., Jr., Regier, D. A., & Rae, D. S. (1990). Age at onset of selected mental disorders in five community populations. *Archives of General Psychiatry, 47*, 511–518.

Calabrese, J. R., Shelton, M. D., Rapport, D. J., Kimmel, S. E., & Elhaj, O. (2002). Long-term treatment of bipolar disorder with Lamotrigine. *Journal of Clinical Psychiatry*, 63(Suppl. 10), 18–22.

Cassano, G. B., Pini, S., Saettoni, M., & Dell'Osso, L. (1999). Multiple anxiety disorder comorbidity in patients with mood spectrum disorders with psychotic features. *American Journal of Psychiatry*, 156, 474–476.

Clark, D. M. (1986). A cognitive approach to panic. *Behaviour Research and Therapy*, 24, 461–470.

Clark, D. M., & Wells, A. (1995). A cognitive model of social phobia. In R. Heimberg, M. Liebowitz, D. A. Hope, & F. R. Schneider (Eds.), *Social phobia: Diagnosis, assessment, and treatment* (pp. 69–93). New York: Guilford Press.

Cochran, S. D. (1984). Preventing medical non-compliance in the outpatient treatment of bipolar affective disorders. *Journal of Consulting and Clinical Psychology*, 52, 873–878.

Colom, F., Vieta, E., Martinez-Aran, A., Rinares, M., Goilolea, J.M., Benabarre A., Torrent, C., Comes, M., Corbella, B., Parramon, G., & Corominas, J. (2003). A randomized trial on the efficacy of group psychoeducation in the prophylaxis of recurrences in remitted bipolar patients. *Archives of General Psychiatry*, 60, 402–407.

Cosoff, S. J., & Hafner, R. J. (1998). The prevalence of comorbid anxiety in schizophrenia, schizoaffective disorder and bipolar disorder. *Australian and New Zealand Journal of Psychiatry*, 32, 67–72.

Fairburn, C. G., Shafran, R., & Cooper, Z. (1998). A cognitive behavioral theory of anorexia nervosa. *Behaviour Research and Therapy*, 37, 1–13.

Faedda, G. L., Tondo, L., Baldessarini, R. J., Suppes, T., & Tohen, M. (1993). Outcome after rapid Vs gradual discontinuation of lithium treatment in bipolar disorders. *Archives of General Psychiatry*, 50, 448–455.

Frank, E. (1999). Interpersonal and social rhythm therapy prevents depressive symptomatology in bipolar 1 patient. *Bipolar Disorder*(Suppl. 1), 13.

Fristad, M. A., Goldberg-Arnold, J. S., & Gavazzi, S. M. (2002). Multifamily psychoeducation groups (MFPG) for families of children with bipolar disorder. *Bipolar Disorders*, 4, 254–262.

Gitlin, M. J., Swendsen, J., Heller, T. L., & Hammen, C. (1995). Relapse and impairment in bipolar disorder. *American Journal of Psychiatry*, 152, 1635–1640.

Goodwin, F. K. (2002). Rationale for long-term treatment of bipolar disorder and evidence for long-term lithium treatment. *Journal of Clinical Psychiatry*, 63(Suppl. 10), 5–12.

Grunze, H., Kasper, D., Goodwin, G., Bowden, C., Baldwin, D., Licht, R., Vieta, E., & Moller, H. J. (2002). World Federation of Societies of Biological Psychiatry guidelines for biological treatment of bipolar disorders. Part I: Treatment of bipolar depression. *World Journal of Biological Psychiatry*, 3, 115–124.

Gupta, R. D., & Guest, J. F. (2002). Annual cost of bipolar disorder to UK society. *British Journal of Psychiatry*, 180, 227–233.

Hornig, A., Hoffman, A., Rozendaal, N., & Dingemans, P. (1997). Psycho-education in bipolar disorder, *Psychiatry Research*, 72, 12–22.

Jauhar, P., & Weller, M. P. I. (1982). Psychiatric morbidity and time zone changes: A study of patients from Heathrow Airport. *British Journal of Psychiatry*, 140, 231–235.

Keck, P. E., & McElroy, S. L. (2002). Carbamazepine and valproate in the maintenance treatment of bipolar disorder. *Journal of Clinical Psychiatry*, 63(Suppl. 10), 13–17.

Keller, M. B. (1985). Chronic and recurrent affective disorders: incidence, course and influencing factors. In K. Kemali & G. Racagu (Eds.), *Chronic treatments in neuropsychiatry* (pp. 111–120). New York: Raven Press.

Klein, M. (1950). *Contributions to psycho-analysis 1921–1945.* London: Hogarth Press.

Kusumakar, V. (2002). Antidepressants and antipsychotics in the long-term treatment of bipolar disorder. *Journal of Clinical Psychiatry, 63*(Suppl. 10), 23–28.

Lam, D. H. (1991). Psycho-social family intervention in schizophrenia: A review of empirical studies. *Psychological Medicine, 21,* 423–441.

Lam, D. H., Bright, J., Jones, S., Hayward, P., Schuck, N., Chisholm, D., & Sham, P. (2000). Cognitive therapy for bipolar illness a pilot study of relapse prevention. *Cognitive Therapy and Research, 24,* 503–520.

Lam, D. H., Jones, S., Bright, J., & Hayward, P. (1999). *Cognitive therapy for bipolar disorder: A therapist's guide to concepts, methods and practice.* Chichester, UK: Wiley.

Lam, D., Watkins, E., Hayward, P., Bight, J., Wright, K., Kerr, N., Parr-Davis, G., & Sham, P. (2003). A randomized controlled study of cognitive therapy of relapse prevention for bipolar affective disorder—Outcome of the first year. *Archives of General Psychiatry, 60,* 145–152.

Lam, D. H., & Wong, G. (1997). Prodromes, coping strategies, insight and social functioning in bipolar affective disorders. *Psychological Medicine, 27,* 1091–1100.

Lam, D. H., Wong, G., & Sham, P. (2001). Prodromes, coping strategies and course of illness in bipolar affective disorders—A naturalistic study. *Psychological Medicine, 31,* 1397–1402.

Lam, D. H., Wright, K., & Sham, P. (2005). Sense of hyper-positive self and response to cognitive therapy for bipolar disorder. *Psychological Medicine, 35,* 69–77.

Lam, D., Wright, K., & Smith N. (2004). Dysfunctional assumptions in bipolar disorder. *Journal of Affective Disorder, 79,* 193–199.

Malkoff-Schwartz, S., Frank, E., Anderson, B., Sherrill, J. T., Siegel, L., Patterson, D., & Kupfer, D. J. (1998). Stressful life events and social rhythm disruption in the onset of manic and depressive bipolar episodes. *Archives of General Psychiatry, 55,* 702–707.

Mansell, W., & Lam, D. (2004). Conceptualizing a cycle of ascent into mania: A case report. *Behavioral and Cognitive Psychotherapy, 31,* 363–367.

McGuffin, P., Rijsdijk, F., Andrew, M., Sham., P., Katz, R., & Cardno, A. (2003). The heritability of bipolar affective disorder and the genetic relationship to unipolar depression. *Archives of General Psychiatry, 60,* 497–502.

Miklowitz, D. J., Goldstein, M. J., Nuechterlein, K. H., Snyder, K. S., & Mintz, J. (1998). Psycho-education in bipolar disorder. *Archives of General Psychiatry, 45,* 225–231.

Miklowitz, D. J., Simoneau, T. L., George, E. L., Richards, J. A., Kalbag, A., & Sachs-Ericsson, S. R. (2000). Family-focused treatment of bipolar disorder: 1-year effects of a psychoeducation program in conjunction with pharmacotherapy. *Biological Psychiatry, 48,* 582–592.

Molnar, G., Fava, G. A., Zielezny, M., Spinks, M. T., & Loretan, A. (1987). Measurement of subclinical changes during lithium prophylaxis: A longitudinal study. *Psychopathology, 20,* 155–161.

Molnar, G. J., Feeney, M. G., & Fava, G. A. (1988). Duration and symptoms of bipolar prodomes. *American Journal of Psychiatry, 145,* 1576–1578.

Moncrieff, J. (1995). Lithium revisited: A re-examination of the placebo-controlled trials of lithium prophylaxis in manic-depressive disorder. *British Journal of Psychiatry, 167,* 569–574.

Moorhead, S. R. J., & Young, A. H. (2003). Evidence for a late onset bipolar-I disorder sub-group from 50 years. *Journal of Affective Disorders, 73,* 271–277.

Perlick, D., Rosenbeck, R. A., Clarkin, J. F., Sirey, J. A., Salahi, J., Struening, E. L., & Link, B. G. (2001). Adverse effects of perceived stigma on social adaptation of persons diagnosed with bipolar affective disorder. *Psychiatric Services, 52,* 1627–1632.

Perry, A., Tarrier, N., Morriss, R., McCarthy, E., & Limb, K. (1998). Randomized controlled trial of efficacy of teaching patients with bipolar disorder to identify early symptoms of relapse and obtain treatment. *British Medical Journal, 318,* 139–153.

Perugi, G., Akiskal, H. S., Ramacciotti, S., Nassini, S., Toni, C., Milanfranchi, A., & Musetti, L. (1999). Depressive comorbidity of panic, social phobic and obsessive–compulsive disorders re-examined: Is there a bipolar II connection? *Journal of Psychiatric Research, 33,* 53–61.

Price, J. (1968). Neurotic and endogenous depression: a phylogenetic view. *British Journal of Psychiatry, 114,* 119–120.

Priebe, S., Wildgrube, C., & Muller-Oerlinghausen, B. (1989). Lithium prophylaxis and expressed emotion. *British Journal of Psychiatry, 154,* 396–399.

Prien, R. F., & Potter, W. Z. (1990). NIMH workshop report on treatment of bipolar disorder. *Psychopharmacology Bulletin, 26,* 409–427.

Rice, D. P., & Miller, L. S. (1995) The economic burden of affective disorders, *British Journal of Psychiatry, 27*(Suppl.), 34–42.

Scott, J., Garland, A., & Moorhead, S. (2001). A pilot study of cognitive therapy in bipolar disorders. *Psychological Medicine, 31,* 459–467.

Smith, J. A., & Tarrier, N. (1992). Prodromal symptoms in manic depressive psychosis. *Social Psychiatry and Psychiatric Epidemiology, 27,* 245–248

Solomon, D. A., Keitner, G. I., Miller, I. W., Shea, M. T., & Keller, M. B. (1995). Course of illness and maintenance treatments for patients with bipolar disorders. *Journal of Clinical Psychiatry, 56,* 5–13.

U.S. Department of Health Education and Welfare Medical Practice Report. (1979). *A State of the Science Report for the Office of the Assistant Secretary for the U.S. Department of Health, Education and Welfare.* Baltimore MD: Policy Research.

Weissman, M. M., Leaf, P. J., Tischler, G. L., & Blazer, D. G. (1988). Affective disorders in five United States communities. *Psychological Medicine, 18,* 141–153.

Winokur, G., Coryell, W., Keller, M., Endicott, J., & Akiskal, H. (1993). A prospective follow-up of patients with bipolar and primary unipolar affective disorder. *Archives of General Psychiatry, 50,* 457–465

World Health Organization. (2002). *World Health Report 2002.* Geneva, Switzerland: Author.

Zaretsky, A. E., Segal, Z. V., & Gemar, M. (1999). Cognitive therapy for bipolar depression: A pilot study. *Canadian Journal of Psychiatry, 44,* 491–494.

8

Eating Disorders

TRACI McFARLANE
JACQUELINE CARTER
MARION OLMSTED

OVERVIEW OF THE DISORDERS

There are two recognized eating disorders, anorexia nervosa (AN) and bulimia nervosa (BN). Recently, a new eating disorder, termed "binge-eating disorder" (BED), has also been proposed. BED is listed as an example of "eating disorders not otherwise specified" and as a provisional disorder requiring further study in the fourth edition of the *Diagnostic and Statistical Manual of Mental Disorders* (DSM-IV; American Psychiatric Association, 1994). Eating disorders mainly affect adolescent and young adult women, although BED affects an older age group and a higher percentage of men.

The clinical features of AN and BN overlap significantly. In both cases, the core psychopathology is a tendency to overvalue shape and weight such that self-worth is mainly, if not exclusively, judged in terms of satisfaction with these aspects of appearance. The defining features of BN include persistent attempts to restrict food intake that are punctuated by recurrent episodes of binge eating and inappropriate compensatory behaviors to prevent weight gain. Binge eating has two defining characteristics: the consumption of a large amount of food given the circumstances and a sense of loss of control. Compensatory behaviors are divided into two categories: purging and nonpurging. Purging techniques include self-induced vomiting and laxative or diuretic misuse. Nonpurging compensatory behaviors include strict dieting, fasting, and excessive exercise. Most individuals with BN are within the normal weight range but exhibit a strong drive for thinness.

The central features of AN include extreme food restriction and a refusal to maintain body weight at or above a minimally normal weight for age and height (i.e., chart average weight less than 85%). To the extent that the pursuit of thinness is successful, this behavior is typically not seen as a problem (i.e., it is ego-syntonic) and individuals with AN are frequently not motivated to overcome the disorder. Approximately half of those presenting with AN describe recurrent episodes of binge eating and/or purging. In some cases, the amount of food eaten during binge-eating episodes in AN is not objectively large.

Symptoms of depression, anxiety, impaired concentration, poor social functioning, and low self-esteem are common to both AN and BN and can be secondary to self-starvation, chaotic eating habits, or weight loss. These symptoms typically improve with the normalization of eating and weight. There is also a subgroup who engage in substance abuse, self-injury, or both (Dansky, Brewerton, & Kilpatrick, 2000; Paul, Schroeter, Dahme, & Nutzinger, 2002; Welch & Fairburn, 1996). In addition, eating disorders are associated with a number of (sometimes serious) medical complications including gastrointestinal problems, hypotension, electrolyte disturbances, dental problems, cardiovascular abnormalities, and osteoporosis (Mitchell, Pyle, Eckert, Hatsukami, & Lentz, 1983; Sharp & Freeman, 1993). The long-term mortality rate is over 10%. Death most commonly results from starvation, suicide, or electrolyte imbalance (American Psychiatric Association, 1994).

BED is characterized by recurrent and persistent binge eating in the absence of compensatory behaviors. Unlike patients with BN who report elevated levels of dietary restriction between binge-eating episodes, patients with BED typically exhibit a general tendency to overeat (Marcus, Wing, & Lamparski, 1985). Several studies have documented that BED patients eat significantly more than weight-matched controls both during and between binge-eating episodes (Yanovski et al., 1992). Consequently, the majority of patients with BED are overweight (i.e., body mass index greater than 27). In comparison with overweight patients without BED, those with BED have significantly more psychiatric comorbidity including depression, anxiety, low self-esteem, impaired social functioning, and personality disorders (Specker, de Zwann, Raymond, & Mitchell, 1994).

OVERVIEW OF EMPIRICALLY SUPPORTED TREATMENTS

Bulimia Nervosa

Cognitive-Behavioral Therapy

Most randomized clinical trials of cognitive-behavioral therapy (CBT) for BN consist of three stages that span 19 sessions or approximately 20 weeks. In the first stage the focus is on behavioral change and includes psychoeducation on normal eating, and the connection between restricting and binge eating. In addition, clients are taught to use behavioral strategies (e.g., meal planning, distraction, and stimulus control) to normalize their eating and to avoid acting on urges to binge, purge, restrict, or exercise. Self-monitoring is used to help clients normalize their eating and to identify triggers for symptoms and eating-disordered thoughts. The second stage involves teaching problem-solving skills, cognitive restructuring, and addressing shape and weight concerns. In the third stage, the focus moves to the use of relapse prevention strategies (Wilson, Fairburn, & Agras, 1997). It may not be possible to consider broader concerns during this limited amount of time; however, addressing motivational issues, underlying issues, and comorbidity are an important part of treatment that can be encompassed into the CBT approach.

More than 50 randomized controlled trials have evaluated treatments for BN. On balance, the evidence suggests that CBT is the most effective treatment for BN that has been studied to date (for a detailed review, see Wilson & Fairburn, 2002). CBT for BN is based on a cognitive model of the maintenance of BN (Fairburn, 1997a). A detailed treatment manual is available (Fairburn, Marcus, & Wilson, 1993; Wilson et al., 1997). Manual-based CBT for BN has been shown to result in clinically significant reductions in binge eating, purging, dietary restraint, and overconcern with weight and shape, as well as improving associated psychopathology including depression and poor self-esteem. However, less than half of clients achieve abstinence from binge eating and purging with CBT and a significant number of those relapse after treatment ends.

Across the available studies, between 40 and 50% of treatment completers are abstinent from binge eating and purging at the end of treatment. Of the remainder, some show partial improvement, some do not benefit, and some drop out of treatment. In one study, it was found that 44% of participants were abstinent from binge eating and vomiting at the end of treatment (Fairburn, Peveler, Jones, Hope, & Doll, 1993). At 1-year follow-up, 27% of those who were abstinent had resumed binge eating and purging. In another study, 4 months after the end of CBT treatment, 44% of 48 clients with BN who had achieved abstinence from bingeing and purging had relapsed (Halmi et al., 2002). In a recent large multicenter study, 60% of CBT completers were not abstinent from binge eating and purging over the previous 4 weeks at follow-up (Agras, Walsh, Fairburn, Wilson, & Kraemer, 2000).

Several recent studies suggest that full CBT is not necessary in all cases of BN; a significant subgroup have been shown to benefit from brief treatments, including cognitive-behavioral self-help (e.g., Carter et al., 2003; Palmer, Birchall, McGrain, & Sullivan, 2002) and psychoeducation (Olmsted et al., 1991).

Interpersonal Therapy

Interpersonal therapy (IPT) is a short-term focal psychotherapy in which the goal is to help patients identify and modify current interpersonal problems. IPT does not address eating or eating disorder symptoms directly (Fairburn,

1997b). Despite this, findings from two studies suggest that IPT may be as effective as CBT for the treatment of BN, although its effects are delayed. Fairburn et al. (1991) compared CBT with IPT. CBT was significantly more effective than IPT at reducing purging, dietary restraint, and overconcern with shape and weight at the end of treatment. At 1-year follow-up, however, clients who had received IPT were doing as well as clients who had received CBT on all outcome measures. A recent randomized controlled trial replicated these results (Agras, Walsh, et al., 2000). These findings suggest that CBT and IPT may achieve their effects through different mechanisms.

Pharmocotherapy

Antidepressant medications, particularly selective serotonin reuptake inhibitors (SSRIs), have been shown to cause a significant decrease in binge eating and purging frequency, but dropout rates are higher and the effects are not well maintained once the drug is stopped (Wilson & Fairburn, 2002). Combining CBT with antidepressant medication has few additional benefits compared with CBT alone in terms of reductions in eating disorder symptoms (Agras et al., 1992; Walsh et al., 1997). However, the combination of CBT and antidepressant medication has been shown to be more effective than CBT alone in reducing comorbid depression and anxiety symptoms (Mitchell, Pyle, Eckert, Hatsukami, & Soll, 1990).

Given the limitations of available treatments for BN, attention has recently turned to improving the effectiveness of CBT and developing alternative treatments for CBT nonresponders (Fairburn, Cooper, & Shafran, 2003; Wilson, 1996, 1999). This area of research is still at an early stage.

Anorexia Nervosa

In contrast to the state of research into treatments for BN, few randomized controlled treatment studies of AN have been published to date, and empirically supported treatments for AN have not yet been established. There is widespread agreement that an initial weight restoration phase typically involving inpatient or day-hospital treatment is vital, and it is evident that such treatments are effective for weight restoration (Olmsted, McFarlane, Molleken, & Kaplan, 2001; Touyz, Beumont, Glaun, Phillips, & Cowie, 1984). Unfortunately, successful weight restoration is associated with high rates of relapse following discharge from the hospital (Carter, Blackmore, Sutander-Pinnock, & Woodside, 2004; Eckert, Halmi, Marchi, Grove, & Crosby, 1995; Herzog et al., 1999). Findings from three studies suggest that there is value in involving family members in the treatment of young patients (Eisler et al., 1997; Eisler et al., 2000; Robin, Siegel, & Moye, 1995), and two published studies support the use of fluoxetine to prevent weight loss once clients are discharged from the hospital (Halmi, Goldberg, Casper, Eckert, & Davis, 1979; Kaye et al., 2001).

Cognitive-Behavioral Therapy

The first phase of CBT for AN consists of building trust and setting treatment parameters. This includes increasing motivation to change; evaluating and treating medical complications; implementing a weight gain meal plan; interrupting bingeing, vomiting and exercise; and introducing initial cognitive interventions and challenging cultural values regarding weight and shape. In phase two the emphasis continues on gaining weight and normalizing eating. In addition, the therapy is broadened to include identifying dysfunctional thoughts, modifying self-concept, developing an interpersonal focus, and involving the family if appropriate. In phase three the focus is on preventing relapse and preparing for termination (Garner, Vitousek, & Pike, 1997). In the only study to evaluate CBT as a posthospital relapse prevention treatment for AN, it was found that CBT was significantly more effective than nutritional counseling in improving outcome and preventing relapse (Pike, Walsh, Vitousek, Wilson, & Bauer, 2003).

Overall, the available studies share several shortcomings, including small sample size and high rates of attrition, which make interpretation of the results difficult. The effectiveness of CBT (or any other treatment) for AN has not yet been established (Garner et al., 1997).

Binge-Eating Disorder

Psychological treatments that have been shown to be effective in the treatment of BED include CBT and IPT (Wilfley & Cohen, 1997). Antidepressant medications (particularly SSRIs) have been shown to produce significant reductions in binge-eating frequency in BED. Across the available studies of CBT, rates of abstinence from binge eating ranging from 40–60% have been reported for treatment completers (Wilfley & Cohen, 1997). Wilfley et al. (1993, 2002) found that IPT was as effective as CBT in reducing binge eating in BED. A recent study comparing group CBT and group IPT for BED obtained abstinence rates of 59% and 62% at 1-year follow-up (Wilfley et al., 2002). Cognitive-behavioral self-help interventions have been shown to produce posttreatment abstinence rates of 40–50% in BED that are maintained at 6-month follow-up (Carter & Fairburn, 1998).

PREDICTORS OF TREATMENT OUTCOME

Bulimia Nervosa

No consistent clinically useful predictors of treatment outcome in BN have been identified. Factors that have been found to be statistically significant predictors in some studies have not been found to be significant predictors in others. Most studies have examined pretreatment client characteristics as predictor variables. A history of low weight has been found to be predictive of a poorer outcome in some studies (Fahy & Russell, 1993; Wilson, Rossiter, Kleifield, & Lindholm, 1986), whereas other studies have found previous low weight to have no effect (Fairburn, Peveler, et al., 1993) or even a positive effect on outcome following CBT (Blouin et al., 1994). Depression (Fairburn et al., 1995), low self-esteem (Fairburn, Peveler, et al., 1993), a higher frequency of binge eating (Wilson et al., 1999), comorbid personality disorder (Fahy & Russell, 1993; Rossiter, Agras, Telch, & Schneider, 1993), a history of substance abuse or dependence (Wilson et al., 1999), and a history of obesity (Bulik, Sullivan, Joyce, Carter, & McIntosh, 1998) have been shown to be predictive of a worse outcome in some studies. Unexpectedly, pretreatment degree of concern about shape and weight has been shown to predict outcome with CBT such that clients with the most severe attitudinal disturbance show greater improvement at posttreatment (Fairburn, Peveler, et al., 1993).

Recently, researchers have begun to examine whether early response to treatment, such as rapid behavioral changes, might provide more useful predictors of treatment outcome. Wilson et al. (1999) reported that a rapid reduction in binge and vomit frequency was associated with a better overall outcome with CBT. Another study showed that 62% of improvement in binge eating and purging occurs by week 6 of CBT and the magnitude of the initial behavioral response is a strong predictor of outcome (Wilson, Fairburn, Agras, Walsh, & Kraemer, 2002). Agras, Crow, et al. (2000) similarly found that early symptom reduction (i.e., at least a 70% reduction in purging by session 6 of CBT) was the most powerful predictor of outcome. These findings suggest that if BN clients do not show a rapid reduction in symptoms early on in the course of outpatient CBT, an alternative treatment should be considered.

Anorexia Nervosa

A range of prognostic variables have been identified in AN, but none has been linked to particular treatment approaches. Certain characteristics of the disorder have been found to predict a poorer outcome including older age at onset (Ratnasuriya, Eisler, Szmukler, & Russell, 1991); longer duration of illness (Herzog, Schellberg, & Deter, 1997; Rosenvinge & Mouland, 1990); history of previous hospitalizations (Halmi et al., 1979; Theander, 1985); lower weight at presentation (Gillberg, Rastam, & Gillberg, 1994; Herzog, Keller, & Lavori, 1988); and the presence of binge eating or purging behavior (Eckert et al., 1995; Herzog et al., 1997). A number of social environmental variables including impaired social functioning (Gillberg et al., 1994); disturbed family relationships (Morgan & Russell, 1975; Ratnasuriya et al., 1991); and the occurrence of stressful life events in the first year after presentation (Sohlberg & Norring, 1992) have also been linked with an unfavorable course. For a detailed review, the reader is referred to Steinhausen (2002).

Binge-Eating Disorder

Little is currently known about predictors of treatment outcome in BED. Wilfley et al. (2000) found that the presence of Cluster B (antisocial, borderline, histrionic, and narcissistic) personality disorder was associated with more frequent binge eating at 1-year following group CBT or group IPT. Carter and Fairburn (1998) reported that initial level of self-esteem predicted response to a cognitive-behavioral self-help program. The nature of the association was unexpected, with those who had higher self-esteem scores responding less well.

DEFINING IMPROVED OUTCOME

Despite their best efforts, some clients will not recover from their eating disorder, and others will not engage in treatment focused on recovery. In an area characterized by ego-syntonic symptoms, denial, and imperfect treatment options, it may be worth considering several different levels of "improved" outcome.

Recovery

Recovery is generally defined as being symptom-free, weight-restored, and eating normally as a first step, with subsequent attention to psychological health (especially self-esteem, identity, and body image) and social adjustment. This is the goal of all published CBT treatment trials and manuals, and movement by clients in this direction is the fundamental definition of improvement.

Harm Reduction

Some clients are unwilling or unable to achieve full symptom control and weight restoration but may accept a specific goal that confers an improved medical status or an improved quality of life. For example, some clients want to withdraw from laxatives or diuretics without focusing on normalized eating or control of other symptoms. A client with AN may be willing to gain 5 or 10 pounds but may refuse complete weight restoration. In our view, achieving any of these goals would constitute an improved outcome. Although care should be taken not to do a disservice to the client by setting the goal too low, some clients are very clear about their current goals and abilities, and it can be more beneficial for the client to make *some* changes than to make no changes at all.

Quality of Life

Clients who are not willing to work toward symptom control or who have exhausted such treatment options without success may benefit from treatment goals that focus on improving their quality of life. Examples include increasing social contact, developing leisure activities or interests, seeking appropriate medical or dental care, and dealing with pressure from family members.

PRACTICAL STRATEGIES FOR IMPROVING OUTCOME

Enhancing Motivation

One important aspect of the treatment of eating disorders is to consider the stages of change in the recovery process (Prochaska & DiClemente, 1984), and to address the ego-syntonic aspects of the disorder (Vitousek, Watson, & Wilson, 1998). This idea is based on the motivational enhancement work in the addictions field that aims to increase intrinsic motivation in an attempt to increase the probability of permanent behavioral change (Miller & Rollnick, 2002). Although most clients and clinicians are aware of the negative consequences of an eating disorder, the benefits are often overlooked. To facilitate change it is helpful to acknowledge that the eating disorder likely also has benefits for the client and may be serving an important function (e.g., protection from failure, distraction from painful memories or emotions, providing a unique identity). Once these functions have been identified, clinicians can address these issues in therapy and help clients find other ways to fulfill these needs. One technique that is useful to help uncover the function of the eating disorder is to use a decisional balance (Miller & Rollnick, 2002). This involves asking a client to record or discuss the costs and the benefits of his or her eating disorder and the costs and benefits of recovery from the eating disorder.

In the transtheoretical approach, behavioral change is described as consisting of five different stages: precontemplation, contemplation, preparation, action, and maintenance (Prochaska & DiClemente 1984). Miller and Rollnick (2002) stress the importance of using therapeutic interventions that are consistent with each individual's stage of change in order to enhance intrinsic motivation and promote change. People who are in the precontemplation stage usually do not think that they have a problem, or they believe their eating disorder is working for them and they are not ready to consider changing. Although most people in this stage do not present for treatment of their eating disorder, clinicians may encounter them in the context of some other presenting problem or when they are referred by medical professionals because of health complications. If clinicians do encounter these individuals it is important to focus their efforts on raising the client's awareness of the eating disorder and the problems associated with it through discussion and psychoeducation. It is also important for clinicians to know that during the initial stages of an eating disorder it is possible that there are very few costs involved. If this is the case, clients may not be ready to consider changing until they start to experience some of the physical and psychological complications that are a result of the eating disorder. At this stage, the goal is to build a therapeutic relationship and for the client to identify the clinician as a potential resource for support or referral should she decide she wants to explore her eating concerns in the future.

During the contemplation stage people are ambivalent about changing. It is important that the therapist avoid arguing in favor of change. Rather than trying to convince clients that they *should* or *must* change, the therapist can provide conditions to allow the client to consider change. The key at this stage is to help the individual weigh the pros and cons carefully, acknowledge the benefits and functions of the disorder, and help to highlight reasons to change. The decisional balance is helpful with this process. Motivational interviewing techniques (e.g., expressing empathy, providing psychoeducational material, exploring personal values, developing discrepancy, using experimental strategies, avoiding argumentation, and supporting self-efficacy) are critical during this stage (Miller & Rollnick, 2002; Vitousek et al., 1998).

The preparation stage is a window of opportunity for clinicians to help clients move into the active stage of recovery. The key to helping clients move into the action stage is to develop a treatment plan that is tailored to the client's needs, which requires collaboration between the clinician and the client. In the action stage, the client may be ready to normalize her eating and to use cognitive-behavioral strategies. Once some of the eating disorder thoughts have been addressed and behavioral symptoms have been interrupted, an individual is considered to be in the maintenance stage of recovery and emphasis can be placed on the prevention of relapse.

One mistake that many clinicians make is to assume that clients are in the action stage when they present for treatment. It is important to assess what is motivating the client and to determine his or her current stage of change so that clinicians can offer appropriate and effective interventions and guidance. For example, if an individual is still contemplating change and a clinician offers active cognitive-behavioral strategies, the transtheoretical model suggests that the client may respond by dropping out of treatment or by complying only temporarily. This can lead to resistance in the client and impatience in the therapist (Miller & Rollnick, 2002). On the other hand, if the clinician directs his or her efforts to trying to increase the client's intrinsic motivation before introducing action strategies the client may be more likely to embrace the strategies and to succeed with permanent behavior change. Matching treatment interventions to a client's stage of change has intuitive appeal and is well received by clients; however, the only study to test it empirically did not find support for it (Treasure et al., 1999). In this study there was no evidence that motivational enhancement therapy led to better outcome than CBT for clients in the contemplation stage of change.

Another way to encourage clients to consider change despite continued ambivalence is to frame recovery as an experiment. Clients already know what it is like to live with an eating disorder; perhaps it is time to find out what their life would be like without an eating disorder. This is not to say that their life will be perfect once they make changes, but it is at least worth finding out. Encourage them to try recovery for 3 months, 6 months, or 12 months. Ask them to collect the data and see. If they decide that they cannot cope without the eating disorder, or they cannot tolerate their body, remind them that they can always go back to the eating disorder. Treating recovery as tentative and experimental often gives an ambivalent client the freedom and the ability to make and maintain changes.

Maximizing the Benefits of Cognitive-Behavioral Therapy for Clients Who Are in the Action Stage of Recovery

Educating Clients and Modeling Normal Eating

Normalizing eating is considered an essential first step in active treatment for an eating disorder. Normal eating for women includes eating around 2,000 calories per day, usually divided into three meals or three meals and snacks. Normal eating also includes eating foods from all food groups, including high-calorie or "forbidden foods." Many clients find this approach contrary to their beliefs about dieting and weight regulation. If binge eating is a symptom of their eating disorder, clients often believe that the only way to control their bingeing is to restrict their eating. In fact the opposite is true, caloric restriction can cause urges to binge eat, and it is important that clients understand this connection between restricting calories and bingeing. Clients may require a great deal of education about the benefits of normalized eating and how it is essential to their recovery from their eating disorder. Because clients have a difficult time trusting normalized eating, it can be helpful for clinicians to model this type of eating if given the opportunity (e.g., the client can bring a risky snack to session as an exposure, and the therapist can eat the same thing).

Preparing Clients for the Washout Phase

When clients start to normalize their eating they are likely to experience a "washout" phase. The washout phase occurs during the initiation of normalized eating. It is typical during this phase for clients to experience an increase in gastrointestinal discomfort and pain (i.e., bloating, gas, constipation, and reflux); to feel more preoccupied with food, more dissatisfied with body image, and more anxious and depressed; and to have increased urges to binge eat. Eventually the physical discomfort will pass, and eating normally helps to reduce urges to binge, but at first clients have to do the eating while enduring an increase in physical and emotional discomfort.

It is best to prepare clients for the washout phase, and to let them know that this is a normal but extremely difficult part of recovery. Clients find it helpful to know that the only way to get to the other side of the washout phase is to eat through the distress and pain until they start to feel better, both physically and emotionally. Coping phrases such as "food is my medicine" and strategies such as mechanical eating (i.e., planning meals and following through despite feelings) can also help with this process.

In addition, there are gastric motility medications (e.g., domperidone) that are available with a prescription that help to speed up the digestive system and can reduce the discomfort and pain associated with the initial process of eating. Another medication in this category is cisapride. However, cisapride is now rarely prescribed for eating disorders because it has been associated with abnormal health rhythms that can lead to death (Molleken, 2000).

Preparing Clients for Weight Restoration

Weight gain is a crucial first step in recovery from AN. Often this work requires intensive therapy in either a day hospital or an inpatient setting. Obstacles to weight gain include extremely negative associations with weight gain and eating, physical activity and exercise, and hypermetabolic responses. Weight gain and eating are often associated with beliefs about failure, laziness, weakness, lack of will power, and loss of control, worth, identity or special status. Strong feelings of disgust, shame, and guilt can also occur. These thoughts and feelings need to be expressed and addressed in therapy. It is often helpful to remind clients of the experimental nature of recovery and weight gain and to use mechanical eating as a strategy.

In addition to the psychological barriers to weight gain there are behavioral and physiological roadblocks. Purposeful exercise to burn calories and nonexercise activity such as standing, tensing, and fidgeting can burn calories and prevent or reduce weight gain. Clients can be taught to use strategies (e.g., distraction, self-talk, and stimulus control) to reduce or eliminate activity and may have to spend some time on bed rest to maximize the probability of weight gain. Clients require gradual increases in calories to support continued weight gain. The body responds to refeeding by increasing resting energy expenditure (Krahn, Rock, Dechert, Nairn, & Hasse, 1993), resting metabolic rate (Obarzanek, Lesem, & Jimerson, 1994), and diet-induced thermogenesis (Moukaddem, Boulier, Apfelbaum, & Rigaud, 1997). This hypermetabolic response results in burning off excess calories rather than supporting weight gain. Therefore, a large number of calories may be required to support weight gain for some clients (e.g., 3,600 calories per day or more). This amount of food is physically difficult to consume. Liquid supplements can be used when meal plans exceed normal calories to reduce the burden of consumption, and to keep meals looking normal. In addition, clients with AN require an initially higher level of maintenance calories (i.e., 300 extra calories per day) in order to maintain weight after weight restoration (Kaye et al., 1986; Weltzin, Fernstrom, Hansen, McConaha, & Kaye, 1991).

Tailoring Strategies

Coping strategies must be individually tailored to each client. What works for some clients will not work for others. For example, encouraging clients to take a walk when they feel like bingeing is not effective if the walk is likely to turn into a trip to the grocery store to buy binge food. Similarly, many people find it easier to eat meals with others, though some clients find this more difficult than eating alone. If clinicians take time to explore and understand individual symptoms and motivators, they can be very creative with strategies that will optimize outcomes for clients. For example, stimulus narrowing can be operationalized by asking clients to limit binges to only one type of food (to reduce the pleasure associated with bingeing) or to exercise only at 5:00 A.M. or buy laxatives at a distant pharmacy (to decrease convenience). Clients can also be coached to use alternative routes to avoid bathrooms to prevent purging, or to incorporate personal goals into coping phrases.

Expanding and Increasing the Comprehensiveness of Cognitive-Behavioral Therapy

Currently, research on the efficacy of CBT focuses on behavioral symptom reduction and weight restoration. Given the time limits of most research protocols, this focus is necessary. However, recent developments in the field are pointing toward ways of expanding and increasing the comprehensiveness of CBT for eating disorders in order to improve outcome.

Tailoring Treatment

Fairburn et al. (2003) have recently written about the need to expand the existing cognitive-behavioral framework for the treatment of eating disorders to include additional treatment components based on individual clients' needs. These modules include clinical perfectionism, core low self-esteem, mood intolerance, and interpersonal difficulties. Fairburn and colleagues recommend a formal assessment of the likely contribution of each of these areas, and the development of an individually tailored treatment intervention that includes both an emphasis on modifying the client's eating disorder psychopathology and attention to these additional maintaining factors.

Decreasing Weight-Based Self-Esteem

The core maladaptive cognition in clients with eating disorders involves weight-based self-esteem (Fairburn, 1985; Fairburn, Marcus, & Wilson, 1993; Vitousek & Hollon, 1990). Clients with AN and BN devalue their entire self-worth because of their dissatisfaction with their weight and shape. This type of evaluation has been identified as a predictor of relapse in both AN and BN (Carter et al., 2004; Fairburn, Peveler, et al., 1993). There are a number of methods described in CBT manuals to challenge and modify these beliefs about weight and shape (e.g., weighing the pros and cons of using this frame of reference, projecting into the future, discussing how this frame of reference fits with personal values and goals, examining the utility of this belief, and behavioral experiments; see Fairburn, Marcus, & Wilson,

1993). Unfortunately, recent studies have indicated that CBT is less effective in reducing clients' excessive concerns about weight and shape than in eliminating symptoms (Walsh et al., 1997). It has therefore been recommended that there needs to be much more emphasis placed on the reduction of weight-related self-esteem in order to improve outcome in eating disorders (Fairburn et al., 2003; Rosen, 1996; Wilson, 1999). Wilson (1999) has indicated the necessity of using more powerful techniques to modify these concerns such as exposure to cues that elicit dysfunctional attitudes combined with emotional processing of associated feelings and/or training in mindfulness where clients are taught to observe rather than judge their body.

Addressing Body-Checking Behaviors

Another way to improve outcome in CBT for eating disorders may be to enhance the treatment procedures for addressing body-checking behaviors (Fairburn, Shafran, & Cooper, 1998). Many clients repeatedly check aspects of their body in highly idiosyncratic ways, including inspecting themselves in the mirror, weighing, pinching skinfolds, and measuring body parts with a measuring tape, hands, or clothing. This process intensifies body concerns and dissatisfaction and can maintain the eating disorder. It is important to assess body checking behavior and to help clients develop strategies to reduce or eliminate this behavior (Rosen, 1997; Wilson, 1999). Clients need to be coached on finding a balance between the extremes of excessive body checking on one hand and body avoidance (e.g., wearing shapeless clothing) on the other (Fairburn, Marcus, & Wilson, 1993).

Combining Cognitive-Behavioral Therapy with Other Treatments

Another way to boost outcome is to combine CBT with other treatments to address aspects of the eating disorder that may be maintaining the disorder and may not be fully addressed within the context of CBT.

Antidepressant Medication

Compared to the treatment of depression, higher doses of SSRIs are required to treat bulimia. Using fluoxetine as an example, a dosage of 60 mg is generally needed and well tolerated. Clients who are prescribed medications need to be educated on the importance of consistent doses and should be warned that vomiting after ingestion of the medication will prevent it from being absorbed properly. Clients can be instructed to take medication at a time of day when they are less likely to vomit. At proper doses, SSRIs can facilitate a better outcome for some clients who are participating in CBT for BN (Zhu & Walsh, 2002). Research suggests that the combination of CBT and SSRIs leads to greater reduction in comorbid anxiety and depressive symptoms, but not bingeing and vomiting (Mitchell et al., 1990).

Currently there are no successful pharmacological interventions for AN (Zhu & Walsh, 2002). It is likely that the neurochemical effects of starvation play a major role in this finding. For example, antidepressants do not seem to work when clients are at a very low weight because they work on serotonin which comes from tryptophan found in food, an insufficient amount of which is being eaten (Molleken, 2000). However, there is some evidence to suggest that fluoxetine may have a positive impact on preventing relapse in weight-restored AN (Kaye et al., 2001). Currently there is a multisite randomized controlled study under way comparing CBT with fluoxetine to CBT with placebo to investigate any added benefits of fluoxetine in preventing relapse in AN (Kaplan & Walsh, 2002).

Mindfulness-Based Stress Reduction

Mindfulness-based stress reduction provides systematic training in mindfulness meditation as a self-regulation approach to stress reduction and management of emotions. Mindfulness is a state in which one is highly aware of, and focused on the present moment, accepting and acknowledging it, without getting caught up in thoughts or emotional reactions to the situation (Kabat-Zinn, 1990, 1994). Recently, a study has shown that adding mindfulness techniques to cognitive therapy helps to prevent relapse in major depressive disorder (Segal, Williams, & Teasdale, 2002). Although still very new in its application to eating disorders, there is some evidence that mindfulness training does reduce binge eating in those diagnosed with BED (Kristeller & Hallett, 1999), and it has been adapted for use in body image work (Wilson, 1999). In addition, mindfulness may help clients disengage from eating-disordered thoughts and aid in the treatment of comorbid conditions (e.g., anxiety, depression, and borderline personality).

Emotion-Focused Therapy

Emotion focused therapy was designed for and shown to be effective with clients who are depressed or anxious, as well as those who suffer from interpersonal problems, childhood maltreatment, and problems in living (Greenberg & Paivio, 1997). Emotion-focused interventions are used to facilitate clients' processing of emotion, to deepen their experience, and to promote the generation of new meaning and a direction for action. The key intervention process involves directing clients' attention to their internal experience (Korman & Greenberg, 1996). Although it has not yet been studied in eating disorder populations, emotion-focused therapy may be a good partner with CBT and may be well suited to helping these clients identify and process their emotional experiences. This may be particularly relevant for clients who have used their eating disorder symptoms to avoid or distract from emotions. Learning to identify and process emotions adaptively may have a positive impact on eating disorder symptoms (i.e., binge, purge, exercise, and restriction) that function to distract an individual from his or her affect. Also, at least for some forms of negative affect, directly experiencing the distress may be a more effective means of coping than either distraction or problem solving, which are typical of CBT (Hunt, 1998; Wilson, 1999).

Addressing Resource Issues

Resource issues include financial costs and psychological costs. Because resources are frequently limited, applying them effectively should improve outcome at both institutional and individual levels.

Matching Clients to Their Optimum Treatment

The premise that some clients may respond to one type of treatment while other clients would respond better to a different type of treatment leads to the goal of matching clients to the type of treatment best suited to them. This strategy should be the most cost-effective and should also minimize client discouragement resulting from ineffective treatment. Unfortunately, treatment-specific predictors of outcome have not been identified. In one study, Wilson (2000) searched for differential predictors of response to IPT and CBT for BN but found none. In another study, Treasure et al. (1999) found no evidence that motivational enhancement therapy was superior to CBT for clients in the contemplation stage of change. Both treatments were associated with reductions in symptoms and increased readiness for action. In short, there is limited evidence for specificity in response to treatments that were designed to work toward different goals. A significant body of research is needed to determine the feasibility of matching clients to their optimum treatment.

Sequencing of Treatments

The primary rationale for sequencing CBT treatments relates to the goal of providing cost-effective treatment; a less intensive and relatively inexpensive intervention is offered initially and only those who fail to respond are offered a more expensive treatment. The potential disadvantage relates to clients becoming discouraged if they do not respond to the initial treatment. The preliminary evidence suggests that prefacing individual CBT with a self-care manual (Treasure et al., 1996) or a brief psychoeducation group (Davis, McVey, Heinmaa, Rockert, & Kennedy, 1999) works well and is cost-effective.

Another type of sequencing strategy is to offer CBT nonresponders a different type of treatment. Walsh et al. (2000) showed that treatment with fluoxetine is better than placebo for BN clients who did not respond to CBT or IPT. In another study, Mitchell et al. (2002) observed a 16% abstinence rate for IPT and a 10% abstinence rate for medication management in BN clients who did not respond to CBT. The treatment effects may be small (and there was not a no-treatment control group), but perhaps this is to be expected with secondary treatments of similar intensity to the initial treatment. Another variation on this sequencing strategy may be to offer CBT nonresponders a different treatment and to follow that offer with another chance at CBT. Anecdotal evidence suggests that diabetic patients with BN who responded poorly to CBT were able to successfully resume CBT after an intervening course of IPT (Peveler & Fairburn, 1992). Being a "nonresponder" to CBT may be a temporary state for some clients, indicating that a second trial may prove useful even if a first trial was not.

Length of Treatment

Most outpatient treatment trials offer 4–5 months of therapy for BN and closer to 1 year for AN. However, for BN, treatment response is usually evident in the first 2–3 weeks (Olmsted, Kaplan, Rockert, & Jacobsen, 1996; Wilson, 1996). In one study Agras, Crow, et al. (2000) identified a reduction in purging of less than 70% by session 6 as a predictor of poor response to CBT. In clinical practice it may be useful to stop the intervention and to consider an alternate if response is poor after 4–6 weeks. There is little evidence that continuing the treatment for BN will improve the outcome in this case. In fact, continuing treatment too long with a nonresponder may sometimes be harmful. Clients can come to feel very negative about therapy, and also about their own ability to change after investing a lot of time and energy in their treatment without seeing much improvement.

On the other hand, it may be that CBT responders can benefit from a lengthened course of treatment. Extending treatment can allow for more work on body image, self-esteem, and other maintaining factors. Although extending treatment duration might be expected to reduce relapse rates, there is currently no evidence one way or the other. For BED there is some indication that the situation may be different. One study showed that extending CBT for BED nonresponders after 12 weeks resulted in clinical improvement during an additional 12 weeks of CBT (Eldredge et al., 1997).

Increasing the Probability of an Early Response

Given that the magnitude of initial behavioral response is a powerful predictor of outcome (Agras, Crow, et al., 2000; Olmsted et al., 1996; Wilson et al., 2002), it is important to maximize the probability that clients will have an early response. Increasing the frequency of contact during the first month of treatment can help to support early behavioral change (e.g., seeing clients twice a week for the initial 4 weeks of outpatient treatment). Also, efforts should be made to ensure that treatment is not interrupted, especially during the initial stages, as even short breaks can result in substantial setbacks (Fairburn et al., 2003).

Responding to Clients Who Do Not Make Behavioral Changes

For a number of different reasons, some clients fail to make any behavioral changes during CBT for eating disorders. For example, some clients make good plans in session to eat more or to take a food risk but do not follow through session after session. Others work on strategies to avoid symptoms or to gain weight and continue to be symptomatic despite well-intentioned plans. The following steps can be very useful with such clients: (1) use motivational strategies to address fears, expectations, cognitions, and other obstacles; (2) negotiate an achievable behavioral goal; (3) make plans and discuss strategies directed toward achieving the goal; (4) review progress toward the goal, and then revisit steps 1 through 4 for any remaining goals. If the client will not participate in steps 2 or 3, or continues to not follow through with plans, clinicians should stop working on behavioral change, process the situation with the client, and return to motivational work. After 6–8 weeks of CBT with no behavioral change, the utility of continuing with more of the same is questionable.

Ongoing Follow-Up

Regardless of whether the client has responded to treatment, it may be useful to offer periodic follow-up contact. For some clients this may reinforce the idea that they will continue working on their problems on their own and check in with a progress report every 6–12 months. For others, the sense of connection and accountability may encourage maintenance of gains. When the client has not responded to treatment and remains ill, being followed periodically provides the opportunity for clients to request additional treatment when they feel ready, or for the clinician to inform them about any new developments in the area which may be of benefit to them.

Adapting Treatments for Specific Disorders

Anorexia Nervosa

In addition to special considerations associated with weight restoration described previously, clients with AN are also more likely to be ambivalent about change. This is particularly true for those diagnosed with the restricting subtype of anorexia (without binge eating or purging). Restricting and exercising are symptoms that are more likely to be ego-syntonic, and clients who are working to suppress their weight are therefore more protective of these behaviors. As a result, these clients require more motivational work, which can include providing psychoeducational material and raising awareness about the future costs and impact of the disorder. It is also helpful to identify the client's personal values and explore how the anorexia fulfills or interferes with these values (Vitousek et al., 1998). Negative beliefs around eating and weight gain are particularly inflexible and rigid in this population, especially when clients are emaciated. Unfortunately, these beliefs do not always respond to regular cognitive restructuring attempts, and clients may require some weight gain before meaningful cognitive work can be accomplished.

Fairburn et al. (1998) recently synthesized and extended the existing accounts of the cognitive-behavioral model of AN and suggested that the theme of self-control needs to be addressed at all stages of treatment in this population. It is essential that the focus of control be shifted away from eating and weight by helping clients derive satisfaction and a sense of achievement from other activities, and by demonstrating that control over eating does not actually provide the control that they are seeking.

Bulimia Nervosa

BN and the bulimic subtype of AN have been associated with an increased risk of reckless or impulsive behaviors involving a lack of consideration of the risks and consequences before taking action (Bell & Newns, 2002). Impulsive behaviors include self-harm behaviors, alcohol and drug abuse, risky sexual activity, compulsive shopping, and shoplifting. Other empirical studies have depicted clients with BN as interpersonally sensitive and low in self-esteem (Wonderlich, 2002). Therefore, careful attention needs to be directed toward fostering a therapeutic relationship, and treatment needs to be tailored to address existing comorbidities and impulsive behaviors.

Binge-Eating Disorder

Treatment considerations related to BED have been described by Marcus (1997). Clients with BED typically present for help with two problems, binge eating and obesity. Eliminating the binge eating and normalizing eating must be achieved before the issue of weight can be addressed. The strategies for the normalization of eating proceed the same as with CBT for BN. Because individuals with BED tend to have a problem with overeating generally, dietary advice that includes recommending a normal degree of restraint over eating should be provided. Even though they do not tend to restrict their eating in the same way as patients with BN, BED patients often share many of the distorted ways of thinking about food and eating, particularly all-or-nothing thinking. This should be addressed using cognitive restructuring procedures. Because overeating can be related to a lack of awareness with regard to eating, training in mindfulness and mindful eating can also be helpful. Many individuals use food to modulate affect and need to learn alternative ways of coping with negative emotional experiences.

When relevant, it is important to provide education about obesity and the outcome of behavioral weight loss programs. A typical dietary/behavioral program results in the loss of about 10% of initial body weight in those who complete treatment (Devlin, Yanovski, & Wilson, 2000). Once treatment is stopped, the lost weight is almost always regained—with about 40% being regained in the first year and the rest over the following 3 years. Devising ways to prevent or minimize weight regain is a great challenge. Research on the behavioral characteristics of people who have experienced minimal weight regain has identified the following characteristics as being important: (1) maintenance of an exercise program; (2) maintenance of a moderate meal plan; and (3) regular monitoring of body weight (Cooper & Fairburn, 2001). It is important to highlight the difference between the goal of continued weight loss (requires maintaining an energy deficit) and the goal of maintaining a stable weight (requires a balance between energy input and output). Many commercial weight-loss programs advocate an energy intake during the maintenance phase that is well below that required to maintain a stable weight. It is also essential to discuss with patients weight-loss goals and expectations (Cooper, Fairburn, & Hawkins, 2003). It is not realistic to expect weight loss greater than 5–10% of current body weight. In addition, it has been documented that modest weight loss is associated with a significant reduction in the health risks associated with obesity (Devlin et al., 2000). There is a tendency for people to become demoralized when unrealistic weight-loss goals are not achieved and to abandon weight-control efforts altogether when this occurs. Because individuals with BED tend to be sedentary, the treatment plan should include a program of regular moderate exercise. It is also important to address shame and negative self-evaluation related to overweight and overeating and the internalization of societal attitudes concerning weight. It is often the case that overcoming BED involves acceptance of a higher than average body weight.

Addressing Comorbidity

Substance Abuse

Compared to individuals without an eating disorder, rates of lifetime substance abuse are significantly higher in individuals with AN or BN, but not among those with BED (Wilson, 2002). There appears to be a relationship between bulimic behavior and substance abuse whether observed in a person with BN or the bulimic subtype of AN (O'Brien & Vincent, 2003). Research has shown that up to 50% of individuals with bulimia also struggle with current substance abuse (Lilenfeld et al., 1997). Substances that are often used by people with eating disorders include alcohol, marijuana, cocaine, MDMA (ecstacy), and items containing ephedra, used to boost metabolism and energy levels and decrease appetite. Besides the dangers associated with regular use of these substances, there are specific concerns related to using these substances in the context of an eating disorder. Alcohol interferes with normal eating because clients tend to count the calories in alcohol as part of their meal plan and skip meals when drinking. Marijuana and cocaine both have an impact on appetite that can interfere with normal eating (i.e., marijuana stimulates whereas cocaine suppresses appetite). Also, when clients are under the influence of a substance, they are less able to use therapeutic strategies and are more vulnerable to symptoms. Both ecstacy and ephedra can contribute to dehydration and electrolyte abnormalities already caused by the eating disorder and can lead to serious physical problems and even death.

Clients are encouraged to remain abstinent from these substances at least until they have successfully tackled their eating disorder symptoms. Motivational interviewing techniques can be used to prepare clients to change their substance use (Miller & Rollnick, 2002). It is important to do a functional analysis of the client's substance use (e.g., weight control, suppression of memories, and escape from life demands), and to address these benefits in treatment. Clients can be educated on the aforementioned concerns, and taught to use behavioral coping strategies to avoid acting on urges to use substances while working on their eating disorder. In cases of substance dependence, specialized treatment aimed at the substance use may be required as a first step.

Depression

Population-based studies have consistently shown that major depression is the most common comorbid condition in women with eating disorders (Bulik, 2002). A recent review documented prevalences of depression ranging from 45% in a sample of women with a variety of eating disorders to 86% in a sample of women with AN (O'Brien & Vincent, 2003). It is helpful to assess whether the depression is a primary disorder or a consequence of the eating disorder. If the depression is a result of the eating disorder, the depression may lift as the client improves her eating and disengages from the eating disorder, although there may be a period of worsening first. If the depression is primary, treatment for the depression will need to continue after the eating disorder has remitted or may need to be pursued prior to eating disorder treatment depending on the severity of the depression and the degree to which it interferes with engagement in therapy focused on the eating disorder. Cognitive-behavioral strategies for depression and antidepressant medication may be used to treat the depression in conjunction with the eating disorder treatment. Depression can either increase or decrease appetite. Therefore, clients who are showing signs of depression should be reminded to plan their meals and to follow through with the plan despite how they are feeling (i.e., mechanical eating), similar to scheduling pleasant events to combat depression.

Anxiety

Research indicates that anxiety disorders occur frequently and usually at a higher rate in individuals with AN and BN (Godart, Flament, Perdereau, & Jeammet, 2002). Specifically, higher levels of social anxiety, generalized anxiety, and obsessive–compulsive disorder have been documented in those with these eating disorders (Godart et al., 2002). Most research indicates that the anxiety disorder usually predates the eating disorder (Bulik, 2002). Some clients report a worsening of anxiety as the eating disorder intensifies, whereas others report an inverse relationship between anxiety symptoms and eating disorder symptoms. In this latter group, some clients report that the eating disorder functions to distract from or relieve anxious thoughts and feelings. Therefore, as the eating disorder improves the anxiety increases and can be an impetus to relapse. In most cases, cognitive-behavioral strategies for anxiety can be used to treat the anxiety in combination with treatment for the eating disorder.

Personality Disorders

Research on the restricting subtype of AN indicates a higher prevalence of avoidant, dependent, and obsessive–compulsive personality disorders (Dennis & Sansone, 1997). On the other hand, individuals diagnosed with BN or the bulimic subtype of AN are more likely to suffer from borderline or histrionic personality disorder. Although prevalence rates range drastically, it is estimated that 34% of those with bulimic symptoms also have borderline personality disorder (BPD) (Dennis & Sansone, 1997).

It is important to recognize with comorbid eating and BPD that the eating disorder symptoms are usually part of a lifelong pattern of self-regulatory deficits and self-destructive behaviors. Treatment of the eating disorder needs to take this context into account and may require more intensive therapy. Dennis and Sansone (1991) have described treatment considerations related to the eating disorder client with BPD, including an emphasis on building the therapeutic relationship; creating a stable treatment environment; setting boundaries and limits; modeling appropriate affect, but remaining neutral during episodes of crisis or self-destructive behaviors to avoid reinforcing the behaviors; teaching new methods of self-regulation; and enhancing self-esteem.

Although dialetical behavior therapy has been shown to be effective for the treatment of BPD (Linehan, Armstrong, Suarez, Allmon, & Heard, 1991; Linehan, Heard, & Armstrong, 1993), there is currently no research that addresses its use in the treatment of BPD and comorbid eating disorders. There is, however, a treatment manual for this population that is currently under development (Chen & Linehan, 2003).

Special Populations

Chronicity

In clients who have undergone a series of treatments for their eating disorder and who have been unable to change or maintain improvements, treatment may be adapted to suit their needs. For example, it is possible to take a harm-reduction approach with weight gain and to agree on a realistic weight goal that still may be below what is recommended for full recovery. Clients may be more likely to maintain this weight and may experience a significant improvement in their quality of life. Clients who are able to maintain this partial weight restoration for a period of time may subsequently be willing to move their weight closer to a healthy range. Some clients tolerate this stepped approach to weight gain better than immediate and complete weight restoration.

Clinicians should guard against setting unrealistic goals that can have the effect of encouraging a sense of failure and hopelessness. On the other hand, clinicians need to find a balance between expecting too much and expecting too little, because therapeutic pessimism can also promote chronicity (Yager, 2002). It is important to develop clear expectations when working with these clients and to use behavioral contracts where appropriate. For example, clinicians may want to negotiate a lowest weight limit, a weight at which the client agrees to hospitalization. It is also important to communicate closely with other providers to coordinate care and avoid splitting (Yager, 2002). Improved quality of life may be very beneficial for the chronic client. This might include increasing social activity, obtaining appropriate medical or dental care, or adding an outside interest to the clients' daily activities.

Type 1 Diabetes Mellitus

The combination of disordered eating and diabetes mellitus (DM) can be especially challenging. Disordered eating has been associated with poor metabolic control (Rydall, Rodin, Olmsted, Devenyi, & Daneman, 1997) which, in turn, has been directly linked with the longer-term medical complications of DM such as retinopathy and neuropathy (Diabetes Control and Complications Trial [DCCT] Research Group, 1993). More immediately, disturbed eating and lack of compliance with a DM management regime may lead to diabetic ketoacidosis or coma, requiring emergency medical treatment. Thus, the reasons for concern about the individual's health and safety are significantly amplified when disordered eating occurs in an individual who has DM. Although health concerns may be a source of motivation to change for some clients with DM, it is a mistake for the clinician to assume that they "must" change because the stakes are so high. Instead, the full range of ambivalence inherent in eating disorders should be expected. The therapist should take care to explore the client's goals for therapy and ensure that behavioral prescriptions address goals that have been endorsed by the client.

The behavioral change plan, designed to interrupt symptoms and normalize eating, must include management of the DM. This means that blood sugar testing and an insulin protocol are part of the plan. If the client does not know how to adjust her insulin dose to match the eating plan, it is important to consult with her endocrinologist. Both the client and the therapist need to understand the insulin protocol, so that both are able to identify any episodes of insulin underdosing or omission as symptoms. A specific plan for dealing with hypoglycemic episodes should be developed as these are a common trigger for bingeing. Self-monitoring should be expanded to include blood sugar levels and insulin administered (or omitted). Some clients resist testing their blood sugars either to avoid confronting upsetting information (e.g., that they are in poor control) or as a way of avoiding responsibility for appropriate action (e.g., taking insulin). In this case, self-monitoring in the form of testing and recording blood sugars, with no expectation of behavioral change, may be an early goal of treatment. The ultimate behavioral treatment goals are cessation of symptoms, normalization of eating, and good DM management with well-controlled blood sugars. However, any improvement in diabetic control is associated with a reduced risk for the medical complications of diabetes (DCCT Research Group, 1993), indicating that a harm reduction model is appropriate when needed.

Therapists should work with clients to explore the functional connection between disordered eating and DM. Women with DM tend to be significantly heavier than their nondiabetic peers, and some may view either the DM or their "defective" body as the source of their weight-related body dissatisfaction. Underdosing insulin, which results in high blood sugars, is an effective method of weight control. In most cases, improved metabolic control comes with the price of weight gain. The dietary focus and restraint imposed by a DM meal plan may set the stage for bulimic episodes. The schedule of eating and insulin administration may evoke issues around control; negligent self-care may be experienced by some clients as being in control and/or appropriate punishment for a defective body. The therapist needs to be aware that the DM may have had a very significant impact on the client's beliefs and feelings about herself. Treating individuals with disordered eating and DM requires that the therapist be knowledgeable about the management of DM and possible specific psychological issues, but CBT is readily tailored for this purpose.

Males

The findings from recent community-based epidemiological studies of AN and BN suggest a ratio of 1 male case to about 6 female cases. In clinical samples, the ratio is somewhat lower with 1 male case to 10 female cases of AN. Although male cases of BN are relatively uncommon, there does not appear to be a gender difference in BED (Andersen, 2002). Although the treatment of eating disorders in males and females is essentially the same, there are some issues that seem to be more relevant to the male population. For example, eating disorders in males are more likely to be related to participation in sports, past obesity, gender identity conflicts, or fear of future medical illness than sociocultural pressures for thinness. The notion of "reverse anorexia nervosa" or body dysmorphic disorder is well established in males. This is characterized by subjective thinness even when highly muscular and it is often associated with the abuse of anabolic steroids (Andersen, 2002). Finally, there is more stigma and shame associated with male eating disorders because eating disorders are often considered to be a female problem.

PREDICTORS OF RELAPSE

Bulimia Nervosa

Employing varying definitions of remission and relapse, estimates of the relapse rates in BN have ranged from 30% (Maddocks, Kaplan, Woodside, Langdon, & Piran, 1992; Olmsted, Kaplan, & Rockert, 1994) to 63% (Field et al., 1997). Several studies have examined the prediction of relapse in BN. Significant predictors include body dissatisfaction at the end of treatment (Freeman, Beach, Davis, & Solyom, 1985), stressful life events (Mitchell, Davis, & Goff, 1985), severity of residual concern about shape and weight at the end of treatment (Fairburn, Peveler, et al., 1993), and younger age and higher pretreatment and posttreatment vomiting frequency (Olmsted et al., 1994). In a recent study, Halmi et al. (2002) examined predictors of relapse in BN clients who had achieved abstinence from binge eating and purging with CBT. It was found that higher posttreatment level of preoccupation and rituals regarding eating, as well as higher posttreatment dietary restraint, predicted relapse. In addition, a shorter duration of abstinence during the course of treatment predicted relapse. Following day hospital treatment, Olmsted et al. (1996) found a much lower rate of relapse in clients who had responded rapidly to the treatment as compared with those who had been "slow" responders.

Anorexia Nervosa

Based on different definitions of relapse and varying lengths of follow-up, relapse rates ranging from 9% (Strober, Freeman, & Morrell, 1997) to 42% (Eckert et al., 1995) have been reported in AN. Few specific predictors of relapse in AN have been identified to date. Deter and Herzog (1994) found that shorter duration of illness, younger age at presentation, and lower purging frequency was associated with a lower risk of relapse. Strober et al. (1997) reported that excessive exercisers were more likely to relapse. Finally, Carter et al. (2004) identified several significant predictors of relapse: a history of suicide attempt(s), excessive exercise (three months after discharge), previous specialized treatment for an eating disorder, severity of obsessive–compulsive symptoms at presentation; and residual concern about shape and weight at discharge.

Binge-Eating Disorder

To our knowledge, only one study has examined predictors of relapse in BED. This study found that early onset of binge eating (before age 16) and higher posttreatment dietary restraint scores predicted relapse in clients who had achieved abstinence with dialectical behavior therapy (Safer, Lively, Telch, & Agras, 2002).

PRACTICAL STRATEGIES FOR PREVENTING
RELAPSE AND REOCCURRENCE

Sticking to the Experiment

It is helpful to remind clients to view recovery as an experiment. We recommend that clients try recovery (i.e., normal eating and being symptom-free) for at least 1 year in order to collect all the necessary data before deciding whether they should continue with recovery or return to the eating disorder. If clients have a slip or a difficult period, remind them that this is not the time to make a decision about recovery.

Addressing Ambivalence

It is important to let clients know that ambivalence is a normal part of recovery and can occur at any time during the recovery process. If a client begins to question whether recovery is worthwhile, or starts to think about what it will take to drop a few pounds, it does not indicate that she is giving up or that she has lost her motivation to recover. Rather, this is a time to return to motivational interviewing techniques in order to explore the ambivalence and the function of the eating disorder. Working through these periods of ambivalence is considered essential work toward permanent change.

Addressing Expectations

Recovery from an eating disorder is difficult work. It is important to educate clients about the process of recovery so that they are able to continue this work despite setbacks and challenges. It is also essential that clients realize that life without an eating disorder will not be perfect and problem free. In fact, without the eating disorder as a coping mechanism many clients will experience increased levels of distress and emotional discomfort. It is not uncommon for underlying issues to begin to surface once eating disorder symptoms stop. Even after clients have developed more adaptive coping methods and have addressed underlying issues, they will be exposed to the hassles, problems, disappointments, and tragedies that are part of the human experience.

Some clients will be lucky enough to have supportive and helpful family members and friends to help them with their recovery. This will not be the case for everyone. Some loved ones may try to be supportive but may in fact be unhelpful because they do not know what to say or do. Also, some family members and friends will not understand or want to be involved in the recovery process at all. Others may have gotten used to their role as caretaker or decision maker and may feel threatened by their loved ones attempting to improve or become more independent. It is helpful to prepare clients for the dynamic in their family to shift, and to recommend family therapy if needed.

Exploring Past Relapses

If this is not the client's first attempt at recovery it can be extremely helpful to explore what led to relapse in the past. It is useful to review these past experiences and to try to identify contributing factors to prevent future relapse. During this discussion it is important to help clients reframe past relapses as valuable learning opportunities rather than personal failures. Clinicians can explore with clients the changes that were made, how long the changes lasted, what factors led to a recurrence of symptoms, and what was learned from the experience that can be applied to the current situation.

Promoting Self-Efficacy

Self-efficacy refers to a person's belief in his or her ability to carry out and succeed with a specific task such as recovery. Although self-efficacy has not been studied in eating disorders, it is a good predictor of outcome in the addictions field and is considered a key element in making and maintaining change (Miller & Rollnick, 2002). There are a number of ways to support self-efficacy, including enhancing confidence talk, reviewing progress and past successes, and highlighting personal strengths and supports.

Enhancing Confidence Talk

One way to enhance confidence talk is to ask open-ended questions aimed at accomplishing this task. Questions include the following: "How might you go about maintaining this change?" "What obstacles do you anticipate, and how will you deal with them?" and "What gives you confidence that you can do this?" Another way to elicit confidence talk is to ask clients to rate how confident they are that they can maintain their recovery using a scale from 0 to 10, where 0 is not at all confident and 10 is extremely confident. Once clients have rated themselves, clinicians can follow up with questions that include the following: "Why are you at a 5 not a 0?" or "What would it take for you to go from a 5 to a 6?" Clinicians need to be careful not to reverse the question and ask "Why are you at a 5 and not a 10?" which would serve to highlight lack of abilities and decrease self-efficacy (Miller & Rollnick, 2002).

Reviewing Progress and Past Successes

At times, clients can get frustrated because they are still struggling with eating-disordered thoughts, urges, or occasional symptoms. It is helpful to reflect on the progress they have made so far. Ask clients to evaluate their progress over a reasonable amount of time by having them reflect on where they were 1 month ago, 6 months ago, or 1 year ago and compare it with where they are right now in terms of their eating disorder symptoms and thoughts. This reminds clients of any progress they have made despite current setbacks or struggles.

Another strategy for enhancing self-efficacy is to identify past successes and to explore these successes with clients. Past successes with regard to the client's eating disorder are relevant, but so are successes related to other areas of her life. Clinicians can look for changes that the client made on her own initiative, particularly ones that are important to her (e.g., finished a degree, stopped smoking, and left an unhealthy relationship). Several examples should be solicited and explored in depth by asking how the client made each change, what worked and did not work, what preparation was involved, what challenges were faced, how obstacles were managed, and how the changes were maintained. Clinicians should look for skills and personal strengths and resources that can be generalized and applied to maintaining the client's recovery from the eating disorder (Miller & Rollnick, 2002).

Avoiding Slips and Coping with Stressors

Slips occur during the recovery process when clients act on an urge for a symptom, often in response to a risky situation. One way to protect against slips is to identify risky situations in advance and to make careful plans to deal with these situations without symptoms. Risky situations include pressures to control weight; unpleasant emotions such as anxiety or depression; pleasant emotions such as wanting to celebrate; physical discomfort such as feeling hungry, full, or sick; being alone and having the opportunity to have symptoms; having conflicts with others; being exposed to certain foods; being in habitual settings; feeling fat; unintentional changes in weight or eating habits (e.g., dental work and illness); and the change of season (i.e., bathing suit season).

Stressors are different from risky situations as they are ongoing and cumulative. Stressors include, but are not limited to, marital or relationship difficulties, personal or family illnesses, time pressure, work or school duties, parenting, financial situations, moving, and daily hassles. In the past, clients may have responded to stressors by engaging in symptoms to relieve stress. It is important that clients learn to cope with stressors in a more adaptive and healthy way through problem solving and communication. Clinicians can also help clients identify and experiment with ways to relax (e.g., listening to music, yoga, taking a vacation, meditating, being involved in nature, gardening, taking a long bath, and creating art).

Dealing with Slips

Clients need to know that slips are a normal part of recovery and are different from relapse. Clients are prone to interpret slips as "erasing all of their hard work toward recovery and putting them back to square one." It is important to address this all-or-nothing thinking in response to a slip to prevent the slip from turning into a complete relapse via the abstinence violation effect (Marlatt & Gordon, 1978). This effect occurs when clients become very symptomatic in response to one symptom because they believe that they no longer have control over any of their symptoms. Although a slip can be very upsetting, it is possible to help clients reframe slips as temporary setbacks and valuable learning experiences. Clinicians can help clients learn from their slips by asking the following questions: What symptoms were involved in the slip? What factors contributed to the slip? What unhelpful thoughts were present? What statements or facts might help to shift unhelpful thoughts to a more realistic view? What stressors are present? What can be done differently in the future to avoid further slips?

After a slip it is important for clients to get back on track immediately. Clinicians should inform clients that this means if they skipped breakfast, they should have a normal lunch; if they binge at lunch, they should have a normal dinner; if they vomit dinner, they should try to replace that dinner. Waiting for the next day or the next week to get back on track can set a client up for more symptoms and may start the slide toward relapse. Clients should also be reminded that if they have a slip it is important to return to strategies that they used in the earlier stages of their recovery (e.g., self-monitoring, mechanical eating, distraction, and avoiding situations that are too risky to manage without symptoms). It is helpful for clients to prepare in advance a plan for managing a slip. The plan should include eating and meal planning; strategies to prevent other eating disorder symptoms; managing thoughts about weight, body image, and slips; and sources of social support.

Addressing Secondary Gain

One function that eating disorder symptoms can fulfill is obtaining attention from others (i.e., family, friends, and health care providers). Therefore, it is important to avoid reinforcing this function by reducing or withdrawing attention once symptoms have abated. It is helpful to reassure clients that therapy and care will continue once symptoms and eating have improved, and to follow through with this plan (Orimoto & Vitousek, 1992).

Continuing Therapeutic Work and Support

Ongoing support with individual or group therapy may help to prevent relapse. Clients may need to continue to explore the function of their eating disorder and to work on finding new ways to meet these needs. In addition, clients may need to continue to work on body image concerns, weight-related self-esteem, underlying issues, and comorbid conditions in an effort to prevent relapse.

CASE EXAMPLE

Aimee was a 23-year-old woman who had a long history of AN, restricting subtype, despite her young age. She had a series of intensive treatments for her AN. Each time she was admitted to hospital she was able to gain weight to a target weight and normalize her eating. Unfortunately, she also had a history of relapsing after each hospital stay. Following her third stay in intensive treatment she was involved in individual CBT aimed at relapse prevention. Despite this focused treatment, within 1 year her weight dropped to a dangerously low level, and she required and agreed to yet another intensive treatment.

During the relapse prevention treatment, Aimee was able to articulate that her eating disorder served many functions, including providing her a unique identity within her family, protecting her from pressures to excel at school, and helping her to manage her social anxiety. On the other hand, she reported that the anorexia was taking a huge toll on her health and her life, and that she was tired of her constant struggle with food and weight. She was also very worried about the stress it was causing to her family and friends. For all these reasons she presented as highly motivated to stay well.

As part of the relapse prevention work, Aimee explored her past relapses and was able to identify pressures related to school as a common factor for each relapse. She had many perfectionistic thoughts about her performance at school, and she strived to achieve the highest grades. These attempts often resulted in sleepless nights of studying and going days without eating. Therefore, it was concerning that she had been accepted to a local university and was scheduled to start a demanding business program within a few months. After a great deal of cognitive work related to these perfectionistic beliefs, she decided to first complete a small related program at another institution before starting at the university in order to gain some experience and practice her new skills. The goal was to complete the program without striving for perfection and to focus on keeping herself well. Once the program started, it became clear that the bigger challenge for Aimee was the anxiety related to being with other students. She reported many anxious thoughts about not fitting in, having nothing to offer socially, and being seen as a loser by others. Aimee was taught to monitor and challenge these thoughts, and some exposure exercises related to her social anxiety were incorporated into the treatment. However, she found that restricting her eating and losing weight were more effective methods of dealing with these distressing thoughts and feelings. Despite being fully aware of this coping reaction she was unable to stop the behavior. Once the psychological and physical complications returned (i.e., isolation, food preoccupation, depression, and lethargy) she was regretful that she was once again severely ill with anorexia and seemed very motivated to improve her condition so that she could attend university. Despite increasing her sessions to twice weekly, and her insistence on setting behavioral goals each week, she continued to lose weight and narrow her eating. Ten months after intensive treatment she was eating very little, exercising 5 hours per day, and spending significant amounts of time checking her body on scales and in mirrors.

A significant precipitating factor to Aimee's relapse was the social anxiety that surfaced when she returned to school. This situation stimulated her core self-esteem deficits beyond a level that she could tolerate or combat with CBT strategies. In retrospect, it appeared that even the easier academic program and its social context were too evocative for Aimee's level of recovery. The new treatment plan included weight restoration followed by individual and group CBT and the strong recommendation that Aimee delay attending university until she had managed an extended period of weight maintenance outside the hospital. This would allow more time to address issues related to self-esteem, social anxiety, and body image in a less stressful environment. Concurrent participation in group therapy was intended to provide more protected opportunities for Aimee to deal with her social anxiety and feelings of being inadequate in comparison to other people. Other behavioral exposure exercises were included in the individual therapy but at an intensity that was therapeutic and not driven by Aimee's feeling that she had to attend university as soon as she left the hospital.

Currently Aimee has regained about half of her recommended weight gain. She is willing to postpone university and continue with the treatment plan. She is hopeful that she will be able to maintain this attempt at recovery, and that she will eventually be able to pursue her dreams of university and a career in business.

CONCLUSION

Eating disorders can be difficult to treat and are associated with high relapse rates. One of the main challenges when working with this population is to appreciate the functions that the disorder serves, as well as its ego-syntonic nature. It is therefore important to be knowledgeable in the area of motivational enhancement as well as CBT. Comorbidity is the norm in this population, and comorbid conditions must be addressed and treated in order to improve outcome and prevent relapse. Treatment needs to be tailored to individual needs including considerations for distinct eating disorders (i.e., AN, BN, and BED) and special populations (i.e., chronic clients, diabetic clients, and males).

Although CBT is the first line treatment for eating disorders, its effectiveness for eating disorders is limited. On average, only 50% of clients with BN stop binge eating and purging, and fewer are able to gain and maintain a healthy weight after AN. This chapter discusses ways to apply existing CBT principles, expand CBT, and combine CBT with other treatments in order to improve short- and long-term outcomes. Issues related to resources, including treatment matching and sequencing, are also discussed in this context. The research in this area is at a relatively early stage and cannot currently provide definitive answers on how to improve the effectiveness of CBT in this population. Ideally, continued work in this area will eventually guide clinical practice focused on maximizing the benefits of CBT and promoting better outcome for clients with eating disorders.

REFERENCES

Agras, W. S., Crow, S. J., Halmi, K. A., Mitchell, J. E., Wilson, G. T., & Kraemer, H. C. (2000). Outcome predictors for the cognitive behavior treatment of bulimia nervosa: Data from a multisite study. *American Journal of Psychiatry, 158*, 1302–1308.

Agras, W. S., Rossiter, E. M., Arnow, B., Schneider, J. A., Telch, C., Raeburn, S., Bruce, B., Perl, M., & Koran, L. M. (1992). Pharmacologic and cognitive-behavioral treatment for bulimia nervosa: A controlled comparison. *American Journal of Psychiatry, 149*, 82–87.

Agras, W. S., Walsh, B. T., Fairburn, C. G., Wilson, G. T., & Kraemer, H. C. (2000). A multicenter comparison of cognitive-behavioral therapy and interpersonal therapy for bulimia nervosa. *Archives of General Psychiatry, 57*, 459–466.

American Psychiatric Association. (1994). *Diagnostic and statistical manual of mental disorders* (4th ed.). Washington, DC: Author.

Andersen, A. E. (2002). Eating disorders in males. In C. G. Fairburn & K. D. Brownell (Eds.), *Eating disorders and obesity* (2nd ed., pp. 188–192). New York: Guilford Press.

Bell, L., & Newns, K. (2002). What is multi-impulsive bulimia and can multi-impulsive patients benefit from supervised self-help? *European Eating Disorders Review, 10*, 413–427.

Blouin, J. H., Carter, J., Blouin, A. G., Tener, L., Zuro, C., & Barlow, J. (1994). Prognostic indicators in bulimia nervosa treated with cognitive-behavioral group therapy. *International Journal of Eating Disorders, 15*, 113–123.

Bulik, C. M. (2002). Anxiety, depression and eating disorders. In C. G. Fairburn & K. D. Brownell (Eds.), *Eating disorders and obesity* (2nd ed., pp. 193–198). New York: Guilford Press.

Bulik, C. M., Sullivan, P. F., Joyce, P. R., Carter, F. A., & McIntosh, V. (1998). Predictors of 1-year treatment outcome in bulimia nervosa. *Comprehensive Psychiatry, 39*, 206–214.

Carter, J. C., Blackmore, E., Sutandar-Pinnock, K., & Woodside, D. B. (2004). Relapse in anorexia nervosa: A survival analysis. *Psychological Medicine, 34*, 671–679.

Carter, J. C., & Fairburn, C. G. (1998). Cognitive-behavioral self-help for binge eating disorder: A controlled effectiveness study. *Journal of Consulting and Clinical Psychology, 66*, 616–623.

Carter, J. C., Olmsted, M. P., Kaplan, A. S., McCabe, R. E., Mills, J., & Aime, A. (2003). Self-help for bulimia nervosa: A randomized controlled trial. *American Journal of Psychiatry, 160*, 973–978.

Chen, E. Y., & Linehan, M. M. (2003). *Manual development for dialectical behavior therapy for clients with borderline personality disorder and eating disorders: A work in progress.* Paper presented at the annual Eating Disorder Research Society Meeting, Ravello, Italy.

Cooper, Z., & Fairburn, C. G. (2001). A new cognitive behavioural approach to the treatment of obesity. *Behaviour Research and Therapy, 39*, 499–511.

Cooper, Z., Fairburn, C. G., & Hawkins, D. M. (2003). *Cognitive-behavioral treatment of obesity: A clinician's guide.* New York: Guilford Press.

Dansky, B. S., Brewerton, T. D., & Kilpatrick, D. G. (2000). Comorbidity of bulimia nervosa and alcohol use disorders: Results for the national women's study. *International Journal of Eating Disorders, 27*, 180–190.

Davis, R., McVey, G., Heinmaa, M., Rockert, W., & Kennedy, S. (1999). Sequencing of cognitive-behavioral treatments for bulimia nervosa. *International Journal of Eating Disorders, 25*, 361–374.

Dennis, A. B., & Sansone, R. A. (1991). The clinical stages of treatment for eating disorder patients with borderline personality disorder. In C. L. Johnson (Ed.), *Psychodynamic treatment of anorexia nervosa and bulimia* (pp. 126–164). New York: Guilford Press.

Dennis, A. B., & Sansone, R. A. (1997). Treatment of patients with personality disorders. In D. M. Garner & P. E. Garfinkel (Eds.), *Handbook of treatment for eating disorders* (2nd ed., pp. 437–449). New York: Guilford Press.

Deter, H. C., & Herzog, W. (1994). Anorexia nervosa in a long-term perspective: Results of the Heidelberg–Mannheim study. *Psychosomatic Medicine, 56*, 20–27.

Devlin, M. J., Yanovski, S. Z., & Wilson, G. T. (2000). Obesity: What mental health professionals need to know. *American Journal of Psychiatry, 157*, 854–866.

Diabetes Control and Complications Trial Research Group. (1993). The effect of intensive treatment of diabetes on the development and progression of long-term complications in insulin-dependent diabetes mellitus. *New England Journal of Medicine, 329*, 977–986.

Eckert, E. D., Halmi, K. A., Marchi, P., Grove, W., & Crosby, R. (1995). Ten-year follow-up of anorexia nervosa: Clinical course and outcome. *Psychological Medicine, 25*, 143–156.

Eisler, I., Dare, C., Hodes, M., Russell, G., Dodge, E., & Le Grange, D. (2000). Family therapy for adolescent anorexia nervosa: The results of a controlled comparison of two family interventions. *Journal of Child Psychology and Psychiatry, 41*, 727–736.

Eisler, I., Dare, C., Russell, G. F. M., Szmukler, G., Le Grange, D., & Dodge, E. (1997). Family and individual therapy in anorexia nervosa: A 5-year follow-up. *Archives of General Psychiatry, 54*, 1025–1030.

Eldredge, K. L., Agras, W. S., Arnow, C. F., Bell, S., Castonguay, L., & Marnell, M. (1997). The effects of extending cognitive-behavioral therapy for binge eating disorder among initial treatment nonresponders. *International Journal of Eating Disorders, 21*, 347–352.

Fahy, T. A., & Russell, G. F. M. (1993). Outcome and prognostic variables in bulimia nervosa. *International Journal of Eating Disorders, 14*, 135–146.

Fairburn, C. G. (1985). Cognitive-behavioral treatment for bulimia. In D. M. Garner & P. E. Garfinkel (Eds.), *Handbook of psychotherapy for anorexia nervosa and bulimia* (pp. 160–192). New York: Guilford Press.

Fairburn, C. G. (1997a). Eating disorders. In D. M. Clark & C. G. Fairburn (Eds.), *Science and practice of cognitive behavior therapy* (pp. 209–241). New York: Guilford Press.

Fairburn, C. G. (1997b). Interpersonal psychotherapy for bulimia nervosa. In D. M. Garner & P. E. Garfinkel (Eds.), *Handbook of treatment for eating disorders* (pp. 278–294). New York: Guilford Press.

Fairburn, C. G., Cooper, Z., & Shafran, R. (2003). Cognitive behaviour therapy for eating disorders: A transdiagnostic theory and treatment. *Behaviour Research and Therapy, 41*, 509–528.

Fairburn, C. G., Jones, R., Peveler, R. C., Carr, S. J., Solomon, R. A., O'Connor, M. E., Burton, J., & Hope, R. A. (1991). Three psychological treatments for bulimia nervosa. *Archives of General Psychiatry, 48*, 463–469.

Fairburn, C. G., Marcus, M. D., & Wilson, G. T. (1993). Cognitive-behavioral therapy for binge eating and bulimia nervosa: A comprehensive treatment manual. In C. G. Fairburn & G. T. Wilson (Eds.), *Binge eating: Nature assessment and treatment* (pp. 361–404). New York: Guilford Press.

Fairburn, C. G., Norman, P., Welch, S. L., O'Connor, M. E., Doll, H. A., & Peveler, R. C. (1995). A prospective study of outcome in bulimia nervosa and the long-term effects of three psychological treatments. *Archives of General Psychiatry, 52,* 304–312.

Fairburn, C. G., Peveler, R. C., Jones, R., Hope, R. A., & Doll, H. (1993). Predictors of 12-month outcome in bulimia nervosa and the influence of attitudes to shape and weight. *Journal of Consulting and Clinical Psychology, 61,* 696–698.

Fairburn, C. G., Shafran, R., & Cooper, Z. (1998). A cognitive behavioral theory of anorexia nervosa. *Behaviour Research and Therapy, 37,* 1–13.

Field, A. E., Herzog, D. B., Keller, M. B., West, J., Nussbaum, K., & Colditz, G. A. (1997). Distinguishing recovery from remission in a cohort of bulimic women: How should asymtomatic period be described? *Journal of Clinical Epidemiology, 50,* 1339–1345.

Freeman, R. J., Beach, B., Davis, R., & Solyom, L. (1985). The prediction of relapse in bulimia nervosa. *Journal of Psychiatric Research, 19,* 349–353.

Garner, D. M., Vitousek, K. M., & Pike, K. M. (1997). Cognitive-behavioral therapy for anorexia nervosa. In D. M. Garner & P. E. Garfinkel (Eds.), *Handbook of treatment for eating disorders* (pp. 94–144). New York: Guilford Press.

Gillberg, I. C., Rastam, M., & Gillberg, C. (1994). Anorexia nervosa outcome: Six-year controlled longitudinal study of 51 cases including a population cohort. *Journal of the American Academy of Child and Adolescent Psychiatry, 33,* 729–739.

Godart, N. T., Flament, M. F., Perdereau, F., & Jeammet, P. (2002). Comorbidity between eating disorders and anxiety disorders: A review. *International Journal of Eating Disorders, 32,* 253–270.

Greenberg, L. S., & Paivio, S. C. (1997). *Working with emotions in psychotherapy.* New York: Guilford Press.

Halmi, K. A., Agras, W. S., Mitchell, J., Wilson, G. T., Crow, S., Bryson, S. W., & Kraemer, H. (2002). Relapse predictors of patients with bulimia nervosa who achieved abstinence through cognitive behavioral therapy. *Archives of General Psychiatry, 59,* 1105–1109.

Halmi, K. A., Goldberg, S. C., Casper, R. C., Eckert, E. D., & Davis, J. M. (1979). Pretreatment predictors of outcome in anorexia nervosa. *British Journal of Psychiatry, 134,* 71–78.

Herzog, D. B., Dorer, D. J., Keel, P. K., Selwyn, S. E., Ekeblad, E. R., Flores, A. T., Greenwood, D. N., Burwell, R. A., & Keller, M. B. (1999). Recovery and relapse in anorexia nervosa and bulimia nervosa: A 7.5-year follow-up study. *Journal of the American Academy of Child and Adolescent Psychiatry, 38,* 829–837.

Herzog, D. B., Keller, M. B., & Lavori, P. W. (1988). Outcome in anorexia nervosa and bulimia nervosa: A review of the literature. *Journal of Nervous and Mental Disease, 176,* 131–143.

Herzog, W., Schellberg, D., & Deter, H. C. (1997). First recovery in anorexia nervosa patients in the long-term course: A discrete-time survival analysis. *Journal of Consulting and Clinical Psychology, 65,* 169–177.

Hunt, M. G. (1998). The only way out is through: Emotional processing and recovery after a depressing life event. *Behaviour Research and Therapy, 36,* 361–384.

Kabat-Zinn, J. (1990). *Full catastrophe living: Using the wisdom of you body and mind to face stress, pain and illness.* New York: Dell.

Kabat-Zinn, J. (1994). *Wherever you go, there you are: Mindfulness mediation in everyday life.* New York: Hyperion.

Kaplan, A., & Walsh, B. T. (2002). *Brief presentation of ongoing treatment research.* Paper presented at the annual Eating Disorders Research Society Meeting. Charleston, SC.

Kaye, W. H., Gwirtsman, H. E., Obarzanek, E., George, T., Jimerson, D. C., & Ebert, M. H. (1986). Caloric intake necessary for weight maintenance in anorexia nervosa: Nonbulimics require greater caloric intake than bulimics. *American Journal of Clinical Nutrition, 44,* 435–443.

Kaye, W. H., Nagata, T., Weltzin, T. E., Hsu, L. K. G., Sokol, M. S., McConaha, C., Plotnicov, K. H., Weise, J., & Deep, D. (2001). Double-blind placebo-controlled administration of fluoxetine in restricting- and restricting-purging-type anorexia nervosa. *Biological Psychiatry, 49,* 644–652.

Korman, L. M., & Greenberg, L. S. (1996). Emotion and therapeutic change. *Advances in Biological Psychiatry, 2,* 1–25.

Krahn, D. D., Rock, C., Dechert, R. E., Nairn, K. K., & Hasse, S. A. (1993). Changes in resting energy expenditure and body composition in anorexia nervosa patients during refeeding. *Journal of the American Dietetic Association, 93,* 434–438.

Kristeller, J. L., & Hallett, C. B. (1999). An exploratory study of a meditation-based intervention for binge eating disorder. *Journal of Health Psychology, 4,* 357–363.

Lilenfeld, L. R., Kaye, W. H., Greeno, C. G., Merikangas, K. R., Plotnicov, K., Pollice, C., Rao, R., Strober, M., Bulik, C. M., & Nagy, L. (1997). Psychiatric disorders in women with bulimia nervosa and their first-degree relatives: Effects of comorbid substance dependence. *International Journal of Eating Disorders, 22,* 253–264.

Linehan, M. M., Armstrong, H. E., Suarez, A., Allmon, D., & Heard, H. L. (1991). Cognitive-behavioral treatment of chronically parasuicidal borderline patients. *Archives of General Psychiatry, 48,* 1060–1064.

Linehan, M. M., Heard, H. L., & Armstrong, H. E. (1993). Naturalistic follow-up of a behavioral treatment for chonically parasuicidal borderline patients. *Archives of General Psychology, 50,* 971–974.

Maddocks, S. E., Kaplan, A. S., Woodside, D. B., Langdon, L., & Piran, N. (1992). Two year follow-up of bulimia nervosa: The importance of abstinence as the criterion of outcome. *International Journal of Eating Disorders, 12,* 133–141.

Marcus, M. D. (1997). Adapting treatment for patients with binge eating disorder. In D. M. Garner & P. E. Garfinkel (Eds.), *Handbook of treatment for eating disorders* (pp. 484–493). New York: Guilford Press.

Marcus, M. D., Wing, R. R., & Lamparski, D. M. (1985). Binge eating and dietary restraint in obese patients. *Addictive Behaviors, 10,* 163–168.

Marlatt, G. A., & Gordon, J. R. (1978). Determinants of relapse: Implications for the maintenance of behavior change. In P. Davison (Ed.), *Behavioral medicine: Changing health lifestyles* (pp. 410–452). New York: Brunner/Mazel.

Miller, W. R., & Rollnick, S. (2002). *Motivational interviewing: Preparing people for change* (2nd ed.). New York: Guilford Press.

Mitchell, J. E., Davis, L., & Goff, G. (1985). The process of relapse in patients with bulimia. *International Journal of Eating Disorders, 4,* 457–463.

Mitchell, J. E., Halmi, K., Wilson, G. T., Agras, W. S., Kraemer, H., & Crow, S. (2002). A randomized secondary treatment study of women with bulimia nervosa who fail to respond to CBT. *International Journal of Eating Disorders, 32,* 271–281.

Mitchell, J. E., Pyle, R. L., Eckert, E. D., Hatsukami, D., & Lentz, R. (1983). Electrolyte and other physical abnormalities in patients with bulimia. *Psychological Medicine, 13,* 273–278.

Mitchell, J. E., Pyle, R., Eckert, E. D., Hatsukami, D., & Soll, E. (1990). The influence of prior alcohol and drug problems on bulimia nervosa treatment outcome. *Addictive Behaviors, 15,* 169–173.

Molleken, L. (2000). Medications and eating disorders. *National Eating Disorder Information Centre Bulletin, 15*(5).

Morgan, H. G., & Russell, G. F. M. (1975). Value of family background and clinical features as predictors of long-term outcome in anorexia nervosa: Four-year follow-up study of 41 patients. *Psychological Medicine, 5,* 355–371.

Moukaddem, M., Boulier A., Apfelbaum M., & Rigaud D. (1997). Increase in diet-induced thermogenesis at the start of refeeding in severely malnourished anorexia nervosa patients. *American Journal of Clinical Nutrition, 66,* 133–140.

Obarzanek, E., Lesem, M. D., & Jimerson, D. C. (1994). Resting metabolic rate of anorexia nervosa patients during weight gain. *American Journal of Clinical Nutrition, 60,* 666–675.

O'Brien, K. M., & Vincent, N. K. (2003). Psychiatric comorbidity in anorexia and bulimia nervosa: Nature, prevalence, and causal relationships. *Clinical Psychology Review, 23,* 57–74.

Olmsted, M. P., Davis, R., Rockert, W., Irvine, M. J. R., Eagle, M., & Garner, D. M. (1991). Efficacy of a brief group psychoeducation intervention for bulimia nervosa. *Behaviour Research and Therapy, 29,* 71–83.

Olmsted, M. P., Kaplan, A. S., & Rockert, W. (1994). Rate and prediction of relapse in bulimia nervosa. *American Journal of Psychiatry, 151,* 738–743.

Olmsted, M. P., Kaplan, A. S., Rockert, W., & Jacobsen, M. (1996). Rapid responders to treatment of bulimia nervosa. *International Journal of Eating Disorders, 19,* 279–285.

Olmsted, M. P., McFarlane, T. L., Molleken, L., & Kaplan, A. S. (2001). Day hospital treatment for eating disorders. In G. O. Gabbard (Ed.), *Treatment of psychiatric disorders* (3rd ed., pp. 2127–2137). Washington, DC: American Psychiatric Press.

Orimoto, L., & Vitousek, K. B. (1992). Anorexia nervosa and bulimia nervosa. In P. Wilson (Ed.), *Principles and practices of relapse prevention* (pp. 85–127). New York: Guilford Press.

Palmer, R. L., Birchall, H., McGrain, L., & Sullivan, V. (2002). Self-help for bulimic disorders: A randomized controlled trial comparing minimal guidance with face-to-face or telephone guidance. *British Journal of Psychiatry, 181,* 230–235.

Paul, T., Schroeter, K., Dahme, B., & Nutzinger, D. O. (2002). Self-injurious behavior in women with eating disorders. *American Journal of Psychiatry, 159,* 408–411.

Peveler, R. C., & Fairburn, C. G. (1992). The treatment of bulimia nervosa in patients with diabetes mellitus. *International Journal of Eating Disorders, 11,* 45–53.

Pike, K. M., Walsh, B. T., Vitousek, K., Wilson, G. T., & Bauer, J. (2003). Cognitive-behavioral therapy in the posthospital treatment of anorexia nervosa. *American Journal of Psychiatry, 160*(11), 2046–2049.

Prochaska, J. O., & DiClemente, C. C. (1984). *The transtheoretical approach: Crossing the traditional boundaries of therapy.* Malabar, FL: Krieger.

Ratnasuriya, R. H., Eisler, I., Szmukler, G. I., & Russell, G. F. M. (1991). Anorexia nervosa: Outcome and prognostic factors after 20 years. *British Journal of Psychiatry, 158,* 495–502.

Robin, A. L., Siegel, P. T., & Moye, A. (1995). Family versus individual therapy for anorexia: Impact on family conflict. *International Journal of Eating Disorders, 17,* 313–322.

Rosen, J. C. (1996). Body image assessment and treatment in controlled studies of eating disorders. *International Journal of Eating Disorders, 20,* 331–343.

Rosen, J. C. (1997). Cognitive-behavioural body image therapy. In D. M. Garner & P. E. Garfinkel (Eds.), *Handbook of treatment for eating disorders* (pp. 188–201). New York: Guilford Press.

Rosenvinge, J. H., & Mouland, S. O. (1990). Outcome and prognosis of anorexia nervosa: A retrospective study of 41 subjects. *British Journal of Psychiatry, 156,* 92–97.

Rossiter, E. M., Agras, W. S., Telch, C. F., & Schneider, J. A. (1993). Cluster B personality disorder characteristics predict outcome in the treatment of bulimia nervosa. *International Journal of Eating Disorders, 13,* 349–357.

Rydall, A. C., Rodin, G. M., Olmsted, M. P., Devenyi, R. G., & Daneman, D. (1997). Disordered eating behavior and microvascular complications in young women with insulin-dependent diabetes mellitus. *New England Journal of Medicine, 336,* 1849–1854.

Safer, D. L., Lively, T. J., Telch, C. F., & Agras, W. S. (2002). Predictors of relapse following successful dialectical behavior therapy for binge eating disorder. *International Journal of Eating Disorders, 32,* 155–163.

Segal, Z. V., Williams, J. M. G., & Teasdale, J. D. (2002). *Mindfulness-based cognitive therapy for depression: A new approach to preventing relapse.* New York: Guilford Press.

Sharp, C. W., & Freeman, C. P. L. (1993). The medical complications of anorexia nervosa. *British Journal of Psychiatry, 162,* 452–462.

Sohlberg, S., & Norring, C. (1992). A 3-year prospective study of life events and course for adults with anorexia nervosa/bulimia nervosa. *Psychosomatic Medicine, 54,* 59–70.

Specker, S., de Zwaan, M., Raymond, N., & Mitchell, J. (1994). Psychopathology in subgroups of obese women with and without binge eating disorder. *Comprehensive Psychiatry, 35,* 185–190.

Steinhausen, H. C. (2002). The outcome of anorexia nervosa in the 20th century. *American Journal of Psychiatry 159,* 1284–1293.

Strober, M., Freeman, R., & Morrell, W. (1997). The long-term course of severe anorexia nervosa in adolescents: Survival analysis of recovery, relapse and outcome predictors. *International Journal of Eating Disorders, 22,* 339–360.

Theander, S. (1985). Outcome and prognosis in anorexia nervosa: Some results of previous investigations, compared with those of a Swedish long-term study. *Journal of Psychiatry Research, 19,* 493–508.

Touyz, S. W., Beumont, P. J., Glaun, D., Phillips, T., & Cowie, I. (1984). A comparison of lenient and strict operant conditioning programs in refeeding patients. *British Journal of Psychiatry, 144,* 517–520.

Treasure, J. L., Katzman, M., Schmidt, U., Troop, N., Todd, G., & de Silva, P. (1999). Engagement and outcome in the treatment of bulimia nervosa: First phase of a sequential design comparing motivation enhancement therapy and cognitive behavioural therapy. *Behaviour Research and Therapy, 37,* 405–418.

Treasure, J. L., Schmidt, U., Troop, N., Tiller, J., Todd, G., & Turnbull, S. (1996). Sequential treatment for bulimia nervosa incorporating a self-care manual. *British Journal of Psychiatry, 168,* 94–98.

Vitousek, K., & Hollon, S. D. (1990). The investigation of schematic content and processing in eating disorders. *Cognitive Therapy and Research, 14,* 191–214.

Vitousek, K., Watson, S., & Wilson, G. T. (1998). Enhancing motivation for change in treatment-resistant eating disorders. *Clinical Psychology Review, 18,* 391–420.

Walsh, B. T., Agras, W. S., Devlin, M. J., Fairburn, C. G., Wilson, G. T., Kahn, C., & Chally, M. K. (2000). Fluoxetine for bulimia nervosa following poor response to psychotherapy. *American Journal of Psychiatry, 157,* 1332–1334.

Walsh, B. T., Wilson, G. T., Loeb, K., Devlin, M. J., Pike, K. M., Roose, S. P., Fleiss, J., & Waternaux, C. (1997). Medication and psychotherapy in the treatment of bulimia nervosa. *American Journal of Psychiatry, 154,* 523–531.

Welch, S. L., & Fairburn, C. G. (1996). Impulsivity or comordity in bulimia nervosa: A controlled study of deliberate self-harm and alcohol and drug misuse in a community sample. *British Journal of Psychiatry, 169,* 451–458.

Weltzin, T. E., Fernstrom, M. H., Hansen, D., McConaha, C., & Kaye, W. H. (1991). Abnormal caloric requirements for weight maintenance in patients with anorexia and bulimia nervosa. *American Journal of Psychiatry, 148,* 1675–1682.

Wilfley, D. E., Agras, W. S., Telch, C. F., Rossiter, E. M., Schneider, J. A., Cole, A. G., Sifford, L. A., & Raeburn, S. D. (1993). Group cognitive-behavioral therapy and group interpersonal psychotherapy for the nonpurging bulimic individual: A controlled comparison. *Journal of Consulting and Clinical Psychology, 61,* 296–305.

Wilfley, D. E., & Cohen, L. R. (1997). Psychological treatment of bulimia nervosa and binge eating disorder. *Psychopharmacology Bulletin, 33,* 437–454.

Wilfley, D. E., Friedman, M. A., Dounchis, J. Z., Stein, R. I., Welch, R. R., & Ball, S. A. (2000). Comorbid psychopathology in binge eating disorder: Relation to eating disorder severity at baseline and following treatment. *Journal of Consulting and Clinical Psychology, 68,* 641–649.

Wilfley, D. E., Welch, R. R., Stein, R. I., Borman Spurrell, E., Cohen, L. R., Saelens, B. F., Dounchis, J. Z., Frank, M. A., Wiseman, C. V., & Matt, G. E. (2002). A randomized comparison of group cognitive-behavioral therapy and group interpersonal psychotherapy for the treatment of overweight individuals with binge-eating disorder. *Archives of General Psychiatry, 59,* 713–721.

Wilson, G. T. (1996). Treatment of bulimia nervosa: When CBT fails. *Behaviour Research and Therapy, 34,* 197–212.

Wilson, G. T. (1999). Cognitive behaviour therapy for eating disorders: Progress and problems. *Behaviour Research and Therapy, 37,* S79–S95.

Wilson, G. T. (2000). *How does cognitive-behavioural therapy work and for whom?* Paper presented at plenary session, 9th International Conference on Eating Disorders, New York.

Wilson, G. T. (2002). Eating disorders and addictive disorders. In C. G. Fairburn & K. D. Brownell (Eds.), *Eating disorders and obesity* (2nd ed., pp. 199–203). New York: Guilford Press.

Wilson, G. T., & Fairburn, C. G. (2002). Treatment for eating disorders. In P. E. Nathan & J. M. Gorman (Eds.), *A guide to treatments that work* (2nd ed., pp. 559–592). New York: Oxford University Press.

Wilson, G. T., Fairburn, C. G., & Agras, W. S. (1997). Cognitive-behavioral therapy for bulimia nervosa. In D. M. Garner & P. E. Garfinkel (Eds.), *Handbook of treatment for eating disorders* (pp. 67–93). New York: Guilford Press.

Wilson, G. T., Fairburn, C. G., Agras, W. S., Walsh, B. T., & Kraemer, H. (2002). Cognitive-behavioral therapy for bulimia nervosa: Time course and mechanisms of change. *Journal of Consulting and Clinical Psychology, 70,* 267–274.

Wilson, G. T., Loeb, K. L., Walsh, B. T., Labouvie, E., Petkova, E., Liu, X., & Waternaux, C. (1999). Psychological versus pharmacological treatments of bulimia nervosa: Predictors and processes of change. *Journal of Consulting and Clinical Psychology, 67,* 451–459.

Wilson, G. T., Rossiter, E., Kleifield, E., & Lindholm, L. (1986). Cognitive-behavioural treatment of bulimia nervosa: A controlled evaluation. *Behaviour Research and Therapy, 24,* 277–288.

Wonderlich, S. A. (2002). Personality and eating disorders. In C. G. Fairburn & K. D. Brownell (Eds.), *Eating disorders and obesity* (2nd ed., pp. 204–209). New York: Guilford Press.

Yager, J. (2002). Management of patients with intractable eating disorders. In C. G. Fairburn & K. D. Brownell (Eds.), *Eating disorders and obesity* (2nd ed., pp. 345–349). New York: Guilford Press.

Yanovski, S. Z., Let, M., Yanovski, J. A., Flood, M., Gold, P. W., Kissileff, H. R., & Walsh, B. T. (1992). Food selection and intake of obese women with binge eating disorder. *American Journal of Clinical Nutrition, 56,* 975–980.

Zhu, A. J., & Walsh, B. T. (2002). Pharmacologic treatment of eating disorders. *Canadian Journal of Psychiatry, 47,* 227–234.

9

Schizophrenia

NICHOLAS TARRIER

OVERVIEW OF THE DISORDER

Descriptions of disordered states that resemble schizophrenia can be found throughout history and as far back as 1400 B.C. in ancient Hindu texts (Kendell, 1993). In the 19th century, Kraepelin divided insanity into two conditions based on their course and outcome. The first, called manic–depression, was an affective disorder of episodic fluctuating course but with full recovery between episodes. The second, termed "dementia praecox," incorporated previously described conditions of catatonia, hebephrenia, and dementia paranoids into a condition with a steadily deteriorating course, or at least incomplete recovery. Kraepelin's classification and assumption that psychosis was a disease of the brain became the accepted convention. In 1911, Bleuler (1911/1978) coined the term "schizophrenia," meaning "split mind" or a loosening of associations between different psychological functions. Debate and confusion continued over the first part of the 20th century, with "various centres and regions developing their own diagnostic modifications and refinements so that the term *schizophrenia* was used throughout the world, but in a bewildering variety of different ways which were rarely made explicit" (Kendell, 1993, p. 398). In 1958, Schneider focused attention on the symptoms present during acute illness and described first-rank symptoms. These included specific auditory hallucinations, thought insertion or withdrawal, thought broadcast, alien control, passivity, and delusional perception. These first-rank symptoms became very influential in standardizing diagnostic systems. Recognition that schizophrenia would be diagnosed much more frequently in some countries than others, especially the United States (Cooper et al., 1972; World Health Organization, 1973), eventually led to concerted attempts to improve on the reliability of the diagnosis and narrow the concept to clearly defined characteristic symptoms. These were established within the third edition, revised and fourth edition of the *Diagnostic and Statistical Manual of Mental Disorders* (DSM-III-R, DSM-IV; American Psychiatric Association, 1987, 1994) and the *International Classification of Diseases: Classification of Mental And Behavioral Disorders* (ICD-10; World Health Organization, 1992). Methods are now available using computer-based algorithms (the OPCRIT system) to make a diagnosis based on multiple criteria (McGuffin, Farmer, & Harvey, 1991).

According to DSM-IV, schizophrenia is diagnosed when two or more symptoms are present that are considered to be characteristic of the disorder. These symptoms are (1) delusions; (2) hallucinations; (3) disorganized speech; (4) grossly disorganized or catatonic behavior; and (5) negative symptoms. It should be noted that only one characteristic symptom is required to make a diagnosis of schizophrenia if the delusions are bizarre, or if hallucinations contain a voice that keeps a running commentary on the person's thoughts or behavior or two or more voices conversing with each other (American Psychiatric Association, 1994).

The first four characteristic symptoms of schizophrenia are considered positive symptoms because they reflect an "excess or distortion of normal functions" (American Psychiatric Association, 1994, p. 274). Delusions are usually defined as "false, unshakeable beliefs, which are out of keeping with the patient's social and cultural background" (Hamilton, 1974, p. 39). Delusions can be of a number of types, such as delusions of reference (a conviction that events have a special personal significance, e.g., seeing a red bus signifies that the person is of special importance), of control (a conviction that the person or his or her thought, speech, or movements are controlled by alien forces), and about possession of thought (a conviction that the person's thoughts are inserted, withdrawn, or broadcast). Other types of delusions are more common, such as delusions of persecution (a conviction that others are acting against the person) and are not specific to schizophrenia.

The second characteristic symptom of schizophrenia is hallucinations. Hallucinations are defined as false perceptions. Although hallucinations can occur in any sensory modality, the most common form is auditory hallucinations, typically experienced as voices, either talking to or about the person. Visual hallucinations are less frequent. Tactile, olfactory, gustatory, and somatic hallucinations are also reported and can involve such things as believing that gas is being pumped into the room or that a device has been inserted into one's body (described as alien insertion).

The third characteristic symptom of schizophrenia is disorganized speech. Disorders of speech are assumed to be a manifestation of underlying thought disorder and can manifest themselves in various ways, including dysfunction in the stream of thought, (e.g., pressure of thought), poverty of thought, and thought blocking. A loosening of associations, or a lack of connection between ideas, is also seen in schizophrenia. This may be apparent in illogical thinking or talking past the point. In its most severe form, the structure and

coherence of thought are lost, so that utterances are jumbled (word salad), or-
dinary words may be used in unusual ways (paraphrasia), or new words in-
vented (neologisms) (Gelder, Gath, & Mayou, 1991).

In contrast to positive symptoms, the negative symptoms of schizophrenia are characterized by an absence of elements normally within the repertoire
of human behavior, function, and experience, such as emotional responsiveness, spontaneous speech, motivation, and self-care. Severe levels of negative
symptoms compromise the individual's ability to engage in general and social
activity, as well as adequately look after him- or herself.

OVERVIEW OF EMPIRICALLY SUPPORTED TREATMENTS

Pharmacotherapy

History is replete with various bizarre and sometimes tortuous treatments of
the unfortunate and the "insane." Prior to the post-World War II pharmacological era, a number of physical treatments were attempted, such as insulin
treatment, neurosurgery, and electroconvulsive treatment (ECT), although
containment and institutionalization were the more usual management. These
physical treatments have been largely discredited and are rarely used today.
ECT still has its advocates for the treatment of refractory cases, although this
remains controversial (Gelder et al., 1991).

Antipsychotic drug treatments (e.g., chlorpromazine, fluphenazine, and
haloperidol) have been the foundation of treatment for schizophrenia since
the early 1950s. Medication is used both in treating the acute stage of the illness, during which the patient may be highly agitated and disturbed, and in
maintenance, during which symptoms are controlled and risk of relapse reduced. With the development of these antipsychotic medications (also termed
"neuroleptics"), considerable progress has been made in treating psychotic
symptoms and reducing the disability of those suffering from schizophrenia.
As discussed further later in this chapter, these medications are associated with
significant side effects, requiring that physicians make a special effort to ensure compliance, thus increasing the likelihood of a good clinical outcome. In
recent years, a number of so-called atypical antipsychotics have been introduced, with risperidone and olanzapine being the most widely used. The atypical antipsychotics have been heavily promoted, touted for their superior side
effect profile and their greater clinical efficacy compared to traditional
antipsychotics. These novel antipsychotics may be more acceptable to patients
because they cause fewer side effects than the older antipsychotic drugs (NHS
Centre for Reviews and Dissemination, 1999).

In spite of the efficacy of antipsychotic medication in reducing symptoms
of schizophrenia, there is an acknowledgment that there are significant disadvantages and weaknesses to these medications, not least the fact that many
patients suffer persistent residual psychotic symptoms (Tarrier, 1987) and that
medication alone is not an adequate treatment (Pilling et al., 2002b). Further-

more, there are reports that a subgroup of patients can do well without antipsychotic medication (Bola & Mosher, 2002).

Psychological Treatments

The traditional alternative to physical treatments was psychodynamic psychotherapy. Mueser and Berenbaum (1990) reviewed studies of psychodynamic therapy for patients with schizophrenia and concluded that there was no evidence to support its use and that it could, in fact, be harmful by causing undue stress. They recommended a moratorium on its use. There have, however, been some recent, but unconvincing, attempts to revive this approach (e.g., Paley & Shapiro, 2002).

Cognitive-Behavioral Therapy

Origins of Cognitive-Behavioral Therapy for Schizophrenia. Cognitive-behavioral therapy (CBT) for schizophrenia, although following a common theme and set of principles, has developed in a number of centers, mostly in the United Kingdom, and been informed by a number of theoretical and conceptual perspectives. A dramatic expansion in the use of CBT in the 1980s and 1990s in the treatment of anxiety and affective disorders influenced clinical psychologists working in the field of schizophrenia, who were trying to understand and treat schizophrenia from a psychological perspective. This was especially true in the United Kingdom where clinical psychologists treated a range of disorders in adult mental health services and were able to transfer their treatment methods across diagnostic groups.

The coping skills approach was developed in Manchester, United Kingdom, drawing on a number of sources. First, empirical findings suggested that many patients with schizophrenia acquired coping strategies to deal with their hallucinations and delusions (Tarrier, 1987). Second, a great deal of research was done on self-regulation (Karoly & Kanfer, 1982), in which target behaviors are identified as problematic and monitored with the purpose of implementing alternative responses. This approach was thought to be especially relevant to schizophrenia as it involved a potential enhancement of executive control through response inhibition, selection, and implementation. Last, central to the coping approach, although not unique to it, the case formulation approach (e.g., developing a detailed individual idiosyncratic assessment) began to be used as a means of understanding the experience of psychosis (Chadwick, Williams, & MacKenzie, 2003; for a detailed account of case formulation in CBT generally see Tarrier & Calam, 2002; for psychosis, see Haddock & Tarrier, 1998; Tarrier, 2002). This allowed a treatment strategy to be formulated based on the clinician's assessment of the determinants of the individual's psychotic symptoms. The aim of the coping-skills approach is in line with a recovery model in which patients learn cognitive and behavioral strategies with which to reduce psychotic symptoms or the distress they cause. This has the advantage of emphasizing coping as a normal reaction to aversive experiences, which aids engagement. Table 9.1 outlines the characteristics and methods used in the coping approach.

Other clinical research groups have modified Beck's cognitive therapy for use with schizophrenic patients (Kingdon & Turkington, 1991). This approach gives central emphasis to the role of beliefs in causing and maintaining psychopathology. Beck first published a case study of cognitive therapy in the treatment of delusions in 1952. Kingdon and Turkington (1994) have also given prominence to the concept of a *normalizing rationale* in providing the patient with an acceptable understanding of his/her disorder. This emphasis on beliefs has been taken a logical step further in analysis of schema or underlying assumptions or beliefs held by the patient (Brabban & Turkington, 2002).

In spite of the variety of clinical models, there are a number of common clinical strategies that underlie all variants of CBT for schizophrenia. These are engagement and establishment of a therapeutic relationship; assessment based on an individualized case formulation which identifies psychotic experience (symptoms) and establishes associations between the patient's cognition, behavior, and affect within the environmental context in response to this experience; an intervention strategy that is based on this formulation and aims to use cognitive and behavioral methods to reduce psychotic symptoms and associated emotional distress. Patients are taught to be aware of their symptoms and learn methods to control them (e.g., learning to control auditory hallucinations by switching their attention away from them). This is usually achieved by breaking coping strategies down into elements that are learned individually and then aggregated into an overall strategy. To ensure that these coping strategies can be implemented, they are overlearned during the therapy session. Learning such control techniques allows the patients to challenge beliefs he or she may have had about the voices, such as "the voices are uncontrollable," "the voices are all powerful," and "I must obey the voices." Thus, by learning to control basic psychological processes such as attention, through attention switching and distraction, patients also learn to challenge their beliefs about their experiences and symptoms. Behavioral experiments and reality tests can also be used to disprove delusional and inappropriate beliefs. Particular attention is paid to identifying avoidance and safety behaviors that reinforce inappropriate beliefs. Changing these behaviors is a powerful method of changing beliefs and delusions. Patients may be assisted in their attempts at behavior change by means of self-instruction and coping strategies that decrease arousal (such as breathing exercises, quick relaxation, guided imagery, and encouraging positive task-oriented internal dialogue). In some refractory cases, the patient's conviction that his or her delusional beliefs are true is unshakable and he or she is unwilling to examine the veracity of this subjective experience. In these cases, the clinician must negotiate treatment goals aimed at reducing distress rather than the symptoms themselves. A failure to do this will probably result in the patient refusing treatment.

TABLE 9.1. Characteristics and Treatment Methods Used in Coping Training

Characteristics

- Emphasizes a normal and general process of dealing with adversity.
- Is carried out systematically through overlearning, simulation, and role play.
- Is additive in that different strategies can be combined in a sequence that progresses to *in vivo* implementation.
- Is based on providing a new response set that will be a method of coping with an ongoing problem rather than being curative.
- The learning of cognitive coping skills occurs through a process of external verbalization that is slowly diminished until the required procedure is internalized under covert control.
- The learning of behavioral coping skills occurs through a process of graded practice or rehearsal.

Treatment methods

- *Attention switching.* A process whereby a patient actively changes the focus of his or her attention from one subject or experience to another. This involves inhibiting an ongoing response and initiating an alternative.
- *Attention narrowing.* A process whereby the patient restricts the range and content of his or her attention. Many patients talk about "blanking" their mind or focusing their attention as a method of coping. Evidence suggests that one problem that patients with schizophrenia face is an inability to adequately filter information input, to distinguish signal from noise, and attention narrowing may alleviate this.
- *Modified self-statements and internal dialogue.* The use of self-statements and internal dialogue.
- *Reattribution.* Patients are asked to generate an alternative explanation for an experience and then utilize re-attributional statements when that experience occurs.
- *Awareness training.* Patients are taught to be aware of and monitor the onset of their positive symptoms as part of self-monitoring and self-regulation.
- *Dearousing techniques.* Patients learn brief arousal reduction techniques, such as quick relaxation and breathing exercises, to use in specific situations.
- *Increased activity levels.* Simple activity scheduling can be a powerful coping strategy, especially if implemented at the onset of the symptom and creates competition for attentional resources.
- *Social engagement and disengagement.* Patients learn to use social engagement and positive social support in a gradual manner and titrate their contact with their level of arousal.
- *Belief modification.* Patients learn to examine their beliefs and challenge them if they are inappropriate by examination of the evidence and generation of alternative explanations.
- *Reality testing and behavioral experiments.* Patients learn to identify specific beliefs and generate competing predictions that can be tested. The failure to do this in real life usually leads to avoidance, which can be reversed to challenge the beliefs that support this behavior.

It is frequently the case that the patient's delusional beliefs persist in spite of evidence to contradict them, including evidence that occurs naturally as well as evidence that is manufactured by the therapist through behavioral experiments and reality testing. To weaken these delusional explanations, the therapist should use all available opportunities, through guided discovery and Socratic questioning, to reappraise the evidence for the patient's explanation of events and thus to weaken the delusions. Pointing out the contradictory evidence in a quizzical and puzzled manner, often known as the "Columbo technique," is advised, so the patient has to account for contradictions and review his or her explanation in light of this new and contradictory evidence. When delusions are strongly held, this can be a slow process, but the weakening of delusional beliefs can occur, or, as happens in some cases, the delusional interpretations remain or return but their importance and distressing nature are greatly reduced. For example, one elderly female patient treated by the author experienced auditory hallucinations that were of a blasphemous and obscene nature. She believed that her brain acted as a transmitter and broadcast her thoughts so that other people in the vicinity could hear her thoughts, which were also blasphemous and obscene. Her main social contact was with her local church and associated social club. One Sunday, during the church service, she heard the voices and became convinced that her own thoughts about the voices were broadcast aloud to the congregation. She was mortified and so ashamed that she left the church and was unable to return or to have any contact with her friends. She was convinced that she had become ostracized by the church congregation. On being asked about the evidence for this, she replied that she had seen other members of the church in town and they had totally ignored her, which had further reinforced her sense of shame and self-disgust. On further questioning, she revealed that she had been walking on the pavement and had seen her friends drive by some distance away. There was a high probability that they had not seen her. Thus the evidence for being ostracized was challenged. A treatment goal was agreed on that would test her interpretation of the situation. If the fear that the church congregation would shun her if she returned was real, then she should expect a negative reaction when she returned to church. If the fear were irrational, there would be no negative reaction; in fact, they should be pleased to see her return. She experienced considerable anxiety at the thought of returning to church, but through being taught methods to cope with both the experience of auditory hallucinations and anxiety, her return was managed. To her surprise, far from being shunned or ostracized, she was greeted with warmth and concern. This experience considerably weakened her beliefs that others could hear her thoughts. Some months later, on being asked about the events, she said that she believed that others could hear her thoughts, but as it did not appear to bother them, she was no longer concerned about it either. In this case, her delusional explanation of past events had returned but no longer caused her any distress or disrupted her social functioning.

Phases of the Disorder and Relationship to Aims of Treatment. Schizophrenia is a complex disorder that may well be lifelong and passes through a number of phases. For example, the prodromal phase that occurs before a full-blown psychotic episode is characterized by nonspecific symptoms and symptoms of anxiety, depression, irritability, insomnia, and quasi-psychotic experience (e.g., magical thinking and feelings of paranoia). The prodromal phase will develop into a psychotic episode, during which the most florid psychotic symptoms are present and seriously interfere with functioning. A psychotic episode usually requires acute management, frequently including hospitalization. Recovery from an acute episode of psychosis is followed by a period of remission or partial remission. It is not uncommon for residual symptoms to remain during the recovery and remission phase, and in some cases, there is little recovery at all. Treatment aims and strategies will vary depending on the phase of the disorder. For example, during the prodromal phase, the aim will be to prevent transition into a full psychotic episode; during an acute episode, the aim will be to speed recovery; during partial remission, the aim will be to reduce residual symptoms and to prevent further relapse; and in full remission, the aim will be to keep the patient well. The specifics of CBT may vary depending on these aims and the phase of the disorder in which it is applied. For example, during an acute admission for a psychotic episode, the patient is often disturbed, distressed, and agitated. Thus, therapy sessions are often brief and frequent, whereas in chronically ill patients living within the community, therapy sessions will follow the normal outpatient format. In all cases, therapy will be tailored to the tolerance of the patient. In all but the most exceptional cases, CBT will be used in addition to appropriate antipsychotic medication.

Speeding Recovery in Acute Illness. Three studies have investigated CBT in addition to treatment as usual (TAU, or standard psychiatric care including antipsychotic medication) with patients hospitalized for an acute psychotic episode. In an innovative study, the Birmingham group reported that CBT was associated with a 25–50% reduction in recovery time compared to activity and recreational therapy (ATY) (Drury, Birchwood, Cochrane, & MacMillan, 1996b). As would be expected during hospital treatment, all patients showed a decline in symptoms, but after 9 months, only 5% of the CBT group displayed moderate to severe residual symptoms, compared to 56% of the ATY group (Drury, Birchwood, Cochrane, & MacMillan, 1996a). This demonstrated that it was feasible to use CBT with acutely ill and disturbed patients. Haddock, McCarron, Tarrier, and Faragher (1999) attempted to replicate these findings but found no significant differences between the groups. Although the relative benefit of CBT over ATY is still unclear, both studies demonstrated that CBT can be carried out with acutely ill and disturbed schizophrenic patients.

In an attempt to answer some of the questions raised by the earlier preliminary studies on acute patients, a large multisite trial (the SoCRATES trial) was carried out. This study recruited 309 recent onset patients from 11 mental health units at three geographically defined catchment centers with a combined population of 2,150,000. Patients were randomly allocated on admission to a 5-week program of CBT and TAU (N = 101), an equivalent program of supportive psychotherapy (SP) and TAU (N = 106), or TAU alone (N = 102). It was hypothesized that the CBT group would have a speedier recovery and would be less likely to relapse compared to the other two groups. SP was hypothesized to be an inactive treatment and to confer no advantage over TAU alone. Patients were assessed throughout the acute phase (for 70 days postadmission) and then again at 18-month follow-up. During the acute phase, all patients improved. This would be expected in recent-onset, mainly drug-naïve patients treated in the hospital with medication (Remington, Kapur, & Zipursky, 1998). As predicted, there were faster improvements in the CBT group, with significant benefits after 4 weeks. However, by the sixth week of the study, group differences were no longer evident (Lewis et al., 2002). Patients who received CBT during the acute phase of illness did show improvements in auditory hallucinations, whereas those who received SP actually experienced a worsening in this symptom, suggesting that SP might have an adverse effect on hallucinations.

It is also important to examine the effects of CBT over the long term. Drury, Birchwood, and Cochrane (2000), who found strong support for the use of CBT with acutely ill patients, also reported on a 5-year follow-up of their study. There were no overall significant differences between treatment groups (CBT vs. ATY) on symptoms or relapse rates. Haddock et al. (1999), who found no differences between CBT and ATY during acute treatment, also found no differences in relapse rates between the two treatments after 2 years. In the SoCRATES trial, the results after 18 months showed that patients who received CBT or SP along with TAU had fewer psychotic symptoms than the patients who received TAU alone. The only difference between the two groups that received some form of psychosocial treatment was that the SP group continued to experience more auditory hallucinations than the CBT group. There were no differences in relapse rates between the three treatment groups (Tarrier et al., 2004).

Symptom Reduction in Chronic Residual Symptoms. The initial application of CBT in psychosis was with chronically ill patients suffering from drug-resistant positive psychotic symptoms. With this population, CBT involves an individualized assessment of the patient's psychotic symptoms, with details of the nature of delusions and hallucinations, usually voices. In assessment of hallucinations, the patient is asked about the content of the voices, what they say, who they are thought to be, and other important characteristics such as their power, malevolence, and omnipotence. The patient's beliefs about the voices frequently determine emotional reactions and behavior in response to these auditory hallucinations. With both delusions and hallucinations, a formulation is built on information regarding the frequency and variation in psychotic symptoms, the antecedent conditions under which they occur, and the behavioral and emotional consequences of the symptoms. The latter include any avoidance or safety behaviors that reinforce abnormal or inappropriate beliefs and any active coping strategies that are used by the patient. Interventions are then devised to assist the patient in coping with the psychotic experience and changing behavior to dispute inappropriate or delusional beliefs, especially about the content of their voices, and more accurately assess the reality of their experiences. Complex behaviors should be broken down into component parts and learned in sequence. For example, in teaching a patient to identify the onset of a hallucination and then switch his or her attention away from it, each stage would be practiced within the therapy session and augmented by self-instruction. Practical exercises would be broken down into their component parts and each part learned before practicing the whole procedure. The therapist would simulate the patient's auditory hallucinations to assist role playing of the scenario. Within the session, repetition and overlearning should be achieved, especially if the exercise will involve exposure to a frightening or threatening situation. For example, the patient who believes he is being potentially attacked and threatened in his house by a gang of Hell's Angels because he hears their voices and only saves himself from harm by shouting back at the voices, must be persuaded to relinquish this safety behavior (shouting back at the voices) which, in his mind, saves him from being attacked. Simply instructing him to do so as a homework exercise is unlikely to be successful. Practicing this exercise in session will increase the patient's confidence in dropping the safety behavior when he tries it out at home.

Fourteen studies have been conducted on the effectiveness of CBT in chronic schizophrenia patients who have drug-resistant positive psychotic symptoms. In these studies, CBT is added to TAU. The results are generally very positive, with studies consistently showing significant symptom reduction in those patients receiving CBT (plus TAU) as compared to those receiving only TAU. There is also good evidence that these benefits were clinically significant. A significantly greater proportion of patients receiving CBT achieved a 50% reduction in symptoms as compared to control patients (Tarrier et al., 1993; Tarrier, Yusupoff, Kinney, et al., 1998). In a logistic regression, Tarrier, Yusupoff, Kinney, et al. (1998) found that patients who received CBT were almost eight times more likely to achieve a 50% improvement in symptoms than those who received TAU alone.

A number of studies have attempted to compare CBT and TAU with another psychological treatment to control for the nonspecific effects of psychological treatment. This nonspecific treatment has most typically been SP and assumed to be therapeutically inactive. When the effect of therapy on positive symptoms has been examined, results from such studies have been inconsistent, with one study failing to find a significant difference between CBT and SP (Tarrier, Yusopoff, & Kinney, et al., 1998), one study showing that CBT (with TAU) was superior to SP (also with TAU) or TAU alone (Durham et al., 2003), and another study also showing superiority of CBT over SP, but only at follow-up (Sensky et al., 2000). The findings become somewhat more consistent when the effects on specific positive symptoms are explored. Tarrier et al. (2001) reported that both CBT and SP had greater effects on delusions than TAU. Whereas CBT decreased the occurrence of hallucinations, SP was found to actually increase their occurrence.

Whether treatment gains are maintained at follow-up after CBT is discontinued is an important question in schizophrenia research. Because schizophrenia is thought to be an enduring disorder, treatments must be evaluated according to their ability to aid recovery and enhance long-term coping with chronic illness. In these follow-up studies, standard psychiatric care, including medication, continues although CBT has been discontinued. Sensky et al. (2000) found that at 9-month follow-up, the CBT group continued to improve, whereas the SP group did not. Thus, over the follow-up period, there was a divergence between the two groups in favor of CBT. Kuipers et al. (1998) reported significantly maintained benefits of CBT over TAU alone at 18 months (9 months after treatment completion), but they did not include a SP control. Wiersma, Jenner, van de Willige, Sparkman, and Nienhuis (2001) reported on a naturalistic follow-up of patients suffering refractory auditory hallucinations 2–4 years after their treatment with CBT. Improvements were sustained in 60% of patients, with one-third showing further improvement after treatment was discontinued. Complete eradication of hallucinations occurred in 18% of patients. Tarrier et al.'s (1999, 2000) results did not suggest a clear benefit for CBT but, rather, showed that the addition of any psychosocial treatment (either CBT or SP) to medication and standard care was superior to medication and standard care alone 2 years after the psychological treatments had been discontinued.

Other Psychosocial Treatments

The other main nondrug interventions are family interventions (these studies are reviewed below), social skills training, and cognitive remediation. Social skills training is a structured psychosocial intervention intended to enhance social performance and reduce distress in difficult social situations. This intervention consists of "behaviorally based assessments of a range of social and interpersonal skills with importance placed on verbal and non-verbal communication, and the individual's ability to perceive and process relevant social cues, and to respond to and provide appropriate social reinforcement" (Pilling et al., 2002a, p. 784). Cognitive remediation consists of intensive training in a series of information-processing tasks with the aim of compensating for putative underlying cognitive deficits. Pilling et al. (2002a), in their meta-analysis of trials of social skills training and cognitive remediation, found that there was no clear evidence for any benefits of social skills training on relapse rates, global adjustment, social functioning, quality of life, or treatment compliance.

They also found no evidence that cognitive remediation had any benefit on attention, verbal memory, visual memory, planning, cognitive flexibility, or mental state. They concluded that "social skills training and cognitive remediation do not appear to confer reliable benefits for patients with schizophrenia and cannot be recommended for clinical practice" (p. 783).

PREDICTORS OF TREATMENT OUTCOME WITH COGNITIVE-BEHAVIORAL THERAPY

Specific Effects

A number of specific factors have been found to be predictive of outcome in patients treated with CBT. In a small trial of CBT with chronically ill patients, Tarrier et al. (1993) found that alogia (cognitive slowing) was significantly associated with poor response to CBT (Tarrier, 1996). In a later study, Tarrier, Yusupoff, Kinney, et al. (1998) reported that a shorter duration of illness and less severe symptoms were predictive of better response. Garety et al. (1997) reported that a higher number of hospital admissions in the preceding 5 years and an acknowledgement that delusional thoughts might be mistaken were significantly and independently associated with good response to CBT. Taken together, these results suggest that greater *cognitive flexibility* might be associated with good treatment response. These indicators are also suggestive that greater severity of illness is associated with poorer outcome, although it is unclear whether cognitive flexibility is independent from, or a product of, severity of illness.

General Factors

Prognostic factors have traditionally been investigated in first-episode cohort studies; that is, the tracking of a representative group of patients from the onset of their illness over a period of time. There are a number of factors that have been found to be predictive of outcome in schizophrenia. These factors, although not specific to CBT, are likely relevant regardless of treatment modality. The duration of untreated psychosis, which refers to the time from the onset of the psychosis until treatment with antipsychotic medication is initiated, has consistently been found to be associated with poorer outcome. Other factors associated with poorer outcome are male gender, earlier age at onset, poor premorbid functioning, executive dysfunction, the use of street drugs, and more negative symptoms at first presentation (Joyce et al., 2002; MacMillan, Crow, Johnson, & Johnstone, 1986).

Cultural Factors

In urban and minority populations, there is an increase in the incidence of schizophrenia (Harrison et al., 1997; Selten et al., 2001; van Os & McGuffin,

2003) and some evidence of increased medication noncompliance (Sellwood & Tarrier, 1994). However, there is a complete dearth of information on CBT for schizophrenia with culturally diverse groups. When CBT is used with diverse groups, it is essential that clinicians understand that the content of delusions can vary across patients from differing cultural, religious, and political backgrounds (Kim et al., 1993) and that family attitudes and values should also be considered (e.g., Wahass & Kent, 1997) in order to optimize treatment outcome.

Life Events

Life events or crises have been demonstrated to cluster in the period prior to illness onset and relapse (Brown & Birley, 1968; Paykel, 1976). This effect is found even when the events can be shown to be independent of the patient's behavior; that is, the patient was unlikely to have caused the event. Thus, exposure to excessive or persistent psychosocial stress is thought to have an adverse effect on the course of schizophrenia, perhaps due to the effect of stress on physiological arousal (Tarrier, Vaughn, Lader, & Leff, 1979; Tarrier & Turpin, 1992). In a CBT treatment program, therapists should be watchful for unexpected life events and stresses and should be flexible in their treatment approach to be able to deal with such eventualities. For example, coping techniques for reducing arousal (e.g., breathing techniques), enhancing self-confidence (e.g., positive self-talk), and general problem-solving skills may be useful in these circumstances.

PRACTICAL STRATEGIES FOR IMPROVING OUTCOME

A major barrier to good outcome in treatment for schizophrenia is attrition—obviously, to benefit from treatment, patients must remain in treatment and be compliant with the treatment plan. Attrition rates can be high in schizophrenia treatment trials. There are clearly practical and ethical difficulties in researching why patients do not want to take part in research, especially when consent has been withdrawn or not given; thus, understanding of this behavior is scant. Tarrier, Yusupoff, McCarthy, Kinney, and Wittkowski (1998) sent a questionnaire to patients who dropped out of a randomized controlled trial of CBT. The response rate to this questionnaire was surprisingly high, at 75%. The most common reason that patients gave for dropping out of treatment was that they believed that therapy would not be useful for their problems. Other common explanations included the belief that nothing had helped them in the past and that talking about their problems would actually make them worse. Patients who dropped out tended to be male, single, and unemployed with a low level of educational attainment and a low premorbid IQ. They had a longer duration of illness than patients who remained in treatment, although at the time of discontinuation, they were not necessarily severely ill, and they could function at a reasonable level. They suffered from both hallucinations and delusions and were likely to be quite depressed and to feel moderately hopeless. They were likely to be paranoid, although not necessarily suspicious of the therapist. Generally, they did not see the point of entering therapy or they were worried that it would make them worse, which suggested that they had not accepted or had not understood the rationale or potential benefits of treatment. It was also observed that in some cases professional staff directly responsible for their care discouraged patients from participating. To decrease attrition, clinicians should be mindful of these factors as they treat patients with schizophrenia. The clinician should consider therapeutic engagement as paramount when embarking on CBT with a patient with schizophrenia. Effort is required to build a therapeutic alliance, and this should involve getting to know the person and his or her goals and interests. This type of personal contact is very important for the patient with schizophrenia, and the clinician should be cautious about commencing with particular therapeutic techniques too quickly and before good engagement has been achieved. Furthermore, there is evidence that the absence of a positive relationship between the clinician and patient with schizophrenia at the beginning of treatment is related to poorer outcome 9 months later (Tattan & Tarrier, 2000).

Typical Obstacles in Pharmacotherapy and Strategies for Overcoming Them

CBT is rarely used in the treatment of schizophrenia without the concurrent use of antipsychotic medication. A major obstacle to pharmacotherapy for schizophrenia is the high incidence of side effects, including sedation, dry mouth, blurred vision, constipation, impotence, dizziness from lowered blood pressure, subjective restlessness (akathisia), involuntary movements of the mouth and face (tardive dyskinesia), and movement disorders resembling Parkinson's Disease (expressionless face, shuffling gait, paucity of movement, and tremor) (American Psychiatric Association, 1992; Grebb, 1995; Kinon & Lieberman, 1996). Physicians have tried to decrease side effects by prescribing antipsychotics at lower doses. This strategy gained support from a meta-analysis examining efficacy and side effect data from drug trials in which antipsychotics were prescribed at either high or low doses (Bollini, Pampallona, Orza, Adams, & Chambers, 1994). The data from these studies suggested that at doses higher than 375 mg of chlorpromazine equivalents, antipsychotics did not yield greater clinical improvement but did lead to significant increases in adverse reactions.

Another concern pertaining to side effects is the issue of medication compliance (Kane, 1983). Patients stop taking medications because side effects are uncomfortable or embarrassing. As a means of increasing compliance, drugs are often administered through regular depot injections with slow release of the medication over a period of weeks or months.

Typical Obstacles in Assessment and Treatment Planning and Strategies for Overcoming Them

Outcome of CBT for schizophrenia will likely be significantly improved if the treatment plan is firmly based on an individualized case formulation or behavioral assessment of the patient's clinical problems. By individualizing the treatment protocol, it is more likely that patients will be engaged with therapy and will be compliant with it. Furthermore, any individualized treatment plan will better accommodate the complex interactions between psychosis, the individual response to illness, and the environmental context (including family and social interactions).

Before devising a treatment plan, it is essential that a careful assessment is completed that covers different types of symptoms, including positive symptoms, negative symptoms, thought disorder, and affective symptoms (see Barnes & Nelson, 1994, for a review of methods for accomplishing these assessment goals). More recently, methods of assessing the multidimensional nature of hallucinations and delusions have been devised, both to understand in more detail the nature of this psychopathology and also to investigate the mechanisms by which psychological treatments have their effects (e.g., Haddock et al., 1999). A detailed assessment of the patient's psychotic symptoms aids the therapist in understanding the patient's experience and in formulating the cognitive-behavioral intervention. Tarrier (1992, 2002) developed a semi-structured interview schedule, the Antecedent and Coping Interview (ACI), based on a psychiatric interview to elicit psychotic symptoms and a behavioral assessment of antecedents and consequences. The ACI was designed to elicit information about psychotic symptoms, their variability under different conditions, and how the patient coped with these experiences. The information derived from this interview describes the configuration and fluctuation in psychotic symptoms and informs intervention by means of enhancing coping skills.

Following a complete evaluation, it is important for clinicians to generate a case formulation (Chadwick & Lowe, 1990; Chadwick et al., 2003; Tarrier, 2002; Tarrier & Calam, 2002), which has been defined as "a hypothesis about the causes, precipitants and maintaining influences of patients' psychological, interpersonal and behavioral problems" (Eels, 1997, p. 1). The case formulation provides a psychological understanding of the patient's clinical problems that will inform treatment or intervention by identifying key targets for change, making it "a central process in the role of the scientific practitioner" (Tarrier & Calam, 2002, p. 311). Some patients may be too distressed or agitated for a comprehensive assessment to be carried out. In these cases, a pragmatic approach to reducing symptoms in the absence of a thorough assessment has to be adopted, although this situation is not optimal.

In conventional psychiatry, psychotic disorders have been thought, erroneously, to be beyond rational explanation. From a CBT viewpoint, a psychological understanding is both possible and necessary for effective treatment.

Thus, a detailed cognitive-behavioral case formulation is important to understand the variability in the patient's symptoms and the meaning attributed to them. Without this understanding, the therapist will be unable to adequately challenge the patient's explanations of events and experience and set up behavioral experiments to test hypotheses. Case formulation allows the therapist and patient to arrive at a shared understanding of the patient's problems, promotes the collaborative approach typically taken in CBT, and enhances engagement. Tarrier and Calam (2002) have advanced three modifications to traditional case formulation that may further improve this process. These modifications are (1) the conceptualization of dysfunctional systems (i.e., a self-maintaining cycle of dysfunctional cognitions, behaviors, and affect in the maintenance of clinical problems); (2) attention to the epidemiological evidence that indicates vulnerabilities underlying the clinical problems; and (3) accommodation for the interpersonal environment of patients and their reactions to key others in this environment within the formulation of the clinical problem.

Matching the Intervention to the Phase of the Disorder

As mentioned earlier, the nature of any CBT intervention and its aims will vary depending on the phase of the disorder. In the residual chronic phase, when symptoms are not responding further to medication, the aim is symptom reduction. In the acute phase, the aim is to speed symptom resolution in tandem with medication. In the remission phase, the aim is to prevent subsequent relapse or deterioration, whereas in the prodromal phase, the aim will be to abort relapse. Table 9.2 outlines these differing options and treatment aims.

Associated Features and Disability

Another way to improve outcome in CBT for schizophrenia is to attend not only to the symptoms of the disorder but also to associated features and com-

TABLE 9.2. Treatment Aims and Methods in Different Phases of the Schizophrenic Illness

Phase	Aim	Treatment method
Preillness prodrome	Prevention of translation into full psychosis	CBT for early signs and prevention of symptom escalation
Acute episode	Speed recovery	CBT and coping training
Partially remitted residual symptoms	Symptom reduction	CBT, coping training, self-esteem enhancement
Remission	Relapse prevention	CBT for staying well and family intervention
Relapse prodrome	Abort relapse	Early signs identification and relapse prevention

plicating factors. These vary from the effects of the disorder on basic psychological processes, such as attention, to clinical issues, such as suicide risk, to social issues such as social deprivation and poor employment opportunities. Table 9.3 outlines these associated features.

The crucial point is that the clinician is aware that these problems can arise. Some of them can be dealt with by keeping the message simple and brief but with plenty of repetition (i.e., using overlearning in the teaching of coping strategies). Writing down simple points for the patient as a memory aid can also be helpful, as can creating a small "workbook" so that the patient has a continuous record of these points. This is usually more effective than providing handouts that are rarely read and frequently lost. It is important to titrate the nature and duration of sessions against the patient's level of tolerance. Initially, it might be best to keep sessions brief or to allow the patient to leave when he or she has had enough. The one-to-one nature of therapy will be highly stressful, so initial sessions may serve merely to provide habituation to

TABLE 9.3. Features to Be Assessed and Considered as Potential Difficulties in the Psychological Treatment of Schizophrenia

Psychological

- Disrupted or slowed thought processes
- Difficulty discriminating signal from noise
- Restricted attention
- Hypersensitivity to social interactions
- Difficulty in processing social signals
- Flat and restricted affect
- Elevated arousal and dysfunctional arousal regulation
- Hypersensitivity to stress and life events
- High risk of depression and hopelessness
- Stigmatization
- Low self-esteem and self-worth
- High risk of substance and alcohol abuse
- High risk of suicide and self-harm
- Interference of normal adolescent and early adult development due to onset of illness

Psychosocial

- Hypersensitivity to family and interpersonal environment (including that created by professional staff)
- Risk of perpetrating, or being the victim of, violence

Social

- Conditions of social deprivation
- Poor housing
- Downward social drift
- Unemployment and difficulty in competing in the job market
- Restricted social network
- Psychiatric career interfering with utilization of other social resources

the social stress of being with the clinician. Teaching the patient simple strategies to deal with tension and anxiety (such as brief relaxation) may be helpful in habituating to the therapy situation and will also provide a concrete task on which to focus attention. Simple attention-focusing tasks, such as focusing on some item in the room for a short period, may be helpful in reducing the effect of irrelevant stimuli on the patient's conscious awareness. It is also important to recognize that the verbal and nonverbal cues that the therapist might expect to indicate severe distress, depression, or suicidality may not be expressed in someone with schizophrenia. Affect may be flat or inappropriate, which could result in the therapist missing important danger signals. This can be avoided, in part, by knowing the person and how he or she reacts, by never making assumptions about mental state, and by agreeing from the outset that the patient will inform the therapist of important changes in his or her life or mood. Unfortunately, there are often some issues, such as social conditions, which are beyond the therapist's power to change. However, there is nothing wrong in assuming an advocacy role or in helping patients to empower themselves by aiding their attempts to improve their own circumstances. Last, it is important that therapists adopt a noncritical approach and learn to accommodate their own frustrations if therapy is progressing more slowly than was hoped. There are aspects of schizophrenia that can make some patients difficult to deal with and the therapist needs to be aware of this and develop a tolerant approach.

The Procedure of Cognitive-Behavioral Therapy

When CBT gets under way, the first objective should be to engage the patient. Patients suffering from schizophrenia, especially those with paranoid or persecutory delusions, can be extremely difficult to engage. The therapist should initially develop a relationship with the patient and verify that the relationship is secure before commencing assessment and therapy. This can be achieved by acknowledging that therapy may be difficult for the patient especially with someone they do not know well. Patients should also be encouraged to raise any problems or insecurities that they may have at any time. This can be included as an agenda item at the beginning of each session. To embark on too detailed an assessment or on treatment strategies before the patient has understood and accepted the rationale risks the patient disengaging if the process seems too intrusive or irrelevant to his or her concerns.

The therapeutic relationship is important, and data from the SoCRATES trial showed that patients' perception of the therapeutic alliance was significantly associated with outcome 18 months later (Bentall et al., 2003). The therapeutic relationship will form a basis on which to establish collaborative treatment goals and strategy. As has been suggested earlier, if the therapist shows an interest in the patient as a person, they are more likely to develop a positive relationship.

Location of Therapy

In some cases, the location of therapy will be determined by other treatment factors, such as whether the patient is receiving inpatient care. When the patient is based within the community, there is potential choice of whether CBT is provided at a hospital, at another health care facility, or in the patient's own home. Practices differ within different countries and health services. In the United Kingdom, where home treatment is common practice, it has been the author's practice to give the patient the choice of where to be seen. This can be at a hospital outpatient clinic, within a community mental health center, or at home. Giving the patient the choice is likely to improve adherence. A distinct advantage of having sessions in a health care setting is that appointments can be combined to address patients' needs. For example, a CBT appointment can be combined with an appointment at the medication clinic. This combined approach might facilitate treatment adherence.

Home visits have numerous advantages as well. Home treatment allows for observation of patients in their own environment and acquisition of coping skills within the environment in which they need to be implemented. Furthermore, home visits allow for increased collaboration with other family members. When appropriate, family members can be informed of the treatment approach and encouraged to facilitate CBT, although issues of confidentiality and consent will need to be addressed. For example, family members can encourage the use of coping strategies, help with rationalizing psychotic experiences through behavioral experiments and reality testing, and provide assistance in a graded practice program by accompanying patients on trips out.

While home visits have numerous advantages, they can be associated with various complications that should be dealt with in order to facilitate good outcome. Therapy sessions might be disturbed by other residents or ambient noise. Requesting that the television is turned off, or at least the volume turned down, is often a prerequisite to therapy. The provision of a quiet and private location for therapy within the household should be the goal.

If embarking on home visits, the therapist should be aware of issues of his or her own personal security. There may be risks from patients themselves, their family or other residents, or the neighborhood in which the patient resides. This can be especially true if the patient is a drug user and has contact with drug dealers or gangs or lives in a neighborhood where drug dealers or gangs are active. There are commonsense precautions that therapists can adopt, and, ideally, there will be security policies and procedures operational within the department in which they work. These policies should include a risk assessment, including the opinion of someone who knows the patient and his or her circumstances well prior to the visit, and a well-learned emergency procedure should a situation become problematic. It can sometimes be advisable for therapists to attend home sessions with a co-therapist, especially where the risks may be elevated or unknown.

Homework

Setting homework tasks is a basic procedure of traditional CBT; however, problems with the assignment and completion of homework tasks regularly occur (Helbig & Fehm, 2004). Similarly, patients suffering from schizophrenia are frequently poor at carrying out homework exercises, including record-keeping and other therapeutic activities. Although some patients are very good at completing homework exercises, homework compliance should not be assumed.

Typical Obstacles in Challenging Delusions and Strategies for Overcoming Them

In some patients, even when receiving medication, delusions can be so severe and intractable that the patient will not tolerate any investigation of their veracity. For example, patients may be so convinced that their beliefs of persecution are true that any suggestion to the contrary will only elicit hostility. Because maintaining engagement is the key factor in successful CBT, it is necessary to find some common ground with which to work. It is possible to suggest to the patient that the delusional thoughts result in considerable distress and that the goal of therapy will be to reduce this distress rather than challenging the delusion itself. Most patients, however disturbed, will agree to this.

Either directly challenging or colluding with delusions is to be avoided in these cases. The validity of the patient's experience should be accepted at all times. Take, for example, a patient who believes with great certainty that her neighbors are part of a government plot against her and are poisoning her water supply. Clearly, such beliefs would cause the patient to feel very distressed. A patient like this can get very upset if the therapist suggests that she is experiencing olfactory and gustatory hallucinations and delusions of persecution. A better strategy is to label the extreme distress experienced as a result of these psychotic experiences as the problem and to engage the patient in a collaborative endeavor to reduce distress. This approach would be less likely to compromise engagement. Furthermore, high levels of arousal accompanying distress can actually maintain symptoms. Reducing distress may also reduce the strength of the experience, allowing the therapist and patient to more directly address the delusion.

If the patient becomes very upset or agitated, it is best to acknowledge this, to terminate the session, and to arrange a later one. Sometimes, auditory hallucinations will instruct patients not to speak to the therapist or to behave in a certain manner. This can be detected by inappropriate behavior, strange twists in the conversation, or behavior that suggests patients are listening to their voices. This can be directly addressed, although the therapist should be aware that on occasion, the voices will threaten some dire consequences if the patient does not obey them. Disjointed interactions can also be the sign of thought disorder and the therapist will need to distinguish this from command hallucinations.

Typical Obstacles in Challenging Thought Disorder and Strategies for Overcoming Them

Thought disorder, typically characterized by disruption to language, makes it difficult to comprehend the meaning that the patient is imparting. However, with experience and patience, it is often possible to follow some internal logic in the patient's speech. This can be accomplished by asking the patient to explain the meaning, by reflecting back the therapist's understanding, and then rephrasing in more coherent language. Progressing through these organized steps in a calm manner can help prevent the patient from feeling overloaded with the emotional content of the discussion, which can happen especially when the material being discussed is emotionally salient (Haddock, Wolfenden, Lowens, Tarrier, & Bentall, 1995).

Modification of Cognitive Content or Cognitive Process

Therapists frequently face the choice of whether to try to modify the content of hallucinations or delusions or the attentional processes that these phenomena have captured. In practice, these tactics can work together. Initial modification of attentional processes through attention switching, for example, can decrease the emotional impact of the experience. A similar effect can be produced by attending to the physical characteristics of a hallucination rather than what the voice actually said. This can provide not only an opening to challenge the truth of the content of the voice or delusional thought but also a sense of control over these experiences. Take, for example, a young man who is experiencing voices that accuse him of having committed a murder and that also say he is Russian. Initially, he can be taught to turn his attention away from the voices in a systematic way to reduce their emotional impact. This technique can be used to elicit a sense of control and to challenge the belief that the voices are all-powerful. With increased self-efficacy and a greater sense of power, the patient can later challenge the content of the voices that accuse him of murder by investigating the objective evidence that a murder has been committed. Furthermore, the untruthfulness of the voices in saying he is Russian can be used to challenge the veracity of the murder accusation; the voices had been wrong about one issue so they could be wrong about the other. Modification of cognitive process and content provides the therapist with two basic routes to intervention and the flexibility to move from one tactic to the other.

Intractable Psychotic Symptoms

Regrettably, there will be cases in which the therapist's best efforts and optimum medication produce little improvement in the patient's symptoms. There are a number of options available in such intractable cases. First, it is necessary to ensure that appropriate support services are in place so that the patient's quality of life is maximized. There should also be regular reviews of treatment, especially of medication and of environmental circumstances, so that excessive stresses are avoided. Finally, it is always worth continuing with a few simple and direct cognitive-behavioral strategies because, over a long period of time, they may begin to have an effect.

Risk of Suicide and Self-Harm

The risk of suicide in patients suffering from schizophrenia is significant. It is estimated that 1 in 10 patients suffering from schizophrenia will successfully kill him- or herself (Caldwell & Gottesman, 1990). Risk factors in patients with schizophrenia include being young and male, chronic illness with numerous exacerbations, high levels of symptomatology and functional impairment, feelings of hopelessness in association with depression, fear of further mental deterioration, and excessive dependence on treatment or loss of faith in treatment (Caldwell & Gottesman, 1990). Tarrier, Barrowclough, Andrews, and Gregg (2004) carried out a path analysis of precursors to suicide risk and found that illness duration independently increased risk. Two other paths to suicide risk, both of which were mediated by hopelessness, were also identified: (1) increased social isolation, to which longer illness duration, more positive symptoms, older age, and being unemployed contributed; and (2) greater negative views of the self, higher frequency of criticism from relatives and more negative symptoms, to which being male, unmarried, and unemployed significantly contributed.

It is important to be aware that suicide attempts are a very real possibility while treating someone suffering from schizophrenia. Unfortunately, patients with schizophrenia often commit suicide impulsively and use lethal methods, such as jumping from heights, immolation, or firearms. The presence of suicidal ideation needs to be assessed and the patient needs to be asked whether any specific plans have been made or actions have been taken. It is necessary to be aware of factors that can elevate risk, including erosion of self-esteem; increased sense of hopelessness and despair especially related to the perception of the patient's illness and recovery; disruptive family or social relationships, and any changes in social circumstances or loss of supportive relationships (e.g., changes in mental health staff or staff holidays or leave). Furthermore, the occurrence of life events, loss or shameful experiences can lead to despondency.

Some factors that can increase risk for suicide are quite unique to the psychotic disorders, such as the experience of command hallucinations. I had a patient who experienced strange physical sensations that he interpreted as the Queen entering his body. As a loyal subject, he thought he should vacate his body to give her sole possession, and he attempted to kill himself by slashing his wrists. This was not the result of a will to die but more driven by some sense of social protocol toward royalty. Fortunately, the attempt was unsuccessful.

Many therapists hypothesize that psychotic symptoms have a protective aspect in masking the harsh realities of the burden of serious mental illness. Improvement in insight and symptomatology can bring with it an increased exposure to this burden and may thus increase the probability of potential escape through suicide. The therapist needs to be aware of all these factors, to know his or her patients well, and to monitor changes in their circumstances or mood that may be problematic. It is important to be aware of predictable changes and plan for them, to establish good communication with other mental health workers, and to address low mood and hopelessness in an open manner. Assessing acute suicide risk is further complicated by patients' flat or incongruous affect, so that the cues that a therapist would look for in a depressed patient may not be exhibited by a patient with schizophrenia. When risk is high, emergency psychiatric services should be called on.

Cognitive-Behavioral Therapy within a Multiagency Mental Health Service

Patients suffering from severe mental illnesses such as schizophrenia usually have access to a range of resources provided by mental health services, and it is generally recognized that psychiatric care should consist of a multifaceted program delivered by different agencies. There is ample evidence indicating that inactivity and neglect have an adverse effect on schizophrenia (e.g., Wing & Brown, 1970). Comprehensive services usually include access to hospital beds and inpatient treatment when necessary or intensive community crisis treatment, day hospital facilities, vocational and occupational activity, medical review, and monitoring within the community, such as assertive outreach from a community mental health team. This would be coordinated through some model of case management. Services would also provide advocacy and crisis intervention. CBT should be delivered as part of a holistic response of the mental health service. It may be that the CBT therapist takes on some aspects of the role of a key worker or advocate or accepts the task of reengaging the patient with mental health services.

The integration of CBT treatment into multiagency services can bring with it a number of logistic and professional problems. The CBT model of treatment may be in conflict with models held by other disciplines or staff members, leading to difficulties in implementation. Unfortunately, these difficulties reflect the realities of multidisciplinary work and need to be addressed and managed. Some of the problems and solutions to introducing psychological treatments into mental health services are covered by Barrowclough and Tarrier (1992). These include the following:

- Do preparatory groundwork, eliciting management support for evidence-based treatments and identifying "product champions" and "opinion setters" in parts of the organization that are the most amenable to introducing the new treatment approach.

- Provide staff training and ongoing supervision to other interested professional staff.
- Ensure that management provides adequate time and resources for the new treatment to be implemented and for staff training and supervision.
- Elicit support from service users and patients to help the new treatment approach become established. Obtain and publicize testaments from past patients who have received the treatment and have been satisfied with it.
- Maintain good public relations within the organization.
- Consider establishing a special CBT service.

Organizational management methods such as these are most likely to ensure that CBT becomes established and delivered to those patients who need it.

Dual Diagnosis: Comorbidity of Alcohol and Substance Use

Comorbid substance use disorders are an escalating problem in patients with schizophrenia. Lehman and Dixon (1995) estimated that comorbid substance use may be present in 60% of patients with schizophrenia. Others believe this to be an underestimate, particularly as the prevalence of substance use among patients with schizophrenia seems to be increasing (Bellack, personal communication, September 2001). Dual-diagnosis patients tend to do worse than patients with schizophrenia alone on a range of outcomes. They tend to be more persistently symptomatic, tend to suffer more frequent and earlier relapse and readmission, are more likely to present to the emergency services, have higher levels of aggression and violence, and are at greater risk of suicide and self-harm (Drake, Osher, & Wallach, 1989; Menezes et al., 1996). In addition, the economic and service burden of dual diagnosis is high. Mental health staff often feel they are unable to cope with the complex needs of these patients and frequently feel unsympathetic toward psychotic patients who use drugs and alcohol contrary to advice (Haddock, Barrowclough, Moring, Tarrier, & Lewis, 2002).

Motivational interviewing has been effectively used to enhance motivation to change substance use behavior in nonpsychotic patients (Miller & Rollnick, 2002), and has been included in an integrated treatment approach in dual-diagnosis patients (Barrowclough et al., 2001; Haddock et al., 2002). Motivational interviewing has been termed a "style" rather than a specific intervention and can be incorporated into a CBT approach in order to increase the patient's motivation to change substance or alcohol use behavior while concurrently addressing the psychosis. It is postulated that there is an important interaction between alcohol or substance use and psychotic symptoms that requires this dual treatment approach. Many patients do not consider their alcohol or substance use a problem and perceive the positive benefits, such as self-medication, peer identification, or enjoyment as outweighing any negative consequences. The aim during the initial sessions is to elicit change or motivational statements from the patient. The therapist uses the motivational interviewing skills of reflective listening, acceptance, and selective reinforcement to elicit such statements. Once the patient identifies substance or alcohol use as a problem and expresses a desire to change, therapy can then progress to practical ways to achieve this goal (see Haddock et al., 2002, for further details).

PREDICTORS OF RELAPSE AND RECURRENCE

The Quality of Interpersonal Relationships and the Home Environment

The distress and burden associated with caring for a mentally ill relative is very high (Schene, Tessler, & Gamache, 1994). Between 29% and 60% of relatives who informally care for relatives with mental illness suffer from significant psychological distress (Barrowclough & Parle, 1997; Birchwood & Cochrane, 1990: McGilloway, Donnelly, & Mays, 1997; Oldridge & Hughers, 1992). The stress of caring for an ill relative can compromise the well-being of the caregiver in many ways (career, other relationships, etc.) and can also have an impact on the course of the illness itself and on the clinical outcome of the patient.

Since the 1960s, research on *expressed emotion* (EE) has demonstrated the importance of the interpersonal environment on the course and outcome of schizophrenia. Families can be classified as either high or low on EE based on the number of critical comments, presence of hostility, and marked emotional overinvolvement (EOI) that occurs during a semistructured interview with the patient's key relative(s) (Leff & Vaughn, 1985). Numerous studies from different countries and cultures have consistently demonstrated that returning to live with a high EE relative after an acute episode is associated with poorer medication compliance (Sellwood, Tarrier, Quinn, & Barrowclough, 2003) and higher rates of relapse (Butzlaff & Hooley, 1998; Kavanagh, 1992; Wearden, Tarrier, Barrowclough, Zastowny, & Rahill, 2000). Interestingly, psychophysiological studies have indicated that the presence of a high-EE relative elevates or maintains high levels of autonomic arousal in the patient, whereas the presence of a low-EE relative appears to be associated with a reduction in arousal (Tarrier & Turpin, 1992).

Further research has suggested that relatives' attributional beliefs were actually more predictive of subsequent relapse than EE (Barrowclough, Johnston, & Tarrier, 1994). High-EE relatives are more likely than low-EE relatives to believe that patients have the potential to control aspects of their illness and behavior (Barrowclough & Hooley, 2003; Hooley, 1985, 1987). These relatives make more attributions to factors internal and personal to, and controllable by, the patient than do low-EE relatives (Barrowclough et al., 1994; Brewin, MacCarthy, Duda, & Vaughn, 1991; Weisman, Nuechterlein, Goldstein, & Snyder, 1998). Barrowclough et al. (1994) suggested that relatives' beliefs may influence patients' methods of coping, and these may be an important focus of intervention.

Self-Esteem

Negative attitudes and beliefs about self-worth are common in those suffering from mental health problems (Silverstone, 1991). Living with critical and hostile family members has been shown to decrease feelings of self-worth and to lead to increased positive schizophrenic symptoms (Barrowclough et al., 2003). Self-esteem may also be depressed by factors outside the immediate home environment, such as poor-quality social relationships, inference arising from poor social comparisons, and the general stigma of severe mental illness. Negative self-esteem is implicated in pathways to elevated suicide risk because it is a precursor to hopelessness (Tarrier et al., 2004).

Nonadherence with Antipsychotic Medication

Deterioration and relapse are associated with poor adherence to maintenance antipsychotic medication (Buchanan, 1996). Although this most often results in symptom exacerbation and loss of treatment gains, not all patients experience these adverse effects. Morrison (1994) described a patient successfully treated with CBT who had previously discontinued antipsychotic medication because of its unpleasant side effects. CBT decreased symptomatology, and these gains were maintained at 3-month follow-up in spite of the absence of antipsychotic medication. Nevertheless, it is important to note that the majority of patients will benefit from strict adherence to maintenance medication, and that nonadherence can have potentially detrimental consequences.

PRACTICAL STRATEGIES FOR PREVENTION OF RELAPSE AND RECURRENCE

Increasing Medication Adherence

Many patients do not adhere to their medication or adhere in a suboptimal way. There is evidence that poor adherence is influenced by the beliefs of patients about their illness and their relationship with their doctor (Buchanan, 1996). Recently, a therapeutic approach termed "compliance therapy" based on motivational interviewing has been shown to improve adherence to medication (Kemp, Kirov, Everitt, Hayward, & David, 1996) while avoiding the confrontation and stalemate of many doctor–patient interactions (Tarrier & Bobes, 2000). This method is consistent with the ethos of CBT and can be integrated with it in a strategic approach as it allows the patient to explore the costs and benefits of medication and encourages guided problem solving.

Although there is a subpopulation of patients suffering from psychotic illnesses who appear to function well without medication, the majority greatly increase their risk of relapse without it. Ideally, pharmacological and psychological treatments would be integrated with the type and dose of medication being adjusted as psychological management progresses. In some patients, especially young patients with recent onset of illness, the use of medication only when symptoms emerge (termed "targeted medication") may be a feasible goal rather than continuous medication. Unfortunately, research is currently lacking to provide detailed guidance on this question.

Family Interventions

The impetus for the development of family interventions to reduce relapse in schizophrenia came from the research on EE and its association with poor outcome. These interventions vary from the behavioral (e.g., Falloon et al., 1985) and cognitive-behavioral (Barrowclough & Tarrier, 1992) to the more eclectic (e.g., Leff, Kuipers, Berkowitz, Eberlein-Vries, & Sturgeon, 1982). There is considerable evidence that family interventions have a preventive effect on relapse and readmission (Pilling et al., 2002b; Pitschel-Walz, Leucht, Bauml, Kissling, & Engel, 2001; Tarrier & Bobes, 2000). Table 9.4 summarizes the results of family intervention studies.

As with all adjunct psychological and psychosocial treatments, family interventions are provided in addition to standard treatment or TAU. Family interventions can be delivered to individual families or in group format. While group formats are effective, individual family intervention results in greater reduction of relapse and better compliance (Pilling et al., 2002b). Significant benefits in terms of reduction in relapse and rehospitalization have been reported in the first 12 and 24 months after admission (Pilling et al., 2002b), with one study reporting significantly lower relapse rates in the treated group after 5 and 8 years compared to those receiving standard care (Tarrier, Barrowclough, Porceddu, & Fitzpatrick, 1994). Support for the effectiveness of family intervention has also been shown when it is provided by mental health service staff under supervision (Barrowclough et al., 1999; Sellwood et al., 2001).

Cognitive-behavioral family intervention consists of three main elements: education, stress management with family members, and goal planning (Barrowclough & Tarrier, 1992). The aim of education is to provide relatives with the information they require to manage and cope with the illness in a member of their family. Education aims to promote positive behavior from relatives by helping them to see the connection between their beliefs about the illness and how they act and behave toward the patient (Barrowclough et al., 1987).

The second element of the intervention aims to identify stress in the lives of family members. The stress may be the patient's illness but can also emanate from other sources. Relatives are then taught appropriate ways to manage stress. A stress inoculation session is included during which relatives prepare to deal with stress arising from a future relapse. Emphasis is placed on the idea that relatives will be much more effective in assisting the patient if they are calm and relaxed themselves and less prone to stress and irritability.

TABLE 9.4. Controlled Studies Comparing Family Intervention with Standard Treatment for Patients with Schizophrenia

Studies	Treatment conditions	N	Type of family intervention	Frequency and duration of treatment	Relapse
Goldstein, Rodnick, Evans, May, and Steinberg (1978)	Moderate dose of fluphenazine decanoate plus FI Moderate fluphenazine dose plus TAU Low fluphenazine dose FI Low fluphenazine does plus TAU	25 28 27 24	Crisis-oriented psychoeducation	6 weekly sessions	6 months: moderate doses plus FI were better than moderate doses without FI; low dose conditions were equal and inferior to the moderate-dose conditions.
Kottgen, Sonnichsen, Mollenhauer, and Jurth (1984)	FI, high EE TAU, high EE TAU, low EE	15 14 20	Psychodynamic; separate groups for patients and relatives	Weekly or monthly up to 2 years	2 years: FI equal to TAU for families with either high or low EE.
Falloon et al. (1982) Falloon et al. (1985)	Behavioral FI Individual management	18 18	Home-based behavioral FI	Weekly for 3 months, biweekly for 6 months, monthly for 15 months	2 years: behavioral FI better than individual management.
Leff, Kuipers, Berkowitz, Eberlein-Vries, and Sturgeon (1982) Leff, Kuipers, Berkowitz, and Sturgeon (1985)	FI TAU	12 12	Psychoeducation to help relatives with high EE model coping of low-EE relatives	Biweekly for relatives' groups for 9 months	2 years: FI better than TAU.
Glick et al. (1985) Glick et al. (1990)	FI TAU	37 55	Crisis-oriented psychoeducation	Average of 8.6 sessions over 5-week inpatient stay	18 months: for women, more improvements in FI group with poor premorbid functioning than in all others; for men, conditions equal.
Tarrier et al. (1988) Tarrier et al. (1989) Tarrier, Barrowclough, Proceddu, and Fitzpatrick (1994)	Behavioral FI, enactive Behavioral FI, symbolic Education only TAU	16 16 25 20	Behavioral FI comprising stress management plus training in goal setting	3 stress-management and 8 goal-setting sessions over 9 months	2 years: behavioural FI better than education or TAU; education and TAU equal. 5–8 years: behavioral FI maintains significant difference.
Vaughn et al. (1992)	Single-family psychoeducation and support TAU	18 18	Psychoeducation	10 weekly sessions	9 months: single-family education and support equal to TAU. (continued)

TABLE 9.4. (*continued*)

Studies	Treatment conditions	N	Type of family intervention	Frequency and duration of treatment	Relapse
Zhang, Hequin, Chengde, and Wang (1993)	Multiple-family psychoeducation and support TAU	2,076 1,016	Clinic-based lectures and discussions	10 lectures and 3 discussion groups over 12 months	1 year: multiple-family education and support better than TAU.
Randolph et al. (1994)	Behavioral FI TAU	21 18	Clinic-based behavioral FI	Weekly for 3 months; biweekly for 3 months, monthly for 6 months	2 years: behavioral FI better than TAU.
Xiong et al. (1994)	Behavioral FI TAU	34 29	Clinic-based psychoeducation, skills training, medication/ symptom management	Bi-monthly for 3 months; family sessions for 2 years (plus individual sessions with family members and patients); maintenance sessions every 2–3 months	18 months: behavioral FI better than TAU.
Zhang, Wang, Li, and Phillips (1994)	Multiple- and single-family psychoeducation and support TAU	39 39	Multiple-family clinic-based psychoeducation, counseling, medication/symptom management	Individual and group counseling sessions every 1–3 months for 18 months	18 months: family education and support better than TAU.
Telles et al. (1995)	Behavioral family management Individual case management	Total $N = 42$; N for individual conditions not listed	Clinic-based behavioral family management	Weekly for 6 months, every 2 weeks for 3 months, monthly for 3 months	12 months: for total group, condition equal; for "poorly acculturate" patients, individual management better; for "highly acculturated" patients, conditions equal.
Leff et al. (1990)	Multiple-family psychoeducation and support Single-family psychoeducation and support	11 12	Multiple-family groups in the clinic; single-family sessions at home	Biweekly for 9 months; varying amounts afterward	2 years: conditions equal.

Study	Conditions	N	Intervention	Schedule	Results
Zastowny, Lehman, Cole, and Kane (1992)	Behavioral FI Single-family psychoeducation and support	13 17	Hospital-based behavioral FI; hospital-based single-family psychoeducation and advice on handling common problems	Weekly for 4 months, monthly for 12 months	16 months: conditions equal.
McFarlane et al. (1995)	Multiple-family psychoeducation and support Single-family psychoeducation and support	83 89	Multiple-family groups or single-family session in the clinic	Bi-weekly sessions for 2 years	2 years: multiple-family condition better than single-family condition.
Schooler et al. (1997)	Applied family management Supportive family management	157 156	Applied family management, comprising home-based behavioral FI sessions plus supportive family management; supportive family management comprising clinic-based multiple-family groups	Applied family management: behavioral FI weekly for 3 months, bi-weekly for 6 months, and monthly for 3–6 months plus concurrent monthly supportive family management for 24–28 months; supportive family management: monthly for 24–28 months	2 years: conditions equal.
Barrowclough et al. (1999)	Needs-based behavioral FI TAU and family support	77	Individual family sessions delivered by specialist and key workers	Depending on needs assessment, 10–20 sessions over 6 months	12 months: behavioral FI better.
Barrowclough et al. (2001)	CBT plus FI plus MI plus family support TAU plus family support	36	Individual family management, individual CBT + motivational interviewing	MI: 5 sessions; CBT: 24 sessions weekly, then fortnightly; FI: 10–16 sessions	Significant improvement in positive symptoms and functioning, reduced relapse and decreased substance abuse in CBT and FI group.

Note. FI, family intervention; TAU, treatment as usual; EE, expressed emotion; CBT, cognitive-behavioral therapy; MI, motivational interviewing.

The final element in the intervention is goal planning. In this phase, relatives and patients identify what they wish to change in their lives. These changes are then translated into feasible goals, and methods for achieving these goals are then planned. These procedures are carried out within family sessions, and the actions required from different family members are operationalized. Specific attention is placed on the alleviation of high EE behavior and attitudes exhibited by the relatives. For example, relatives are taught to praise the patient for success rather than criticize him or her for failure. Overinvolved relatives are instructed to do less for the patient so he or she can become more independent. It is anticipated that increased activity and independence on the part of the patient will elicit less criticism and hostility from the relatives, while also being more positive and reinforcing for the patient.

The therapist must be alert to a number of potential problems when working with the families of patients who have schizophrenia. First, it is important that relatives accept that there are some situations that they can do very little to change. In these situations they are better advised to manage their reactions rather than continually trying to change the situation. Second, as relatives become more aware of their own reactions and become less critical, there is a risk that they will become overinvolved and overprotective. They may also feel guilty for having been critical in the past. It is useful to forewarn them that this is a common reaction and that they were attempting to cope with a difficult situation as best they could at the time. Relatives can set goals to reduce any overprotective or overinvolved behavior and encourage independent behavior in the patient. Last, there are relatives who are very difficult to engage or who wish to maintain the situation as it is. Behavioral analysis can be used to understand which factors will increase or decrease the probability that families will adhere to the treatment plan (see Barrowclough & Tarrier, 1992). The three major factors that can affect adherence are characteristics of the relative, characteristics of the treatment, and characteristics of the interaction between the family and mental health services.

In terms of family characteristics, poor outcome is predicted by older age, poor physical health, competing demands and lack of resources, a lack of understanding about the illness or inappropriate health beliefs, apathy and pessimism, residential instability, dispositional characteristics, dissatisfaction with the therapist or the treatment approach, and inappropriate expectations and attitudes toward treatment. Important characteristics of the treatment include how much it contrasts with the relatives' current behavior. The relative will have more difficulty changing their behavior if it has become entrenched over time or if it differs greatly from the target behavior. Furthermore, the more intrusive and complex the intervention program, the lower the adherence, with adherence also showing a decrease over time. In family interventions it is important that adherence is maintained over time and behavior change is sustained. Adherence is usually improved if the family is recruited during an acute crisis when they are amenable to advice and assistance. Adherence is less likely if recruitment occurs during a chronic and stable period when an attitude of "nothing can be done" has developed. Relatives who are subject to disruptive or aggressive behavior from the patient may not be inclined to seek help through fear of making the situation worse. Relatives may also be difficult to engage if they are very dissatisfied with their experience with mental health services or they feel stigmatized by mental illness within the family. For example, theories on the family pathogenesis of schizophrenia have been widespread and many families feel blamed by mental health professionals for causing the illness.

For the therapist, it is important to elicit the beliefs held by the family members about the illness and aspects of the patient's behavior. This includes both specific beliefs as to causality and the emotional reactions that aspects of the patient's illness or behavior evoke in the relative. The semistructured interview, the Relative Assessment Interview, was designed for this purpose (Barrowclough & Tarrier, 1992). There is little point in providing education to relatives without knowing their current beliefs because if the new information is in conflict with the relative's health belief model it is unlikely to be assimilated and to influence the relative's behavior (Tarrier & Barrowclough, 1986).

Identification of Early Signs of Relapse

Relapses rarely occur without any forewarning. They are usually preceded by a period of prodromal symptoms that can last days, or more usually weeks, and in some cases, months. Common prodromal signs and symptoms, such as insomnia, irritability, mood fluctuations, and magical thinking, can be used as prompts. Specific assessment instruments (e.g., Birchwood et al., 1989) have been designed to identify the characteristics of prodromes and can be helpful. Patients can be asked to recall prodromal signs and symptoms that preceded previous episodes and relapses. Each can be written on a card and the patient asked to arrange them in temporal order of occurrence. In this way the patient's prodomal signature, that is the individual set of signs and symptoms that characterized the patient's prodrome and its time course, can be identified. The patient needs to be able to discriminate between an actual relapse prodrome and mood fluctuations that do not signal a relapse. This is done through a process of discrimination training, whereby the patient monitors mood and experiences over a number of weeks, with a goal of learning to distinguish a real prodrome from a false alarm.

The next stage is to formulate a "game plan" to deal with a prodrome should one occur. Coping strategies can be formulated and rehearsed, the help of others can be elicited, and the assistance of psychiatric services can be requested, which may include an increase or change in medication. With an understanding of the time course of their prodrome, different actions for different phases of the prodrome can be identified. Such a program has been found to successfully reduce manic episodes in patients suffering from bipolar affective disorders (Perry, Tarrier, Morriss, McCarthy, & Limb, 1999).

Enhancing Self-Esteem

Anecdotal observation suggests that low self-esteem can persist despite improvements in symptoms. This may be because self-esteem is affected by a broad range of factors (family factors, other social factors) in addition to the experience of having a chronic mental illness. As a preliminary attempt to address this problem, a treatment technique to enhance self-esteem was developed (Tarrier, 2002). The technique involves asking patients to generate a number of their positive attributes (e.g., being generous or helpful). They are then asked to rate on a 0–100 scale how much they believe they possess this attribute. Typically the strength of belief rating is low. They are then asked to give as many concrete examples as possible of times when they behaved in a manner that indicated that they possess this attribute. For example, they are asked to give examples of times when they were generous. Once a list has been generated, they are asked to go over each example in detail in their mind, reproducing an image of what occurred, the positive emotions that it elicited, and the reactions they received from others. After patients have done this for all the examples for that attribute, they are asked to rerate the belief that they actually possess this attribute. Typically the strength of the belief increases significantly. Patients are helped to see that the belief increased when they focused their attention on positive behavior. This is repeated through a list of attributes. For homework, patients are asked to select an attribute and to monitor examples of times when they behaved in a way that is congruent with that attribute. For example, patients can monitor times when they behave in a generous manner. The aim of homework is to focus on positive attributes and also to create reactance. When patients are asked to be more aware of generosity, they tend to act more generously, which can serve to increase self-esteem.

A feasibility trial using this approach was carried out with chronic inpatients. The approach resulted in improved self-esteem and reductions in positive and negative psychotic symptoms (Hall & Tarrier, 2003). Although there were a number of methodological flaws in this trial, the preliminary evidence suggests that this approach is beneficial and should be further investigated.

Importantly, patients like this approach because it focuses on positives rather than negatives (Hall & Tarrier, 2003). There are the usual difficulties with this approach as there are with other psychological approaches. The major difficulty is eliciting from patients their positive attributes. It is important not to set too high an expectation. Patients will find it discouraging if they are asked for 10 attributes but can only think of 2. Goals, therefore, should be realistic and achievable. A second problem is that patients can put a negative connotation on a positive quality. For example, the patient who thinks he is a good father because he cares for his children can come to a negative conclusion if he focuses too much on the fact he is separated from his wife and not providing a stable family home. Care has to be taken to avoid these situations or to counter them should they occur. In this example, the patient could be asked how many marriages end in divorce and how many separated fathers retain such good relationships with their children.

Our knowledge about self-esteem is rudimentary at present and we do not know whether its enhancement will result in improved clinical outcomes for patients with schizophrenia. Furthermore, our research on the mediating role of negative self-esteem between relatives' criticism and positive symptoms would suggest that intervention should focus more on reducing negative views of the self rather than increasing positive aspects. These issues remain to be addressed.

CONCLUSION

There is accumulating evidence that CBT is effective for reducing psychotic symptoms when used in conjunction with medication. However, much work is still needed. The future will require further research into psychological and psychosocial models that increase our understanding of factors that maintain schizophrenic symptoms. The results of these investigations should further inform and refine psychological treatments. Further research needs to inform our understanding of depression and anxiety disorders that are often comorbid with schizophrenia and reduce the quality of life of the sufferer and how these comorbid disorders can be treated.

As for the current state of our knowledge, there is good evidence that family interventions reduce relapse and that these effects can be relatively long lasting. Combining CBT with family interventions should have significant clinical benefits in reducing ongoing symptomatology and reduction in relapse risk.

There are many areas in which further research is required. The evidence that CBT prevents subsequent schizophrenic relapse is lacking. We also know little about accurate predictors of good treatment response or about how to work with different ethnic or minority groups. Further research is needed on how to adapt CBT to diverse cultural groups and to patients with dual diagnoses, particularly substance use disorders. The inclusion of motivational interviewing techniques is a potentially beneficial strategy. The problem of high suicide rates in this population needs to be investigated further, and methods must be devised to alleviate this serious problem. Once clinically efficacious treatments have been devised, they need to be disseminated so that there is increased and appropriate access to these treatments. This in itself is a major challenge.

In spite of these many omissions in our knowledge and understanding, the advances that have been made in the development of psychosocial treatments such as CBT and the benefits for many persons who suffer with schizophrenia should not be underestimated.

REFERENCES

American Psychiatric Association. (1987). *Diagnostic and statistical manual of mental disorders* (3rd ed., rev.). Washington, DC: Author.

American Psychiatric Association. (1992). *Tardive dyskinesia: A task force report of the American Psychiatric Association*. Washington, DC: Author.

American Psychiatric Association. (1994). *Diagnostic and statistical manual of mental disorders* (4th ed.). Washington, DC: Author.

Barnes, T. R. E., & Nelson, H. E. (1994). *The assessment of psychoses*. London: Chapman & Hall Medical.

Barrowclough, C., Haddock, G., Tarrier, N., Lewis, S., Moring, J., O'Brian, R., et al. (2001). Randomised controlled trial of motivational interviewing and cognitive behavioral intervention for schizophrenia patients with associated drug or alcohol misuse. *American Journal of Psychiatry, 158,* 1706–1713.

Barrowclough, C., & Hooley, J. (2003). Attributions and expressed emotion: A review. *Clinical Psychology Review, 23,* 649–880.

Barrowclough C., Johnston C., & Tarrier, N. (1994). Attribution, expressed emotion and patient relapse: An attributional model of relatives' response to schizophrenic illness. *Behavior Therapy, 25,* 67–88.

Barrowclough, C., & Parle, M. (1997). Appraisal, psychological adjustment and expressed emotion in relatives of patients suffering from schizophrenia. *British Journal of Psychiatry, 171,* 26–30.

Barrowclough, C., & Tarrier, N. (1992). *Families of schizophrenic patients: A cognitive-behavioural intervention*. London: Chapman & Hall.

Barrowclough, C., Tarrier, N., Humphreys, L., Ward, J., Gregg, L., & Andrews, B. (2003). Self esteem in schizophrenia: The relationships between self evaluation, family attitudes and symptomatology. *Journal of Abnormal Psychology, 112,* 92–99.

Barrowclough, C., Tarrier, N., Sellwood, W., Quinn, J., Mainwaring, J., & Lewis, S. (1999). A randomised controlled effectiveness trial of a needs-based psychosocial intervention service for carers of schizophrenic patients. *British Journal of Psychiatry, 174,* 506–511.

Barrowclough, C., Tarrier, N., Watts, S., Vaughn, C., Bamrah, J. S., & Freeman, H. L. (1987). Assessing the functional value of relatives' reported knowledge about schizophrenia: A preliminary report. *British Journal of Psychiatry, 151,* 1–8.

Beck, A. T. (1952). Successful out-patient psychotherapy of a chronic schizophrenic with delusions based on borrowed guilt. *Psychiatry, 15,* 305–312.

Bentall, R. P., Lewis, S., Tarrier, N., Haddock, G., Drake, R., & Day, J. (2003). Relationships matter: The impact of the therapeutic alliance on outcome in schizophrenia. *Schizophrenia Research, 60*(Suppl. 1), 319.

Birchwood, M., & Cochrane, R. (1990). Families coping with schizophrenia: Coping styles, their origins and correlates. *Psychological Medicine, 20,* 857–865.

Birchwood, M., Smith, J., MacMillan, F., Hogg, B., Prasad, R., Harvey, C., et al. (1989). Predicting relapse in schizophrenia: The development and implementation of an early signs monitoring system using patients and families as observers. *Psychological Medicine, 19,* 649–656.

Bleuler, M. (1978). *The schizophrenic disorders* (M. Clemens, Trans.). New Haven, CT: Yale University Press. (Original work published 1911)

Bola, J. R., & Mosher, L. R. (2002). Predicting drug-free treatment response in acute psychosis from the Soteria project. *Schizophrenia Bulletin, 28,* 559–576.

Bollini, P., Pampallona, S., Orza, M. J., Adams, M. E., & Chambers, T. C. (1994). Antipsychotic drugs: Is more worse? A meta-analysis of the published randomised controlled trials. *Psychological Medicine, 24*, 307–316.

Brabban, A., & Turkington, D. (2002). The search for meaning: Detecting congruence between life events, underlying schema and psychotic symptoms. In A. Morrison (Ed.), *A casebook of cognitive therapy for psychosis* (pp. 59–75). Cambridge, UK: Cambridge University Press.

Brewin, C. R., MacCarthy, B., Duda, K., & Vaughn, C. E. (1991). Attributions and expressed emotion in the relatives of patients with schizophrenia. *Journal of Abnormal Psychology, 100*, 546–554.

Brown, G. W., & Birley, J. L. T. (1968). Crisis and life change at the onset of schizophrenia. *Journal of Health and Social Behaviour, 9*, 203–224.

Buchanan, A. (1996). *Compliance with treatment in schizophrenia.* (Maudsley Monograph No. 37). London: Psychiatry Press.

Butzlaff, R. L., & Hooley, J. M. (1998). Expressed emotion and psychiatric relapse: A meta-analysis. *Archives of General Psychiatry, 55*, 547–552.

Caldwell, C. B., & Gottesman, I. I. (1990). Schizophrenics kill themselves too: A review of risk factors for suicide. *Schizophrenia Bulletin, 16*, 571–589.

Chadwick, P. D., & Lowe, C. F. (1990). Measurement and modification of delusional beliefs. *Journal of Clinical and Consulting Psychology, 58*, 225–232.

Chadwick, P. D., Williams C., & MacKenzie, J. (2003). Impact of case formulation in cognitive behaviour therapy for psychosis. *Behaviour Research and Therapy, 41*, 671–680.

Cooper, J. E., Kendell, R. E., Gurland, B. J., Sharpe, L., Copeland, J. R. M., & Simon, R. (1972). *Psychiatric diagnosis in New York and London* (Maudsley Monograph No. 20). London: Oxford University Press.

Drake, R. E., Osher, F. C., & Wallach, M. A. (1989). Alcohol use and abuse in schizophrenia: A prospective community study. *Journal of Nervous and Mental Disease, 277*, 408–414.

Drury, V., Birchwood, M., & Cochrane, R. (2000). Cognitive therapy and recovery from acute psychosis: A controlled trial. III: Five year follow-up. *British Journal of Psychiatry, 177*, 8–14.

Drury, V., Birchwood, M., Cochrane, R., & MacMillan, F. (1996a). Cognitive therapy and recovery from acute psychosis: A controlled trial. I: Impact on psychotic symptoms. *British Journal of Psychiatry, 169*, 593–601.

Drury, V., Birchwood, M., Cochrane, R., & MacMillan, F. (1996b). Cognitive therapy and recovery from acute psychosis: A controlled trial. II: Impact on recovery time. *British Journal of Psychiatry, 169*, 602–607.

Durham, R. C., Guthrie, M., Morton, R. V., Reid, D. A., Treliving, L. R., Fowler, D., et al. (2003). Tayside–Fife clinical trial of cognitive-behaviour therapy for medication-resistant psychotic symptoms: Results to three month follow-up. *British Journal of Psychiatry, 182*, 303–311.

Eels, T. (1997). *Handbook of psychotherapy case formulation.* New York: Guilford Press.

Falloon, I. R., Boyd., J. L., McGill, C. W., Razani, J., Moss, H. B., & Gilderman, A. M. (1982). Family management in the prevention of exacerbations of schizophrenia: A controlled study. *New England Journal of Medicine, 306*, 1437–1440.

Falloon, I. R., Boyd, J. L., McGill, C. W., Williamson, M., Razani, J., Moss, H. B., et al. (1985). Family management in the prevention of morbidity of schizophrenia: Clinical outcome of a two-year longitudinal study. *Archives of General Psychiatry, 42,* 887–896.

Garety, P. A., Fowler, D., Kuipers, E., Freeman, D., Dunn, G., Bebbington, P. E., et al. (1997). London–East Anglia randomised controlled trial of cognitive-behavioural therapy for psychosis. II: Predictors of outcome. *British Journal of Psychiatry, 171,* 420–426.

Gelder, M., Gath, D., & Mayou, R. (1991). *Oxford textbook of psychiatry* (2nd ed.). Oxford, UK: Oxford University Press.

Glick, I., Clarkin, J., Spencer, J., Haas, G. L., Lewis, A. B., Peyser, J., et al. (1985). A controlled evaluation of inpatient family intervention, I: Preliminary results of a 6-month follow-up. *Archives of General Psychiatry, 42,* 882–886.

Glick, I., Spencer, J., Clarkin, J., Haas, G. L., Lewis, A. B., Peyser, J., et al. (1990). A randomized trial of inpatient family intervention, IV: Follow-up results for subjects with schizophrenia. *Schizophrenia Research, 3,* 187–200.

Goldstein, M. J., Rodnick, E. H., Evans, J. R., May, P. R., & Steinberg, M. R. (1978). Drug and family therapy in the aftercare of acute schizophrenics. *Archives of General Psychiatry, 35,* 1169–1177.

Grebb, J. (1995). *Movement induced disorders.* New York: Williams & Wilkins.

Haddock, G., Barrowclough, C., Moring, J., Tarrier, N., & Lewis, S. (2002). Cognitive behaviour therapy for patients with co-existing psychosis and substance use problems. In A. P. Morrison (Ed.), *A casebook of cognitive therapy for psychosis* (pp. 265–280). Hove, UK: Brunner-Routledge.

Haddock, G., McCarron, J., Tarrier, N., & Faragher, B. (1999). Scales to measure dimensions of hallucinations and delusions: The Psychotic Symptom Rating Scales (PSYRATS). *Psychological Medicine, 29,* 879–890.

Haddock, G., & Tarrier, N. (1998). Assessment and formulation in the cognitive behavioural treatment of psychosis. In N. Tarrier, A. Wells, & G. Haddock (Eds.), *Treating complex cases: The cognitive behavioural therapy approach* (pp. 155–175). Chichester, UK: Wiley.

Haddock, G., Wolfenden, M., Lowens, I., Tarrier, N., & Bentall, R. P. (1995). The effect of emotional salience on the thought disorder of patients with a diagnosis of schizophrenia. *British Journal of Psychiatry, 167,* 618–620.

Hall, P. H., & Tarrier, N. (2003). The cognitive-behavioural treatment of low self-esteem in psychotic patients: A pilot study. *Behaviour Research and Therapy, 41,* 317–332.

Hamilton, M. (1974) *Fish's clinical psychopathology.* Bristol: John Wright & Sons.

Harrison, G., Glazebrook, C., Brewin, J., Cantwell, R., Dalkin, T., Fox, R., et al. (1997). Increased incidence of psychotic disorders in migrants from the Caribbean to the United Kingdom. *Psychological Medicine, 27,* 799–806.

Helbig, S., & Fehm, L. (2004). Problems with homework in CBT: Rare exception or rather frequent? *Behavioural and Cognitive Psychotherapy, 32,* 291–301.

Hooley, J. M. (1985). Expressed emotion: A review of the critical literature. *Clinical Psychology Review, 5,* 119–139.

Hooley, J. M. (1987). The nature and origins of expressed emotion. In M. J. Goldstein & K. Hahlweg (Eds.), *Understanding major mental disorders: The contribution of family interaction research* (pp. 176–194). New York: Family Process Press.

Joyce, E., Hutton, S., Mutsatsa, S., Gibbins, H., Webb, E., Paul, S., et al. (2002). Executive functioning in first episode schizophrenia and relationship to duration of untreated psychosis: The West London study. *British Journal of Psychiatry, 181*(Suppl. 43), 38–44.

Kane, J. M. (1983). Problems with compliance in the outpatient treatment of schizophrenia. *Journal of Clinical Psychiatry, 44,* 3–6.

Karoly, P., & Kanfer, F. H. (1982). *Self-management and behaviour change: From theory to practice.* New York: Pergamon.

Kavanagh, D. J. (1992). Recent developments in expressed emotion and schizophrenia. *British Journal of Psychiatry, 160,* 601–620.

Kemp, R., Kirov, G., Everitt, B., Hayward, P., & David, A. (1998). Randomised controlled trial of compliance therapy: 18 month follow-up. *British Journal of Psychiatry, 172,* 413–419.

Kendell, R. E. (1993). Schizophrenia. In R. E. Kendell & A. K. Zealley (Eds.), *Companion to psychiatric studies* (5th ed., pp. 397–426). Edinburgh, Scotland: Churchill-Livingstone.

Kim, K., Li, D., Liang, Z., Cui, X., Lin, L., Kang, J., et al. (1993). Schizophrenic delusions among Korean, Korean-Chinese and Chinese: A transcultural study. *International Journal of Social Psychiatry, 39,* 190–199.

Kingdon, D. G., & Turkington, D. (1991). The use of cognitive behaviour therapy with a normalising rationale in schizophrenia. *Journal of Nervous and Mental Disease, 179,* 207–211.

Kingdon, D. G., & Turkington, D. (1994). *Cognitive behavioural therapy of schizophrenia.* New York: Guilford Press.

Kinon, B., & Lieberman, J. (1996). Mechanisms of action of atypical antipsychotic drugs: A critical analysis. *Psychopharmacology, 24,* 2–34.

Kottgen, C., Sonnichsen, I., Mollenhauer, K., & Jurth, R. (1984). Group therapy with the families of schizophrenic patients: Results of the Hamburg Camberwell-Family-Interview Study, III. *International Journal of Family Psychiatry, 5,* 84–94.

Kuipers, E., Fowler, D., Garety, P., Chisholm, D., Freeman, D., Dunn, G., et al. (1998). London-East Anglia randomised controlled trial of cognitive-behavioural therapy for psychosis. III: Follow-up and economic evaluation at 18 months. *British Journal of Psychiatry, 173,* 61–68.

Leff, J. P., Berkowitz, R., Shavit, N., Strachan, A., Glass, I., & Vaughn, C. (1990). A trial of family therapy versus a relatives' group for schizophrenia: Two year follow-up. *British Journal of Psychiatry, 157,* 571–577.

Leff, J., Kuipers, L., Berkowitz, R., Eberlein-Vries, R., & Sturgeon, D. (1982). A controlled trial of social intervention in the families of schizophrenic patients. *British Journal of Psychiatry, 141,* 121–134.

Leff, J., Kuipers, L., Berkowitz, R., & Sturgeon, D. (1985). A controlled trial of social intervention in the families of schizophrenic patients: A two year follow-up. *British Journal of Psychiatry, 146,* 594–600.

Leff, J., & Vaughn, C. (1985). *Expressed emotion in families: Its significance for mental illness.* New York: Guilford Press.

Lehman, A. F., & Dixon, L. B. (1995). *Double jeopardy: Chronic mental illness and substance abuse disorders.* Chur, Switzerland: Harwood Academic Press.

Lewis, S. W., Tarrier, N., Haddock, G., Bentall, R., Kinderman, P., Kingdon, D., et al. (2002). Randomised controlled trial of cognitive-behaviour therapy in early schizophrenia: Acute phase outcomes. *British Journal of Psychiatry, 181*(Suppl. 43), 91–97.

MacMillan, F., Crow, T. J., Johnson, A. L., & Johnstone, E. (1986). The Northwick Park study of first episodes of schizophrenia. *British Journal of Psychiatry, 148,* 128–133.

McFarlane, W. R., Lukens, E., Link, B., Dushay, R., Deakins, S. A., Newmark, M., et al. (1995). Multiple-family groups and psychoeducation in the treatment of schizophrenia. *Archives of General Psychiatry, 52,* 679–687.

McGilloway, S., Donnelly, M., & Mays, N. (1997). The experience of caring for former long-stay psychiatric patients. *British Journal of Clinical Psychology, 36,* 149–151.

McGuffin, P., Farmer, A., & Harvey, I. (1991). A polydiagnostic application of operational criteria in studies of psychotic illness: Development and reliability of the OPCRIT system. *Archives of General Psychiatry, 48,* 764–770.

Menezes, P. R., Johnson, S., Thornicroft, G., Marshall, J., Prosser, D., Bebbington, P., et al. (1996). Drug and alcohol problems among individuals with severe mental illnesses in South London. *British Journal of Psychiatry, 168,* 612–619.

Miller, W. R., & Rollnick, S. (2002). *Motivational interviewing: Preparing people for change* (2nd ed.). New York: Guilford Press.

Morrison, A. P. (1994). Cognitive behaviour therapy for auditory hallucinations without concurrent medication: A single case. *Behavioural and Cognitive Psychotherapy, 22,* 259–264.

Mueser, K. T., & Berenbaum, H. (1990). Psychodynamic treatment of schizophrenia: Is there a future? *Psychological Medicine, 20,* 253–262.

NHS Centre for Reviews and Dissemination. (1999). Drug treatment for schizophrenia. *Effective Health Care, 5,* 1–11.

Oldridge, M. I., & Hughes, I. C. T. (1992). Psychological well-being in families with a member suffering from schizophrenia: An investigation into longstanding problems. *British Journal of Psychiatry, 161,* 249–251.

Paley, G., & Shapiro, D. A. (2002). Lessons from psychotherapy research for psychological interventions for people with schizophrenia. *Psychology and Psychotherapy: Theory, Research and Practice, 75,* 5–18.

Paykel, E. S. (1976). Life stress, depression and attempted suicide. *Journal of Human Stress, 2,* 3–12.

Perry, A., Tarrier, N., Morriss, R., McCarthy, E., & Limb, K. (1999). A randomised controlled trial of teaching bipolar disorder patients to identify early symptoms of relapse and obtain early treatment. *British Medical Journal, 318,* 149–153.

Pilling, S., Bebbington, P., Kuipers, E., Garety, P., Geddes, J., Martindale, B., et al. (2002a). Psychological treatments in schizophrenia: II. Meta-analysis of randomised controlled trials of social skills training and cognitive remediation. *Psychological Medicine, 32,* 783–792.

Pilling, S. Bebbington, P., Kuipers, E., Garety, P., Geddes, J., Orbach, G., et al. (2002b). Psychological treatments in schizophrenia: I. Meta-analysis of family intervention and cognitive behaviour therapy. *Psychological Medicine, 32,* 763–782.

Pitschel-Walz, G., Leucht, S., Bauml, J., Kissling, W., & Engel, R. R. (2001). The effect of family intervention on relapse and rehospitalisation in schizophrenia: A meta-analysis. *Schizophrenia Bulletin, 27,* 73–92.

Randolph, E. T., Eth, S., Glynn, S. M., Paz, G. G., Leong, G. B., Shaner, A. L., et al. (1994). Behavioural family management in schizophrenia: Outcome of a clinic-based intervention. *British Journal of Psychiatry, 164,* 501–506.

Remington, G., Kapur, S., & Zipursky, R. B. (1998). Pharmacotherapy of first-episode schizophrenia. *British Journal of Psychiatry, 172*(Suppl. 33), 66–70.

Schene, A. H., Tessler, R. C., & Gamache, G. M. (1994). Instruments measuring family or caregiver burden in severe mental illness. *Social and Psychiatric Epidemiology, 24,* 228–240.

Schneider, K. (1958). *Klinische psychopathologie* (Trans., M. W. Hamilton). New York: Grune & Stratton.

Schooler, N. R., Keith, S. J., Severe, J. B., Matthews, S. M., Bellack, A. S., Glick, I. D., et al. (1997). Relapse and rehospitalisation during the maintenance treatment of schizophrenia: The effects of dose reduction and family treatment. *Archives of General Psychiatry, 54,* 453–463.

Sellwood, W., Barrowclough, C., Tarrier, N., Quinn, J., Mainwaring, J., & Lewis, S. (2001). Needs-based cognitive-behavioural family intervention for carers of patients suffering from schizophrenia: Twelve month follow-up. *Acta Psychiatrica Scandinavica, 104,* 346–355.

Sellwood, W., & Tarrier, N. (1994). Demographic factors associated with extreme noncompliance in schizophrenia. *Social Psychiatry and Psychiatric Epidemiology, 29,* 172–177.

Sellwood, W., Tarrier, N., Quinn, J., & Barrowclough, C. (2003). The family and compliance in schizophrenia: The influence of clinical variables, relatives' knowledge and expressed emotion. *Psychological Medicine, 33,* 91–96.

Selten, J. P., Veen, N., Feller, W., Blom, J. D., Schols, D., Camoenie, W., et al. (2001). Incidence of psychotic disorders in immigrant groups to the Netherlands. *British Journal of Psychiatry, 178,* 373–377.

Sensky, R., Turkington, D., Kingdon, D., Scott, J. L., Scott, J., Siddle, R., et al. (2000). A randomised controlled trial of cognitive-behavioural therapy for persistent symptoms in schizophrenia resistant to medication. *Archives of General Psychiatry, 57,* 165–172.

Silverstone, P. H. (1991). Low self esteem in different psychiatric conditions. *British Journal of Clinical Psychology, 30,* 185–188.

Tarrier, N. (1987). An investigation of residual psychotic symptoms in discharged schizophrenic patients. *British Journal of Clinical Psychology, 26,* 141–143.

Tarrier, N. (1992). Modification and management of residual psychotic symptoms. In M. Birchwood & N. Tarrier (Eds.), *Psychological approaches to schizophrenia: Innovations in assessment and treatment and services* (pp. 147–169). Chichester, UK: Wiley.

Tarrier, N. (1996). A psychological approach to the management of schizophrenia. In M. Moscarelli & N. Sartorius (Eds.), *The economics of schizophrenia* (pp. 271–285). Chichester, UK: Wiley.

Tarrier, N. (2002). The use of coping strategies and self-regulation in the treatment of psychosis. In A. Morrison (Ed.), *A casebook of cognitive therapy for psychosis* (pp. 79–107). Cambridge, UK: Cambridge University Press.

Tarrier N., & Barrowclough, C. (1986). Providing information to relatives about schizophrenia: Some comments. *British Journal of Psychiatry, 149,* 458–463.

Tarrier, N., Barrowclough, C., Andrews, B., & Gregg, L. (2004). Suicide risk in recent onset schizophrenia: The influence of clinical, social, self-esteem and demographic factors. *Social Psychiatry and Psychiatric Epidemiology, 39,* 927–937.

Tarrier, N., Barrowclough, C., Porceddu, K., & Fitzpatrick, E. (1994). The Salford Family Intervention project for schizophrenic relapse prevention: Five- and eight-year accumulating relapses. *British Journal of Psychiatry, 165,* 829–832.

Tarrier, N., Barrowclough, C., Vaughn, C., Bamrah, J. S., Porceddu, K., Watts, S., et al.

(1988). The community management of schizophrenia: A controlled trial of a behavioural intervention with families. *British Journal of Psychiatry, 153,* 532–542.

Tarrier, N., Barrowclough, C., Vaughn, C., Bamrah, J. S., Porceddu, K., Watts, S., et al. (1989). The community management of schizophrenia: A controlled trial of a behavioural intervention with families: Two year follow-up. *British Journal of Psychiatry, 154,* 625–628.

Tarrier, N., Beckett, R., Harwood, S., Baker, A., Yusupoff, L., & Ugarteburu, I. (1993). A controlled trial of two cognitive behavioural methods of treating drug-resistant residual psychotic symptoms in schizophrenic patients: 1. Outcome. *British Journal of Psychiatry, 162,* 524–532.

Tarrier, N., & Bobes, J. (2000). The importance of psychosocial interventions and patient involvement in the treatment of schizophrenia. *International Journal of Psychiatry in Clinical Practice, 4*(Suppl. 1), 35–52.

Tarrier, N., & Calam, R. (2002). New developments in cognitive-behavioural case formulation: Epidemiological, systemic and social context: An integrative approach. *Behavioural and Cognitive Psychotherapy, 30,* 311–328.

Tarrier, N., Kinney, C., McCarthy, E., Humphreys, L., Wittkowski, A., & Morris, J. (2000). Two year follow-up of cognitive-behavior therapy and supportive counselling in the treatment of persistent positive symptoms in chronic schizophrenia. *Journal of Consulting and Clinical Psychology, 68,* 917–922.

Tarrier, N., Kinney, C., McCarthy, E., Wittkowski, A., Yusupoff, L., Gledhill, A., et al. (2001). Are some types of psychotic symptoms more responsive to CBT? *Behavioural and Cognitive Psychotherapy, 29,* 45–55.

Tarrier, N., Lewis, S. W., Haddock, G., Bentall, R., Drake, R., Dunn, G., et al. (2004). 18 month follow-up of a randomised, controlled clinical trial of cognitive-behavior therapy in first episode and early schizophrenia. *British Journal of Psychiatry, 184,* 231–239.

Tarrier, N., & Turpin, G. (1992). Psychosocial factors, arousal and schizophrenic relapse: A review of the psychophysiological data. *British Journal of Psychiatry, 161,* 3–11.

Tarrier, N., Vaughn, C., Lader, M. H., & Leff, J. P. (1979). Bodily reactions to people and events in schizophrenia. *Archives of General Psychiatry, 36,* 311–315.

Tarrier, N., Wittkowski, A., Kinney, C., McCarthy, E., Morris, J., & Humphreys, L. (1999). The durability of the effects of cognitive behaviour therapy in the treatment of chronic schizophrenia: Twelve months follow-up. *British Journal of Psychiatry, 174,* 500–504.

Tarrier, N., Yusupoff, L., Kinney, C., McCarthy, E., Gledhill, A., Haddock, G., et al. (1998). A randomised controlled trial of intensive cognitive behaviour therapy for chronic schizophrenia. *British Medical Journal, 317,* 303–307.

Tarrier, N., Yusupoff, L., McCarthy, E., Kinney, C., & Wittkowski, A. (1998). Some reason why patients suffering from chronic schizophrenia fail to continue in psychological treatment. *Behavioural and Cognitive Psychotherapy, 26,* 177–181.

Tattan, T., & Tarrier, N. (2000). The expressed emotion of case managers of the seriously mentally ill: The influence of EE and the quality of the relationship on clinical outcomes. *Psychological Medicine, 30,* 195–204.

Telles, C., Karno, M., Mintz, J., Paz, G., Arias, M., Tucker, D., et al. (1995). Immigrant families coping with schizophrenia: Behavioral family intervention vs. case management with a low-income Spanish-speaking population. *British Journal of Psychiatry, 167,* 473–479.

van Os, J., & McGuffin, P. (2003). Can the social environment cause schizophrenia? *British Journal of Psychiatry, 182*, 291–292.

Vaughn, K., Doyle, M., McConaghy, N., Blaszczynski, A., Fox, A., & Tarrier, N. (1992). The Sydney Intervention Trial: A controlled trial of relatives' counselling to reduce schizophrenic relapse. *Social Psychiatry and Psychiatric Epidemiology, 27*, 16–21.

Wahass, S., & Kent, G. (1997). The modification of psychological interventions for persistent auditory hallucinations to an Islamic culture. *Behavioural and Cognitive Psychotherapy, 25*, 351–364.

Wearden, A., Tarrier, N., Barrowclough, C., Zastowny, T. R., & Rahill, A. A. (2000). A review of expressed emotion research in health care. *Clinical Psychology Review, 20*, 633–666.

Weisman, A., Nuechterlein, K. H., Goldstein, M. J., & Snyder, K. S. (1998). Expressed emotion, attributions and schizophrenia symptom dimensions. *Journal of Abnormal Psychology, 107*, 355–359.

Wiersma, D., Jenner, J. A., van de Willige, G., Spakman, M., & Nienhuis, F. J. (2001). Cognitive behaviour therapy with coping training for persistent auditory hallucinations in schizophrenia: A naturalistic follow-up study of the durability of effects. *Acta Psychiatrica Scandinavica, 103*, 393–399.

Wing, J. K., & Brown, G. W. (1970). *Institutionalism and schizophrenia*. London: Cambridge University Press.

World Health Organization. (1973). *Report on the international pilot study of schizophrenia*. Geneva, Switzerland: Author.

World Health Organization. (1992). *The ICD-10 Classification of Mental and Behavioural Disorders*. Geneva, Switzerland: Author.

Xiong, W., Phillips, M. R., Hu, X., Wang, R., Dai, Q., Kleinman, J., et al. (1994). Family-based intervention for schizophrenic patients in China: A randomized controlled trial. *British Journal of Psychiatry, 165*, 239–247.

Zastowny, T. R., Lehman, A. F., Cole, R. E., & Kane, C. (1992). Family management of schizophrenia: A comparison of behavioral and supportive family treatment. *Psychiatric Quarterly, 63*, 159–186.

Zhang, M., Heqin, Y., Chengde, Y., & Wang, G. (1993). Effectiveness of psychoeducation of relatives of schizophrenic patients: A prospective cohort study in five cities of China. *International Mental Health, 22*, 47–59.

Zhang, M., Wang, M., Li, J., & Phillips, M. R. (1994). Randomised-control trial of family intervention for 78 first-episode male schizophrenic patients: An 18 month study in Suzhou, Jiangsu. *British Journal of Psychiatry, 165*(Suppl. 24), 96–102.

10

Alcohol Use Disorders

FREDERICK ROTGERS
LAURA SHARP

> To cease smoking is the easiest thing I ever did. I ought to
> know because I've done it a thousand times.
> —attributed to MARK TWAIN

The maintenance of behavior change following treatment of substance use disorders has been one of the major conundrums in the addictions treatment field. In this chapter we review approaches to the enhancement of outcomes and behavior change maintenance (relapse prevention) in the treatment of persons with alcohol problems. A number of issues cloud the consideration of these topics, not the least of which revolves around the sorts of behavior changes that should be considered a positive outcome, and the definition of relapse (or, its mirror image, maintenance). At the outset, we should warn the reader that much of what we write will seem to contradict "standard" clinical belief on this arena. However, we have taken an approach that we believe is solidly based in the research on treatment of alcohol problems.

We would also point out that despite our focus on alcohol problems, much of what we write can be applied to treatment and change maintenance in the treatment of users of other drugs, both legal and illegal. From a behavioral theory perspective, there is no inherent difference in the learning processes that occur in effective treatment of problem use of various substances. Therefore, we adopt alcohol as a "prototype," and certainly as the drug with which the largest percentage of the population experiences problems. We will also, for the sake of ease, use the term "relapse prevention" (RP) synonymously with the term "maintenance of change." This corresponds with common usage in the addictions treatment field, although as we shall see, the term "relapse prevention" is fraught with definitional difficulties.

This chapter addresses several important issues in the enhancement of outcomes and RP. First, we provide a brief overview of the diagnostic criteria for alcohol problems following the perspective of DSM-IV-TR (American Psychiatric Association, 2000). We then consider the problems in defining positive treatment outcome and relapse in the treatment of alcohol problems. Then we turn to a discussion of approaches that are effective for enhancing treatment outcome as defined in the previous section, followed by a similar discussion of approaches to RP. It should be noted that because of the definitional problems we discuss, enhancement of outcomes and RP in addictions treatment are often taken to be synonymous. We attempt here to clearly separate them, but the inherently fuzzy nature of the difference between them may result in occasional overlapping of categories.

DIAGNOSTIC CRITERIA

DSM-IV-TR (American Psychiatric Association, 2000) places alcohol problems within the category of psychoactive substance use disorders. This category describes two "generic" categories that can be applied, with varying degrees of fit, to problem use of a variety of psychoactive substances. Two types of alcohol use disorders are defined: alcohol abuse and alcohol dependence.

The diagnostic criteria for alcohol abuse require that the individual display a maladaptive pattern of alcohol use that leads to clinically significant impairment or distress. This is manifested by one or more of the following occurring within a 12-month period: (1) recurrent alcohol use resulting in a failure to fulfill major role obligations at work, school, or home; (2) recurrent alcohol use in situations in which use is physically hazardous; (3) recurrent alcohol-related legal or interpersonal problems; and (4) continued alcohol use despite having persistent or recurrent social or interpersonal problems caused or exacerbated by the effect of alcohol. To qualify for the diagnosis of alcohol abuse, the individual must not have had symptoms that have met the criteria for alcohol dependence (American Psychiatric Association, 2000).

At this point we begin to encounter some of the definitional difficulties alluded to previously. This is reflected in a somewhat different set of criteria for diagnosing a similar disorder (an alcohol use disorder that is less severe than alcohol dependence) in the *International Classification of Diseases–10* (ICD-10; World Health Organization, 1992). The corresponding category in the ICD-10 to the DSM-IV-TR's alcohol abuse is the harmful use of alcohol. In the ICD-10, harmful use of alcohol is described by a pattern of alcohol use that is causing actual harm to the individual's physical or psychological health. To qualify for the diagnosis of harmful use of alcohol the individual must not have a concurrent diagnosis of alcohol dependence syndrome (World Health Organization, 1992). Although there are subtle differences between

ICD-10 and DSM-IV-TR alcohol use disorders, there is one substantial difference. The DSM-IV-TR abuse category includes social, legal, and occupational consequences of the use of alcohol, where the ICD-10 harmful use category includes only physical or psychological harm (Hasin, 2003). The alcohol abuse and the harmful use of alcohol categories account for very different types of substance-related consequences and may be responsible for some of the cross-system disagreement that has been found (Rounsaville, Bryant, Babor, Kranzler, & Kadden, 1993).

DSM-IV-TR provides for a second, more severe diagnosis: alcohol dependence. A diagnosis of alcohol dependence is assigned when an individual's symptoms have met three or more of the following criteria in a 12-month period: (1) tolerance for alcohol; (2) withdrawal syndrome for alcohol or using alcohol to relieve or avoid withdrawal symptoms; (3) taking alcohol in increased amounts or over a longer period than intended; (4) any unsuccessful effort or persistent desire to cut down or control the use of alcohol; (5) spending a great deal of time in activities necessary to obtain alcohol, drink alcohol, or recover from alcohol use; (6) giving up or reducing important social, occupational, or recreational activities because of alcohol use; and (7) continued use of alcohol despite knowing of a persistent or recurrent problem(s) that is caused or exacerbated by alcohol use (American Psychiatric Association, 2000).

Under ICD-10, a diagnosis of alcohol dependence is assigned when the individual displays at least three of six symptoms. The symptoms are (1) a strong desire or sense of compulsion to use alcohol; (2) impaired capacity to control the use of alcohol; (3) evidence of a withdrawal state from alcohol or the use of alcohol to relieve or avoid withdrawal symptoms with an awareness of the effectiveness of such behavior; (4) evidence of tolerance to alcohol; (5) progressive neglect of alternative pleasures, behaviors, or interests in favor of alcohol use; and (6) continued use of alcohol despite clear evidence of harmful consequences (World Health Organization, 1992). Despite the somewhat different criteria, there appears to be reasonable agreement between DSM and ICD systems for diagnosing alcohol use disorders.

A careful review of both sets of criteria reveals a somewhat startling omission: In neither definitional set does alcohol use per se play more than a foundational role in the definition of the disorder (i.e., one cannot suffer from an alcohol use disorder unless one actually uses alcohol). Yet, in clinical practice, the use of alcohol itself has come to assume a touchstone role in the assessment of both treatment outcome and relapse. This disconnect between research-based diagnostic systems and clinical practice has been at the center, in our view, of the controversial nature of many approaches to the treatment of alcohol use disorders (Roizen, 1987) that have nonetheless been well supported by research (Miller, Wilbourne, & Hettema, 2003; Walters, 2000). Our position in this controversy is solidly on the side of the research-based diagnostic systems. The import of this position will become clearer as this chapter unfolds.

DEFINING TREATMENT OUTCOME AND RELAPSE

Unlike other psychiatric disorders in which positive treatment outcome is typically defined as symptom reduction or resolution, and relapse a reappearance of symptoms, in the arena of alcohol and other drug use disorders, symptom reduction has never been the primary criterion used by clinicians to assess treatment outcomes, despite much urging from the research and academic communities (e.g., Maltzman, 1994). Nor has relapse typically been defined as a reappearance of symptoms previously resolved or the appearance of new symptoms that now requalifies the individual for the substance use disorder diagnosis.

Rather, the touchstone outcome pursued both clinically and in ancillary support groups (with one exception) for treatment of substance use disorders has been complete abstinence from the use of the substance. Likewise, a return to any use of the substance has often been considered clinically to be indicative of a relapse. Traditional lore has held for years "once an alcoholic, always an alcoholic," and this view is reflected in DSM-IV-TR criteria for outcome specifiers. The latter allow for, at best, "sustained full remission," but never for a "cure" or complete resolution of the disorder such that the individual no longer carries the diagnosis in any form. In fact, in the substance use disorders, the clinical course has been made a part of the criteria for the disorder. Contrast this with other highly prevalent disorders such as anxiety disorders in which the course of the disorder, although noted in the descriptive material accompanying the criteria, is not embodied in the diagnostic criteria themselves (certain mood and psychotic disorders also contain course specifiers in the diagnostic criteria for the disorder, e.g., major depressive episode and manic episode).

Coupled with the extensive focus on the single, dichotomous criterion of substance use or abstinence as an indicator of treatment outcome and relapse, this process places substance use disorders squarely among a group of disorders presumed to have a largely physiological basis. Although the debate regarding whether "addiction is a brain disease" (Leshner, 1997) is beyond the scope of this chapter, it should be noted that there is a persistent (and perhaps incorrect) emphasis in both the clinical and research literatures (until recently) on abstinence as the touchstone outcome. Thus, the touchstone outcome for substance use disorders is a behavior that does not, itself, form a part of the diagnostic criteria for the disorders, nor is it mentioned in the diagnostic manuals other than as a foundational aspect of the disorders in question.

Following from this theoretical position (e.g., that abstinence is the defining positive outcome of treatment for substance use disorders) is the prevalent clinical view, at least in the United States (Rosenberg & Davis, 1994), that the primary goal of treatment should be to initiate and maintain abstinence from not only the substance that created the problems that led to a diagnosis but often from all other substances as well. Consistent with this latter view, the definition of relapse becomes somewhat problematic, particularly in the context of a diagnostic system that excludes substance use itself as a diagnostic criterion.

In the context of this clinical position, the definition of relapse has become quite problematic. Depending on the theoretical views of the writer, and his or her familiarity with the broad research on the epidemiology of substance use disorders, relapse may be defined variously as (1) any substance use at all; (2) any use of the substance that caused the problems leading to a diagnosis; (3) persistent substance use with no symptoms present (a condition the DSM refers to as "full" remission); (4) persistent substance use with some symptoms, but not enough to qualify for the diagnosis (a condition the DSM refers to as "partial" remission); or (5) persistent use with a sufficient symptoms to qualify for the diagnosis.

We adopt a model in which substance use itself is not necessarily indicative of a poor outcome, nor is it, following treatment, necessarily an indication of relapse. Marlatt and Gordon (1985), the authors who first systematized a cognitive-behavioral approach to RP, specified degrees of return to substance use following adoption and achievement of an abstinence goal in treatment (this notion—of whether abstinence is the goal adopted by the patient—becomes a critical consideration in enhancing treatment outcomes and reducing relapse, as we demonstrate later on). A *lapse* is defined as a short-term return to drinking that may extend itself temporally and greatly increases the likelihood of abandonment of the abstinence goal, and a full blown relapse. *Relapse* itself is defined as "a return to uncontrolled drinking and abandonment of the abstinence goal" (Larimer, Palmer, & Marlatt, 1999, p. 153).

In addition to the substance use-focused approach of Marlatt, we also adopt a symptom-based criterion for relapse similar to that of DSM-IV-TR's qualifiers of "partial" and "full" remission in which a return to drinking with or without symptoms is considered. In fact, recent research suggests that a common outcome of abstinence focused treatment is a return to substance use without accompanying symptoms (Miller, Walters, & Bennett, 2001). From the perspective of DSM-IV-TR, this approach is more consistent with the descriptive and diagnostic views of substance use disorders than is an exclusive focus on the presence or absence of abstinence.

FACTORS ASSOCIATED WITH OUTCOMES

It is clear from the foregoing discussion, that the major outcome focused on by most treatment is a cessation of drinking behavior. In fact, few clinicians would say that the ultimate goal of treatment is anything other than lifelong abstinence from alcohol. The question is whether or how to approach this goal, given research suggesting that abstinence is only one of several outcomes (as discussed previously), and that positive outcomes (at least in terms of symptom and negative consequence reduction) are often achieved by reductions in use to levels short of abstinence (Fletcher, 2001).

However, here we encounter another conundrum. As exemplified by Mark Twain's quip cited at the beginning of the chapter, quitting or reducing use is, in fact, quite easy for problem drinkers and drug users. What is difficult is expanding the duration of the change beyond a few hours, days, or weeks. Thus, in a sense, positive treatment outcome in treating alcohol and drug problems depends almost entirely on RP. In that sense, substance use disorders may require more of a combined approach to outcome enhancement and RP than other disorders. This seems to be so for several reasons.

Alcohol and substance use disorders are complex phenomena and extremely variable both between and across individuals. It is important to remember when considering treatment that unlike many other psychiatric disorders, substance use has a distinct appetitive component. That is, substance users perceive some positive benefit from what becomes over time for many, a problematic behavior. Thus, problem users of alcohol and other drugs find themselves in a distinct approach–avoidance conflict. Research clearly indicates that positive expectancies for substance use are firmly established for legal drugs such as alcohol, at a very early age (Leigh & Stacy, 2004). These expectancies persist into adulthood and form a significant factor driving substance use if once initiated. Positive drinking expectancies often revolve, for problem users, around a belief that alcohol relaxes them, that they function better socially and otherwise with alcohol in their bodies, and that as substance use increases, alcohol is a rapid, convenient medication for hangovers and aftereffects of drinking. In persons with co-occurring psychiatric disorders such as depression, anxiety, or schizophrenia, alcohol use expectancies may revolve around a belief that symptoms are alleviated by drinking, and drinking may become a form of "self-medication" (Khantzian, 1985). Expectancies have been shown to be strongly predictive of drinking behavior, and in order for treatment to be successful, expectancies must be addressed.

In problem users of alcohol and other drugs, the behavior of using itself often becomes automatized (Tiffany, 1990). That is, chains of behavior leading ultimately to drinking unfold often without conscious awareness in the presence of overlearned environmental and external cues to drink that are strongly associated with drinking outcome expectancies. Paying attention to one's behavior in a way that disrupts the automatic nature of many drinking behaviors also becomes a central part of successful behavior change (Marlatt & Gordon, 1985).

However, expectancies are not the entire story, and the role of expectancies in maintaining drinking varies significantly across drinkers. Many other factors associated with drinking problems develop gradually over the individual's lifetime and are not easily resolved in a period of brief treatment. In fact, treatment outcome research has demonstrated repeatedly that length of treatment involvement (whether treatment is defined as professional intervention or attendance at support groups) is associated with better substance use and other outcomes (Simpson, Joe, & Broome, 2002). Thus, it has become something of a truism in the clinical arena, a truism apparently supported by research, that longer treatment involvement is associated with consistently better outcomes, in terms of both substance use and other associated outcomes such as improved vocational, family, and health status. There are, however, varied interpretations of the meaning of this relatively consistent finding. One, perhaps most apropos here, was advanced by Miller (2000), who suggested that a third variable—degree of motivation for change—was the key to explaining the length-of-treatment-to-outcome relationship. That is, the more motivated (for change, for treatment, or for a particular treatment goal) an individual was, and the more closely treatment fit with that person's goals, the greater the likelihood of longer treatment retention and positive outcomes. Following from this view, procedures that enhance motivation should enhance treatment outcomes.

Commitment to a particular substance use goal (in the research cited, usually abstinence) has also been shown to be highly predictive of treatment outcome and likelihood of relapse. In both smokers and diverse groups of other substance users, a patient's degree of commitment to abstinence has been shown to be a strong predictor of abstinence at outcome, regardless of the nature of treatment or the degree to which the patient engaged in treatment or change-related behaviors (e.g., attendance at self-help support groups during or after treatment) (Hall, Havassy, & Wasserman, 1990; Morgenstern, Frey, McCrady, Labouvie, & Neighbors, 1996). Thus procedures that enhance goal commitment also should enhance outcomes.

In addition to motivational factors, outcomes of treatment and likelihood of relapse appear to be influenced by the number and variety of high-risk situations a particular patient reports as being associated with substance use, the patient's style of coping with these situations, and patient self-efficacy with respect to enacting an appropriate coping response in a high-risk situation (Annis & Graham, 1995; Marlatt & Gordon, 1985).

Researchers (Marlatt & Gordon, 1985) have identified a variety of high-risk situations that encompass both external factors (interpersonal conflict, social pressure to use, etc.) and internal factors (both negative and positive affective states, coping skill levels, etc.) that appear to be differentially associated with both treatment outcome and likelihood of relapse. There are also assessment instruments designed to describe these situations (e.g., Inventory of Drug Taking Situations; Annis, Martin, & Graham, 1992). The dilemma for treatment provision is that there is extreme variability across patients with respect to the number and type of high-risk situations associated with a particular patient's substance use. This means that effective treatment must, at some level, be tailored to each individual's particular profile of high-risk situations.

Coping style has also been implicated in treatment outcome and relapse potential. Much of this research has been based on Lazarus's notion that there are two styles of coping with stressors: emotional and behavioral. Persons who use predominantly emotional coping styles tend to focus on suppression of negative affect as a way of dealing with stressors (Lazarus & Folkman, 1984). Often, these coping efforts are somewhat passive and have little effect on the cause of the stress itself but, rather, serve as temporary palliatives. In contrast, persons who use predominantly behavioral coping styles focus on active problem solving and engagement in behaviors designed not only to alleviate stress but to alter the likelihood of its recurrence (e.g., developing and implementing a plan for how to refuse the offer of alcohol in a drinking situation). Behavioral coping seems to be associated with improved treatment outcomes and reduced likelihood of relapse posttreatment.

Coping style is important; however, it operates hand in hand with the patient's belief that not only is coping possible but he or she can actually implement the coping response effectively. Knowing how to "just say no" when offered drugs has little impact if the individual does not believe that he or she can effectively say "no" or that so doing will result in the desired outcome (avoidance of a slip or lapse). The degree to which a patient reports high self-efficacy with respect to coping with his or her unique high-risk situations appears to be a strong predictor of actual successful coping and avoidance of relapse (Rychtarik, Prue, Rapp, & King, 1992). As with high-risk situations, there are a number of instruments available to measure self-efficacy with respect to high-risk situations (Situational Confidence Questionnaire; Annis & Graham, 1988; Drug Avoidance Self Efficacy Scale; Martin, Wilkinson, & Poulos, 1995). Use of these instruments can alert clinicians to likely stumbling blocks on a patient's path to goal attainment and maintenance.

It would seem, then, that positive treatment outcome and RP for alcohol and other drug problems depend broadly on several factors:

1. Treatment retention, defined as persistence in change efforts
2. Motivation for change
3. Development of strategies for coping with expectancies and other factors maintaining substance use (i.e., co-occurring psychiatric disorder) that counter the automatic nature of many of these behavior chains
4. Commitment to particular change goals
5. Identification of high-risk situations and development of strategies for coping with them
6. Enhancing patient self-efficacy with respect to implementation of strategies for coping with high-risk situations

This is not an exhaustive list of factors that need to be considered when addressing the issues of improving outcomes and preventing relapse in substance use disorders. However, a broad reading of the research literature points increasingly to these three factors as having significant implications for outcomes in many treatment and behavior change contexts.

There are other more patient-focused factors that have been proposed by clinicians as associated with treatment outcomes. Age, gender, socioeconomic status, problem duration, and severity have all been suggested as patient factors that might be associated with outcomes and relapse potential. Despite the intuitive appeal of these, mostly static factors, research findings have often been contradictory with respect to the role these factors play in treatment outcome and maintenance. Thus, depending on the population, the drug of choice, and perhaps other factors, research has shown both early onset of problems and later onset of problems to be associated with treatment outcomes (Crits-Christoph et al., 2003). Thus, it seems clinically most appropriate to adopt a largely idiographic approach to assessment and intervention with substance users as more global factors seem to have little value in predicting treatment outcome and relapse potential with any particular individual.

The presence of untreated co-occurring psychiatric disorder is associated with poorer outcomes. This finding likely relates to the strong implication of negative affect in relapse to substance use outlined earlier. To the extent that an individual experiences repeated and intense negative affect due to co-occurring psychopathology, the likelihood of relapse increases if the co-occurring disorder is not treated along with the substance use disorder (Rosenthal & Westreich, 1999). Given the high degree of comorbidity between substance use and other psychiatric disorders, this factor is one that needs to figure prominently in assessment and treatment planning for most patients entering treatment for substance use disorders, and it bears addressing should outcomes be less than what is hoped for with a particular patient (Regier et al., 1990).

Contextual factors such as employment, stable family, and living environment also seem associated with better outcomes. To the extent that patients have supports in their natural environment, they will be more likely to be able to make lasting changes in substance use behavior. Recent research has begun to strongly support the role of self-help support group affiliation and attendance in maintaining treatment gains (Gossop et al., 2003). Although much of the reporting of these findings focuses on affiliation with 12-step groups such as Alcoholics Anonymous, there is no reason to believe that affiliation with other support groups whose philosophies are consistent with the patient's substance use goals would not also have a similar effect on maintenance of change. In fact, some research suggests that pushing patients who do not endorse a "disease" view of their substance use problems to attend 12-step groups, may be counterproductive (Crits-Christoph et al., 2003). As it is, a variety of alternative support groups have developed in recent years that are consistent in philosophy with both cognitive-behavioral models of substance use disorders (e.g., S.M.A.R.T.; Recovery, Horvath & Velten, 2000) and that support nonabstinence goals (Moderation Management; Rotgers & Kishline, 1999). In addition, there is an increasing availability of support on the Internet in the form of discussion groups that adhere to the tenets of various support groups, and which provide ready access to support "from the comfort of one's home" (Humphreys & Klaw, 2001). Given the strong research support for the benefit of support group affiliation on maintenance of behavior changes, this should be a component of any effort to enhance treatment outcomes.

A final consideration, but one only tentatively supported by research, is the "fit" between a patient's readiness to change (stage of change) and the intervention(s) made available to him or her (DiClemente & Prochaska, 1998). DiClemente and Prochaska (1998) have suggested that a mismatch of intervention to stage of change (i.e., providing an "action" oriented intervention to patients in the precontemplation or contemplation stages) may be a major cause of treatment failure. Given their findings that the majority of persons in treatment or change-focused programs report being in one of the preaction stages, this may be an important, but largely ignored, factor in treatment retention and outcome. A recent study of patients in mandated drug treatment found that pretreatment motivation was highly predictive of treatment engagement and retention (Hiller, Knight, Leukefeld, & Simpson, 2002). Specifically, those patients who indicated a readiness for treatment at entry did better than those whose degree of readiness was less or who indicated a reluctance to be part of a treatment program.

It is important to recognize at this juncture that patient motivation may be somewhat deceptive, and it is important that the clinician thoroughly assess motivation before launching into a particular therapeutic course. It is clear, with respect to stage of change, that patients can be in multiple stages depending on the particular behavior that is the change target. For example, a patient may be ready to change substance use behavior but not ready to do so using a proffered treatment program. Or, a patient may be ready for treatment but not the particular type of treatment that is offered.

OVERVIEW OF EMPIRICALLY SUPPORTED TREATMENTS

Despite strong evidence that substance users are a diverse group on a variety of characteristics, and that substance use problems fall along a continuum rather than being dichotomous ("you're an alcoholic or you're not"), traditional treatments have tended to provide a "one size fits all" approach, with little emphasis on individualized problem and skills assessment or interventions (Hester & Miller, 2003; Marlatt, Blume, & Parks, 2001). Yet, the research on treatment outcomes suggests that a number of these approaches are effective when delivered with a high degree of treatment integrity, and that treatment retention and completion are among the strongest predictors of sustained behavior change (e.g., Project MATCH Research Group, 1997).

In recent years, there have been a number of reviews of effective treatments for alcohol problems (e.g., Miller et al., 1995; Miller et al., 2003; Walters, 2000). These reviews have focused on cognitive-behavioral approaches as having the most empirical evidence of efficacy and have identified a number of specific approaches as having research support for their efficacy. The approaches reviewed include both behavioral and pharmacological approaches. Specific approaches that have strong evidence for their efficacy in treating problem drinkers include (1) brief intervention; (2) motivational enhancement; (3) pharmacotherapy with gamma aminobuytric acid (GABA) agonist or opioid antagonist; (4) community reinforcement and behavioral contracting; (5) behavioral self-control training; (6) social skills training; and (7) behavioral marital therapy (Miller et al., 2003). This list is not exhaustive, but clearly cognitive-behavioral and behavioral techniques have significant empirical support. However, it should be noted that these reviews focused, with few exceptions (e.g., behavioral self-control training, community reinforcement, and behavioral marital therapy) on specific techniques rather than on the sort of combination technologies that typically make up a treatment "program." Treatment is more often delivered using combinations of approaches in a programmatic fashion. Thus, for example, a specific program may combine aspects of social skills training, problem solving (itself not well supported in these reviews), and community reinforcement or contingency management. Until recently. most studies had been conducted in clinical research settings, and there has been little research supporting the efficacy of these combinations of techniques as delivered in the real world.

Recently, a number of studies have begun to muddy the waters somewhat by seeming to demonstrate positive outcomes from more traditional 12-step-based approaches and other approaches that, in the reviews just discussed, did not fare well. Particularly when the approach is well designed and delivered, there is growing evidence that cognitive and behavioral approaches may not maintain the superiority they have shown in outcome research to date. The prototypical example of this "muddying of the waters" is the multisite Project MATCH study sponsored by the National Institute on Alcohol Abuse and Alcoholism (Project MATCH Research Group, 1997). In a randomized comparison of three manualized approaches: 12-session cognitive-behavioral and 12-step facilitation (most like the predominant treatment approach currently used in the United States) treatments, and a four-session motivational enhancement treatment, treatment outcomes differed little across the treatments, with all treatments producing positive results. Of note, however, was the fact that the four-session motivational enhancement treatment performed as well at follow-up as did the other two more lengthy treatments. This would seem to contradict the notion that length of treatment is the main reason for successful outcomes in this study, but to reinforce Miller's hypothesis noted earlier, the critical variable is motivation itself.

In the treatment of other drug problems, a major multisite study conducted by the National Institute on Drug Abuse, the Drug Abuse Treatment Outcome Study (DATOS), has found positive outcomes, typically associated with high levels of treatment retention and motivation to change, across a variety of treatment modalities used to treat users of illegal drugs (Simpson et al., 2002).

Finally, research on therapeutic communities (French, Sacks, DeLeon, Staines, & McKendrick, 1999) has typically found very high rates of success (defined as abstinence from substances) among program completers (although these studies typically have very low rates of program completion). In fact, data from this research and the DATOS study appear to define a retention period of 90 days as being a critical dividing line between those who achieve and maintain abstinence and those who do not (Simpson et al., 2002).

Thus, a broad reading of the treatment outcome literature suggests that rather than a focus on specific techniques as being better than others at fostering lasting change in substance use, clinicians might better focus on enhancing broader treatment engagement and process. This might best be done through implementation of motivational strategies and the use of techniques that facilitate specific strategies taught by a particular treatment modality (including enhancement of commitment to use goals endorsed by the treatment modality) rather than a focus on specific techniques themselves. In the section that follows, we consider how this might be done most effectively. The model we present is one in which outcomes and RP are enhanced by embedding the teaching of specific, individualized coping strategies within a treatment context that address the factors of motivation, commitment, and retention and on countering the automaticity of substance use behavior particularly where that automaticity is associated with identifiable environmental and internal cues associated with substance use. We describe in some detail four approaches that have been shown, either with substance users directly or with other patients facing issues similar to substance users, to either enhance motivational and treatment retention or facilitate the process of "deautomatizing" individual substance use behavior chains. Of the four approaches we focus on, three are behavioral: motivational interviewing, community reinforcement/contingency management, and mindfulness training. The fourth is pharmacological but works best when used in combination with the other approaches.

Before we discuss these approaches, however, a brief aside is necessary to reinforce what cognitive-behavioral therapists already know but sometimes neglect: the importance of a comprehensive assessment as a guide to treatment interventions. It is clear that the processes associated with both successful treatment and relapse prevention are complex and highly individual specific. For the clinician to be able to most effectively implement the global strategies discussed below, he or she must have a fairly detailed understanding of these factors. Although it is beyond the scope of this chapter to discuss assessment fully, its omission as a major focus is not meant to diminish in any way the important, indeed often crucial, role that a thorough assessment can play in enhancing outcomes and maintenance (e.g., Tucker, Vuchinich, & Murphy, 2002).

ENHANCING MOTIVATION AND RETENTION

Enhancement of motivation to change addictive behavior is a complex phenomenon that has been treated, until very recently, as if it were a simple matter of "breaking through denial" (Metzger, 1988). There has been a pervasive assumption in the substance abuse treatment field that persons with alcohol and drug use problems suffer from a stable, internal characteristic of the "disease" of addiction that makes them engage in various forms of rationalization and evasion when confronted with evidence that their substance use is problematic. According to this view, "denial" is such a powerful internal mechanism that treatment cannot succeed unless "denial" is broken down and overcome. This has resulted in treatment approaches that have tended to be confrontational, highly prescriptive, and rule-focused (in order to get better you must attend 90 support group meetings in 90 days, avoid "people, places and things" associated with substance use, abstain from all mood altering substances, etc.).

In recent years, however, this view of the main obstacle to motivating change as being "in denial," has begun to erode. Starting with Miller's (1985) analysis of denial in terms of the interpersonal process that occurs between a substance user and others who view that person's substance use as problematic, there has been a gradual shift in perspective on motivation from a purely internal characteristic of the person to an interactional process that occurs between the person and the environment. In Miller's analysis, "denial" is conceived of as a normal human response to directive behavior change messages delivered by one person (e.g., a counselor or therapist) to another person who is ambivalent about the behavior toward which the change message is aimed.

Motivational Interviewing

Based on this analysis, Miller and Rollnick developed an approach to enhancing change motivation called "motivational interviewing" (MI; Miller & Rollnick, 1991, 2002). In this approach, the clinician's approach to the patient, while directive, is gently so. Although confrontational, the confrontation is not between the clinician's view and the patient's but between the poles of the patient's ambivalence about his or her substance use. The clinician acts, in effect, as a mirror into which the patient can gaze and observe his or her ambivalence. Thus, patients are encouraged to examine both sides of their ambivalence (both the "good" and "not so good" things about using substances) about their substance use and are aided (this is the directive part) toward a resolution of ambivalence by systematic, carefully selected reflections from the clinician of the patient's own words and ideas.

In addition to Miller's motivational analysis, a large body of research spanning more than three decades has examined the conditions under which motivation is most likely to be increased and sustained. Beginning with early analyses of the factors that appeared to motivate learning among schoolchildren, and with subsequent investigation of motivation in a variety of other groups and contexts, Ryan and Deci (2000) developed "self-determination theory" (SDT). SDT provides a theoretical explanation for why approaches such as MI exert a salutary effect on motivation to change. According to SDT, when certain conditions exist in a learning or behavior change situation, the likelihood of any new behavior being a result of intrinsic motivation is greatly increased. In their larger analysis of motivation, Ryan and Deci postulate that the more intrinsically motivated a behavior—that is, the greater the degree to which the behavior is engaged in for its own sake (i.e., is inherently reinforcing)—the more likely it is that the behavior will persist over time. This analysis has clear implications for treatments aimed at changing substance use as that behavior is, itself, highly intrinsically motivated, and one goal of treatment is to make a life with either no substance use or greatly reduced substance use intrinsically motivating.

Ryan and Deci (2000) propose that when a context is created in which the person feels that his or her behavior is self-governed (autonomous) rather than coerced or externally imposed, there is a relationship with others that is respectful, caring, and supportive of autonomy, and the means for enhancing competency (skills training and practice) are provided (if the individual requests or needs it to initiate and maintain behavior changes), there will be a greater likelihood of both initial and lasting behavior change. This analysis has been validated across a variety of behaviors, settings, and populations, including substance users entering treatment. Though often overlooked by clinicians, there are numerous studies in the research literature that support this analysis, particularly the focus on subjective autonomy as a key factor in motivating treatment entry and participation.

Practically, an emphasis on patient autonomy in treatment boils down to such things as permitting patients to have a strong say in selecting their own substance use goals (abstinence or reduced use), establishing a strong working relationship based on respect for the patient as an autonomous individual, and working with the patient toward goals to which the patient is committed.

Research has strongly supported taking such a stance in substance abuse treatment. For example, in a randomized trial in which patients seeking help for alcohol problems were assigned a group that chose its own goals (abstinence vs. moderation) or to one in which the goal, itself, was randomly assigned (in essence, chosen for the patient and imposed, albeit gently, but the clinician), results indicated that patients who chose their own goals did better than those who had a goal assigned, regardless of whether the goal was abstinence or moderation (Sanchez-Craig & Lei, 1986).

Miller and colleagues have reported similar findings when using MI as a "treatment induction" procedure. Patients who receive a single session of MI prior to entering treatment seem to do better regardless of the type or focus of treatment. In addition, behavioral self-control training, which is highly autonomy supportive and patient-directed, has been shown to be an extremely effective approach to the treatment of alcohol problems across a number of studies (see Walters, 2000, for a review). For example, in a study of cocaine users entering a detoxification program, Stotts, Schmitz, Rhoades, and Grabowski (2001) found that a single MI session not only enhanced the likelihood of program completion (with the effect being most pronounced with patients who were unsure of their commitment to the detoxification program in the first place) but also enhanced the use of more effective behavioral (as opposed to emotional) coping strategies postdetoxification.

Motivational Interviewing Technique

MI consists of a style of interacting with patients that permits the clinician to establish a therapeutic climate in the session that is consistent with Ryan and Deci's three conditions for enhancing motivation and behavior change. Miller and Rollnick (2002) have summarized the characteristics of MI in the acronym FRAMES (i.e., Feedback; Responsibility; Advice; Menu; Empathic; Self-Efficacy).

In doing MI, the clinician provides objective, nonjudgmental *Feedback* to the patient using both the patient's own reported experiences and objective information (case histories, assessment data) that may be available. The style of presentation of feedback revolves around reflection of patient concerns, with a particular emphasis on helping the patient recognize, consider, and resolve ambivalence about change.

Responsibility for change is acknowledged to rest with the patient, and the clinician explicitly acknowledges that he or she can only suggest courses of action. It is the patient's responsibility to decide whether to use the behavior change methods that might be developed or suggested by the clinician. This aspect of MI is the most clearly supportive of the patient's sense of autonomy, one of the three critical conditions identified by Ryan and Deci (2000).

While acknowledging that the responsibility for change rests squarely on the patient, the clinician using MI is also not hesitant to give specific *Advice* to the patient as to what change strategies have, in the clinician's experience, worked with other patients, and to suggest that the patient consider using these strategies as well. It is important to note that this advice is not presented as a prescription or as the "right" way for the patient to achieve his or her goals. Rather, advice is presented in a collaborative fashion with a willingness on the part of the clinician to take an "experimental" attitude toward recommendations and advice. That is, the clinician explicitly acknowledges that there may be other ways to proceed with the process of behavior change and is open to consider them based on the patient's experience with attempts to implement those the clinician suggests.

A *Menu* of change options is explicitly presented and discussed, with the patient again being the final determiner of which of a variety of change options are selected and implemented. In a manner that is highly consistent with basic tenets of cognitive-behavioral practice, the approach to intervention selection is collaborative rather than paternally descriptive as is often the case in substance abuse treatment programs. One goal of the clinician is to help the patient to "own" or make a strong commitment to a behavior change approach and then to work in a supportive way with the patient to implement that approach.

Perhaps the central aspect of MI is an Empathic approach by the clinician. The clinician acknowledges that the person with the best knowledge of the patient is the patient and attempts to engage the patient from a perspective of understanding the patient's perspective, even while exploring alternatives to that perspective. In MI, the clinician attempts to see the world through the patient's eyes and then to reflect back that vision while highlighting discrepancies and contradictions, particularly where the patient's view is truncated or incomplete. Often this takes the form of emphasizing positive aspects of the patient's behavior or situation that the patient may not have recognized. The centrality of empathy to MI cannot be emphasized too much, and it is in this technical aspect of MI that the second of Ryan and Deci's (2000) factors for promoting motivation—a caring, respectful working therapeutic relationship—is most clearly realized.

Finally, in doing MI, the clinician makes every attempt to foster Self-efficacy. This takes the form with very discouraged patients of helping the patient recognize that change is possible (instilling hope), and with patients who are actively working on change, designing behavioral experiences and experiments that will produce success experiences that can augment the patient's belief that he or she is capable of affecting the changes he or she desires. This aspect of MI maps most closely onto the last of Ryan and Deci's (2000) factors—competency enhancement or skills training. However, it should be noted that skills training is most effective when it is the patient who is making the argument for engaging in new learning, not when the clinician is the primary impetus for the new behaviors.

Contingency Management/Community Reinforcement

MI focuses on enhancing intrinsic motivation by working with patient ambivalence within a supportive, respectful therapeutic relationship. Contingency management approaches (Budney & Higgins, 1998; Meyers & Smith, 1995) take a different, though complementary, approach to enhancing and maintaining change motivation. We briefly discuss two contingency management systems here: the therapist/treatment center-administered approach outlined by Budney and Higgins (1998), and the community reinforcement approach (CRA; Meyers & Smith, 1995), which makes use of supportive significant others in the patient's environment to implement change-supportive contingencies under the guidance of a clinician (often in conjunction with the use of medications such as disulfiram). Both of these approaches attempt to structure aspects of the patient's environment to be supportive of healthy changes in substance use, typically abstinence. They can be particularly helpful for patients who have chosen abstinence as their substance use goal but who lack ongoing incentives to maintain it (Mark Twain would seem to fall into this group). We start the discussion with a consideration of CRA.

CRA was originally developed by Azrin and colleagues (Hunt & Azrin, 1973) as a means of encouraging and sustaining the use of disulfiram (an emetic medication that produces severe vomiting and other negative physiological changes upon consumption of even small amounts of alcohol) by alcohol-dependent patients in treatment. CRA trains and makes use of concerned significant others (CSOs) in the patient's life to administer, monitor, and reinforce the taking of disulfiram as an aid to maintaining abstinence. For many patients with drinking problems, the buffer that disulfiram provides can be of assistance in "buying time" during which other treatment strategies such as skills training, RP, and so on can be implemented.

By making use of persons already in the patient's environment to reorient contingencies away from those that support problem substance use to ones that support healthy change behaviors, CRA builds in a motivational component to the patient's life that in other approaches is generally done in a somewhat haphazard fashion (e.g., telling patients that they need to affiliate with Alcoholics Anonymous and attend so many meetings in so many days, but providing no incentive other than the patient's own desire to be abstinent for doing so). Of note in CRA is that the CSOs are worked with to change their behavior in response to other substance use-related behaviors by the patient. For example, a spouse who previously had cleaned up the vomit after the drinking spouse arrived home drunk is taught to shift that task to the drinking spouse, and to provide positive social reinforcement for the drinking spouse beginning to take responsibility for remediating the negative effects of his or her drinking.

As an overview (a more detailed discussion is available in Meyers & Smith, 1995), the CSO is taught, in collaboration with the patient, a routine set of instructions for administering disulfiram and reinforcing the patient for taking it. There is no reason, in principle, why this approach could not be extended to other change-supportive medications, including psychotropic medications that may help reduce symptoms and the likelihood of slips or relapse in patients with co-occurring Axis I disorders. The CSO is also taught how to respond in an appropriate, nonconfrontational, nonconflictual fashion the patient's refusal to take a dose of the medication, should that occur. In addition, the CSO is taught basic contingency management and reinforcement application techniques that focus on positively reinforcing change behaviors and withdrawing attention from behaviors that inhibit change. In many cases it is these latter behaviors that have previously drawn the most attention from CSOs, thus setting up a cycle of negative reinforcement in which the patient withdraws from the CSO or uses substances in response to the negative affect triggered by the CSO's positive attention to change-inhibiting behaviors.

While CRA has focused mainly on alcohol users (recent studies have applied it to other types of drug users, particularly as part of the community reinforcement and family training [CRAFT] approach to encouraging drug using persons to enter treatment), other contingency management (CM) approaches have focused on the implementation of change-supporting contingencies by clinicians. These approaches have been shown to be particularly effective in enhancing both treatment retention and participation and in supporting reduced substance use (e.g., Higgins et al., 1994). The most typical use of CM in this regard provides token or voucher reinforcers to patients contingent upon targeted change-supportive behaviors and actual behavior change indicators. The model is quite similar to the token economy model developed for the treatment of chronic psychiatric patients by Ayllon and Azrin (1968) in the early 1970s. In conjunction with the patient, the clinician develops and implements a set of reinforcement contingencies that involve both positive reinforcement of change positive behaviors (e.g., attendance at treatment sessions or provision of drug-free urine specimens) and response costs (e.g., loss of "points" in a point reinforcer system for provision of a urine specimen containing drugs). The research suggests that the use of these latter contingencies may be counterproductive, however, in that particularly early in treatment (before abstinence has been established), patients may experience far more response cost contingencies than change-reinforcing ones. This can often backfire and produce discouragement and treatment dropout. Therefore, care is needed in the design and implementation of contingencies to ensure that patients have the opportunity to experience positive reinforcement for change behaviors early in treatment (Budney & Higgins, 1998).

Care also needs to be exercised in the selection of the form of positive reinforcers. In particular, monetary reinforcers or vouchers that are negotiable, like cash, should be avoided as it is possible that patients, particularly when under stress, will convert their cash to alcohol or drugs, thus defeating the purpose of the reinforcement contingency, at least temporarily. Thus, nonnegotiable vouchers or tokens that can be exchanged in a controlled fashion for a variety of nonsubstance primary reinforcers (e.g., food and shelter) appear to be the best way to implement positive contingencies.

CM approaches have been shown to significantly enhance treatment engagement and outcomes in a number of well-controlled studies (Budney & Higgins, 1998). The major obstacles to implementing them appear to be both philosophical and pragmatic. The philosophical objections, typically from proponents of traditional, nonbehavioral approaches to treatment, focus on the belief that all treatment motivation should be intrinsic, and that provision of external reinforcers undermines what is believed to be a necessary aspect of change in substance use—personal commitment to change. Other objections focus on concerns that "paying" addicts to be in treatment will undermine the message that patients must change because they want to, not because of external contingencies. However, the use of external contingencies on a broader and less systematic basis is common in our society's approach to substance users. That is, external coercion and negative contingencies in the form of intervention by the legal system is common. In fact, some research suggests that legal coercion actually operates as a negative reinforcer (the patient avoiding incarceration by participating in treatment) and enhances treatment retention (Hiller, Knight, Broome, & Simpson, 1998).

The second major obstacle to implementation of CM approaches seems to be financial. Most treatment providers have little or no budget to provide access to positive reinforcers for which vouchers or tokens can be exchanged. Some researchers have circumvented this obstacle by working with community merchants, transportation systems, and so forth to provide access to reinforcers in return for vouchers as one form of public service (Budney & Higgins, 1998).

Despite these obstacles, the use of CM approaches and CRA has been repeatedly demonstrated to enhance treatment engagement and retention, and thereby improve outcomes.

ENHANCING MAINTENANCE OF BEHAVIOR CHANGE

Thus far we have focused our discussion on methods for enhancing treatment engagement and retention. We now turn to two methods for enhancing the likelihood of behavior change maintenance: mindfulness training (MT) and the use of medications in support of cognitive-behavioral treatment. Although we have grouped these approaches under the heading of enhancing maintenance, both approaches are useful adjuncts to treatment itself, which reflects the blurring of the distinction between treatment outcome and RP in the treatment of substance use disorders.

In our earlier discussion of factors associated with increased risk of relapse, we highlighted two aspects of substance use behavior that we propose as obstacles to change maintenance: the automatic nature of many of the thoughts and behaviors associated with relapse and the use of substances to cope with negative affective states. MT and the use of medications both address these concerns, but from different perspectives. MT addresses the automaticity of behavior, especially as it relates to coping effectively and adaptively with negative affect, from a skill perspective. That is, MT provides the patient with a set of skills that allows the patient to become more aware of automatic thoughts and resulting behaviors, and to accept and tolerate negative affect long enough to implement appropriate but relatively newly learned behavioral coping strategies. Medications address these issues by affecting neurochemical changes that either suppress automatic behaviors or negative affect or reduce the reinforcing properties of substances when used to cope with negative affects or to enhance positive ones.

Mindfulness

As noted in an earlier discussion, one of the major difficulties facing persons attempting to reduce or stop using alcohol or other drugs is defeating the overlearned automaticity of behavioral sequences conditioned to a variety stimuli, both internal and external. In addition, the ability to forestall the unfolding of these behavioral sequences in response to strong affective states, particularly negative ones, exacerbates the difficulty faced by many substance-dependent persons in maintaining changes in substance use. MT represents a

potential strategy to help patients cope with both of these threats to maintenance of changes in substance use.

MT and meditation have long been proposed as useful adjuncts in the
treatment of substance use disorders (Breslin, Zack, & McMain, 2002), and
they have a significant history in the treatment of other disorders in which the
ability to tolerate intense negative affect and inhibit maladaptive coping responses is an important aspect of treatment and maintenance of change. Thus,
mindfulness and other forms of meditation-based practice have been used successfully to help patients with chronic pain (Kabat-Zinn, Lipworth, Burney, &
Sellers, 1986), anxiety (Miller, Fletcher, & Kabat-Zinn, 1995), and recurrent
major depression (Segal, Williams, & Teasdale, 2002).

The focus of MT and related approaches such as radical acceptance as
taught in dialectical behavior therapy (DBT; Linehan, 1994) and acceptance
and commitment therapy (ACT; Hayes, Strosahl, & Wilson, 1999) is on helping patients accomplish two main tasks: (1) a global and full awareness of experience, and (2) an acceptance that experience is what it is, and is neither
good nor bad in itself. That is, the patient is taught to "have" experiences
rather than to "evaluate" and attempt to alter them. Learning the latter assists
patients in a third focus: inhibition of behaviors aimed at changing or eliminating experiences that the patient evaluates as negative.

MT has its origins in Eastern philosophies, most notably Buddhism. In
MT, patients are taught various techniques for focusing attention on what
William James (1892/2001) called the stream of consciousness. In addition to
becoming aware of conscious experience, patients are also taught to take a
particular psychological stance toward their experiences—one of uncritical
acceptance of experience as it is. MT is based on the premise that these two
abilities, awareness and nonjudgmental acceptance, can be taught in much the
same fashion as other skills. MT provides a variety of exercises and approaches, many based in Buddhist meditation practices, for learning these two
important skills. While often perceived as religious or spiritual in nature, MT
is actually neither of these, in and of itself. Rather, its focus is on helping
patients learn to attend to and accept aspects of experience over which they
exercise no direct control but which can be modified by a shift in the way in
which experience is (or is not) evaluated.

A number of manuals have been written in recent years that set forth basic training programs to teach mindfulness. These manuals provide an excellent basis for integrating MT into treatment, and therefore the specifics of MT
are not reviewed here in more than a cursory fashion using one or two examples. The reader is referred to volumes by Kabat-Zinn (1990) and Segal et al.
(2002) for a detailed discussion of the specifics of MT.

Aspects of MT have been incorporated for some time into the cognitive-
behavioral treatment of substance use disorders in the form of training in
"urge surfing" to help people cope with intense urges and desires to use their
substance of choice (Larimer et al., 1999). In urge surfing the patient is instructed to attend to and observe the cognitive and affective states associated

with urges and to "ride them out" rather than to attempt to suppress them. Although not as extensive or intensive as MT, urge surfing aims to accomplish the same goal—help the patient to inhibit impulsive, maladaptive behavioral responses to affect (e.g., using substances to suppress the affect). Urge surfing is premised on a large body of research that clearly demonstrates that efforts to suppress automatic thoughts and feelings typically leads to their exacerbation (Muraven, Collins, & Nienhaus, 2002). For example, trying to follow the instruction "don't think about pink elephants" results in an increased frequency of thoughts about pink elephants.

With respect to assisting in the maintenance of changes in substance use, Breslin et al. (2002) presented an excellent analysis of a rationale for the inclusion of MT in the toolkits of clinicians treating substance users. This rationale focuses specifically on the identification and interruption of automatic processes, both cognitive and behavioral, and on tolerance of negative affect. By becoming fully and nonjudgmentally aware of one's entire experience, and accepting it as real and not something to be eliminated (e.g., by self-medication with psychoactive substances), the patient in essence "buys time" in which it then becomes possible to both short-circuit drug-seeking behaviors and implement other cognitive and behavioral strategies for coping with the attended to experience and for avoiding an escalation of negative affect that might otherwise come about as a result of efforts to suppress it (Breslin et al., 2002).

In addition to urge surfing, examples of MT techniques that have been used with substance users include exercises that teach the patient to focus on his or her breathing. When attention wanders, rather than reacting with a sense of failure or dismay, the patient is taught to notice the wandering of attention and then to gently refocus on the breath. Each time attention wanders, as it almost inevitably will, the patient is taught to react to this fact as an interesting phenomenon to be noticed, observed, and then allowed to recede back into the stream of consciousness. Negative emotions that occur as part of the process are addressed in the same way—observed, accepted, and allowed (as they typically do when efforts to suppress or control them are avoided) to recede from awareness.

In the context of cognitive-behavioral treatment, MT provides the patient with a tool that allows a deescalation of negative affect and a concomitant implementation of cognitive and behavioral coping strategies that maintain changes. For example, if a patient is able to observe anger, accept it, and resist urges to suppress it in the moment by heading to the nearest bar and having a few drinks, he or she then buys time in which to refocus and implement more effective problem-solving and behavioral coping strategies. By defusing the immediate escape response when negative affect occurs, MT facilitates more appropriate coping.

Depending on the specific program of MT being used, MT itself can place somewhat onerous requirements on a patient. For example, the MT program developed by Kabat-Zinn (1990) and applied with success to the prevention of relapse in major depressive disorder by Segal et al. (2002) requires 8 weeks of intensive practice (45 minutes daily, 6 days per week) in addition to attending MT sessions. In contrast, the mindfulness and radical acceptance strategies that form a core component of Linehan's (1993) DBT are presented in a fashion that places fewer practice demands on the patient. Although there have been no studies comparing more intensive training and practice with the less intensive approach espoused by Linehan, it is reasonable to assume that many substance-dependent patients will have difficulty adhering to the sort of intensive practice schedule demanded in Kabat-Zinn's and Segal's MT programs. Until such research is done, it remains a clinical decision and contracting issue between clinician and patient that determines which of these approaches will best fit in with the demands of a particular patient's lifestyle.

Medication

While the use of medication is viewed by many clinicians as a primary treatment modality for many Axis I disorders, its status as an adjunct to treatment has been somewhat controversial in the case of substance use disorders. In this field the use of medications has been largely neglected, due in part to a therapeutic ideology that has held that the use of any psychoactive substances is inappropriate by persons attempting to overcome substance use problems. Thus, for many years, despite pleas and counter arguments from the central force in the recovery movement in the United States, Alcoholics Anonymous World Service Organization (Alcoholics Anonymous, 1984), there has been a belief that in order for a person to fully recover from a substance use disorder, he or she must abandon the use of all psychoactive substances, even those prescribed for treatment of other psychiatric disorders such as depression, anxiety, or schizophrenia (Rychtarik, Connors, Derman, & Stasiewicz, 2000).

As a result of this ideology, the use of medications as an adjunct in treating substance use disorders has been largely neglected by mainstream treatment providers, despite strong research support for their efficacy (Volpicelli, Pettinati, McLellan, & O'Brien, 2001; Ward, Mattick, & Hall, 1998). In fact, on one reading of the research literature, the approach to treating substance use disorders with the most empirical support is, in fact, a pharmacological one—opioid replacement (until recently, primarily in the form of methadone maintenance).

Although the use of medications in conjunction with psychosocial treatments for patients who suffer from co-occurring serious Axis I disorders such as major depression, bipolar disorder, or schizophrenia is rapidly becoming the standard of practice (Rosenthal & Westreich, 1999), the use of medication in less complicated cases is not as widely accepted. In addition to the ideological reasons for this lacuna in our therapeutic toolkit, the fact that there are relatively few substance-specific medications available has made the use of medications for the primary treatment of substance use disorders less widespread than the research suggests it should be. With the exception of alcohol and opioids, there are no medications currently approved for the treatment of substance use disorders. However, for both alcohol use and opioid use disorders, medications are available that can play a prominent role in treatment, and for some patients may be sufficient treatments in and of themselves. We review these medications in the sections that follow.

Alcohol Use Disorders

There are currently two medications approved by the Food and Drug Administration for the treatment of alcohol use disorders: disulfiram (marketed under the brand name Antabuse) and naltrexone (marketed under the brand name ReVia). Disulfiram acts to initiate a response cost contingency that occurs only when alcohol is consumed, and as such, for persons who experience the reaction triggered by disulfiram (approximately one-third of patients do not experience this reaction or they experience a reaction that produces only minor discomfort), it can act as a support to both the initiation and maintenance of abstinence, if abstinence is the patient's goal. As previously discussed, disulfiram seems to work best in conjunction with behavioral approaches such as the CRA, where the biochemical contingencies produced by disulfiram are bolstered by other psychosocial contingencies applied by significant others in the patient's environment (Meyers & Smith, 1995). When used in conjunction with other CM, disulfiram has been shown to be an effective means of preventing relapse to drinking, particularly in patients who demonstrate a "binge" pattern of drinking (i.e., a pattern characterized by long periods of abstinence interspersed with periods of intense alcohol consumption). The main issue with disulfiram, as with all medications, is adherence to the prescribed regimen of dosing. In the case of CRA, the medication and psychosocial interventions provide a mutually supportive set of contingencies that enhances the efficacy of both.

The other medication currently approved for treatment of alcohol use disorders is naltrexone. An opioid antagonist, naltrexone has been shown in two randomized clinical trials to be useful in preventing relapse in patients who are undergoing concurrent psychosocial treatment (O'Malley, Jaffe, Chang, Schottenfeld, Meyer, & Rounsaville, 1992; Volpicelli, Alterman, Hayashida, & O'Brien, 1992). Recent studies have also shown that naltrexone can be of use in assisting persons whose drinking goal is moderation rather than abstinence. Administered intermittently in anticipation of situations with a high drinking risk (e.g., a daughter's wedding) and in conjunction with a behaviorally focused moderation plan, naltrexone seems to be useful for helping "put the brakes" on drinking once it starts. Naltrexone appears to accomplish this by reducing the reinforcing effect of alcohol in patients taking it (Volpicelli, Watson, King, Sherman, & O'Brien, 1995).

Opioid Use Disorders

Until recently there were only a few pharmacological options in the treatment of opioid dependence, though the empirical support for the efficacy of these options was quite strong (Ward et al., 1998). Opioid replacement therapy (ORT) or the substitution of a legal, prescribed opioid for an illegal one (typically heroin, but often codeine or other prescription opioids) has been a mainstay of the treatment of opioid dependence, particularly with patients who have been unable to maintain abstinence following purely psychosocial treatments.

ORT, in the form of methadone maintenance, was often a burdensome treatment, requiring daily visits to a clinic to obtain the medication, a process that made it an onerous option for many patients. In 2003, however, the Food and Drug Administration approved an additional replacement medication, the partial agonist buprenorphine either alone (marketed as Subutex) or in combination with the antagonist naloxone (marketed as Suboxone), with provisions for office-based dispensing of these medications by physicians who have received specialized training (Fiellin & O'Connor, 2002). The provision to permit office-based prescription of these medications has broadened their acceptability to patients who might be resistant to the more stringently controlled methadone maintenance therapy. Clinical trials suggest that the buprenorphine preparations are as effective as methadone maintenance in preventing relapse to opioid use (Strain, Stitzer, Liebson, & Bigelow, 1994).

The use of ORT as an adjunct to cognitive-behavioral treatments is most reasonable with patients whose ultimate goal is to become drug free. Although there is no evidence-based reason to promote becoming drug free (in fact, the research on methadone maintenance therapy shows that patients who are on the treatment longer, do better on a variety of outcome indicators), patients often desire this outcome in the long run. For these patients, the use of ORT in conjunction with a cognitive-behavioral skills training program that incorporates the other adjuncts to enhancing outcomes discussed earlier, provides a window of opportunity for learning new skills without having to cope with the discomfort associated with opioid withdrawal or protracted withdrawal (Ward et al., 1998).

CASE EXAMPLE

It is often helpful to consider a clinical case example in understanding the process of integrating these approaches into a coherent treatment strategy. In the following case, we discuss how and where some of the aforementioned techniques were implemented with a particularly difficult client.

Rachel is a 41-year-old married woman with a 4-year-old daughter who was referred for aftercare following completion of a traditional, 12-step-oriented treatment program for treatment of alcohol dependence. With respect to education, Rachel had completed all but three courses toward a bachelor's degree. She had worked at a variety of sales jobs over the course of her life, before marrying and leaving the workforce to stay at home with her child. Her marriage was particularly rocky at the time she was referred. Her husband, a highly successful financial manager, had grown increasingly distant from

Rachel since the birth of their daughter, upon whom Rachel dotes. Although she had always been a heavy drinker, and intermittent user of other drugs (primarily marijuana and cocaine) Rachel's drinking only began to become a problem, in her view, following her marriage. Although she stopped drinking during her pregnancy, the year prior she had been consuming a bottle of wine or more nightly, and she recounted how, while pregnant, she counted the days until she could drink again. Once her daughter was born, her drinking gradually returned to her prepartum level and then escalated even further to the point where she would consume a quart of vodka every other day.

Rachel's entry into the rehab had been prompted by an incident in which she had a verbally violent argument with her husband, who she suspected of seeing other women, and who had continued to use both alcohol and cocaine, sometimes at home in front of Rachel. Following the argument Rachel had consumed nearly an entire quart of vodka and had been found passed out, partially clothed, on the lawn in front of her home. She did not remember any of the details of what happened but realized that she needed help and signed herself in to treatment.

When first seen for aftercare, Rachel was highly motivated to abstain and had committed herself to attending the 90 Alcoholics Anonymous (AA) meetings in 90 days that the rehab had recommended. We began work on identifying specific high-risk situations, most of which revolved around either conflicts with her husband or feelings of loneliness and inadequacy. Rachel was also seriously considering a divorce action but was concerned that her husband would gain custody of their daughter by pointing to Rachel's problems with alcohol. She was also totally dependent on her husband financially, and following her admission to rehab, and worried about Rachel driving under the influence with their daughter, he had taken away the car keys. Fortunately for Rachel, she was an avid cyclist, and she would ride to appointments and to other errands close to home.

After identifying high-risk situations and developing strategies to cope with them, Rachel began to experience difficulties. After nearly 6 months of abstinence, she resumed drinking to help relax following an argument with her husband. A functional analysis of the resumption of drinking revealed that Rachel had attempted to call her AA sponsor but could not connect. She had attempted to use urge surfing but had "talked herself out of it (continued abstinence)" when she realized that her husband would not be home and she could drink alone. She described her mood just prior to this slip, which had escalated into a full-blown lapse quite quickly, as one of depression and anger. The more she tried to suppress these feelings, the stronger the urge to drink became. Rachel reported strong expectancies that having a drink would be both self-indulgent and pleasant, and that it would not lead to further drinking. The next morning she awoke with a terrible hangover, and when her husband arrived home later that day, she was still feeling under the weather. He suspected that she had been drinking and verbally abused her as a result, threatening to leave with their daughter.

Although Rachel remained motivated toward abstinence, she was greatly discouraged by this lapse. We addressed it in several ways. First, we reinstituted and reviewed a decisional balance exercise she had been taught early in treatment for assisting in maintaining her commitment to abstinence. Rachel, herself, broached the idea of medication, saying she had heard of a drug (disulfiram) that "stops people from drinking by making them sick" but had never been willing to take it (due largely to the philosophy that had been instilled in her at the rehab that should only be "truly sober" if she was completely drug free).

In addition to the decisional balance, and a review of the utility of taking disulfiram (which Rachel decided to do), we also discussed and implemented a plan to have her taking of the disulfiram monitored by a close friend and neighbor who was supportive of Rachel's decision and who was taught how to verbally reinforce Rachel each time she took a dose of disulfiram.

Finally, based on Rachel's description of her unsuccessful attempts to rid herself of the depression and anger she felt (and continued to feel following her initial slip and lapse), we began MT aimed at enhancing Rachel's ability to tolerate negative affect and strong positive outcome expectancies for drinking without taking action on them. Cognitive restructuring and expectancy challenge via Socratic questioning of the validity of the thoughts leading up to her initial and subsequent drinks also helped Rachel to begin to develop another, more active coping mechanism for delaying action to suppress negative affect.

As of this writing, Rachel had been able to reestablish abstinence but still experienced periodic slips. Helping her "get back on the wagon" following a slip, and honing her affect tolerance and problem-solving skills, as well as addressing some of her depressogenic and anger generating thinking, has helped her lengthen the periods of abstinence and keep the length of slips/lapse limited. In addition, treatment has begun to focus on helping Rachel make plans for how she could enhance her ability to leave her troubled marriage, which she has concluded is not salvageable. Rachel continues to find support through AA and is also still taking disulfiram, which she has always discontinued prior to a slip but has always resumed subsequently, once her current feelings of depression, anger, and shame at slipping have been reduced.

CONCLUSION

The effective treatment of substance use disorders, regardless of the specific treatment approach, depends heavily on maintaining patient motivation and commitment to reduced use or abstinence, and to facilitating the implementation of adaptive coping strategies that are taught in treatment. We have discussed a number of approaches that have shown promise in recent research for helping accomplish these goals. Despite significant progress in this area, much remains to be done to improve treatment outcomes and behavior change maintenance in patients treated for substance use disorders.

Unlike most other psychiatric disorders, substance use disorders often carry with them a complex of nonclinical "baggage" that often interferes with effective treatment, despite the decades-long attempt to shift societal attitudes about these disorders from one of moral and legal opprobrium to a focus on substance use disorders as a health issue. An example of such "baggage" is the fact that the very behavior that initiates substance use disorders is illegal for the vast majority of citizens. This means that in addition to confronting the behavioral difficulties that persons suffering from these disorders must face in order to change their behavior, clinicians are often confronted with patients who come to them as a result of involvement in the criminal justice system. This involvement brings with it a degree of constraint and difficulty in clinical practice that is absent in the treatment of most other Axis I disorders, with rare exceptions (e.g., situations in which patients are a danger to self or others). The criminal justice system often sets as the only acceptable goal for substance using offenders complete and total abstinence from all nonprescribed psychoactive substances. Any slip or lapse at all is often responded to with zero tolerance, despite that fact that decades of clinical research has shown both that occasional slips are highly likely and not necessarily indicative of failure, and that substance use disorders are, by their very nature, highly variable. This constraint often makes it difficult for clinicians to adopt the most clinically reasonable approach to working with a particular client.

This difficulty is particularly marked when using approaches such as those described in this chapter (e.g., MI, CRA, MT) which by their nature are patient focused, often relying on slips to enhance motivation or to address critical issues that were not apparent early in treatment, or which may, in some circumstances actually "program" a slip as a way of enhancing coping skills (Marlatt & Gordon, 1985). Although we have no ready remedy for the difficulties presented by such patients, we do suggest that clinicians make every attempt to justify clinically and research supported interventions, even when these interventions appear to conflict with the agenda of other systems in which the patient may be involved. To society's credit, there are some jurisdictions in which there is greater recognition of the clinical realities that affect patient efforts to reduce or stop their use of psychoactive substances, particularly with the advent of the drug court approach to drug offenders (Shavelson, 2001). We hope that these shifts in the approach to dealing with substance users will continue to grow and expand.

Finally, we want to mention the emerging philosophy of harm reduction with respect to substance use and its consequences (Marlatt, 1998). Much of what we have written about in this chapter is highly consistent with a gradualist, patient-focused philosophy such as harm reduction. A shift from a dominant focus on a single behavior—substance use—to a broader consideration of patient needs, strengths, and weaknesses, seems to us to be much more consistent with the dominant medical/disease model of substance use disorders in the United States than is the current practice. We believe that if we can work to move substance use disorders squarely into the realm of health-related behaviors and begin to think about them in terms similar to those we adopt in addressing other chronic health conditions, we will do our patients and society a great service (O'Brien & McLellan, 1996).

REFERENCES

Alcoholics Anonymous. (1984). *The A.A. member: Medications and other drugs.* New York: AA World Service Organization.

American Psychiatric Association. (2000). *Diagnostic and statistical manual of mental disorders* (4th ed., text rev.). Washington, DC: Author.

Annis, H. M., & Graham, J. M. (1988). *Situational Confidence Questionnaire (SCQ-39) user's guide.* Toronto, Ontario, Canda: Alcoholism and Drug Addiction Research Foundation.

Annis, H. M., & Graham, J. M. (1995). Profile types on the Inventory of Drinking Situations: Implications for relapse prevention counseling. *Psychology of Addictive Behaviors, 9,* 176–182.

Annis, H., Martin, G., & Graham, J. M. (1992). *Inventory of Drug-Taking Situations: Users' guide.* Toronto, Ontario, Canada: Addiction Research Foundation.

Ayllon, T., & Azrin, N. H. (1968). *The token economy: A motivational system for therapy and rehabilitation.* East Norwalk, CT: Appleton-Century-Crofts.

Breslin, F. C., Zack, M., & McMain, S. (2002). An information-processing analysis of mindfulness: Implications for relapse prevention in the treatment of substance abuse. *Clinical Psychology: Science and Practice, 9,* 275–299.

Budney, A. J., & Higgins, S. T. (1998). *A community reinforcement plus vouchers approach: Treating cocaine addiction* (National Institute on Drug Abuse Therapy Manuals for Addiction, Manual 2; NIH Publication Number 98-4309). Rockville, MD: National Institutes of Health.

Crits-Christoph, P., Gibbons, M. B. C., Barber, J. P., Gallop, R., Beck, A. T., Mercer, D., Tu, X., Thase, M. E., Weiss, R. D., & Frank, A. (2003). Mediators of outcome of psychosocial treatments for cocaine dependence. *Journal of Consulting and Clinical Psychology, 71,* 918–925.

DiClemente, C. C., & Prochaska, J. O. (1998). Toward a comprehensive, transtheoretical model of change: Stages of change and addictive behaviors. In W. R. Miller & N. Heather (Eds.), *Treating addictive behaviors* (2nd ed., pp. 3–24). New York: Plenum Press.

Fiellin, D. A., & O'Connor, P. G. (2002). Office-based treatment of opioid dependent patients. *New England Journal of Medicine, 347,* 817–823.

Fletcher, A. M. (2001). *Sober for good: New solutions for drinking problems—Advice from those who have succeeded.* Boston: Houghton Mifflin.

French, M. T., Sacks, S., De Leon, G., Staines, G., & McKendrick, K. (1999). Modified therapeutic community for mentally ill chemical abusers: Outcomes and costs. *Evaluation and the Health Professions, 22,* 60–85.

Gossop, M., Harris, J., Best, D., Man, L., Manning, V., Marshall, J., & Strang, J. (2003). Is attendance at Alcoholics Anonymous meetings after inpatient treatment related to improved outcomes? A 6-month follow-up study. *Alcohol and Alcoholism, 38,* 421–426.

Hall, S. M., Havassy, B. E., & Wasserman, D. A. (1990). Commitment to abstinence and acute stress in relapse to alcohol, opiates and nicotine. *Journal of Consulting and Clinical Psychology, 58,* 175–181.

Hasin, D. (2003). Classification of alcohol use disorders. *Alcohol Research and Health, 27,* 5–17.

Hayes, S. C., Strosahl, K. D., & Wilson, K. G. (1999). *Acceptance and commitment therapy: An experiential approach to behavior change.* New York: Guilford Press.

Hester, R. K., & Miller, W. R. (2003). Preface. In R. K. Hester & W. R. Miller (Eds.), *Handbook of alcoholism treatment approaches: Effective alternatives* (3rd ed., pp. ix–x). Boston: Allyn & Bacon.

Higgins, S. T., Budney, A. J., Bickel, W. K., Foerg, F. E., Donham, R., & Badger, G. J. (1994). Incentives improve outcome in outpatient behavioral treatment of cocaine dependence. *Archives of General Psychiatry, 51,* 568–576.

Hiller, M. L., Knight, K., Broome, K. M., & Simpson, D. D. (1998). Legal pressure and treatment retention in a national sample of long-term residential programs. *Criminal Justice and Behavior, 25,* 463–482.

Hiller, M. L., Knight, K., Leukefeld, C., & Simpson, D. D. (2002). Motivation as a predictor of therapeutic engagement in mandated residential substance abuse treatment. *Criminal Justice and Behavior, 29,* 56–75.

Horvath, A. T., & Velten, E. (2000). Smart Recovery®?: Addiction recovery support from a cognitive-behavioral perspective. *Journal of Rational-Emotive and Cognitive-Behavior Therapy, 18,* 181–191.

Humphreys, K., & Klaw, E. (2001). Can targeting nondependent problem drinkers and providing internet-based services expand access to assistance for alcohol problems? A study of the moderation management self-help/mutual aid organization. *Journal of Studies on Alcohol, 62,* 528–532.

Hunt, G. M., & Azrin, N. H. (1973). A community-reinforcement approach to alcoholism. *Behaviour Research and Therapy, 11,* 91–104.

James, W. (2001). *Psychology: The briefer course.* Mineola, NY: Dover. (Original work published 1892)

Kabat-Zinn, J. (1990). *Full catastrophe living: Using the wisdom of your body and mind to face stress, pain and illness.* New York: Dell.

Kabat-Zinn, J., Lipworth, L., Burney, R., & Sellers, W. (1986). Four-year follow-up of a meditation-based program for self-regulation of chronic pain: Treatment outcomes and compliance. *Clinical Journal of Pain, 2,* 159–173.

Khantzian, E. J. (1985). The self-medication hypothesis of addictive disorders: Focus on heroin and cocaine dependence. *American Journal of Psychiatry, 142,* 1259–1264.

Larimer, M. E., Palmer, R. S., & Marlatt, G. A. (1999). Relapse prevention: An overview of Marlatt's cognitive behavioral model. *Alcohol Research and Health, 23,* 151–160.

Lazarus, R., & Folkman, S. (1984). Stress, appraisal, and coping. New York: Springer.

Leigh, B. C., & Stacy, A. W. (2004). Alcohol expectancies and drinking in different age groups. *Addiction, 99,* 215–227.

Leshner, A. I. (1997). Addiction is a brain disease, and it matters. *Science, 278,* 45–47.

Linehan, M. M. (1993). *Cognitive-behavioral treatment of borderline personality disorder.* New York: Guilford Press.

Linehan, M. M. (1994). Acceptance and change: The central dialectic in psychotherapy. In S. C. Hayes, N. S. Jacobson, V. M. Follette, & M. J. Dougher (Eds.), *Acceptance and change: Content and context in psychotherapy,* (pp. 73–86). Reno, NV: Context Press.

Maltzman, I. (1994). Why alcoholism is a disease. *Journal of Psychoactive Drugs, 26,* 13–31.

Marlatt, G. A. (Ed.). (1998). *Harm reduction: Pragmatic strategies for managing high-risk behaviors.* New York: Guilford Press.

Marlatt, G. A., Blume, A. W., & Parks, G. A. (2001). Integrating harm reduction therapy and traditional substance abuse treatment. *Journal of Psychoactive Drugs, 33,* 13–21.

Marlatt, G. A., & Gordon, J. G. (Eds.). (1985). *Relapse prevention: Maintenance strategies in the treatment of addictive behaviors.* New York: Guilford Press.

Martin, G. W., Wilkinson, D. A., & Poulos, C. X. (1995). The Drug Avoidance Self-Efficacy Scale. *Journal of Substance Abuse, 7,* 151–163.

Metzger, L. (1988). *From denial to recovery: Counseling problem drinkers, alcoholics and their families.* San Francisco: Jossey-Bass.

Meyers, R., J., & Smith, J. E. (1995). *Clinical guide to alcohol treatment: The community reinforcement approach.* New York: Guilford Press.

Miller, J. J., Fletcher, K., & Kabat-Zinn, J. (1995).Three-year follow-up and clinical implications of a mindfulness meditation-based stress reduction intervention in the treatment of anxiety disorders. *General Hospital Psychiatry, 17,* 192–200.

Miller, W. R. (1985). Motivation for treatment: A review with special emphasis on alcoholism. *Psychological Bulletin, 98,* 84–107.

Miller, W. R. (2000). Rediscovering fire: Small interventions, large effects. *Psychology of Addictive Behaviors, 14,* 6–18.

Miller, W. R., Brown, J. M., Simpson, T. L., Handmaker, N. S., Bien, T. H., Luckie, L. F., Montgomery, H. A., Hester, R. K., & Tonigan, J. S. (1995). What works? A methodological analysis of the alcohol treatment outcome literature. In R. K. Hester & W. R. Miller (Eds.), *Handbook of alcoholism treatment approaches: Effective alternatives* (2nd ed., pp. 12–44). Boston: Allyn & Bacon.

Miller, W. R., & Rollnick, S. (1991). *Motivational interviewing: Preparing people to change addictive behavior.* New York: Guilford Press.

Miller, W. R., & Rollnick, S. (2002). *Motivational interviewing: Preparing people to change* (2nd ed.). New York: Guilford Press.

Miller, W. R., Walters, S. T., & Bennett, M. E. (2001). How effective is alcoholism treatment in the United States? *Journal of Studies on Alcohol, 62,* 211–220.

Miller, W. R., Wilbourne, P. L., & Hettema, J. E. (2003). What works? A Summary of alcohol treatment outcome research. In R. K. Hester & W. R. Miller (Eds.), *Handbook of alcoholism treatment approaches: Effective alternatives* (3rd ed., pp. 13–63). Boston: Allyn & Bacon.

Morgenstern, J. M., Frey, R., McCrady, B., Labouvie, E., & Neighbors, C. (1996). Mediators of change in traditional chemical dependency treatment. *Journal of Studies on Alcohol, 57,* 53–64.

Muraven, M., Collins, R. L., & Nienhaus, K. (2002). Self-control and alcohol restraint: An initial application of the self-control strength model. *Psychology of Addictive Behaviors, 16,* 113–120.

O'Brien, C. P., & McLellan, A. T. (1996). Myths about the treatment of addiction. *The Lancet, 347,* 237–240.

O'Malley, S. S., Jaffe, A. J., Chang, G., Schottenfeld, R. S., Meyer, R. E., & Rounsaville, B. (1992). Naltrexone and coping skills therapy for alcohol dependence. *Archives of General Psychiatry, 49,* 881–887.

Project MATCH Research Group. (1997). Matching alcoholism treatments to client heterogeneity: Project MATCH posttreatment drinking outcomes. *Journal of Studies on Alcohol, 58*, 7–29.

Regier, D. A., Farmer, M. E., Rae, D. S., Locke, B. Z., Keith, S. J., Judd, L. L., & Goodwin, F. K. (1990). Comorbidity of mental disorder with alcohol and other drug abuse: Results from the Epidemiologic Catchment Area (ECA) Study. *Journal of the American Medical Association, 264*, 2511–2518.

Roizen, R. (1987). The great controlled-drinking controversy. In M. Galanter (Ed.), *Recent Developments in Alcoholism* (Vol. 5, pp. 245–279). New York: Plenum Press.

Rosenberg, H., & Davis, L. A. (1994). Acceptance of moderate drinking by alcohol treatment services in the United States. *Journal of Studies on Alcohol, 55*, 167–172.

Rosenthal, R. N., & Westreich, L. (1999). Treatment of persons with dual diagnosis of substance use disorder and other psychological problems. In B. S. McCrady & E. E. Epstein (Eds.), *Addictions: A comprehensive guidebook* (pp. 439–476). New York: Oxford University Press.

Rotgers, F., & Kishline, A. (1999). Moderation Management®: A support group for persons who want to reduce their drinking, but not necessarily abstain. *International Journal of Self Help and Self Care, 1*, 145–158.

Rounsaville, B. J., Bryant, K., Babor, T., Kranzler, H., & Kadden, R. (1993). Cross system agreement for substance use disorders: DSM-III-R, DSM-IV and ICD-10. *Addiction, 88*, 337–348.

Ryan, R. M., & Deci, E. L. (2000). Self-determination theory and the facilitation of intrinsic motivation, social development and well-being. *American Psychologist, 55*, 68–78.

Rychtarik, R. G., Connors, G. J., Derman, K. H., & Stasiewicz, P. R. (2000). Alcoholics Anonymous and the use of medication to prevent relapse: A anonymous survey of member attitudes. *Journal of Studies on Alcohol, 61*, 134–138.

Rychtarik, R. G., Prue, D. M., Rapp, S. R., & King, A. C. (1992). Self-efficacy, aftercare and relapse in a treatment program for alcoholics. *Journal of Studies on Alcohol, 53*, 435–440.

Sanchez-Craig, M., & Lei, H. (1986). Disadvantages to imposing the goal of abstinence on problem drinkers. *British Journal of Addiction, 81*, 505–512.

Segal, Z. V., Williams, J. M. G., & Teasdale, J. D. (2002). *Mindfulness-based cognitive therapy for depression: A new approach to preventing relapse.* New York: Guilford Press.

Shavelson, L. (2001). *Hooked: Five addicts challenge our misguided drug rehab system.* New York: Free Press.

Simpson, D. D., Joe, G. W., & Broome, K. M. (2002). A national 5-year follow-up of treatment outcomes for cocaine dependence. *Archives of General Psychiatry, 59*, 538–544.

Stotts, A. L., Schmitz, J. M., Rhoades, H. M., & Grabowski, J. (2001). Motivational interviewing with cocaine-dependent patients: A pilot study. *Journal of Consulting and Clinical Psychology, 69*, 858–862.

Strain, E. C., Stitzer, M. L., Liebson, I. A., & Bigelow, G. E. (1994). Comparison of buprenorphine and methadone in the treatment of opioid dependence. *American Journal of Psychiatry, 151*, 1025–1030.

Tiffany, S. T. (1990). A cognitive model of drug urges and drug-use behavior: Role of automatic and nonautomatic processes. *Psychological Review, 97*, 147–168.

Tucker, J. A., Vuchinich, R. E., & Murphy, J. G. (2002). Substance use disorders. In M.

M. Antony & D. H. Barlow (Eds.), *Handbook of assessment and treatment planning for psychological disorders* (pp. 415–452). New York: Guilford Press.

Volpicelli, J. R., Alterman, A. A., Hayashida, M., & O'Brien, C. P. (1992). Naltrexone in the treatment of alcohol dependence. *Archives of General Psychiatry, 49*, 876–880.

Volpicelli, J. R., Pettinati, H. M., McLellan, A. T., & O'Brien, C. P. (2001). *Combining medication and psychosocial treatments for addictions: The BRENDA approach.* New York: Guilford Press.

Volpicelli, J. R., Watson, N. T., King, A. C., Sherman, C., & O'Brien, C. P. (1995). Effect of naltrexone on alcohol "high" in alcoholics. *American Journal of Psychiatry, 152*, 613–615.

Walters, G. D. (2000). Behavioral self-control training for problem drinkers: A meta-analysis of randomized control studies, *Behavior Therapy, 31*, 135–149.

Ward, J., Mattick, R. P., & Hall, W. (1998). *Methadone maintenance treatment and other opioid replacement therapies.* Amsterdam: Harwood Academic Publishers.

World Health Organization. (1992). *International statistical classification of diseases and related health problems, 1989 revision.* Geneva, Switzerland: Author.

11

Couple Distress

MARK A. WHISMAN
MARGARET L. McKELVIE
YAEL CHATAV

OVERVIEW OF THE DISORDER

Couple or relationship distress (or "discord" or "dissatisfaction") is a common problem encountered by many people. In the fourth edition of *Diagnostic and Statistical Manual of Mental Disorders* (DSM-IV; American Psychiatric Association, 1994), relationship distress is discussed as one of the "other conditions that may be a focus of clinical attention" (i.e., a V code). Specifically, "partner relational problem" is used to define a pattern of interaction between spouses or partners that is characterized by negative communication, distorted communication, or noncommunication. Although there have been some recent attempts to develop diagnostic interviews for classifying relationship distress similar to methods used for making other DSM-IV diagnoses (Heyman, Feldbau-Kohn, Ehrensaft, Langhinrichsen-Rohling, & O'Leary, 2001), the most frequent method for determining couple distress is to use a cutoff score on one of the commonly used self-report measures of relationship distress. For example, cutoffs of 100 on the Marital Adjustment Test (Locke & Wallace, 1959), 97 on the Dyadic Adjustment Scale (Spanier, 1989), or a *T* score of 59 on the Global Distress Scale of the Marital Satisfaction Inventory—Revised (Snyder, 1997) are frequently used to define relationship distress.

Potential exposure to relationship distress and other negative relationship outcomes, such as divorce, is very widespread. For example, it has been estimated that within the United States, most people (> 90%) will marry by the end of their lives (Kreider & Fields, 2001), that many people who do not marry will live with a partner in nonmarital (e.g., cohabiting) familial relationships (Seltzer, 2000), that approximately 16–20% of individuals are dissatisfied with their marriage or cohabiting relationship at any given time (e.g., Hjemboe & Butcher, 1991; Ren, 1997), and that nearly 50% of recent marriages may end in separation or divorce (Kreider & Fields, 2001)—20% will end in separation or divorce within the first 5 years of marriage, and 33% will end within the first 10 years (Bramlett & Mosher, 2001). The rate of divorce is also high in Europe, with divorce rates of approximately 40–50% in Northern European countries such as Norway, Sweden, Denmark, and Finland, and 30–40% for France, Germany, and other Western European countries (Bodenmann, 1997).

There is also a large body of literature suggesting that the presence of relationship distress is associated with a variety of negative outcomes. For example, relationship distress has been shown to be associated with physical (for a review, see Kiecolt-Glaser & Newton, 2001) and mental health problems (for a review, see Whisman & Uebelacker, 2003). In addition, relationship distress is associated with elevated rates of physical aggression (for a review, see Holtzworth-Munroe, Smutzler, Bates, & Sandin, 1997), and with mental health and adjustment problems in children (for a review, see Cummings & Davies, 2002). Furthermore, it has been shown that relationship distress is associated with work loss, particularly among men in their first 10 years of marriage, and that this work loss translates into a loss of approximately $6.8 billion per year in the United States (Forthofer, Markman, Cox, Stanley, & Kessler, 1996). Thus, it is not surprising that relationship problems are one of the most common reasons for people to seek services from mental health practitioners.

OVERVIEW OF EMPIRICALLY SUPPORTED TREATMENTS

Behavioral Couple Therapy

Behavioral couple therapy (BCT) is a social learning-based approach for treating relationship distress that views distress in terms of behavioral patterns that are rewarded and punished (Jacobson & Margolin, 1979). BCT is a skills-oriented approach to couple counseling that emphasizes three sets of skills to improve distressed relationships. The first set of skills are "behavioral exchange" strategies, which focus on helping each person pinpoint specific positive behaviors (i.e., "caring behaviors") and negative behaviors that are associated with their partner's level of satisfaction. Both partners are encouraged to increase the frequency of positive behaviors and decrease the frequency of negative behaviors. The second set of skills are expressive and receptive communication skills. Therapists provide specific guidelines for couples on ways to communicate without accusations and blame, and how to use active (i.e., empathic) listening skills. The third set of skills are those needed for effective problem solving or problem resolution. The problem-solving process is broken down into several steps, including problem definition, brainstorming, decision making, and implementation. Couples use these skills to work with problems in their relationship, starting with smaller problems and moving through to larger problems.

The effectiveness of BCT in improving relationship distress has been documented in both narrative (Baucom, Shoham, Mueser, Daiuto, & Stickle, 1998; Christensen & Heavey, 1999) and meta-analytic reviews (Dunn & Schwebel, 1995; Hahlweg & Markman, 1988; Shadish et al., 1993). Although the reviews have differed somewhat in the criteria used for evaluating efficacy, they converge in concluding that BCT is efficacious in the treatment of relationship distress. For example, in a meta-analysis of 17 BCT studies conducted between 1976 and 1984, Hahlweg and Markman (1988) reported a mean effect size of 0.95. These authors discuss how this effect size translates into a 67% improvement rate for BCT, compared to a 33% improvement rate for people not in treatment. In addition, there was no significant difference in the effect size for studies conducted in the United States versus those conducted in Europe, which supports the cross-cultural generalizability of the efficacy of BCT.

Building on the initial results by Hahlweg and Markman (1988), Dunn and Schwebel (1995) examined the findings of 11 studies published between 1980 and 1993 that investigated the effectiveness of BCT as compared to control conditions. Results showed that BCT promoted significant changes in observed behavior and self-reported measures of relationship quality, with a weighted mean effect size of 0.79 and 0.78, respectively. Thus, based on these meta-analyses, BCT appears to be an efficacious treatment for distressed couples. According to the criteria discussed by Chambless and Hollon (1998) for defining empirically supported therapies, BCT meets criteria for an efficacious and specific treatment for relationship distress (Baucom et al., 1998).

It is important to note that the criteria for establishing efficacy, which emphasize statistically significant differences between groups in mean levels of satisfaction, provide little information as to the percentage of people who are likely to improve following therapy. In comparison, clinical significance focuses on change at the level of the individual (or, in the case of couple therapy, the couple). Although there are several methods for defining clinical significance (Jacobson & Revenstorf, 1988), the method reported by Jacobson and colleagues (Jacobson, Follette, & Revenstorf, 1984; Jacobson & Truax, 1991) is perhaps the most commonly employed. According to this perspective, clinically significant change is defined as having occurred when a couple (or individual) moves from the distressed population at the beginning of treatment to the nondistressed population at the end of treatment, as defined by one of the following criteria: at least two standard deviations above the mean for the distressed group, within two standard deviations of the mean for the nondistressed group, or closer to the mean of the nondistressed group than the mean of the distressed group. Furthermore, Jacobson and colleagues underscored that clinically significant change should also be statistically reliable change. Consequently, they developed the "reliable change index," often described in terms of "improvement," which is defined as having occurred when dividing the difference between the pre- and posttest scores by the standard error of the difference scores is greater than 1.96. When criteria for both clinical significance and reliable change have been met, recovery is said to have occurred. According to these criteria, approximately one-third to one-half of couples are likely to recover following treatment (Baucom et al., 1998; Jacobson, Follette, Revenstorf, et al., 1984).

In discussing the efficacy of couple therapy, it is important to note that in the assessment of treatment outcome, an increase in relationship satisfaction is used to measure a treatment's success, whereas the termination of the relationship is judged to be a negative outcome (Baucom et al., 1998). However, many investigators acknowledge that divorce or relationship dissolution can, in some cases, be a mutually agreed upon positive resolution to an unhealthy relationship. It is difficult to come up with a reasonable alternative to the classification of divorce as a negative treatment outcome in the evaluation of couples therapy (for a discussion on one method of evaluating individualized outcomes such as deciding whether to end a relationship, see Whisman & Snyder, 1997). To date, investigators have been unable to effectively deal with this conundrum. Thus, until investigators come up with a viable alternative, the criteria for successful treatment of couple distress will remain an increase in marital adjustment, whereas the dissolution of a relationship will continue to be classified as a negative outcome.

Cognitive-Behavioral Couple Therapy

Based on the finding that not all couples improve with BCT, investigators have attempted to incorporate a cognitive intervention to BCT to strengthen its effectiveness (Baucom et al., 1998). The resulting treatment—cognitive-behavioral couple therapy (CBCT)—incorporates an emphasis on the identification of unrealistic and maladaptive beliefs and expectations in the relationship, and their replacement with more realistic and helpful beliefs (Epstein & Baucom, 2002). The goal of cognitive interventions is to enable partners to identify and modify maladaptive relationship cognitions.

To date, there have been three studies that have assessed whether CBCT produces enhanced treatment outcome compared to BCT alone. In the first study, Baucom and Lester (1986) randomly assigned 24 couples to three experimental conditions: BCT alone, BCT plus cognitive restructuring, and a wait-list control group. The cognitive component of the combined treatment focused on partners' attributions and expectations. Results indicated that couples who were randomly assigned to the two treatment conditions demonstrated significant improvements on levels of marital satisfaction at the termination of the 12-week treatment and at 6-month follow-up. A direct comparison of the two treatment groups, however, indicated that there were no significant differences on outcome measures between BCT alone and the enhanced BCT treatment.

In a subsequent study, Baucom, Sayers, and Sher (1990) compared a BCT alone condition to BCT plus cognitive restructuring (CR), BCT plus emotional expressiveness training (EET), BCT plus CR and EET, and a wait-list control group among 60 couples. The CR component focused on attributions and unrealistic standards, and the EET component focused on the expression of emotion and the development of effective listening skills. After 12 weeks of treatment, results indicated that couples assigned to all four treatment groups demonstrated greater improvement in marital adjustment as compared to couples in the control condition. However, comparisons between treatment conditions indicated that the addition of CR and EET did not appear to enhance BCT effectiveness, in terms of either statistical or clinical significance.

Within a similar research paradigm as described earlier, Halford, Sanders, and Behrens (1993) compared BCT alone to an enhanced BCT (EBCT) condition among 26 couples. The EBCT evolved from the studies that had been conducted by Baucom and colleagues in that it incorporated their CR techniques and a component that focused on affect exploration. Halford et al. found that BCT and EBCT were equally effective in demonstrating significant increases in self-reported marital satisfaction, as well as decreases in interactional negativity, unrealistic cognitions, and negative affect. Moreover, the effects of both treatments appeared to generalize to the home environment (as measured by the coding of couple interactions in the home).

In addition to evaluating the efficacy of combining cognitive interventions with BCT, investigators have also explored the efficacy of cognitive therapy alone in the treatment of relationship distress. In one such study, Huber and Milstein (1985) compared a CR-only treatment for relationship distress to a wait-list control group. The investigators found that interventions directed at modifying unrealistic beliefs about marriage, the self, and one's partner were effective in increasing satisfaction. In a similar study, Emmelkamp et al. (1988) compared CR alone to a communication skills training condition. The CR focused on the identification of causal attributions that distressed couples gave for relationship problems, as well as on the correction of maladaptive attributions. Emmelkamp et al. reported that both treatments were equally effective in decreasing target problems identified by the couples at pretreatment.

As evidenced by this review of the literature, various cognitive approaches for the treatment of relationship distress have been investigated with equivocal success. Given the diversity of approaches described previously, it is difficult to form firm conclusions regarding cognitive approaches for relationship distress. However, two conclusions seem apparent. First, CBCT and cognitive therapy for couples appear to be effective in improving relationship distress. This was the conclusion reached by Dunn and Schwebel (1995) in their meta-analytic review of couple therapy. Specifically, they found that CBCT produced significant effects on behavior, with a weighted mean effect size of 0.54 at posttreatment and 0.75 at follow-up. Significant treatment effects were also demonstrated by CBCT on relationship satisfaction measures, with an effect size of 0.71 at posttreatment and 0.54 at follow-up. According to the criteria discussed by Chambless and Hollon (1998) for defining empirically supported therapies, CBCT and cognitive therapy for couples meet criteria for possibly efficacious treatments (Baucom et al., 1998). A second conclusion that can be drawn from the research conducted to date suggests that CBCT does not seem to be more effective than BCT in improving relationship distress.

In interpreting the apparent comparative efficacy of CBCT and BCT, it is also important to note the substantial overlap that might result from both cognitive and behavioral approaches. The findings of equal efficacy described previously may very likely reflect the reciprocal relationship between cognition and behavior. In fact, results from the studies conducted by Baucom and colleagues (Baucom & Lester, 1986; Baucom et al., 1990) indicated that women in behavioral treatment only demonstrated significant change in both behavior *and* cognition at posttreatment. Moreover, Emmelkamp et al. (1988) reported changes in both cognition and behavior among couples enrolled in a strict cognitive condition and for those enrolled in a communication skills training condition. Additional focus on the specificity of cognitive therapy and its effects should attempt to generate greater understanding of its use for the treatment of relationship distress.

Finally, investigators have noted that random assignment of participants to study groups within the investigations described earlier might have resulted in diluted treatment effects. That is, random assignment restricts the matching of client needs to a specific treatment, as is employed in most treatment settings. Anecdotal evidence suggests that certain couples might benefit more from an approach that includes a cognitive component whereas others might benefit more from a strict behavioral approach (Baucom & Lester, 1986; Baucom et al., 1990). Additional efficacy studies will be necessary to identify moderating factors and to determine their impact on an effective cognitive approach to couple therapy.

Because both early (Jacobson & Margolin, 1979) and recent (Epstein & Baucom, 2002) treatment manuals have included cognitive interventions in their descriptions of the treatment, the term "cognitive behavioral couple therapy" (or CBCT) is used in the remainder of this chapter to describe the general treatment. However, "behavioral couple therapy" (or BCT) is used to refer to interventions that exclusively focus on behavioral aspects of relationship functioning.

Couple Therapy in the Treatment of Mental or Physical Health Problems

Although originally developed as a treatment for relationship distress, CBCT has also been shown to be effective in treating a variety of adult mental health problems, which are typically discussed in terms of "individual" psychiatric disorders (for a review, see Baucom et al., 1998). Couple-based treatment strategies for individual disorders are based on the assumption that distressed couples' functioning may contribute to the development or maintenance of an individual's symptoms. According to this logic, individual psychopathology should be addressed in the context of one's relationship because stressors within the relationship could lead to or aggravate an individual's psychological difficulties.

The efficacy of CBCT as the sole treatment for distressed couples in which the wife is clinically depressed has been evaluated in two investigations (Jacobson, Dobson, Fruzzetti, Schmaling, & Salusky, 1991; O'Leary & Beach, 1990). In terms of alleviating depression, both studies found that CBCT was as effective as cognitive therapy, which is currently the "gold" standard individual treatment for depression (Hollon, Thase, & Markowitz, 2002). Furthermore, O'Leary and Beach found that CBCT was more effective than a wait-list condition in alleviating depression. However, CBCT was less effective than cognitive therapy for couples who were not distressed (Jacobson et al., 1991). Finally, both studies found that couple therapy was more effective than individual cognitive therapy in terms of improving relationship satisfaction.

As reviewed by Epstein and McCrady (1998) and O'Farrell and Fals-Stewart (2000), BCT has also been shown to be effective in the treatment of alcoholism and drug abuse. Specifically, results from clinical trials of BCT for alcoholism and for drug abuse indicate that BCT "produces more abstinence and fewer substance-related problems, happier relationships, fewer couple separations and lower risk of divorce than does individual-based treatments" (O'Farrell & Fals-Stewart, 2000, p. 51). In addition, BCT has also been shown to reduce domestic violence in alcohol- and drug-abusing individuals (O'Farrell & Fals-Stewart, 2000). Finally, cost outcomes for BCT are favorable for both alcoholism and drug abuse and are superior to individual-based treatment for drug abuse (O'Farrell & Fals-Stewart, 2000).

Finally, couple therapists have more recently begun to develop couple-based approaches to other Axis I disorders, Axis II (i.e., personality) disorders, cognitive disorders secondary to aging, and a variety of physical health problems (Gurman & Jacobson, 2002; Schmaling & Sher, 2000; Snyder & Whisman, 2003). With knowledge of these most recent developments, couple therapists can be equipped to work with a wide range of mental and physical health problems that are likely to co-occur with relationship distress.

PREDICTORS OF TREATMENT OUTCOME

In evaluating predictors of treatment outcome, investigators have evaluated a range of predictor variables. As a heuristic for organizing these predictor variables, we have categorized the various predictors in one of three sets of variables: demographic characteristics, relationship characteristics, and individual characteristics. We turn now to a brief review of these three sets of predictor variables.

Demographic Characteristics

The first set of variables that has been evaluated in predicting outcome includes demographic characteristics of the couples in therapy. Some studies have found that younger couples respond more favorably to couple therapy (Baucom, 1984; Hahlweg, Schindler, Revenstorf, & Brengelmann, 1984; Turkewitz & O'Leary, 1981), whereas other studies have found no association between age and treatment outcome (Crowe, 1978; Jacobson, Follette, & Pagel, 1986). In addition, Crowe (1978) found that education was negatively correlated with outcome.

Relationship Characteristics

A second set of variables that has been evaluated in predicting outcome includes characteristics of the relationship. For example, it seems reasonable that couples that are having the greatest difficulties in their relationship may be least likely to benefit from treatment. As discussed in the following paragraphs, there is partial support for this hypothesis across various measures of relationship functioning.

One variable that has been evaluated with respect to relationship functioning is steps taken to divorce. The reasoning behind evaluating this variable is that people with the highest divorce potential may be least likely to be invested in therapy. Some studies have found that lack of commitment and behavioral steps taken toward divorce were negatively associated with outcome to treatment (Beach & Broderick, 1983; Hahlweg et al., 1984), whereas other studies have found no association between divorce potential and outcome to treatment (Jacobson et al., 1986).

A related variable that has been evaluated with respect to relationship functioning and treatment outcome is relationship quality. As with steps taken toward divorce, people with lower satisfaction may be less willing to commit to and less actively involved with therapy. Indeed, Snyder, Mangrum, and Wills (1993) found that poor outcome to couple therapy was predicted by lower relationship quality, greater negative relationship affect and disengagement, and greater desired change in the relationship. Similarly, Hawhleg et al. (1984) found that treatment outcome was predicted by negative communication behavior (but not by other measures designed to measure quality or quantity of conflict resolution or by measures designed to assess emotional affection).

A final construct that has been evaluated with respect to relationship functioning and outcome to treatment is relationship power. Although the concept of power in relationships has a long history, it has been a history characterized by many different conceptualizations and measures of power (for a review, see Gray-Little & Burks, 1983). Differences in defining and measuring power have also characterized the two studies that have evaluated the association between power and treatment outcome. Whisman and Jacobson (1990) operationalized power in terms of communication processes (i.e., asymmetry in relative frequencies of talking time) and found that greater inequality (i.e., greater asymmetry) was associated with better outcome at the end of treatment and at follow-up. More recently, Gray-Little, Baucom, and Hamby (1996) operationalized power in terms of who had the final say in a problem-solving interaction (i.e., which spouse's original position was accepted as the final solution to the problem proposed). Results indicated that wife-dominant couples improved the most in therapy, in terms of increased marital satisfaction and improved communication.

Individual-Difference Characteristics

A third set of variables that has been evaluated in predicting outcome to BCT consists of individual difference variables. Baucom and Aiken (1984) evaluated the association between gender roles measured prior to therapy and change in marital satisfaction from pre- to posttreatment for 54 couples that received BCT. Results indicated that wives' level of femininity was positively associated with increases in wives' and husbands' level of marital satisfaction. It certainly seems plausible that greater femininity, which has been associated with greater interpersonal sensitivity and emotional expressiveness, would predict better outcome to couple therapy. Femininity may not be a very robust predictor of outcome, however, as Jacobson et al. (1986) and Snyder et al. (1993) did not find an association between femininity and treatment outcome.

A second individual difference variable evaluated with respect to outcome was differences between partners in their preferences for closeness and intimacy versus independence and interpersonal distance. Jacobson et al. (1986) hypothesized that when people who are mismatched on these preferences marry, conflict is inevitable and self-perpetuating: "The more contact is sought by the affiliative partner, the more the autonomous partner withdraws; the more the autonomous partner withdraws, the more pressure the affiliative partner applies" (Jacobson et al., 1986, p. 518). Consistent with this perspective, results indicated that couples with a higher degree of traditionality (i.e., higher affiliation in the wife and higher independence in the husband) were less likely to benefit from CBCT. Interestingly, however, the absolute difference in affiliation and independence between partners was not associated with outcome. Therefore, it appears that a particular pattern of differences in affiliation and independence is predictive of outcome (i.e., a pattern that follows traditional relationship roles) and not degree of difference per se. As noted by the authors, insofar as CBCT tends to promote egalitarianism through its emphasis on collaboration and compromise, it may be that "couples with relatively traditional marriages are simply not likely to respond positively to such a perspective" (Jacobson et al., 1986, p. 522). Unfortunately, because this pattern of affiliation and independence has not been evaluated as a predictor of outcome in other approaches to couple therapy, it is unknown whether poor outcome is specific to the behavioral model.

A third individual difference variable that has been evaluated as a predictor of outcome is depression severity. As with several of the other variables already discussed, evidence for an association between depression severity and outcome is mixed. Jacobson et al. (1986) found that severity of depression at baseline was positively associated with outcome at the end of treatment, whereas Snyder et al. (1993) found that severity of depression was negatively related to outcome. The differences between these studies may be due, at least in part, to differences in methodology. In the Jacobson et al. study, depression severity was measured with seven items from a checklist of presenting psychiatric symptoms that was used by the training clinic at the University of Washington. No psychometric information was provided for the resulting scale, and level of depression was operationally defined as reflecting the score of the partner who endorsed the most number of symptoms. In comparison, the Snyder et al. study measured depression severity for each spouse with Scale 2 of the Minnesota Multiphasic Personality Inventory (MMPI).

Summary

It is difficult to draw firm conclusions regarding the studies that have evaluated predictors of outcome to CBCT in the treatment of relationship distress. Some results have been inconsistent, with certain variables (e.g., age and femininity) predicting outcome in some studies but not others. Other variables (e.g., depression) have predicted positive outcome in some studies and negative outcome in others. Still other variables (e.g., traditionality in preferences for closeness and intimacy vs. independence and interpersonal distance, and power) have been evaluated in only one study. Furthermore, the use of different measures for assessing variables across studies (e.g., different methods for operationalizing power and different measures for assessing depression severity) further complicates the interpretation of existing findings. Therefore, perhaps the most conservative conclusion indicates that there are no firmly established constructs that have been consistently associated with posttreatment outcome following CBCT in the treatment of relationship distress.

PRACTICAL STRATEGIES FOR IMPROVING OUTCOME

There are many potential directions that can be pursued in improving couple therapy. In this section, we describe a variety of methods that could be employed to improve outcome. For those strategies that have been subjected to empirical evaluation, we discuss the results from studies that have evaluated the impact that the strategy had on improving outcome.

One potential strategy for improving outcome that has been evaluated in prior studies is to modify parameters of treatment that do not have to do with the content of treatment (Baucom & Hoffman, 1986). For example, perhaps lengthening the course of treatment might help improve outcome. This is a variation of the familiar dose–response perspective, which holds that people are likely to improve to the extent that they receive greater amounts of treatment. The available evidence, however, suggests that increasing the length of treatment by itself does not result in improved outcome. In their meta-analysis of the effectiveness of BCT, Hahlweg and Markman (1988) reported that there was no significant difference in effect sizes between "older" treatment studies (i.e., those published before 1980) and more recent treatment studies (i.e., those published since 1980), although there was a significant difference between the two sets of studies in terms of mean duration of treatment (8 vs. 13 sessions, respectively). Other methods for varying the parameters of treatment would be to compare the effectiveness of treating couples one at a time versus in a group, and treating couples with one therapist versus co-therapists. It could be hypothesized that in comparison to a single couple in treatment with a single therapist, either group therapy or co-therapists might result in improved outcome, because either of these options would allow for greater modeling of the skills covered in therapy. Although limited in number, studies that have varied these parameters have found no significant differences in comparing individual versus group format (Revenstorf, Schindler, & Hahlweg, 1983; Wilson, Bornstein, & Wilson, 1988) and individual versus co-therapist (Mehlman, Baucom, & Anderson, 1983). In summary, the available evidence suggests that varying the noncontent parameters of treatment does not result in significant differences in outcome.

A second strategy for improving outcome that has been evaluated in prior studies is varying the content parameters of treatment by adding interventions to the "standard" treatment. The rationale for this approach is that adding interventions that target different areas of couple's relationship should have a larger impact than focusing on fewer areas. Although reasonable, the existing research does not suggest that "enhanced" treatments that incorporate multiple forms of treatment result in better outcome than treatments that focus on the core behavioral skills included in "standard" BCT (Baucom & Lester, 1986; Baucom et al., 1990; Halford et al., 1993). Although it is possible that some "additive" treatment or intervention will improve outcome, the existing findings offer little evidence for such an additive effect.

A third strategy for improving outcome that has been evaluated in prior studies is tailoring treatment to the specific needs of the couple. Jacobson et al. (1989) assigned 30 couples to one of two treatment groups. In the first group, couples received a structured (i.e., research based) version of CBCT, whereas in the second group, couples received a clinically flexible version in which treatment plans were individually based and there was no set number of sessions. Specifically, the flexible version "allowed for individually-tailored treatment plans, where the number of session could vary as clinically indicated, and the particular modules employed, as well as their length, were determined on a case-by-case basis" (Jacobson et al., 1989, p. 174). Thus, the flexible version of CBCT that was evaluated in this study was viewed as more similar to the practice of CBCT in settings other than a research study. Results indicated that whereas the two groups did not differ in efficacy at posttreatment, couples that had received the flexible version of CBCT maintained their treatment gains better than the couples that had received the structured version of treatment at a 6-month follow-up. These findings suggest that tailoring treatment to the specific needs of a particular couple should result in improved outcome.

A fourth strategy for improving outcome would be to focus on getting couples actively involved in therapy. In the only study that has investigated change processes in CBCT, Holtzworth-Munroe, Jacobson, DeKlyen, and Whisman (1989) had therapists and clients report, session by session, on their reactions to the session and their observations of husband, wife, and therapist behaviors. Results indicated that client behaviors were better predictors of outcome than therapist behaviors, with the strongest associations with improvement being obtained for client in-session and out-of-session involvement.

Given that better outcome appears to be associated with greater client involvement, how can therapists work to enhance involvement in therapy? One method would be to provide clear explanations for the topics and skills covered in couple therapy. Couples are more likely to engage in therapy if they understand what it is that they are being asked to do and why they are being asked to do it. Therapists can also work to structure therapy sessions to maximize efficient use of session time. Estrada and Holmes (1999) conducted a study involving couples who were in couple therapy regarding their perceptions of helpful and hindering aspects of couple therapy. Although the therapy received was not CBCT per se, the model of therapy employed draws on behavioral and communication approaches (as well as psychodynamic models). Results indicated that couples in therapy expected their therapist to be active and direct, and that therapist "mistakes" included such things as wasting time and being unclear in therapy. These results provide indirect support for the importance of therapists being active and clear in their involvement in the session.

Another method for enhancing outcome through increasing client involvement would be to increase adherence to homework assignments. A basic tenet of CBCT is that couples need to practice the skills learned during treatment sessions in their natural environments between sessions. The most common way of promoting generalization of skill acquisition is through homework assignments. Although there is little written about methods for enhancing homework adherence for couple therapy specifically, there are many recommendations that have been made for enhancing homework adherence for cognitive and behavioral therapies for individual problems. Detweiler and Whisman (1999) reviewed a variety of methods for enhancing homework adherence for cognitive therapy, which may also apply to enhancing homework adherence in CBCT. For example, adherence may be enhanced through methods such as covering specific details regarding the homework (e.g., how, when, for how long, and under what circumstances is homework to be done), through starting with smaller assignments and gradually building to more demanding or complicated assignments, and through providing a written description of the homework assignment. Detweiler and Whisman also recommend that therapists discuss potential barriers that may get in the way of doing homework and problem solve methods for overcoming these barriers. For example, a couple who often receives phone calls during the evening when they are trying to practice communication skills could decide to turn off their phone before they begin so as not to be interrupted. Detweiler and Whisman also discuss how adherence may be enhanced by elaborating on the benefits of doing homework rather than on the costs of not doing it. For example, focusing on how an assignment is going to improve a couple's satisfaction is more likely to result in adherence than focusing on how not doing the assignment (i.e., maintaining the status quo) is going to result in continued dissatisfaction. Finally, Detweiler and Whisman recommend that therapists provide choices among various homework alternatives and encourage clients to be actively involved in deciding on the assignment. Following these types of suggestions is likely to enhance homework adherence, which in turn, should result in improved outcome.

The methods for improving outcome thus far reviewed have largely focused on improving conflict resolution or reducing the frequency or impact of negative relationship factors. However, insofar as relationship functioning includes both positive and negative components (Fincham & Linfield, 1997), these strategies may have limited impact in improving positive relationship functioning. Therefore, another strategy for improving outcome following couple therapy would be to include interventions designed to increase positive feelings about the partner or the relationship. In identifying strategies that could enhance positive feelings, it may be instructive to consider the literature on emotional aspects of relationship functioning. According to Berscheid's (1983, 1991) analysis of emotions in relationships, emotions are often precipitated by unanticipated events or outcomes—namely, situations in which the partner unexpectedly does something that he or she "should" not do or by not doing something that he or she "should" do. This model suggests that therapeutic interventions designed to encourage couples to engage in more frequent activities together is likely to result in more frequent opportunities for strong emotional reactions. For example, encouraging couples to go out on dates or other couple activities is not only pleasant in and of itself but also increases the likelihood of interpersonal influence and therefore increases the likelihood of strong emotional reactions. Furthermore, encouraging couples to engage in novel activities together enhances the likelihood of new information and new outcomes, including unanticipated outcomes. For example, encouraging a couple to learn a new sport or hobby together allows for opportunities to see one's partner in a new light (e.g., "I never knew you were so talented at this"), which may elicit strong emotional responses. This application is also consistent with Aron and Aron's (1996) self-in-expansion theory of love, which posits that novel or exciting activities allow for greater self-expansion and, therefore, increases in subjective feelings of love. In support of this perspective,

Reissman, Aron, and Bergen (1993) found that over a 10-week period, couples who were encouraged to engage in activities that they had identified as "exciting" reported in greater increases in satisfaction than couples who engaged in activities identified as pleasant or couples who participated in a wait-list control group. Similarly, relative to engaging in a mundane task, participating in a 7-minute novel and arousing task has been shown to result in greater increases in relationship quality (Aron, Norman, Aron, McKenna, & Heyman, 2000). Therefore, encouraging novel and exciting activities may have a bigger impact on improving positive feelings in a relationship than would be obtained if couples are encouraged only to engage in routine or pleasant activities (as is typical of behavioral exchange strategies).

PREDICTORS OF RELAPSE AND RECURRENCE

Unlike many other problems treated by therapy, couple distress does not have clear boundaries in defining relapse. For example, there is no counterpart to "number of days abstinent" or "time until first drink" in the relationship area as there is in the alcohol field. Many couples cannot pinpoint a specific change in their relationship that they can use to "define" their distress. Defining relapse of relationship distress can, however, be achieved using the criteria for clinical significance set forth by Jacobson and colleagues (Jacobson, Follette, & Revenstorf, 1984; Jacobson & Truax, 1991). Using these criteria, relapse can be defined by a movement in relationship quality that is both statistically reliable and that moves the couple from above the cutoff for defining relationship distress at the end of treatment to below the cutoff for defining distress at follow-up. For example, using the cutoff on the Dyadic Adjustment Scale (DAS; Spanier, 1989) that was identified by Jacobson, Follette, and Revenstorf (1984), a couple (or a partner, if the focus was on each individual in a relationship) would be defined as relapsed if they scored above 97 on the DAS at the end of treatment and 97 or below on the DAS during follow-up. The use of clinical significance statistics aids in the operationalization of the potentially ambiguous constructs of relationship distress and relapse following initial recovery. Moreover, consistent use of these definitions of relapse would allow for comparisons to be made across studies.

Results from prior studies suggest that approximately 28% of couples that meet clinical significance criteria for recovery at the end of treatment will meet clinical significance criteria for relapse at short-term follow-up (Jacobson, Follette, Revenstorf, et al., 1984), whereas 30–40% of couples will relapse at long-term follow-up (Jacobson, Schmaling, & Holtzworth-Munroe, 1987; Snyder, Wills, & Grady-Fletcher, 1991). Therefore, although initial gains seem to be fairly well maintained during short-term follow-up, a significant proportion of couples will be expected to relapse several years after treatment.

Predictor Variables

The most detailed analyses of long-term relapse comes from a study by Jacobson et al. (1987), who conducted a 2-year follow-up study of couples that had participated in BCT. Particularly germane to the present discussion, couples participated in a 30-minute structured telephone interview. Included in the interview were questions designed to identify, among other things, variables that predicted long-term outcome. Comparisons were made between participants that had relapsed ("relapsers") versus those who had maintained their gains ("maintainers"). Results from the study indicated that there were no differences between the two groups in terms of their use of the skills learned in therapy. The two groups also did not differ in their impressions of therapy or their therapist. The groups did, however, differ in their experience of major life changes or stressors subsequent to the end of therapy. Specifically, relapsers reported more stressors than maintainers. Relapsed couples also reported the impact of stressors differently than the couples that did not relapse, with 11% of the relapsers reporting a positive impact of stressors on the marriage, and 79% of the maintainers reporting a positive impact of stressors on the marriage. Jacobson (1989) interpreted these findings to suggest that as time since treatment increases, stressful events become increasingly likely to take center stage, while skills garnered during treatment become less likely to be utilized.

Snyder et al. (1993) also evaluated predictors of long-term outcome, defined in terms of level of satisfaction or divorce 4 years after completing either CBCT or insight-oriented couple therapy. Results indicated that couples were more likely to be distressed or divorced at follow-up if "spouses' intake measures reflected high levels of negative marital affect, poor problem-solving skills, low psychological resilience, high levels of depression, low emotional responsiveness, or if neither spouse was employed at a semiskilled or higher level position" (p. 61); negative outcome at follow-up was predicted by negative affect and poor communication skills at the end of treatment. Similarly, Hahlweg et al. (1984) reported that follow-up outcome to BCT was not predicted by the quality or quantity of conflict but was predicted by the degree of emotional affection of partners for each other: Long-term outcome was poor if partners reported infrequent sexual intercourse and scored low in tenderness.

PRACTICAL STRATEGIES FOR PREVENTING RELAPSE AND RECURRENCE

Booster Sessions and Treatment Fading

The Jacobson et al. (1987) 2-year follow-up of people who had received CBCT included an assessment of participants' perspective as to what could be done to enhance the effectiveness of therapy or make the positive effects of therapy last longer. The most common response, offered by 20% of couples formerly in treatment, was the suggestion for booster maintenance sessions.

Moreover, those who did not spontaneously recommend the use of booster sessions were asked directly, and 90% responded positively. In a review of treatment of marital conflict, Bray and Jouriles (1995) also recommend the use of booster sessions. Furthermore, they calculated the cost-effectiveness of increasing number of sessions of treatment and found that despite the increase in cost due to booster sessions, these costs were still lower than that of divorce, due to expenses such as medical costs often incurred following divorce or separation, legal fees, and the like.

There are several reasons that booster sessions might be expected to prevent relapse and recurrence (Jacobson, 1989; Whisman, 1990). First, the promise of booster sessions may decrease couples' anxiety regarding treatment termination. Frequently, couples express the fear that their relationship will deteriorate once therapy ends, and knowing that therapist contact will continue should mitigate the concerns associated with termination. Second, the expectancy of booster sessions may extend the stimulus control of therapy, at least for the duration of the maintenance treatment. Couples will know that they will be seeing their therapist again, and this knowledge may act as a prompt, increasing the likelihood that they will implement the skills acquired during therapy. Third, booster sessions themselves may aid in the consolidation of skills learned during therapy, thereby facilitating their maintenance. Booster sessions also provide an opportunity for solving problems that emerge with the passing of time that had not been anticipated during the course of treatment. In sum, couples may benefit from both the anticipation and the experience of booster sessions.

Although prior studies indicate that a treatment protocol including booster sessions is predictive of lower rates of relapse following behavior therapy (for a review, see Whisman, 1990), there have been few empirical evaluations of booster sessions following couple therapy. In one unpublished study, Whisman (1991) evaluated the relative efficacy of a booster session protocol (consisting of two scheduled and three optional booster sessions during the 6 months following active treatment) with a standard CBCT protocol that did not include booster sessions in a sample of 27 couples. Results during follow-up favored the group that received booster sessions, although the differences did not reach conventional levels of statistical significance, owing in large part to the small sample and resulting low statistical power. The fact that the therapists in the study were graduate students with minimal experience in couple therapy, and that booster sessions were offered for only 6 months following initial treatment, makes it difficult to generalize these results to what would be obtained with experienced couple therapist offering such sessions over a longer duration. Additional support for the potential efficacy of booster sessions comes from a study by Braukhaus, Hahlweg, Kroeger, Groth, and Fehm-Wolfsdorf (2003), who evaluated the impact of adding two booster sessions to a cognitive-behavioral psychoeducational prevention program for couples that were committed to their relationship. Compared to couples who did not receive the additional sessions, couples who received booster sessions reported significantly higher marital satisfaction and fewer problem areas at a 1-year follow-up. Taken together, these findings provide preliminary support for the notion that including booster maintenance sessions following therapy may be an effective means for enhancing the long-term effectiveness of CBCT.

There are several factors to consider in using booster sessions. One consideration has to do with the role of the therapist in initiating these sessions. Specifically, the question centers on whether booster sessions should be initiated by the therapist or by the client. Jacobson (1989) recommended the use of booster sessions as both checkups by the therapist and client-initiated sessions. Concerning therapist-initiated sessions, the use of scheduled booster sessions could be introduced drawing an analogy with car maintenance or dental maintenance. Similar to how one has regularly scheduled appointments for getting an oil change or a dental cleaning, so also could a couple have regularly scheduled appointments for a relationship "checkup." These sessions could be framed as ways to "polish" the skills learned in therapy and, in so doing, ensure that the relationship continues to "run smoothly." In addition to regular scheduled booster sessions initiated by the therapist, Jacobson (1989) also recommends that booster sessions could be initiated by either partner during stressful times when the couple may benefit from guidance on coping. Again, drawing on the analogy with car or dental maintenance, one schedules an appointment with the mechanic or dentist if there are problems encountered between routine appointments. For example, a couple may be having a difficult time figuring out a solution to a problem in their relationship and would benefit from the therapist's perspective as to where they are getting stuck in resolving the problem. The important point regarding booster sessions is that just as one would not expect to master any complex set of skills (such as learning a new sport or learning how to play an instrument) without extended practice and continued lessons, continued contact with the therapist following the initial set of sessions may be required to master complex relationship skills.

Another consideration in the use of booster sessions has to do with the content of the sessions. Most commonly, the content of booster sessions is likely to be similar to the content of the initial therapy sessions. For example, a therapist might check in with a couple to see how they are doing with maintaining their level of positive behavioral exchanges and problem-solving difficulties in their relationship. In other cases, however, circumstantial changes in the relationship or in either partner may require that the booster sessions focus on new material not covered in the initial treatment. For example, for a couple whose initial therapy focused on communication and problem-solving training but who are now approaching retirement, booster sessions might have a cognitive focus in which partners talk about their expectations about each other and about their relationship after retirement.

Another option for improving maintenance that shares some features with booster maintenance sessions is "fading" the frequency of therapy sessions over time. For example, couple therapy could proceed weekly for a period of time, which could be followed by biweekly and then monthly sessions. Similar to booster sessions, the rationale behind fading the frequency of sessions is that it allows couples greater opportunity to practice and master the skills learned in therapy on their own, while still being able to periodically check in with their therapist to get feedback and guidance in areas in which they are experiencing difficulties. Bögner and Zielenbach-Coenen (1984) evaluated the impact of fading sessions by comparing two groups of couples that received BCT. The first group received nine sessions over 8 weeks, whereas the second group received nine sessions over 13 weeks. The group that received sessions on a fading schedule had better outcomes at the end of treatment and at 2- and 8-month follow-up. Although limited to only one study, these results are promising in suggesting that relapse may be less frequent for couples who receive initial sessions scheduled closely together, followed by a period of fading contact with the therapist. Insofar as this study is one of the few empirically documented procedures for maintaining therapeutic effects for couple distress, routinely incorporating session fading seems to be a worthy recommendation for the practice of CBCT.

Relapse Prevention

One of the most popular models for preventing relapse for a variety of problem behaviors is based on the techniques advanced by Marlatt and Gordon (1985) in their relapse prevention program. Although a detailed description of this program is beyond the scope of this chapter, some key elements of their program may be helpful to consider in preventing relapse of relationship distress.

One important component of Marlatt and Gordon's (1985) relapse prevention program is identifying high-risk situations and developing ways of coping with these situations before they occur. A therapist who was interested in applying this relapse prevention strategy in couple therapy would, toward the end of therapy, discuss with a couple specific kinds of situations that they might anticipate encountering in the future that could pose a challenge to their rediscovered happiness in their relationship. For example, one couple identified the wife's upcoming promotion as a potentially high-risk situation. Although the promotion would mean an increase in pay and recognition, which the couple viewed very favorably, it would also entail longer hours and greater responsibility and, therefore, greater stress. Both partners were concerned that this might have an impact on the amount and quality of their time together, which was one of the issues that brought them to therapy. Once high-risk situations are identified, the therapist would work with the couple on ways of coping with the situation. In this example, the couple discussed the importance of regularly checking in with each other regarding their perception as to how things were going with their relationship, and they targeted ways in which they could reserve certain hours of the week for the two of them to spend together.

In addition to individualized high-risk situations that might be specific to a particular couple, therapists might be well advised to consider more "generic" high-risk situations that are likely to be problems for many couples. One such example is the birth of a child. Research has shown that relationship satisfaction tends to decline following the birth of a child, particularly following the birth of a first child (e.g., Belsky & Kelly, 1994; Cowan & Cowan, 1992). Several factors have been identified as contributing to this decline in satisfaction. For example, research has shown that there is a significant change in the number and timing of daily events done as a couple following the birth of a child (Monk et al., 1996), suggesting that positive exchanges are likely to decrease during the postpartum period. Therefore, a therapist helping a couple to anticipate changes following birth of a child might underscore the importance of maintaining the level of positive behavioral exchanges. Similarly, research has shown that unmet expectations are associated with declines in marital satisfaction following birth of a child (Ruble, Fleming, Hackel, & Stangor, 1988). Therefore, a therapist working with a couple who is pregnant or planning on becoming pregnant may want to encourage the couple, prior to the birth of the child, to discuss their expectations of each other and their relationship to reduce the likelihood and resulting impact of unmet expectations. In addition, therapists may want to provide information regarding other types of adjustments that the couple will likely encounter following the child's birth (e.g., changes in sexual functioning; Massil, 1995), in order to reduce likelihood of unrealistic expectations in these areas as well. Including cognitive and behavioral relapse prevention foci such as these for commonly experienced high-risk situations is likely to reduce the impact that life changes—such as having a child—may have on relapse of relationship distress.

There are no published studies thus far that have compared groups of people who have received relapse prevention versus those who have not, in terms of the impact of such sessions on preventing relapse of relationship distress. However, the use of relapse prevention in couple therapy for alcoholism lends empirical support for its efficacy. In a study by Maisto, McKay, and O'Farrell (1995), males who completed BCT for treatment of alcoholism with and without relapse prevention were followed in the year following the course of treatment. Compared to those who had not received any additional treatment, participants who had received relapse prevention treatment had an equal number of relapse episodes, but their relapses were of shorter duration. Furthermore, O'Farrell, Choquette, and Cutter (1998) found that even after 30 months posttreatment, participants who received the additional relapse prevention sessions reported greater relationship adjustment and maintained their improved relationships longer than those who did not receive relapse prevention sessions; those who received the additional relapse prevention also reported more days of alcohol abstinence. These findings, coupled with the findings regarding the efficacy of relapse prevention strategies for other problems treated with cognitive and behavioral therapies, suggest that incorporating relapse prevention strategies may be effective in preventing relapse of relationship distress.

Based on the foregoing reviewed findings, learning to cope with stressful life events may be particularly important for the health of a relationship. Although avoidance of stressful events is not a feasible recommendation, awareness of the impact stressful events may have on an intimate relationship may allow couples to cope more effectively by way of using maintenance work during these periods. Bodenmann (1997) has developed a program called couples coping enhancement training (CCET). According to this perspective, "the enhancement of dyadic coping in marriage includes four primary issues: (a) improvement of one's own stress communication in such a way that the partner is able to respond to one's needs; (b) improvement concerning the perception of stress signals given by the partner; (c) adequate supportive dyadic coping; and (d) the practice of common dyadic coping or the delegation of coping tasks" (pp. 184–185). The first two of these issues represent important extensions of communication skills training of standard BCT. In comparison, learning and practicing coping strategies is not typically covered in BCT. These kinds of strategies include such skills as "tension reduction methods, helping the partner to reframe the situation, solidarizing with the partner" (p. 186). Although the efficacy of CCET has yet to be evaluated, a similar program that focuses on individual coping has been shown to have positive outcomes that were evident even two years after treatment (Bodenmann, Perrez, Cina, & Widmer, 2002). Therefore, the CCET approach appears to be a very promising method for inoculating couples against the potential deleterious effects of stress on their relationship.

Other Strategies

Based on Snyder et al.'s (1993) findings that depression is associated with poorer outcome to couple therapy, measured at the end of treatment and at follow-up, an additional strategy for maintaining long-term gains for couple therapy would be to incorporate interventions for targeting depression among couples that present with both relationship distress and either clinical or subclinical depression. Although CBCT has been shown to be effective in treating depression, and although interventions that are described in treatment manuals for working with couples with a depressed partner are largely similar to those for distressed couples in general, there may be other strategies that could be added to "standard" CBCT in working with couples with a depressed partner. For example, in working with couples with a depressed partner, Whisman and Uebelacker (1999) suggested that the effectiveness of CBCT could be enhanced by combining it with cognitive interventions (e.g., focusing on depressogenic cognitions that interact with relationship distress, such as the belief that "to be a worthwhile person I need to be approved of and accepted by others"), behavioral interventions (e.g., increasing the frequency of positive behaviors done for oneself as well as for one's partner), interpersonal interventions (e.g., resolving other interpersonal issues, such as grief or role transitions), or antidepressant medications. Integrating couple therapy with other interventions, therefore, may enhance the short- and long-term effectiveness of CBCT.

CASE EXAMPLE

Tim and Jenny are in their early 30s, and they have been married for nearly 5 years. Tim is a white-collar worker in a high-profile business, whereas Jenny works part time at a local bookstore. This is the first marriage for both Tim and Jenny, and they do not have any children. The couple stated that their major reason for requesting therapy was that they "fight all the time."

During the initial consultation, Tim and Jenny presented as partners who were very distant and detached from one another. Tim worked 60 hours or more a week, and when he wasn't working, he liked to hang out with his friends at a local sports bar. Jenny worked part time and spent much of the rest of her time either working out at the gym or reading at home. The couple agreed that whenever they would spend any time together, they would end up in a heated argument. They had learned to live parallel lives and to minimize the friction by limiting their contact with one another. Their major goals for therapy were to learn to communicate better and to rekindle the positive feelings they once had for one another.

Jenny and Tim were initially seen for 12 sessions of weekly therapy. Therapy began with a focus on the couple's primary complaint, which was communication. Both Tim and Jenny were very skilled at communicating with the therapist and with other people. Therefore, it was determined that neither partner lacked the skills necessary for effective communication. Therefore, rather than focusing on communication skill acquisition, therapy focused on getting the couple to practice the same kinds of communication with each other as they did with other people. The couple brainstormed a list of neutral topics about which they could talk with one another. First in session with feedback from the therapist, and later for homework, the couple took turns sharing their thoughts and feelings about these neutral topics. The couple complained that this seemed stilted at first, but over the course of a few sessions, they reported that they felt that they were benefiting from this, and that they were beginning to reconnect with one another.

The focus of therapy then shifted to problem solving. Tim quickly picked up on the problem-solving framework, stating that it was very similar to how problems were handled at his place of employment. Jenny was slower to warm to the notion of problem solving, stating that it felt too structured. The therapist worked with them in tailoring the format to something that they both felt comfortable doing. Over the next several sessions, they practiced the modified format with some ongoing problems in their relationship. For example, the couple was in the process of finding a new home, and they used the problem-solving format to resolve some of the differences they had as to the ideal home with respect to location and size. They then tackled some of their more difficult problems, namely, their differences in how they liked to spend their free time. Jenny didn't like some of Tim's friends and didn't want to join him in the sports bar, whereas Tim felt bored spending time at home. Rather than choosing an option that didn't suit either one, the couple decided instead to look into something new that they could both enjoy. Although they had both enjoyed biking while in college, they had not been biking for some time. They began biking together, and found that this new activity brought them enjoyment and resulted in bringing them closer together. Although they continued to spend time pursuing their own interests, they began spending more time together on biking trips. On one bike trip, they rode through a part of town that they didn't frequent and found a new restaurant that was offering cooking classes. They signed up for the classes and enjoyed spending time together in this new setting.

Although the couple was spending more time together as a result of their problem solving, the therapist also discussed with the couple the importance of caring behaviors. Each person first generated a list of things he or she could do for the partner and then tried them out during the week. This self-focus was followed by generating lists of things that the other person could do to improve the quality of the relationship. Although behavioral exchange strategies are often presented at the beginning of therapy, Tim and Jenny were spending so little time together when they first came in for therapy that it was determined that they had little opportunity for changing their levels of rewarding behaviors. Instead, by introducing behavioral exchange toward the later stages of therapy, the couple was spending more time together and could therefore have a greater impact on improving each other's satisfaction with the relationship.

As Tim and Jenny were getting along much better, the therapist raised the issue of ending weekly sessions. The notion of high-risk situations was introduced, and the couple was encouraged to think of any difficulties that they anticipated in the near future. One consideration was the coming of winter, which would make it more difficult for them to continue with their bike riding. They decided to look into cross-country skiing, which they were both interested in learning. They also discussed how selling their house and moving could be stressful, and expressed their fears of getting back into their old habits of fighting if things didn't go well with the move. They decided that there wasn't anything they wanted to do in reference to the move other than be aware of the warning signs that they were falling back into their old routine. The therapist discussed the idea of booster sessions, and Jenny and Tim both expressed a strong interest in doing these sessions. It was decided that the therapist would call to schedule the first booster session in 3 months, and that either Tim or Jenny could initiate a session before then if needed.

At the first (3-month) booster session, the couple was doing well. They had looked into cross-country skiing but decided against pursuing it as a shared activity. Instead, Tim had joined the gym that Jenny belonged to, and they were taking a swimming class together. They admitted that they hadn't done as well with continuing the problem-solving format, and the therapist focused on modifying the format further to come up with a framework that they would be more likely to use. The couple also sheepishly reported that they had forgotten about trying to do "nice things" for one another until the therapist called, but that they had been trying to do more of this during the previous week. A second booster session was scheduled for 3 months later.

A month later Jenny called and asked to have a session right away. When they came to the session, Tim and Jenny seemed very upset with one another and it was clear that Jenny had been crying. She had found out that Tim had had sex with a colleague at a conference he had attended earlier that year. Although Tim reported that he was very sorry that he had done this, and that he would never do it again, Jenny was very hurt and angry. She reported that she wanted to leave him but that they had signed the papers for a new house and she had too much invested in the new house to leave him.

It was decided that the couple would reenter weekly therapy, focusing on working through the disclosure of the affair. The couple met with the therapist for an additional eight sessions, which were spent helping the couple deal with the crisis of the disclosed affair following the treatment guidelines discussed in Gordon and Baucom (1999). At the end of this time, they were seen for three more booster sessions, at which time they decided they were ready to continue working on their own, knowing that they could contact the therapist if needed.

This case example of couple therapy illustrates many of the topics covered in this chapter. The initial treatment, although "traditional" in the sense of the core components of treatment, was tailored with respect to the topics and sequencing of interventions. The couple also had a very favorable response to the idea of adding some novel and exciting new activities in their relationship (biking and taking a cooking class), which worked better for them than adopting one or the other's interests at the time. They were able to continue building on this notion by adding another activity (swimming) after they finished with weekly therapy sessions. The first booster session seemed helpful in reminding the couple of the importance of maintaining the skills they learned in therapy. However, despite these gains, the couple had a major setback with the disclosure of the affair. Because the couple was in continued contact with the therapist, the therapist was quickly able to meet with the couple and assist them in repairing their relationship. At the end of the maintenance phase of treatment, the couple expressed optimism that they could continue on their own, particularly in light of having weathered such a difficult blow to their relationship.

CONCLUSION

In this chapter, we reviewed the literature on improving outcome and preventing relapse for couple distress with behavioral and cognitive-behavioral couple therapy. Existing findings suggest that BCT and CBCT are effective in improving relationship distress. In addition, preliminary evidence suggests that CBCT may also be effective (alone or as part of a comprehensive treatment package) in the treatment of some individual disorders (depression and alcohol abuse/dependence) among distressed couples. A limited number of studies have evaluated demographic, relationship, and individual difference predictors of treatment outcome, and results have been inconclusive. The chapter also examined methods of improving short-term outcomes, such as modifying noncontent parameters of treatment, enhancing current treatments, tailoring treatments to couples' specific needs, encouraging greater client involvement in the therapeutic process, and incorporating interventions designed to improve positive affect in the relationship. We also discussed predictors of relapse and recurrence of couple distress following CBCT. Predictors include stressful life events, high baseline levels of negative marital or individual affect, poor resiliency, and deficiencies in problem-solving skills. Suggested strategies for preventing relapse and recurrence include booster sessions and treatment fading. Further, incorporation of relapse prevention techniques, as in couple therapy for alcoholism, may be effective in preventing relapse of relationship distress. Despite evidence for positive outcomes of couple therapy for relationship distress, continued exploration of strategies geared toward improving treatment to enhance the short- and long-term effectiveness of CBCT remains a task for future research.

REFERENCES

American Psychiatric Association. (1994). *Diagnostic and statistical manual of mental disorders* (4th ed.). Washington, DC: Author.

Aron, A., Norman, C. C., Aron, E. N., McKenna, C., & Heyman, R. E. (2000). Couples' shared participation in novel and arousing activities and experienced relationship quality. *Journal of Personality and Social Psychology, 78,* 273–284.

Aron, E. N., & Aron, A. (1996). Love and expansion of the self: The state of the model. *Personal Relationships, 3,* 45–58.

Baucom, D. H. (1984). The active ingredients in behavioral marital therapy: The effectiveness of problem-solving/communication training, contingency contracting, and their combination. In K. Hahlweg & N. S. Jacobson (Eds.), *Marital interaction: Analysis and modification* (pp. 73–88). New York: Guilford Press.

Baucom, D. H., & Aiken, P. A. (1984). Sex role identity, marital satisfaction, and response to behavioral marital therapy. *Journal of Consulting and Clinical Psychology, 52,* 438–444.

Baucom, D. H., & Hoffman, J. A. (1986). The effectiveness of marital therapy: Current status and application to the clinical setting. In N. S. Jacobson & A. S. Gurman (Eds.), *Clinical handbook of marital therapy* (pp. 597–620). New York: Guilford Press.

Baucom, D. H., & Lester, G. W. (1986). The usefulness of cognitive restructuring as an adjunct to behavioral marital therapy. *Behavior Therapy, 17,* 385–403.

Baucom, D. H., Sayers, S. L., & Sher, T. G. (1990). Supplementing behavioral marital therapy with cognitive restructuring and emotional expressiveness training: An outcome investigation. *Journal of Consulting and Clinical Psychology, 58,* 636–645.

Baucom, D. H., Shoham, V., Mueser, K. T., Daiuto, A. D., & Stickle, T. R. (1998). Empirically supported couple and family interventions for marital distress and adult mental health problems. *Journal of Consulting and Clinical Psychology, 66,* 53–88.

Beach, S. R., & Broderick, J. E. (1983). Commitment: A variable in women's response to marital therapy. *American Journal of Family Therapy, 11,* 16–24.

Belsky, J., & Kelly, J. (1994). *The transition to parenthood.* New York: Dell.

Berscheid, E. (1983). Emotion. In H. H. Kelly, E. Berscheid, A. Christensen, J. H. Harvey, T. L. Huston, G. Levinger, E. McClintock, L. A. Peplau, & D. R. Peterson (Eds.), *Close relationships* (pp. 110–168). San Francisco: Freeman.

Berscheid, E. (1991). The emotion-in-relationships model: Reflections and update. In W. Kessen, A. Ortony, & F. Craik (Eds.), *Memories, thoughts, and emotions: Essays in honor of George Mandler* (pp. 323–335). Hillsdale, NJ: Erlbaum.

Bodenmann, G. (1997). Can divorce be prevented by enhancing the coping skills of couples? *Journal of Divorce and Remarriage, 27,* 177–194.

Bodenmann, G., Perrez, M., Cina, A., & Widmer, K. (2002). The effectiveness of a coping-focused prevention approach: A two-year longitudinal study. *Swiss Journal of Psychology, 61,* 195–202.

Bögner, I., & Zielenbach-Coenen, H. (1984). On maintaining change in behavioral marital therapy. In K. Hahlweg & N. S. Jacobson (Eds.), *Marital interaction: Analysis and modification* (pp. 27–35). New York: Guilford Press.

Bramlett, M. D., & Mosher, W. D. (2001). First marriage dissolution, divorce, and remarriage: United States. In *Advance Data from Vital and Health Statistics, No. 323.* Hyattsville, MD: National Center for Health Statistics.

Braukhaus, C., Hahlweg, K., Kroeger, C., Groth, T., & Fehm-Wolfsdorf, G. (2003). The effects of adding booster sessions to a prevention training program for committed couples. *Behavioural and Cognitive Psychotherapy, 31,* 325–336.

Bray, J. H., & Jouriles, E. N. (1995). Treatment of marital conflict and prevention of divorce. *Journal of Marital and Family Therapy, 21,* 461–473.

Chambless, D. L., & Hollon, S. D. (1998). Defining empirically supported therapies. *Journal of Consulting and Clinical Psychology, 66,* 7–18.

Christensen, A., & Heavey, C. L. (1999). Interventions for couples. *Annual Review of Psychology, 50,* 165–190.

Cowan, C. P., & Cowan, P. (1992). *When partners become parents: The big life change for couples.* New York: Basic Books.

Crowe, M. J. (1978). Conjoint marital therapy: A controlled outcome study. *Psychological Medicine, 8,* 623–636.

Cummings, E. M., & Davies, P. T. (2002). Effects of marital conflict on children: Recent advances and emerging themes in process-oriented research. *Journal of Child Psychology and Psychiatry and Allied Disciplines, 43,* 31–63.

Detweiler, J. B., & Whisman, M. A. (1999). The role of homework assignments in cognitive therapy for depression: Potential methods for enhancing adherence. *Clinical Psychology: Science and Practice, 6,* 267–282.

Dunn, R. L., & Schwebel, A. I. (1995). Meta-analytic review of marital therapy outcome research. *Journal of Family Psychology, 9,* 58–68.

Emmelkamp, P. M. G., van Linden van den Heuvell, C., Ruphan, M., Sanderman, R., Scholing, A., & Stroink, F. (1988). Cognitive and behavioral interventions: A comparative evaluation with clinically distressed couples. *Journal of Family Psychology*, 1, 365–377.

Epstein, E. E., & McCrady, B. S. (1998). Behavioral couples treatment of alcohol and drug use disorders: Current status and innovations. *Clinical Psychology Review*, 18, 689–711.

Epstein, N. B., & Baucom, D. H. (2002). *Enhanced cognitive-behavioral therapy for couples*. Washington, DC: American Psychological Association.

Estrada, A. U., & Holmes, J. M. (1999). Couples' perceptions of effective and ineffective ingredients of marital therapy. *Journal of Sex and Marital Therapy*, 25, 151–162.

Fincham, F. D., & Linfield, K. J. (1997). A new look at marital quality: Can spouses feel positive and negative about their marriage? *Journal of Family Psychology*, 11, 489–502.

Forthofer, M. S., Markman, H. J., Cox, M., Stanley, S., & Kessler, R. C. (1996). Associations between marital distress and work loss in a national sample. *Journal of Marriage and the Family*, 58, 597–605.

Gordon, K. C., & Baucom, D. H. (1999). A multitheoretical intervention for promoting recovery from extramarital affairs. *Clinical Psychology: Science and Practice*, 6, 382–399.

Gray-Little, B., Baucom, D. H., & Hamby, S. L. (1996). Marital power, marital adjustment, and therapy outcome. *Journal of Family Psychology*, 10, 292–303.

Gray-Little, B., & Burks, N. (1983). Power and satisfaction in marriage: A review and critique. *Psychological Bulletin*, 93, 513–538.

Gurman, A. S., & Jacobson, N. S. (Eds.). (2002). *Clinical handbook of couple therapy* (3rd ed.). New York: Guilford Press.

Hahlweg, K., & Markman, H. J. (1988). Effectiveness of behavioral marital therapy: Empirical status of behavioral techniques in preventing and alleviating marital distress. *Journal of Consulting and Clinical Psychology*, 56, 440–447.

Hahlweg, K., Schindler, L., Revenstorf, D., & Brengelmann, J. C. (1984). The Munich marital therapy study. In K. Hahlweg & N. S. Jacobson (Eds.), *Marital interaction: Analysis and modification* (pp. 3–26). New York: Guilford Press.

Halford, W. K., Sanders, M. R., & Behrens, B. C. (1993). A comparison of the generalization of behavioral marital therapy and enhanced behavioral marital therapy. *Journal of Consulting and Clinical Psychology*, 61, 51–60.

Heyman, R. E., Feldbau-Kohn, S. R., Ehrensaft, M. K., Langhinrichsen-Rohling, J., & O'Leary, K. D. (2001). Can questionnaire reports correctly classify relationship distress and partner physical abuse? *Journal of Family Psychology*, 15, 334–346.

Hjemboe, S., & Butcher, J. N. (1991). Couples in marital distress: A study of personality factors as measured by the MMPI-2. *Journal of Personality Assessment*, 57, 216–237.

Hollon, S. D., Thase, M. E., & Markowitz, J. C. (2002). Treatment and prevention of depression. *Psychological Science in the Public Interest*, 3, 39–77.

Holtzworth-Munroe, A., Jacobson, N. S., DeKlyen, M., & Whisman, M. A. (1989). Relationship between behavioral marital therapy outcome and process variables. *Journal of Consulting and Clinical Psychology*, 57, 658–662.

Holtzworth-Munroe, A., Smutzler, N., Bates, L., & Sandin, E. (1997). Husband violence: Basic facts and clinical implications. In W. K. Halford & H. J. Markman (Eds.), *Clinical handbook of marriage and couples interventions* (pp. 129–156). New York: Wiley.

Huber, C. H., & Milstein, B. (1985). Cognitive restructuring and a collaborative set in couples' work. *American Journal of Family Therapy, 13,* 17–27.

Jacobson, N. S. (1989). The maintenance of treatment gains following social learning-based marital therapy. *Behavior Therapy, 20,* 325–336.

Jacobson, N. S., Dobson, K., Fruzzetti, A. E., Schmaling, K. B., & Salusky, S. (1991). Marital therapy as a treatment for depression. *Journal of Consulting and Clinical Psychology, 59,* 547–557.

Jacobson, N. S., Follette, W. C., & Pagel, M. (1986). Predicting who will benefit from behavioral marital therapy. *Journal of Consulting and Clinical Psychology, 54,* 518–522.

Jacobson, N. S., Follette, W. C., & Revenstorf, D. (1984). Psychotherapy outcome research: Methods for reporting variability and evaluating clinical significance. *Behavior Therapy, 15,* 336–352.

Jacobson, N. S., Follette, W. C., Revenstorf, D., Baucom, D. H., Hahlweg, K., & Margolin, G. (1984). Variability in outcome and clinical significance of behavioral marital therapy: A reanalysis of outcome data. *Journal of Consulting and Clinical Psychology, 52,* 497–504.

Jacobson, N. S., & Margolin, G. (1979). *Marital therapy: Strategies based on social learning and behavior exchange principles.* New York: Brunner/Mazel.

Jacobson, N. S., & Revenstorf, D. (1988). Statistics for assessing the clinical significance of psychotherapy techniques: Issues, problems, and new developments. *Behavioral Assessment, 10,* 133–145.

Jacobson, N. S., Schmaling, K. B., & Holtzworth-Munroe, A. (1987). Component analysis of behavioral marital therapy: 2-year follow-up and prediction of relapse. *Journal of Marital and Family Therapy, 13,* 187–195.

Jacobson, N. S., Schmaling, K. B., Holtzworth-Munroe, A., Katt, J. L., Wood, L. F., & Follette, V. M. (1989). Research-structured vs clinically flexible versions of social learning-based marital therapy. *Behaviour Research and Therapy, 27,* 173–180.

Jacobson, N. S., & Truax, P. (1991). Clinical significance: A statistical approach to defining meaningful change in psychotherapy research. *Journal of Consulting and Clinical Psychology, 59,* 12–19.

Kiecolt-Glaser, J. K., & Newton, T. L. (2001). Marriage and health: His and hers. *Psychological Bulletin, 12,* 472–503.

Kreider, R. M., & Fields, J. M. (2001). *Number, timing, and duration of marriages and divorces: Fall 1996* (Current Population Reports, P70-80). Washington, DC: U.S. Census Bureau.

Locke, H. J., & Wallace, K. M. (1959). Short marital adjustment and prediction tests: Their reliability and validity. *Marriage and Family Living, 21,* 251–255.

Maisto, S. A., McKay, J. R., & O'Farrell, T. J. (1995). Relapse precipitants and behavioral marital therapy. *Addictive Behaviors, 20,* 383–393.

Marlatt, G. A., & Gordon, J. R. (Eds.). (1985). *Relapse prevention: Maintenance strategies in the treatment of addictive behaviors.* New York: Guilford Press.

Massil, H. (1995). Postpartum sexual function: What is the norm? *Sexual and Marital Therapy, 10,* 263–276.

Mehlman, S. K., Baucom, D. H., & Anderson, D. (1983). Effectiveness of cotherapists versus single therapists and immediate versus delayed treatment in behavioral marital therapy. *Journal of Consulting and Clinical Psychology, 51,* 258–266.

Monk, T. H., Essex, M. J., Smider, N. A., Klein, M., Lowe, K. L., & Kupper, D. J. (1996). The impact of the birth of a baby on the time structure and social mixture of a couple's daily life and its consequences for well-being. *Journal of Applied Social Psychology, 26,* 1237–1258.

O'Farrell, T. J., Choquette, K. A., & Cutter, H. S. G. (1998). Couples relapse prevention session after behavioral marital therapy for male alcoholics: Outcomes during the three years after starting treatment. *Journal of Studies on Alcohol, 59,* 357–370.

O'Farrell, T. J., & Fals-Stewart, W. (2000). Behavioral couples therapy for alcoholism and drug abuse. *Journal of Substance Abuse Treatment, 18,* 51–54.

O'Leary, K. D., & Beach, R. H. (1990). Marital therapy: A viable treatment for depression and marital discord. *American Journal of Psychiatry, 147,* 183–186.

Reissman, C., Aron, A., & Bergen, M. R. (1993). Shared activities and marital satisfaction: Causal direction and self-expansion versus boredom. *Journal of Social and Personal Relationships, 10,* 243–254.

Ren, X. S. (1997). Marital status and quality of relationships: The impact on health perception. *Social Science and Medicine, 44,* 241–249.

Revenstorf, D., Schindler, L., & Hahlweg, K. (1983). Behavioral marital therapy applied in a conjoint and a conjoint-group modality: Short and long-term effectiveness. *Behavior Therapy, 14,* 614–625.

Ruble, D. N., Fleming, A. S., Hackel, L. S., & Stangor, C. (1988). Changes in the marital relationship during the transition to first time motherhood: Effects of violated expectations concerning division of household labor. *Journal of Personality and Social Psychology, 55,* 78–87.

Schmaling, K. B., & Sher, T. G. (Eds.). (2000). *The psychology of couples and illness: Theory, research, and practice.* Washington, DC: American Psychological Association.

Seltzer, J. A. (2000). Families formed outside of marriage. *Journal of Marriage and the Family, 62,* 1247–1268.

Shadish, W. R., Montgomery, L. M., Wilson, P., Wilson, M. R., Bright, I., & Okwumabua, T. (1993). Effects of family and marital psychotherapies: A meta-analysis. *Journal of Consulting and Clinical Psychology, 61,* 992–1002.

Snyder, D. K. (1997). *Manual for the Marital Satisfaction Inventory—Revised.* Los Angeles: Western Psychological Services.

Snyder, D. K., Mangrum, L. F., & Wills, R. M. (1993). Predicting couples' response to marital therapy: A comparison of short- and long-term predictors. *Journal of Consulting and Clinical Psychology, 61,* 61–69.

Snyder, D. K., & Whisman, M. A. (Eds.). (2003). *Treating difficult couples: Helping clients with coexisting mental and relationship disorders.* New York: Guilford Press.

Snyder, D. K., Wills, R. M., & Grady-Fletcher, A. (1991). Long-term effectiveness of behavioral versus insight-oriented marital therapy. *Journal of Consulting and Clinical Psychology, 59,* 138–141.

Spanier, G. B. (1989). *Dyadic Adjustment Scale manual.* North Tonawanda, NY: Multi-Health Systems.

Turkewitz, H., & O'Leary, K. D. (1981). A comparative outcome study of behavioral marital therapy and communication therapy. *Journal of Marital and Family Therapy, 7,* 159–169.

Whisman, M. A. (1990). The efficacy of booster maintenance sessions in behavior therapy: Review and methodological critique. *Clinical Psychology Review, 10,* 155–170.

Whisman, M. A. (1991). The use of booster maintenance sessions in behavioral marital therapy. *Dissertation Abstracts International, 51*(11-B), 5598–5599.

Whisman, M. A., & Jacobson, N. S. (1990). Power, marital satisfaction, and response to marital therapy. *Journal of Family Psychology, 4,* 202–212.

Whisman, M. A., & Snyder, D. K. (1997). Evaluating and improving the efficacy of conjoint marital therapy. In W. K. Halford & H. J. Markman (Eds.), *Clinical handbook of marriage and couples intervention* (pp. 679–693). New York: Wiley.

Whisman, M. A., & Uebelacker, L. A. (1999). Integrating couple therapy with individual therapies and antidepressant medications in the treatment of depression. *Clinical Psychology: Science and Practice, 6,* 415–429.

Whisman, M. A., & Uebelacker, L. A. (2003). Comorbidity of relationship distress and mental and physical health problems. In D. K. Snyder & M. A. Whisman (Eds.), *Treating difficult couples: Helping clients with coexisting mental and relationship disorders* (pp. 3–26). New York: Guilford Press.

Wilson, G. L., Bornstein, P. H., & Wilson, L. J. (1988). Treatment of relationship dysfunction: An empirical evaluation of group and conjoint behavioral marital therapy. *Journal of Consulting and Clinical Psychology, 56,* 929–931.

Author Index

Abel, J. L., 78, 89
Abraham, K., 249
Abramowitz, J. S., 132, 133, 134, 136, 139, 140, 141
Abramson, L. Y., 226
Ackerman, S. J., 223
Adams, M. E., 319
Addis, M. E., 12, 213, 219
Agnew-Davies, R., 213
Agras, W. S., 44, 139, 270, 271, 273, 291
Ahearn, E., 184
Aiken, P. A., 388
Akiskal, H. S., 129, 246
Albano, A. M., 61, 62, 109
Albrecht, J. W., 87
Alexander, L., 223
Alford, B. A., 208
Allan, T., 89, 107
Allen, L. B., 19
Allmon, D., 288
Alloy, L. B., 226
Altamura, A. C., 43
Alterman, A. A., 370
Altman, E. S., 258
Alvarez-Conrad, J., 181
Andersen, A. E., 290
Anderson, D. J., 78, 390
Anderson, L. P., 205
Anderson, P. K., 225
Andrade, C., 207
Andreski, P., 175
Andrews, B., 327
Andrews, G., 132
Annis, H. M., 354, 355
Antia, S. X., 43

Antony, M. M., 3, 4, 8, 16, 19, 20, 21, 38, 39, 62, 110, 120, 221, 225, 229
Apfelbaum, M., 278
Apiquian, R., 227
Armstrong, H. E., 288
Arntz, A., 140, 186
Aron, A., 392, 393
Aron, E. N., 392, 393
Arts, W., 141
Astin, M. C., 174, 182
Auer, C., 8
Ayllon, T., 365
Azrin, N. H., 363, 365

Babor, T., 350
Back, S. E., 189
Baer, B. A., 211
Baer, L., 139, 140
Baity, M. R., 223
Baker-Morissette, S. L., 15
Bakker, A., 4
Baldessarini, R. J., 259
Ball, J., 210
Ballenger, J. C., 4, 85
Bang, L. O. M., 137
Barkham, M., 213
Barlow, D. H., 2, 3, 4, 5, 6, 8, 9, 19, 20, 21, 61, 77, 78, 79, 80, 82, 84, 85, 89, 104, 109, 113, 114, 120, 174, 177, 186
Barnes, T. R. E., 320
Barouche, F., 211
Barrett, P. M., 108, 109, 110
Barrowclough, C., 327, 328, 329, 330, 331, 332, 336, 337

Barsky, A. J., 21
Barton, B., 210
Başoğlu, M., 19, 21, 129, 139, 140, 141
Bates, L., 381
Bates, M. J., 7, 21
Baucom, D. H., 382, 383, 384, 385, 387, 388, 389, 390, 402
Bauer, J., 272
Bauer, M. S., 230, 261
Baugher, M., 206
Bauml, J., 332
Beach, B., 291
Beach, R. H., 386
Beach, S. R., 387
Beck, A. T., 9, 82, 89, 91, 96, 97, 178, 182, 208, 210, 214, 261, 264, 310
Beck, J. G., 80
Beck, J. S., 218, 219, 227, 228
Becker, R. E., 39, 40, 48, 49, 50, 55, 56, 61
Beebe, K. L., 183
Behrens, B. C., 384
Beidel, D. C., 41, 44, 61, 62
Bell, L., 285
Belsher, G., 210
Belsky, J., 398
Bennett, M. E., 352
Bentall, R. P., 323, 326
Berenbaum, H., 309
Bergen, M. R., 393
Berkowitz, R., 332
Berlanga, C., 227
Berman, J. S., 207, 213
Berman, R. M., 207
Bernstein, D. A., 81
Bernstein, G. A., 108
Bertelsen, A., 246
Best, C. L., 175, 177
Beumont, P. J., 271
Bezchlibnyk-Butler, K. Z., 207
Bieling, P. J., 9, 19, 221, 225, 229
Bigelow, G. E., 371
Biggs, M. M., 227
Billardon, M., 87
Birchall, H., 270
Birchwood, M., 313, 314, 330, 337
Birley, J. L. T., 318
Birmaher, B., 206
Biswas, A., 107
Blaauw, B. M. J. W., 4
Black, D. W., 140
Blackmore, E., 271
Blagys, M. D., 223
Blanchard, E. B., 104
Blanco, C., 43

Blatt, S. J., 211
Blazer, D. G., 78, 206, 246
Bleuler, M., 306
Block, P., 211
Blouin, J. H., 273
Blume, A. W., 357
Boardman, C., 216
Bobes, J., 331, 332
Bodenmann, G., 381, 399
Bögner, I., 397
Bola, J. R., 309
Bollini, P., 319
Bolwig, T. G., 225
Bond, A. J., 88
Borchardt, C. M., 108
Borison, R. L., 87
Borkovec, T. D., 78, 79, 80, 81, 82, 84, 85, 89, 91, 103, 104, 106, 111, 112, 120
Bornstein, P. H., 390
Boulier, A., 278
Boulougouris, J. C., 134
Boyer, W. F., 87
Brabban, A., 310
Brady, K. T., 184, 189
Brady, S. M., 18
Bramlett, M. D., 381
Brannemann, B. D., 209
Braukhaus, C., 395
Bravo, M. F., 210
Brawman-Mintzer, O., 79
Bray, J. H., 395
Brechman-Toussaint, M., 61, 108
Breitholtz, E., 41, 86, 113
Bremner, J. D., 177
Brengelmann, J. C., 387
Brent, D. A., 206
Breslau, N., 175, 176, 188
Breslin, F. C., 367, 368
Brett, E., 177
Brewerton, T. D., 269
Brewin, C. R., 19, 330
Bridge, J., 206
Bright, J., 251
Bright, P., 20
Broadhead, W. E., 206
Broderick, J. E., 387
Bromet, E., 175
Broome, K. M., 354, 365
Brown, E., 191
Brown, E. J., 46
Brown, G., 261
Brown, G. K., 9, 21, 210
Brown, G. W., 318, 328

Brown, S. A., 184
Brown, T. A., 5, 6, 8, 9, 20, 78, 79, 80, 82, 84, 85, 89, 95, 104, 105, 106, 107, 109, 113, 114, 120, 174
Browne, G., 208
Bruch, M. A., 44
Bryant, K., 350
Bryant, M. J., 213, 219
Buchanan, A., 331
Buckminster, S., 44
Buddeberg, C., 10
Budney, A. J., 363, 365, 366
Bufka, L. F., 18
Bulik, C. M., 273, 287
Burks, N., 387
Burney, R., 367
Burns, D. D., 212, 213
Bushnell, W. D., 137
Butcher, J. N., 381
Butler, G., 80, 107, 112, 113
Butzlaff, R. L., 330
Bux, D. A., 136

Caballero, A., 227
Cahalane, J., 218
Cahill, S. P., 188, 190, 191
Calabrese, J. R., 249
Calam, R., 309, 320, 321
Caldwell, C. B., 327
Campbell, L. A., 79
Caputo, G. C., 20
Carpenter, D., 131
Carpenter, K. M., 12
Carroll, K. M., 189
Carter, F. A., 273
Carter, J. C., 270, 272, 274, 279
Casacalenda, N., 206
Case, G., 87, 113
Casper, R. C., 271
Cassano, G. B., 256
Castle, D. J., 140
Castonguay, L. G., 85, 213
Chadwick, P. D., 309, 320
Chambers, T. C., 319
Chambless, D. L., 8, 9, 20, 46, 55, 58, 59, 133, 139, 141, 382, 385
Charney, D. S., 183
Chattopadhyay, P. K., 107
Chemtob, C. M., 187
Chen, E. Y., 288
Cheslow, D., 130
Choate, M. L., 19
Choquette, K. A., 398
Chorpita, B. F., 77, 79

Christensen, A., 382
Chudzik, S. M., 8, 19, 221
Cina, A., 399
Clark, D., 22, 178
Clark, D. A., 208, 227
Clark, D. B., 44
Clark, D. M., 3, 42, 43, 49, 54, 55, 57, 58, 60, 62, 71, 178, 179, 256, 264
Clark, L. A., 79
Clarke, G. N., 210, 225
Clary, C. M., 184
Cobb, J., 133
Cochran, S. D., 250
Cochrane, R., 313, 314, 330
Cohen, A. S., 104
Cohen, E. M., 85
Cohen, L. R., 272
Cohen, M., 223
Cohn, J. B., 87
Coles, M. E., 45, 54
Colin, V., 87
Collins, K. A., 9
Collins, R. L., 368
Colom, F., 250
Compton, S. N., 109
Connor, K. M., 183, 184
Connors, G. J., 369
Cooley, M. R., 41
Cooley-Quille, M. R., 41
Cooper, J. E., 306
Cooper, Z., 264, 271, 280, 286
Corda, B., 61
Cormier, H. J., 8
Corominas, A., 5, 7
Coryell, W., 211, 227, 246
Cosoff, S. J., 256
Costello, C. G., 210
Costello, E., 80, 84, 112
Costello, F., 210, 225
Côté, G., 8
Cottraux, J., 137
Cournoyer, L. G., 213
Cowan, C. P., 398
Cowan, P., 398
Cowie, I., 271
Cowley, D. S., 4, 86, 87
Cox, M., 381
Craighead, L. W., 227
Craighead, W. E., 227
Craske, M. G., 3, 5, 6, 20, 77, 78, 79, 80, 84, 85, 89, 90, 92, 94, 95, 98, 99, 100, 104, 105, 107, 110, 112, 120

Crino, R., 132
Crits-Christoph, P., 223, 356
Crosby, R., 271
Crow, T. J., 317
Crowe, M. J., 387
Crowe, R. R., 78
Cummings, E. M., 381
Curran, H. V., 88
Curry, J. F., 139
Cutter, H. S. G., 398

Dadds, M. R., 108
Dahme, B., 269
Daiuto, A. D., 382
Daley, S. E., 226, 227
Dan, E., 183
Dancu, C. V., 174, 177, 179, 180, 189, 190, 193
Daneman, D., 289
Dansky, B. S., 175, 189, 269
David, A., 331
Davidson, J., 183, 184
Davidson, J. R. T., 43, 45, 88, 183, 184
Davidson, P. R., 183
Davies, P. T., 381
Davis, G. C., 175
Davis, J. M., 271
Davis, L., 291
Davis, L. A., 351
Davis, M. J., 206
Davis, R., 282, 291
Deale, A., 135
de Araujo, L. A., 135, 140, 141
de Beurs, E., 8
de Boer, A. G., 77
Dechert, R. E., 278
Deci, E. L., 360, 361, 362
de Haan, E., 140
DeKlyen, M., 391
Dell'Osso, L., 256
Delsignore, A., 10
DeMartinis, N., 87
den Boer, J. A., 4
Dennis, A. B., 288
Derman, K. H., 369
DeRubeis, R. J., 208, 210, 213, 214
Deter, H. C., 273, 291
Detweiler, J. B., 391, 392
DeVeaugh-Geiss, J., 137
Devenyi, R. G., 289
Devilly, G. J., 182
Devins, G. M., 39
Devlin, M. J., 285, 286
Dewhurst-Savellis, J., 210

Di Nardo, P. A., 78
Diamond, B. I., 87
DiBernardo, C., 141
DiClemente, C. C., 9, 10, 217, 275, 357
Diehl, L., 79
Dimeo, F., 230
Dingemans, P., 258
Dixon, L. B., 329
Dobson, K. S., 209, 210, 211, 386
Doll, H., 270
Donnelly, M., 330
Donovan, C., 61, 108
Doubleday, E. K., 214
Dow, B. M., 184
Downing, R. W., 87
Dozois, D. J. A., 9, 10, 11
Drake, R. E., 329
Dreessen, L., 140
Drury, V., 313, 314
Du Rand, C., 18
Duda, K., 330
Duffy, A. L., 108
Duggan, C. F., 210
Dunn, R. L., 382, 384
DuPont, R. L., 88
Dupuis, G., 2, 7
Durham, R. C., 89, 91, 107, 111, 316
Dyck, I. R., 4, 8, 20, 91, 139

Eaton, W. W., 1, 2, 39
Eaves, G. G., 209
Eberlein-Vries, R., 332
Eckert, E. D., 269, 271, 273, 291
Edelman, R. E., 9, 46, 59
Eels, T., 320
Ehlers, A., 21, 58, 178, 179
Ehrensaft, M. K., 380
Eisen, J., 139
Eisler, I., 271, 273
Eldredge, K. L., 283
Elhaj, O., 249
Elkin, I., 208, 214, 216, 230
Emery, G., 82, 91, 96, 97, 178, 264
Emmelkamp, P. M. G., 134, 384
Endicott, J., 184, 211, 227, 246
Eng, W., 45, 61
Engel, R. R., 332
Enns, M. W., 209
Epstein, E. E., 386
Epstein, N. B., 385
Epstein, N., 261
Epstein, S., 178
Erwin, B. A., 46, 47, 63

Estrada, A. U., 391
Everitt, B., 331
Ezquiaga, E., 210, 211

Fabbri, S., 230
Faedda, G. L., 259, 260
Fahy, T. A., 273
Fairburn, C. G., 139, 264, 269, 270, 271, 272, 273, 274, 279, 280, 283, 285, 286, 291
Falloon, I. R., 332
Falsetti, S. A., 190
Fals-Stewart, W., 132, 140, 386
Faragher, B., 185, 313
Faravelli, C., 20
Farmer, A., 307
Fava, G. A., 20, 230, 258, 259
Feeney, M. G., 258
Feeny, N. C., 136, 174, 177, 181, 185, 188
Fehm, L., 325
Fehm-Wolfsdorf, G., 395
Feighner, J. P., 87
Feixas, G., 212
Feldbau-Kohn, S. R., 380
Fennell, M. J., 80, 213
Fernstrom, M. H., 278
Ferreri, M., 87
Feske, U., 22, 46
Feuer, C. A., 174
Fichter, M. M., 8
Fiegenbaum, W., 3
Field, A. E., 291
Fields, J. M., 380, 381
Fiellin, D. A., 371
Fieve, R. R., 211
Fincham, F. D., 392
Fink, M., 207
First, M. B., 174, 193, 194
Fischer, S. C., 135
Fitzgibbons, L. A., 177, 186
Fitzpatrick, E., 332
Flament, M. F., 287
Fleming, A. S., 398
Fletcher, A. M., 353
Fletcher, K., 367
Foa, E. B., 41, 45, 51, 59, 60, 63, 71, 128, 129, 130, 131, 132, 133, 135, 137, 138, 139, 140, 174, 176, 177, 178, 179, 180, 181, 186, 187, 188, 189, 190, 191, 193
Folkman, S., 355
Follette, W. C., 382, 383, 387, 393
Forthofer, M. S., 381

Frances, A., 131
Frank, E., 210, 214, 224, 249
Frank, J. B., 183
Frank, M., 3
Franklin, M. E., 41, 45, 131, 133, 135, 136, 137, 138, 139, 140, 141, 158, 174, 177
Freeman, C. P. L., 269
Freeman, R. J., 291
Freeston, M. H., 138
French, M. T., 358
Fresco, D. M., 54, 84
Frey, R., 354
Fridman, R., 87
Friedman, B. H., 81
Fristad, M. A., 257
Fruzzetti, A. E., 386
Fung, T. S., 9
Furlong, M., 211
Furr, J. M., 138, 140, 189, 190
Fyer, A. J., 71

Gagnon, R., 213
Gale, C., 86
Gallagher, D., 213
Gallagher, R., 20
Gamache, G. M., 330
Garcia, A., 210
Garety, P. A., 317
Garland, A., 251
Garner, D. M., 272
Garry, J. K. F., 9
Gaston, L., 213
Gath, D., 308
Gatz, M., 107
Gauthier, J. G., 8
Gavazzi, S. M., 257
Gelder, M., 80, 308
Gelenberg, A. J., 88
Gelernter, C. S., 44
Gelfand, L. A., 208, 213
Gelhart, R. P., 209, 210
Geller, A. M., 87
Geller, D. A., 137
Gemar, M., 226, 251
George, L. K., 78, 206, 207
George, M. S., 207
Gershuny, B. S., 177, 186
Gibbon, M., 193
Giles, D. E., 227
Gillberg, C., 273
Gillberg, I. C., 273
Giller, E. L., 183

Gitlin, M. J., 246, 258
Glass, C. R., 46, 55
Glassco, J. D., 80
Glaun, D., 271
Godart, N. T., 287
Goering, P., 39
Goff, D. C., 18
Goff, G., 291
Goldapple, K., 220
Goldberg, S. C., 271
Goldberg-Arnold, J. S., 257
Goldfried, M. R., 213
Goldstein, A., 46
Goldstein, M. J., 258, 330
Goldstein, S. G., 60
Gollan, J. K., 209
Goodman, W., 130
Goodwin, F. K., 248
Gordon, J. G., 352, 353, 354, 374
Gordon, J. R., 294, 397
Gordon, J. S., 212
Gordon, K. C., 402
Gorman, J. M., 3, 4, 71
Gormley, N., 225
Gorski, T., 112
Gortner, E. T., 209
Gossop, M., 356
Gottesman, I. I., 327
Gould, R. A., 4, 6, 19, 44
Goyer, L. R., 7
Grabowski, J., 361
Gracely, E. J., 20
Grady, D. A., 187
Grady-Fletcher, A., 393
Graham, J. M., 354, 355
Gray-Little, B., 387, 388
Grayson, J. B., 133, 135
Grebb, J., 319
Greenberg, D., 177
Greenberg, L. S., 281
Greenberg, R. L., 82, 178
Greenberger, D., 218, 219, 232
Greenwald, S., 2
Gregg, L., 327
Greist, J. H., 43, 137, 139
Grilo, C. M., 9
Grisham, J. R., 79
Groth, T., 395
Grove, W., 271
Grunze, H., 248
Guerrero, T., 5
Guest, J. F., 247
Gurman, A. S., 386
Guzick, D. S., 227

Haaga, D. A., 214
Hackel, L. S., 398
Hackett, C. A., 89
Hackman, A., 54
Haddock, G., 309, 313, 314, 320, 326, 329, 330
Hafner, R. J., 256
Hahlweg, K., 3, 8, 382, 387, 390, 394, 395
Hakstian, A. R., 209
Halford, W. K., 384, 390
Hall, P. H., 338
Hall, S. M., 354
Hall, W., 369
Hallett, C. B., 281
Halmi, K. A., 270, 271, 273, 291
Halter, U., 230
Hamada, R. S., 187
Hamby, S. L., 388
Hamilton, K. E., 209, 210, 211
Hamilton, M., 307
Hammen, C., 225, 226, 246
Hansen, D., 278
Hantouche, E. G., 87
Harap, S., 140
Harden, T., 218
Hardy, G. E., 210, 211, 213, 223
Harrison, G., 317
Hart, A. B., 227
Harvald, B., 246
Harvey, A. G., 58, 71
Harvey, I., 307
Hasin, D., 350
Haskins, J. T., 88
Hasler, G., 10
Hasse, S. A., 278
Hatsukami, D., 269, 271
Hauge, M., 246
Havassy, B. E., 354
Hawkins, D. M., 286
Hayashida, M., 370
Hayes, A. M., 213
Hayes, S. C., 367
Hayward, C., 61
Hayward, P., 251, 331
Hazlett, R. L., 78, 79
Hazlett-Stevens, H., 81
Heard, H. L., 288
Hearst-Ikeda, D., 187
Heavey, C. L., 382
Hedegaard, K., 137
Hedges, D., 88
Heide, F. J., 103, 104

Heimberg, R. G., 7, 8, 38, 39, 40, 41,
    44, 45, 46, 48, 49, 50, 51, 54, 55,
    56, 59, 60, 61, 71, 84
Heinmaa, M., 282
Heinrichs, N., 3
Heinze, G., 227
Helbig, S., 325
Heller, T. L., 246
Hellstrøm, K., 41
Helzer, J. E., 183
Hembree, E. A., 181, 186, 188
Herbel, B., 135
Herbert, J. D., 46, 60, 140
Hersen, M., 108
Herzog, D. B., 271, 273
Herzog, W., 273, 291
Hester, R. K., 357
Hettema, J. E., 350
Heyman, R. E., 380, 393
Higgins, S. T., 363, 365, 366
Hiller, M. L., 357, 365
Hilsenroth, M. J., 223
Hirsch, C. R., 54
Hirschfeld, R. M. A., 210
Hjemboe, S., 381
Hodgson, R., 134, 135
Hoehn-Saric, R., 78, 79, 81, 88
Hoekstra, R., 140
Hoffman, A., 258
Hoffman, J. A., 389
Hofmann, S. G., 2, 3, 18, 46, 55
Hohagen, F., 137
Holaway, R. M., 40
Hollon, S. D., 279, 382, 385, 386
Holmes, J. M., 110, 391
Holt, C. S., 38, 61
Holtzworth-Munroe, A., 381, 391, 393
Hoogduin, K., 141
Hoogduin, C. A. L., 7, 9, 139
Hooley, J. M., 330
Hope, D. A., 38, 41, 44, 46, 51, 56, 66,
    71
Hope, R. A., 270
Hopkins, M., 78
Hornig, A., 258
Hornig, C. D., 39
Horowitz, L. M., 211
Horowitz, M. J., 178, 187, 188
Horvath, A. O., 213
Horvath, A. T., 356
Horwath, E., 205
Houck, C., 88
Howard, B. L., 108, 109
Hu, S., 79, 84

Huber, C. H., 384
Hughes, D., 78
Hughes, M., 175
Humphreys, K., 356
Hunt, G. M., 363
Hunt, M. G., 282
Huppert, J. D., 8, 15, 41, 47, 59, 158
Huta, V., 39

Ingram, R. E., 226
Insel, T. R., 129
Ito, L. M., 135, 140

Jackel, L., 77
Jacob, R. G., 44
Jacobsen, M., 283
Jacobson, N. S., 209, 213, 219, 381, 382,
    383, 385, 386, 387, 388, 389,
    390, 391, 393, 394, 395, 396
James, W., 367
Janoff-Bulman, R., 178
Jaremko, M. E., 85, 113
Jarrett, R. B., 209, 210, 227, 228
Jasin, S. E., 20
Jauhar, P., 258
Jaycox, L. H., 41, 186
Jeammet, P., 287
Jefferson, J. W., 43
Jeffries, J. J., 207
Jenike, M. A., 137, 140
Jenner, J. A., 316
Jerremalm, A., 40
Jimerson, D. C., 278
Joe, G. W., 354
Johansson, J., 40
Johnson, A. L., 317
Johnson, J., 2, 39, 205
Johnson, T., 107
Johnston, C., 330
Johnstone, E., 317
Joiner, T. E., 212
Jones, E. E., 214
Jones, R., 270
Jones, S., 251
Jouriles, E. N., 395
Joyce, A. S., 214
Joyce, E., 317
Joyce, P. R., 273
Judd, L. L., 206
Juster, H. R., 41, 46, 51

Kabat-Zinn, J., 94, 231, 281, 367, 368
Kadden, R., 350
Kahn, D., 131

Kalsy, S., 138
Kampman, M., 9
Kanai, T., 227
Kane, J. M., 319
Kane, M., 108
Kanfer, F. H., 309
Kaplan, A. S., 271, 281, 283, 291
Kapur, S., 314
Karkowski, L. M., 225
Karoly, P., 309
Kasper, S., 137
Kasvikis, Y., 139
Katon, W., 77, 214
Katz, R., 226
Katzelnick, D. J., 43
Kaufman, N. K., 210
Kavanagh, D. J., 330
Kaye, W. H., 271, 278, 281
Kazdin, A. E., 108
Kearney, B., 210
Keck, P. E., 248
Keijsers, G. P. J., 7, 8, 9, 139, 141, 186
Keitner, G. I., 248
Keller, M. B., 2, 20, 77, 91, 108, 205,
    207, 211, 224, 227, 246, 248,
    273
Kellogg, S., 189
Kelly, J., 398
Kemp, R., 331
Kendall, P. C., 108, 109
Kendell, R. E., 306
Kendler, K. S., 225
Kendren, J. M., 8
Kennedy, S., 282
Kent, G., 318
Kerig, P. K., 214
Kessing, L. V., 225
Kessler, R. C., 1, 39, 77, 175, 176, 188,
    381
Khantzian, E. J., 353
Kiecolt-Glaser, J. K., 381
Kilic, C., 19
Kilpatrick, D. G., 175, 177, 269
Kim, H. Y., 58
Kim, K., 318
Kimmel, S. E., 249
King, A. C., 355, 370
King, H. L., 209, 210
King, P., 214
Kingdon, D. G., 310
Kinney, C., 315, 317, 318
Kinon, B., 319
Kirov, G., 331
Kirsch, I., 206

Kishline, A., 356
Kissling, W., 332
Klaw, E., 356
Kleifield, E., 273
Klein, D. F., 2, 71
Klein, D. N., 205
Klein, E., 87
Klein, M., 249
Klein, R. G., 61
Klerman, G. L., 2, 205
Kline, N. A., 184
Klocek, J., 212
Knight, K., 357, 365
Kobak, K. A., 43, 139
Koch, W. J., 8, 176, 210, 221
Koenen, K., 187
Koke, S., 183, 191
Kolko, D., 206
Korman, L. M., 281
Kosten, T. R., 183
Kozak, M. J., 41, 129, 131, 132, 133,
    135, 139, 140, 178
Kraemer, H. C., 139, 270, 273
Krahn, D. D., 278
Kranzler, H., 350
Kreider, R. M., 380, 381
Kristeller, J. L., 281
Kroeger, C., 395
Krupnick, J. L., 213, 214
Kuipers, E., 316
Kuipers, L., 332
Kulka, R. A., 176
Kurinji, S., 207
Kurzer, N., 210
Kusumakar, V., 249
Kuyken, W., 210

Laberge, B., 8
Labouvie, E., 354
Ladak, Y., 20
Lader, M. H., 88, 318
Ladouceur, R., 120
Lam, D. H., 249, 251, 252, 256, 258, 259
Lambert, M. J., 206
Lamparski, D. M., 269
Langdon, L., 291
Lange, A., 8
Langhinrichsen-Rohling, J., 380
Larimer, M. E., 352, 367
Last, C. G., 108, 109
Latimer, P., 133
Lavori, P. W., 273
Lax, T., 139, 141
Lazarus, R., 355

Leaf, P. J., 246
Leahy, R. L., 96
Lee, A. S., 210, 214
Leff, J., 330, 332
Lehman, A. F., 329
Lehman, C. L., 79
Lei, H., 361
Leigh, B. C., 353
Lelliott, P. T., 129, 139
Lenane, M., 130
Lenox, R. H., 87
Lentz, R., 269
Leonard, H. L., 130
Lerner, J., 71
Lesem, M. D., 278
Leshner, A. I., 351
Leskin, G. A., 2
Lester, G. W., 383, 385, 390
Leucht, S., 332
Leukefeld, C., 357
Leung, A. W., 46, 59
Levitt, A., 207
Levitt, J., 133
Levy, S. J., 9
Lew, A., 212
Lewinsohn, P. M., 210, 225
Lewis, S., 314, 329
Lieberman, J., 319
Liebowitz, M. R., 38, 39, 43, 44, 46, 52,
    71, 79, 85, 89, 109, 120
Liebson, I. A., 371
Lilenfeld, L. R., 286
Limb, K., 249, 337
Lindholm, L., 273
Lindsay, M., 132, 141
Lindwall, R., 41
Linehan, M. M., 288, 367, 369
Linfield, K. J., 392
Lipworth, L., 367
Livanou, M., 174, 185
Lively, T. J., 291
Lizardi, H., 205
Locke, H. J., 380
Londborg, P. D., 191
Looper, K., 206
Loretan, A., 259
Lovell, K., 174
Lowe, C. F., 320
Lowens, I., 326
Lowry-Webster, H., 110
Luborsky, L., 223
Lucas, R. A., 41
Lucente, S., 140
Lucki, I., 87

Lundh, L. G., 58
Lyonfields, J. D., 79
Lytle, R., 91

MacCarthy, B., 330
Machan, J. T., 20
MacKenzie, J., 309
MacMillan, F., 313, 317
Maddocks, S. E., 291
Magee, W. J., 1, 39, 63
Mainguy, N., 7
Maisto, S. A., 398
Malik, M. L., 183
Malkoff-Schwartz, S., 249
Mallinckrodt, B., 223
Maltzman, I., 351
Mancill, R. B., 79
Mandos, L., 87
Manes, F., 207
Mangrum, L. F., 387
Mannu, P., 43
Mansell, W., 256
March, J. S., 131, 135, 137, 139, 143,
    160
Marchand, A., 2, 7
Marchi, P., 271
Marcus, M. D., 269, 270, 279, 280, 285
Margolin, G., 381, 385
Margolis, M., 223
Margraf, J., 3
Markman, H. J., 381, 382, 390
Markowitz, J. C., 386
Marks, A. P., 132
Marks, I. M., 19, 129, 133, 134, 135,
    137, 139, 140, 141, 174, 180,
    181, 189, 190
Marlatt, G. A., 294, 352, 353, 354, 357,
    374, 397
Marshall, R. D., 183, 186
Marten, P. A., 61, 78
Martenyi, F., 183, 191
Martin, G., 354
Martin, G. L., 229
Martin, G. W., 355
Masia, C. L., 61
Massie, E. D., 188
Massil, H., 398
Massion, A. O., 7, 77, 79
Mataix-Cols, D., 139, 140
Matas, M., 87
Mathews, A., 54
Matloff, J. L., 184
Mattick, R. P., 369
Mawson, D., 133

Mayou, R., 308
Mays, N., 330
McCabe, R. E., 3, 8, 19, 20, 221
McCallum, M., 214
McCarron, J., 313
McCarthy, E., 249, 318, 337
McConaha, C., 278
McConnaughy, E. A., 11
McCrady, B. S., 354, 386
McDonald, R., 133
McDougle, C. J., 183
McElroy, S. L., 248
McEvoy, L., 183
McFarlane, T. L., 271
McGeary, J., 218
McGilloway, S., 330
McGinn, L. K., 89
McGonagle, K. A., 39
McGrain, L., 270
McGuffin, P., 307, 317
McIntosh, V., 273
McKay, J. R., 398
McKendrick, K., 358
McKenna, C., 393
McLean, P. D., 8, 138, 209, 210, 221
McLean, R. Y., 4
McLellan, A. T., 369, 375
McLeod, D. R., 78, 81, 88
McMain, S., 367
McManus, F., 54
McVey, G., 282
Meadows, E. A., 179
Mehlman, S. K., 390
Meichenbaum, D. S., 85, 113
Menezes, P. R., 329
Mennin, D. S., 7, 8, 84, 120
Mercer, C., 87
Merrill, K. A., 210
Metalsky, G. I., 212, 226
Metzger, L., 360
Meyers, R. J., 363, 364, 370
Michelson, L. K., 8
Miklowitz, D. J., 250, 252, 254, 258
Miller, I. W., 248
Miller, J. J., 367
Miller, L. S., 247
Miller, M., 112
Miller, W. R., 10, 11, 217, 275, 276,
    287, 293, 294, 329, 350, 352,
    354, 357, 360, 362
Milos, G., 10
Milstein, B., 384
Mindlin, M., 46
Mineka, S., 79

Minichiello, W. E., 140
Mintz, J., 258
Mitchell, J. E., 271, 281, 282,
    291
Mohlman, J., 108
Mohr, D. C., 211
Molleken, L., 271, 278, 281
Molnar, G. J., 258, 259
Moncrieff, J., 248
Monk, T. H., 398
Monroe, S. M., 8, 212
Monteiro, W. O., 129, 139
Montgomery, S. A., 137
Moore, T. J., 206
Moorey, S., 221, 222
Moorhead, S. R. J., 251, 257
Moran-Tynski, S., 216
Morgan, H. G., 273
Morgenstern, J. M., 354
Moring, J., 329
Morrell, W., 291
Morris, T. L., 61
Morrison, A. P., 331
Morrison, K., 6
Morriss, R., 249, 337
Mortensen, P. B., 225
Moser, J., 45, 138, 174
Mosher, L. R., 309
Mosher, W. D., 381
Moukaddem, M., 278
Mouland, S. O., 273
Moye, A., 271
Mueller, T. I., 214
Mueser, K. T., 309, 382
Muldar, R., 187
Mulle, K., 135, 143, 160
Mulrow, C. D., 206
Muraoka, M. Y., 187
Muraven, M., 368
Murdock, T., 174, 176
Murphy, J. G., 359
Murray, R. M., 210, 214

Nairn, K. K., 278
Nasser, E. H., 80, 112, 113
Neighbors, C., 354
Neimeyer, R. A., 212, 213
Nelson, A. H., 137
Nelson, C. B., 175
Nelson, H. E., 320
Nelson, M. L., 223
Newman, C. F., 9
Newman, E., 183
Newman, H., 89

Newman, M. G., 83, 91, 92, 93, 95, 98, 99, 100, 111
Newns, K., 285
Newton, T. L., 381
Nicholls, S. S., 206
Nienhaus, K., 368
Nienhuis, F. J., 316
Ninan, P. T., 184
Nishith, P., 174
Norcross, J. C., 9
Norman, C. C., 393
Norring, C., 273
Noshirvani, H. F., 129, 139, 174
Noyes, R., 43, 78
Nuechterlein, K. H., 258, 330
Nutzinger, D. O., 269

Oakley-Browne, M., 86
Obarzanek, E., 278
O'Brien, C. P., 369, 370, 375
O'Brien, K. M., 286, 287
O'Connor, P. G., 371
Oei, T. P. S., 211
O'Farrell, T. J., 386, 398
Oldham, M., 183
Oldridge, M. I., 330
O'Leary, D., 210, 225
O'Leary, K. D., 380, 386, 387
O'Leary, T. A., 82, 84
Olfson, M., 47
Ollendick, T. H., 20
Olmsted, M. P., 270, 271, 283, 289, 291
Oosterbaan, D. B., 43
Orimoto, L., 295
Orsillo, S. M., 20, 103, 120, 178
Orza, M. J., 319
Osher, F. C., 329
Öst, L. G., 40, 41, 80, 82, 86, 113, 134, 190
O'Sullivan, G., 139, 141
Otto, M. W., 4, 19, 22, 44
Ouellette, R., 2
Ouimette, P. C., 205
Overholser, J. C., 80, 112, 113

Padberg, F., 208
Padesky, C. A., 218, 219, 232
Pagel, M., 387
Paivio, S. C., 281
Paley, G., 309
Pallares, T., 210
Palmer, R. L., 270
Palmer, R. S., 352
Pampallona, S., 319

Pande, A. C., 43
Papageorgiou, C., 54, 214
Parker, K. C. H., 183
Parks, G. A., 357
Parle, M., 330
Paterniti, S., 20
Paul, G. L., 209
Paul, T., 269
Paunovic, N., 190
Paykel, E. S., 318
Pecknold, J. C., 87
Penkower, A., 183
Pepper, C. M., 205
Perdereau, F., 287
Perlick, D., 256
Perloff, J. M., 212
Perrez, M., 399
Perrin, S., 108
Perry, A., 249, 259, 337
Perry, J. C., 206
Perry, K. J., 46
Persons, J. B., 212, 213, 218, 222
Perugi, G., 256
Peselow, E. D., 211
Peterson, E., 175
Peterson, R. A., 7, 20
Pettinati, H. M., 369
Peveler, R. C., 270, 273, 279, 283, 291
Phillips, T., 271
Phoenix, E., 217
Pike, K. M., 272
Pilgrim, H., 185
Pilkonis, P. A., 210, 211
Pilling, S., 308, 316
Pincus, A. L., 91
Pini, S., 256
Pioli, R., 43
Piper, W. E., 214
Piran, N., 291
Pitschel-Walz, G., 332
Plamondon, J., 8
Pollack, M. H., 2, 4, 19, 20, 44
Pollack, R. A., 2
Porceddu, K., 332
Post, R. M., 226
Potter, W. Z., 248
Poulos, C. X., 355
Power, K. G., 7, 8, 88
Powers, M. B., 22
Prakash, A., 183, 191
Prescott, C. A., 225
Price, J., 246
Price, L., 130
Priebe, S., 250, 258

Prien, R. F., 248
Prochaska, J. O., 9, 10, 11, 217, 275, 357
Proest, G., 230
Prue, D. M., 355
Prusoff, B. A., 205
Putnam, F. W., 187
Pyle, R., 271

Quinlan, D. M., 211
Quinn, J., 330

Rabavilas, A. D., 134
Rachman, S., 134, 135, 160
Rae, D. S., 246
Raffa, S. D., 85
Rahill, A. A., 330
Rao, U., 226
Rapaport, M. H., 184
Rapee, R. M., 40, 54, 58, 60, 71, 77, 78, 79, 80, 85, 107, 108
Rapoport, J. L., 130
Rapp, S. R., 355
Rapport, D. J., 249
Rasmussen, S., 130, 139
Rastam, M., 273
Ratnasuriya, R. H., 273
Rauch, S. A., 188
Rauch, S. L., 137
Raue, P. J., 213
Ravindran, A. V., 208
Raymond, N., 269
Rector, N. A., 213
Regier, D. A., 246, 356
Reiss, S., 7, 20
Remington, G., 314
Ren, X. S., 381
Renneberg, B., 46
Renshaw, K. D., 141
Resick, P. A., 174, 178, 179, 181, 189, 190, 191
Resnick, H. S., 175, 176, 177, 190
Revenstorf, D., 382, 383, 387, 390, 393
Reynolds, C. F.,III, 208, 228
Rheingold, A. A., 60
Rhoades, H. M., 361
Rice, D. P., 247
Rickels, K., 22, 87, 88, 109, 113
Riddle, M. A., 137
Rief, W., 8
Rigaud, D., 278
Riggs, D. S., 138, 174, 176, 177, 178, 186, 187, 188, 193
Robin, A. L., 271

Robins, C., 211
Robins, L. N., 183
Robinson, L. A., 213
Robson, P., 80
Rock, C., 278
Rockert, W., 282, 283, 291
Rodebaugh, T. L., 40, 44, 58
Rodin, G. M., 289
Roemer, L., 20, 103, 120
Rohde, P., 210, 225
Roitblat, H. L., 187
Roizen, R., 350
Rollnick, S., 10, 217, 275, 276, 287, 293, 294, 329, 360, 362
Rosen, J. C., 280
Rosenbaum, J. F., 2
Rosenberg, H., 351
Rosenberg, S. E., 211
Rosenthal, R. N., 356, 369
Rosenvinge, J. H., 273
Ross, C. A., 87
Rossiter, E. M., 273
Rotgers, F., 356
Roth, D. A., 38, 39, 41, 59, 158
Roth, S., 183
Rothbaum, B. O., 63, 174, 176, 177, 178, 179, 182, 184, 186, 187, 188, 189, 190, 193
Rounsaville, B. J., 205, 350, 370
Rowa, K., 20
Roy-Byrne, P. P., 4, 77, 86, 87
Rozendaal, N., 258
Ruble, D. N., 398
Ruscio, A. M., 80, 82, 103, 106
Rush, A. J., 178, 209, 227, 264
Russell, G. F. M., 273
Ryan, M. A., 109
Ryan, R. M., 360, 361, 362, 363
Rychtarik, R. G., 355, 369
Rydall, A. C., 289

Sacks, S., 358
Saettoni, M., 256
Safer, D. L., 291
Safran, J. D., 213, 215, 216, 232
Safren, S. A., 45, 46
Salusky, S., 386
Sanchez-Craig, M., 361
Sanders, M. R., 384
Sanderson, W. C., 89
Sandin, E., 381
Sansone, R. A., 288
Santiago, H., 8, 22
Santor, D. A., 225

Saunders, B. E., 175, 177
Sayers, S. L., 384
Scarpato, A., 20
Schaap, C. P. D. R., 7, 139
Schaap, G., 141
Schafer, J., 132
Schellberg, D., 273
Schene, A. H., 330
Schindler, L., 387, 390
Schmaling, K. B., 386, 393
Schmidt, N. B., 3, 7, 8, 16, 21, 22
Schmitz, J. M., 361
Schneider, J. A., 273
Schneider, K., 306
Schneier, F. R., 38, 39, 43, 46
Schnicke, M. K., 178, 181, 190
Schnyder, U., 10
Schroeder, B., 3
Schroeter, K., 269
Schut, A. J., 85
Schwartz, S. A., 140
Schwebel, A. I., 382, 384
Schweizer, E., 22, 87, 88, 113
Scoboria, A., 206
Scott, J., 251, 259
Sedvall, H., 41
Seeley, J. R., 210, 225
Segal, Z. V., 207, 213, 215, 216, 225, 226,
    230, 231, 232, 251, 281, 367, 368
Seivewright, H., 107
Sellers, W., 367
Sellwood, W., 318, 330, 332
Selten, J. P., 317
Seltzer, J. A., 381
Sensky, R., 316
Setzer, N. J., 109
Severeijns, R., 141
Shadick, R., 78
Shafran, R., 264, 271, 280
Sham, P., 249, 252
Shapiro, D. A., 213, 309
Shapiro, F., 182
Shapiro, R. W., 205
Sharp, C. W., 269
Sharp, D. M., 7, 8
Shavelson, L., 374
Shaw, B. F., 178, 226, 264
Shay, J., 183
Shea, M. T., 210, 211, 214, 224, 248
Shear, M. K., 3, 20, 22
Sheikh, J. I., 2
Sheldon, C., 39
Shelton, M. D., 249
Sher, T. G., 384, 386

Sherman, C., 370
Shoham, V., 382
Shokomskas, D., 205
Shuttlewood, G. J., 211
Siegel, P. T., 271
Silverstone, P. H., 331
Simon, G. E., 207
Simons, A. D., 208, 212, 213, 218
Simpson, D. D., 354, 357, 358, 359, 365
Simpson, H. B., 141
Simpson, R. J., 88
Siqueland, L., 108, 109
Skoog, G., 161
Skoog, I., 161
Slaap, B. R., 4
Sloan, T. B., 22
Smith, J. A., 258
Smith, J. E., 363, 364, 370
Smith, N., 251, 258
Smits, J. A. J., 22
Smoller, J. W., 20
Smutzler, N., 381
Snyder, D. K., 380, 383, 386, 387, 388,
    389, 393, 394, 399
Snyder, K. S., 258, 330
Sohlberg, S., 273
Soll, E., 271
Solomon, D. A., 248
Solyom, L., 291
Sommerfield, C., 185
Sonino, N., 230
Sonnega, A., 175
Sotsky, S. M., 209
Southam-Gerow, M. A., 109
Southwick, S. M., 183
Spangler, D. L., 212
Spanier, G. B., 380, 393
Specker, S., 269
Spence, S. H., 61, 108, 182
Spiegel, D. A., 3
Spinhoven, P., 4
Spinks, M. T., 259
Spitzer, R. L., 38, 193
Spurr, J. M., 54
Stacy, A. W., 353
Staines, G., 358
Stangor, C., 398
Stanley, M. A., 80, 108
Stanley, S., 381
Stasiewicz, P. R., 369
Steer, R. A., 261
Stefanis, C., 134
Steil, R., 179
Stein, D. J., 137

Steiner, M., 137
Steinhausen, H. C., 273
Steketee, G. S., 8, 9, 133, 135, 139, 140, 141, 177
Stern, R. S., 133
Stewart, B. L., 214
Stickle, T. R., 382
Stiles, W. B., 213
Stitzer, M. L., 371
St. James, R. L., 183
Stolk, J., 87
Stopa, L., 54
Storch, E. A., 61
Stotts, A. L., 361
Strain, E. C., 371
Street, G. P., 139
Street, L., 80
Strober, M., 291
Strosahl, K. D., 367
Strupp, H. H., 224
Stuart, G. L., 3, 5, 18
Sturgeon, D., 332
Sturpe, D. A., 19
Suarez, A., 288
Sullivan, P. F., 273
Sullivan, V., 270
Suppes, T., 259
Sutherland, S. M., 183
Swanson, V., 88
Swedo, S. E., 130
Swendsen, J., 246
Swinson, R. P., 3, 4, 8, 16, 19, 20, 38, 39, 221
Symonds, B. D., 213
Szmukler, G. I., 273

Tang, T. Z., 208
Tarrier, N., 180, 181, 185, 249, 258, 308, 309, 313, 314, 315, 316, 317, 318, 319, 320, 321, 326, 327, 328, 329, 330, 331, 332, 336, 337, 338
Tattan, T., 319
Taylor, S., 3, 8, 20, 44, 174, 176, 180, 182, 185, 210, 221
Teasdale, J. D., 213, 226, 231, 232, 281, 367
Telch, C. F., 273, 291
Telch, M. J., 3, 5, 22, 41
Tessler, R. C., 330
Thase, M. E., 205, 207, 209, 210, 212, 213, 214, 218, 386
Thayer, J. F., 81
Theander, S., 273

Thomas, J. C., 133
Thomas, L., 184
Thompson, L., 213
Thomsen, P. H., 137
Thrasher, S., 174
Tiffany, S. T., 353
Tischler, G. L., 246
Tkachuk, G. A., 229
Tohen, M., 259
Tolbert, V. E., 210
Tolin, D. F., 178
Tollefson, G. D., 137
Tondo, L., 259
Toni, C., 4
Torres, M., 227
Touyz, S. W., 271
Trakowski, J., 8, 22
Tran, G. Q., 46, 139
Treasure, J. L., 276, 282
Treat, T. A., 3, 5
Trenkamp, S., 8
Triffleman, E., 189
Truax, P., 382, 393
Tse, C. K., 206
Tuby, K. S., 4
Tucker, J. A., 359
Tucker, P., 183
Tupler, L. A., 183
Turgeon, L., 2
Turk, C. L., 41, 51, 54, 71, 84
Turkewitz, H., 387
Turkington, D., 310
Turner, R. M., 133, 135
Turner, S. M., 41, 44, 61
Turpin, G., 318, 330
Tyrer, P., 107

Uebelacker, L. A., 381, 399
Ureno, G., 211

Vallejo, J., 5
van Balkom, A. J. L. M., 4, 8, 19, 43, 137
van de Willige, G., 316
van der Does, A. J. W., 21
van der Kolk, B. A., 183
van Dyck, R., 4, 8, 43
van Kraanen, J., 134
van Minnen, A., 186
van Oppen, P., 43
van Os, J., 317
Varahram, I., 230
Vasey, M., 22
Vaughn, C. E., 330

Velicer, W. F., 11
Veljaca, K., 54
Vella, D. D., 226
Velten, E., 356
Velting, O. N., 109
Versiani, M., 43, 88
Villaseñor, V. S., 211
Vincent, N. K., 286, 287
Vincent, P., 207, 230
Vitousek, K., 272, 275, 276, 279, 295
Vitto, M., 43
Volpicelli, J. R., 369, 370
von Witzleben, I., 3
Vuchinich, R. E., 359

Wade, S. L., 8
Wade, W. A., 3, 5, 210
Wahass, S., 318
Walker, J., 61
Wallace, K. M., 380
Wallace, L. A., 88
Wallach, M. A., 329
Walsh, B. T., 270, 271, 272, 273, 280,
    281, 282
Walsh, W., 176
Walters, G. D., 350, 357, 361
Walters, S. T., 352
Ward, J., 369, 371
Warren, R., 133
Warshaw, M., 77, 91, 139
Wasserman, D. A., 354
Watson, D., 79
Watson, N. T., 370
Watson, S., 275
Wearden, A., 330
Weaver, T., 174, 177
Webb, M., 225
Weisberg, R. B., 20
Weisler, R. H., 184
Weisman, A., 330
Weiss, D. D., 109
Weiss, S., 22
Weissman, A. M., 4, 19, 211
Weissman, M. M., 39, 205, 246
Welch, S. L., 269
Weller, M. P. I., 258
Wells, A., 54, 60, 71, 86, 96, 101, 102,
    120, 256
Weltzin, T. E., 278
Westen, D., 6
Westra, H. A., 9, 216, 217
Westreich, L., 356, 369
Wetherell, J. L., 107, 108, 109, 111,
    112

Wheadon, D. E., 137
Whisman, M. A., 39, 211, 381, 383, 386,
    387, 391, 392, 395, 399
White, C., 46
Widmer, K., 399
Wiersma, D., 316
Wilbourne, P. L., 350
Wildgrube, C., 250
Wilfley, D. E., 272, 274
Wilhelm, K., 210
Wilkinson, D. A., 355
Williams, C., 20, 309
Williams, J. B. W., 193
Williams, J. M. G., 226, 231, 232, 281,
    367
Williams, K. E., 8
Williams, R., 54
Williams, S., 226
Wills, R. M., 387, 393
Wilson, G. L., 390
Wilson, G. T., 139, 270, 271, 272, 273,
    275, 279, 280, 281, 282, 283,
    285, 286
Wilson, K. G., 367
Wilson, L. J., 390
Wilson, R., 63
Wing, J. K., 328
Wing, R. R., 269
Wingrove, J., 88
Winokur, G., 246
Wiser, S. L., 79, 213
Wittchen, H. U., 1, 39, 77, 78,
    89
Wittkowski, A., 318
Wolfenden, M., 326
Wonderlich, S. A., 285
Wong, C., 183
Wong, G., 249, 258
Woods, C. M., 9
Woods, S. W., 3
Woodside, D. B., 271, 291
Woody, S. R., 8, 41, 55, 221
Woolaway-Bickel, K., 16, 22
Woolfolk, R. L., 187
Wright, K., 251, 252, 258

Yager, J., 289
Yanovski, S. Z., 269, 285
Yap, L., 44
Yarczower, M., 188
Yehuda, R., 183
Yonkers, K. A., 2, 77, 91
Young, A. H., 257
Yusupoff, L., 315, 317, 318

Zack, M., 367
Zaider, T. I., 44
Zaninelli, R., 183
Zaretsky, A. E., 251
Zastowny, T. R., 330
Zavodnick, S., 22
Zhang, H., 183, 191
Zhao, S., 77
Zhu, A. J., 280, 281

Zielenbach-Coenen, H., 397
Zielezny, M., 259
Zimmerli, W. D., 78, 88
Zinbarg, R., 186
Zipursky, R. B., 314
Zlotnick, C., 214
Zoellner, L. A., 136, 141, 174, 177, 181
Zuroff, D. C., 213

Subject Index

Abstinence, as outcome in alcohol abuse, 351
Acceptance and commitment therapy, 367
Activity and recreational therapy, for schizophrenia, 313
Adolescents
  GAD in, 108–110
  social anxiety disorder in, 61–62
Agoraphobia. *See also* Panic disorder/agoraphobia
  characteristics, 1
Alcohol dependence
  definitions of, 349–350
  with social anxiety disorder, 63
Alcohol use, bipolar disorder and, 255
Alcohol use disorders, 348–379
  abstinence as touchstone outcome, 351
  behavioral couple therapy for, 386
  case example, 371–373
  contextual factors in, 356
  co-occurring psychiatric disorders and, 356
  coping style and, 354–355
  defining treatment outcome/relapse, 351–352
  diagnostic criteria, 349–350
  empirically supported treatments, 357–359
  enhancing maintenance of behavior change, 366–371
  enhancing motivation and retention, 359–366
  external/internal factors in, 354
  factors associated with outcomes, 352–357
  length of treatment, 354
  mindfulness training in, 366–369

with panic disorder/agoraphobia, 19
patient-focused factors, 355–356
physiological basis, 351
and positive drinking expectancies, 353
self-help groups and, 356–357
treatment of, patient autonomy in, 361–362
All-or-nothing thinking, 98
Alogia, in schizophrenia, 317
Alprazolam, for panic disorder/agoraphobia, 21
Anger, in PTSD, 187–189
Anorexia nervosa, 268
  characteristics, 268–269
  motivational work in, 284–285
  outcome predictors, 273
  relapse predictors, 291
  reverse, 290
  treatments for, 271–272
Antabuse. *See* Disulfiram (Antabuse)
Antianxiety medications, 113
Antidepressants
  for bipolar disorder, 248
  for dysthymia, 207
  for eating disorders, 280–281
  for GAD, 87–88
Antipsychotic medications
  for bipolar disorder, 248
  nonadherence with, 331
  for schizophrenia, 308, 319
Anxiety. *See also* Generalized anxiety disorder; Social anxiety disorder
  with depression, 210
  with eating disorders, 287–288
  in PTSD, 187
  relaxation-induced, 103–104

Anxiety Disorders Interview Schedule–IV, 114–115
Automatic thoughts, 14
    in social anxiety disorder, 56–57

Behavior therapy, for depression, 208–209
Behavioral couple therapy, 381–383
    efficacy of, 403
Behavioral exchange strategies, 381
Benzodiazepines
    for GAD, 86–87
    interference with CBT, 19
Binge-eating disorder, 268
    characteristics, 269
    mindfulness-based stress reduction in, 281
    outcome predictors, 274
    relapse predictors, 291
    treatment adaptations in, 285–286
    treatment of, 272, 283
Bipolar disorder, 246–267
    case example, 261–263
    diagnostic criteria, 247
    economic costs, 247
    empirically supported treatments, 248–251
    etiology, 249
    family involvement in, 254–255
    genetic factors in, 246
    high goal-attainment beliefs in, 252–253
    mixed episodes, 247–248
    natural course, 246–247
    outcome improvement, 252–258
    outcome predictors, 252
    overview, 246–248
    pharmacotherapy for, 248–249
    psychotherapy for, 249–251
    relapse/recurrence predictors, 258–259
    relapse/recurrence prevention, 259–260
    subtypes, 247–248
    valuing highs in, 253–254
Body scan, 231–232
Body-checking behaviors, 280
Borderline personality disorder, with eating disorders, 288
Breathing retraining, for panic disorder/agoraphobia, 15–16
Breathing techniques, for alcohol use disorders, 368–369
Bulimia nervosa, 268
    CBT for, 269–270
    interpersonal therapy for, 270–271
    outcome predictors, 272–273
    pharmacotherapy for, 271

relapse predictors, 291
    treatment adaptations in, 285
Buprenorphine (Subutex), 371
Buspirone, for GAD, 87

Carbamazepine, for bipolar disorder, 248–249
Catastrophizing, 98
Checking rituals, 130
    in OCD, 164
Children
    exposure therapy for, 136
    GAD in, 108–110
    OCD in, 128, 130–131
    social anxiety disorder in, 61–62
Clozapine, for bipolar disorder, 249
Cognitive behavioral therapy, with medications, 64
Cognitive distortions
    in GAD, 115
    recognizing, 98
Cognitive flexibility, 317
Cognitive processing therapy, for PTSD, 179, 181
Cognitive remediation, in schizophrenia, 316
Cognitive restructuring
    in couple therapy, 384
    for panic disorder/agoraphobia, 3
    for PTSD, 179–180, 189–190
    for social anxiety disorder, 50–51
Cognitive therapies
    for bipolar disorder, 263–264
    for depression, 208
    mindfulness-based, for depression, 230–231
    for OCD, 138
    for PTSD, 178, 181
Cognitive vulnerability, depression and, 211–212, 226
Cognitive-behavioral couple therapy, 383–385, 403
Cognitive-behavioral group therapy, for social anxiety disorder, 56
Cognitive-behavioral therapy
    for bipolar disorder, 250–251
    for eating disorders, 277–290
        tailoring strategies, 278–279
    for panic disorder/agoraphobia, 1–37, 2–3, 4
    for persons with cognitive/language difficulties, 222–223
    principles of, 93
    for PTSD, 179–184

for schizophrenia, 309–316
for social anxiety disorder, 38–76
Columbo technique, 312
Communication, in couple distress, 381, 400
Community reinforcement and family training, 364–366
Community reinforcement approach, 363–366
disulfiram used with, 370
Comorbidity
with bipolar disorder, 256
with depression, 209–210, 220–221, 227
with eating disorders, 286–288
with GAD, 111
in generalized anxiety disorder, 89–90
with OCD, 139–140
in panic disorder/agoraphobia, 18–20
with PTSD, 188–189
in social anxiety disorder, 63
Compliance therapy, 331
Compulsions. *See also* Obsessive-compulsive disorder
defined, 128
Concerned significant others, 364
Contingency management, 364–366
Coping Cat Program, 108
Coping skills, alcohol use and, 354–355
Coping skills approach, for schizophrenia, 309–310, 311
Couple distress, 380–408
case example, 400–402
emotional aspects of, 392
empirically supported treatments, 381–386
individual-difference characteristics in, 388–389
outcome improvements, 389–393
outcome predictors, 386–389
overview, 380–381
relapse/recurrence predictors, 393–394
relapse/recurrence prevention, 394–400
relationship characteristics in, 387–388
Couple therapy, for mental/physical health problems, 385–386
Couples coping enhancement training, 399
Cultural factors, in schizophrenia, 317–318

Delusions
challenging, 325–326
defined, 307
in schizophrenia, 312, 314–315, 319

Dementia praecox, 306
Depression, 204–245
case example, 232–235
CBT for comorbid conditions, 220–221
CBT rationale in, 219–220
cognitive theory of, 178
cognitive-behavioral couple therapy for, 399
comorbidity with, 209–210, 227
couple therapy for, 386
demographic variables in, 210–211
double, 205, 210
with eating disorders, 287
empirically supported treatments, 206–209
interpersonal factors in, 215–216
medications for, 206–207
with OCD, 139
outcome improvement, 214–224
outcome predictors, 209–214
overview, 204–206
psychological treatments for, 208–209
realistic, 221–222
relapse prevention, 227–232
relapse/recurrence predictors, 224–227
severity/chronicity of, 209
with social anxiety disorder, 63, 68
stimulant treatment for, 207–208
subsyndromal/minor, 205
Diabetes mellitus, with eating disorders, 289–290
Dialectical behavioral therapy, 367, 369
Disulfiram (Antabuse), for alcohol abuse, 370
Divalproex, for bipolar disorder, 249
Double depression, 205, 210
Dual diagnosis. *See also* Comorbidity
with schizophrenia, 329–330
Dyadic Adjustment Scale, 393
Dysfunctional Attitudes Scale, 211, 252
Dysthymia
CBT for, 208
pharmacotherapy for, 207
Dysthymic disorder, characteristics, 205

Eating disorders, 268–305. *See also*
Anorexia nervosa; Bulimia nervosa
case example, 295–297
defining characteristics, 268–269
with depression, 210
empirically supported treatments, 269–272
in males, 290

Eating disorders (*continued*)
    outcome improvement, 274–290
        defining, 274–275
        strategies, 275–290
    outcome predictors, 272–274
    overview, 268–269
    relapse predictors, 291
    relapse/recurrence prevention, 292–295
    secondary gain from, 295
Electroconvulsive therapy
    for depression, 207
    for schizophrenia, 308
EMDR. *See* Eye movement desensitization
        and reprocessing
Emotional expressiveness training, 384
Emotional numbing, 186–187
    in PTSD, 175
Emotional processing theory, 178–179
Emotion-focused therapy, for eating disor-
        ders, 281–282
Exposure strategies, 131–136
    for children, 136
    duration, 134–135
    gradual versus abrupt, 135
    imaginal, 135–136
    imaginal versus *in vivo*, 131
    for panic disorder/agoraphobia, 15–16
    with pharmacotherapy, 137–138
    for PTSD, 177, 180–182, 188
    for social anxiety disorder, 51–61
    therapist-assisted versus self, 134
    variations in, 133–136
Exposure/ritual prevention therapy
    collaborative approach to, 142–145, 147
    homework, 158–159
    imaginal, 154–155, 166
    rationale for, 145–146
    ritual prevention, 155–158
    therapist questions in, 148–149
    in vivo, 152–154, 166
Expressed emotion
    bipolar disorder and, 252, 258
    schizophrenia and, 330
Eye movement desensitization and repro-
        cessing, for PTSD, 179, 182–183

Family
    attributional beliefs of, 330–331
    of bipolar client, 254–255
    of children with GAD, 109
    of client with schizophrenia, 330–331
    of OCD client, 142
Family interventions, in schizophrenia,
        316, 332, 336–337, 339

Family-focused treatment, for bipolar
        disorder, 250, 252
Fear
    pathological, 178
    two-factor theory of, 177
Flashbacks, in PTSD, 175, 187
Fluoxetine
    for client with eating disorder, 280–282
    for PTSD, 184
FRIENDS program, 110

GAD. *See* Generalized anxiety disorder
Generalized anxiety disorder, 77–127
    case example, 113–119
    cognitive therapy for, 82–84
    comorbidity in, 79, 89–90
    diagnostic criteria, 77
    diagnostic history of, 78–79
    with eating disorders, 288
    empirically supported treatments for, 79–88
    evidence-based pharmacological treat-
        ment for, 86–88
    evidence-based psychological treatment
        for, 79–86
    factors affecting outcomes, 88–110
        client, 89–92
        treatment, 92–110
    overview, 77–79
    with panic disorder, 104
    psychoeducation in, 80
    relapse/recurrence, 111–113
    relaxation training for, 81–82
    self-monitoring in, 80–81
    treatment adaptation in, 107–110
    treatment outcomes, 119–120
    worry imagery exposure for, 84–85

Hallucinations
    command, 327
    defined, 307
    in schizophrenia, 319
Hoarding, in OCD, 130
Hydroxyzine, for GAD, 87
Hypomania, DSM-IV-TR criteria for, 247

Imipramine, for panic disorder/
        agoraphobia, 21
Interpersonal and social rhythm therapy,
        249
Interpersonal functioning
    depression and, 215–216
    in GAD, 91–92
Interpersonal relationships, of client with
        schizophrenia, 330–331

Interpersonal therapy, for depression, 208, 230
Interviewing, motivational. *See* Motivational interviewing techniques

Lamotrigine, for bipolar disorder, 249
Lapse, defined, 352
Liebowitz Social Anxiety Scale, 52
Lifestyle
    depression and, 229–230
    panic disorder/agoraphobia and, 22
Lithium, for bipolar disorder, 248–249

Major depressive disorder. *See also* Depression
    characteristics, 204–205
Mania. *See also* Bipolar disorder
    DSM-IV-TR criteria for, 247
Manic depression, 306. *See also* Bipolar disorder
Medication compliance therapy, for bipolar disorder, 250
Mental health services, CBT for schizophrenia in, 328–329
Mental illness, historical perspective, 306
Mental rituals, in OCD, 129, 163
Metacognitive processes, in GAD, 101–102
Metaworries, in GAD, 101–102, 110
Methadone maintenance, 371
    for alcohol abuse, 369–370
Mindfulness training, for alcohol use disorders, 366–369
Mindfulness-based cognitive therapy, for depression, 230–231
Mindfulness-based meditation, 231
    in treatment of GAD, 94
Mindfulness-based stress reduction, for client with eating disorder, 281
Mirtazapine, for PTSD, 184
Monoamine oxidase inhibitors, for depression, 206–207
Mood stabilizers, for bipolar disorder, 248–249
Motivation
    in addiction treatment, 359–366
    for changing alcohol use, 354
    in depression treatment, 217–218
    in eating disorder treatments, 275–277
    in OCD treatment, 141
    in panic disorder treatment, 9–10
Motivational enhancement therapy, 217
    for eating disorders, 282
    for panic disorder/agoraphobia, 10

Motivational interviewing techniques, 362–363
    in alcohol abuse treatment, 360–366
    and contingency management/ community reinforcement, 363–366
    for eating disorders, 276, 287
    and medication compliance, 331–332
    and substance abuse, 329–330

Naloxone (Suboxone), 371
Naltrexone (ReVia), for alcohol abuse, 370
Neuroleptics
    adverse effects, 86
    for generalized anxiety disorder, 86
    for schizophrenia, 308
Noradrenergic-specific serotonergic antidepressants, for depression, 206
Norepinephrine dopamine reuptake inhibitors, for depression, 206
Numbing, emotional. *See* Emotional numbing

Obsessions. *See also* Obsessive-compulsive disorder
    defined, 128
Obsessive–compulsive disorder, 128–173
    case example, 163–166
    in children, 128, 130–131
    cognitive therapy for, 138
    with eating disorders, 288
    empirically supported treatments, 131–138
    exposure and ritual prevention in, 131–159
    externalizing, 143, 164
    lifestyle changes and, 162–163, 166
    outcome improvement, 142–159
    outcome predictors, 139–142
    overview, 128–131
    pharmacotherapy for, 136–137
        with exposure/ritual prevention, 137–138
    posttreatment obsessions, normalizing, 160–161
    preventing relapse/recurrence, 159–163
    subtypes, 129–130
    symptom severity, 140–141
Olanzapine, for bipolar disorder, 249
Older adults, bipolar disorder in, 257–258

Opioid replacement therapy, 371
  for alcohol abuse, 369–370
Opioid use disorders, 370–371

Panic control treatment, 3
Panic disorder
  characteristics, 1
  fluctuating course of, 5–6
Panic disorder/agoraphobia, 1–37
  breathing retraining for, 16
  case example, 22–30
  cognitive strategies in, 13–15
  cognitive-behavioral therapy for, 3
  cognitive-behavioral therapy versus
      pharmacotherapy for, 4
  comorbid conditions, 18–20
  depression and, 8
  empirically supported treatments, 2–6
  exposure strategies in, 15–16
  homework compliance, 16–17
  motivation for treatment, 9–11
  outcome improvement, 5–6, 9–20
  outcome predictors, 6–9
  overview, 1–2
  personality/personality disorders and, 7
  pharmacotherapy for, 3–4
  psychoeducation about, 13
  relapse predictors, 20–21
  relapse prevention, 5–6, 21–22
  symptom severity, 7–8
  therapist qualities and, 8
  therapy rationale in, 11–12
  treatment goals, 12–13
Personality, depression and, 226
Personality disorders
  couple-based approaches to, 386
  with depression, 210
  with eating disorders, 288
  with OCD, 139–140
  panic disorder/agoraphobia and, 7
Pharmacotherapy
  for alcohol abuse, 369–370
  for bipolar disorder, 248–249
  for depression, 206–207, 230
  with exposure/ritual prevention, 137–
      138
  for GAD, 113
  for OCD, 136–137
  for panic disorder/agoraphobia, 2–4
  for PTSD, 183–184
  for schizophrenia, 308–309, 319
Phobias, treatment of, 177
Pie chart technique, 99–101, 116, 117

Posttraumatic stress disorder, 174–203
  case example, 192–196
  client worldview and, 178–179, 183
  cognitive-behavioral therapies for, 179–
      183
  conceptualizations of, 177–179
  defined, 175
  diagnostic criteria, 175–176
  empirically supported treatments, 179–
      184
  natural recovery patterns, 176–177
  outcome improvement, 186–190
  outcome predictors, 185–186
  outcomes, 174
  overview, 175–177
  pharmacotherapy for, 183–184
  prevalence, 175
  preventing relapse, 190–192
Probability overestimation, 98
Problem-solving techniques
  in couple distress, 381, 400–401
  in GAD, 118
Prochaska–diClemente transtheoretical
    model, 10
Prodromes
  in bipolar disorder, 258, 259
  relapse, in schizophrenia, 337
Project MATCH study, 358
Prolonged exposure therapy, for PTSD,
    179–182, 189–190
Psychoeducation
  in GAD treatment, 80, 112–113, 115
  for panic disorder/agoraphobia, 13
  for social anxiety disorder, 49–50
Psychopathology, role of beliefs in, 310
Psychotherapy
  for bipolar disorder, 249–251, 263
  for schizophrenia, 309
  supportive, 314

Raisin exercise, 231
Rational response, 50, 56–57
Reframing, 50
  in eating disorders, 276–277
Relapse
  defined, 20, 352
  symptom-based criterion for, 352
Relapse prevention. See also "relapse/
    recurrence prevention" under
    specific disorders
  in alcohol use disorders, 355
  cognitive-behavioral approach to, 352
  defined, 348

Relationships. *See also* Couple distress
  high-risk situations in, 401–402
Relaxation training
  for GAD, 81–82, 102–104, 118
  for PTSD, 182
Relaxation-induced anxiety, 103–104
Repetitive checking, 130
ReVia. *See* Naltrexone (ReVia)
Ritual prevention, 131–136
  implementing, 136
  with pharmacotherapy, 137–138
  strategies for, 132
  variations in, 133–136
Ritualistic washing, 129–130
Roll with resistance strategy, 11–12

Safety behaviors
  in panic disorder/agoraphobia, 15–16
  in social anxiety disorder, 55, 68
Schizophrenia, 306–347
  cognitive-behavioral therapy for, 309–
    316
    challenging delusions, 325–326
    challenging thought disorder, 326–
      327
    with dual diagnosis, 329–330
    location, 324–325
    matching with phase of disorder,
      321–323
    with mental health service, 328–329
    procedure, 323
    and suicide/self-harm risk, 327–328
  cultural factors in, 317–318
  delusions/hallucinations in, 307, 312, 319
  diagnostic characteristics, 307
  disorganized speech in, 307–308
  dual diagnosis and, 329–330
  empirically supported treatments, 308–
    317
  family interventions versus standard
    treatments for, 333–336
  intractable symptoms in, 326–327
  other psychosocial treatments, 316–
    317
  outcome improvement, 318–330
  outcome predictors, 317–318
  overview, 306–308
  with panic disorder/agoraphobia, 18
  pharmacotherapy for, 308–309, 319
  relapse prodrome, 337
  relapse/recurrence predictors, 330–331
  relapse/recurrence prevention, 331–339
Schizotypal trait, with OCD, 140

Selective serotonin norepinephrine
    reuptake inhibitors, for depression,
    206
Selective serotonin reuptake inhibitors
  for bipolar disorder, 248
  for depression, 206–207
  for panic disorder/agoraphobia, 3–4
  for PTSD, 184
Self-determination theory, 360–361
Self-esteem
  of client with schizophrenia, 331, 338–
    339
  weight-based, 279–280
Self-help groups, for recovery from alco-
    hol abuse, 356–357
Self-image, in social anxiety disorder, 54–
    55
Self-in-expansion theory of love, 392
Self-monitoring
  in GAD, 115
  purpose of, 93
Sensation-focused intensive therapy, for
    panic disorder/agoraphobia, 3
Sense of Hyper-Positive Self Scale, 252
Serotonin-$_2$ antagonists-reuptake inhibi-
    tors, for depression, 206
Sertraline, for PTSD, 184
Sexual assault
  pharmacotherapy for victims of, 183–
    184
  therapies for victims of, 182
  women's risk for, 175
Sleep–wake routines, in bipolar disorder,
    258, 260
Social anxiety
  bipolar disorder and, 255–256
  with eating disorders, 288
Social anxiety disorder, 38–76
  case example, 67–71
  characteristics, 38
  in children/adolescents, 61–62
  Clark's cognitive therapy for, 41–42
  cognitive restructuring obstacles in, 50–
    51
  comorbid conditions in, 63
  exposure therapy obstacles in, 51–61
  Foa's comprehensive CBT for, 41
  Heimberg's cognitive-behavioral therapy
    for, 40–41
  outcome improvement, 47–61
  overview, 38
  pharmacotherapy for, 43–44
  psychoeducation obstacles in, 49–50

Social anxiety disorder (*continued*)
  psychosocial approaches to, 39–42
  relapse/recurrence predictors, 64
  relapse/recurrence prevention, 65–67
  treatment efficacy, 44–45
  treatment obstacles, 47–61
  treatment outcome predictors, 45–47
Social skills training
  for children with social anxiety
      disorder, 61
  in schizophrenia, 316–317
  in social anxiety disorder, 60–61
SoCRATES trial, 314
Speech, disorganized, in schizophrenia,
      307–308
SST. *See* Social skills training
Stimulant treatments, for depression,
      207–208
Stress inoculation training, for PTSD,
      179–182
Stressful life events
  depression and, 225–226
  in GAD, 90–91
Subjective Units of Discomfort Scale, 52
  in social anxiety disorder, 66
Subjective Units of Distress Scale
  in GAD, 117
  in OCD, 150, 158
Suboxone. *See* Naloxone (Suboxone)
Substance abuse disorders
  behavioral couple therapy for, 386
  with depression, 210
  with eating disorders, 286–287
  motivational interviewing and, 329–330
Subutex. *See* Buprenorphine (Subutex)
SUDS. *See* Subjective Units of Discomfort
      Scale
Suicide risk
  of client with schizophrenia, 339
  in schizophrenia, 327–328
Supportive counseling, for PTSD, 179
Supportive psychotherapy, for schizophre-
      nia, 314–316

Therapeutic alliance, with depressed
      client, 223–224
Therapeutic relationship
  with client with schizophrenia, 310
  with depressed client, 213
  in eating disorder treatments, 275–
      276
  with OCD client, 141–142, 145
  panic disorder/agoraphobia and, 8
Thinking
  all-or-nothing, 98
  distorted, correcting, 96
Thinking patterns, flexible, 99–101
Thought disorder, challenging, 326
Thought suppression, 146
Thought–action fusion, 146, 150
Thoughts
  automatic. *See* Automatic thoughts
  countering/generative alternative, 98–101
  identifying and pursuing, 96–98
Transcranial magnetic stimulation, for
      depression, 207–208
Tricyclic antidepressants
  for bipolar disorder, 248
  for depression, 206–207
  for OCD, 137
  for PTSD, 184

Urge surfing, 367–368

Valproate, for bipolar disorder, 248–249
Video, in social anxiety disorders, 62
Video feedback, in social anxiety disorder,
      56–58
Violence, women's risk for, 175

Washing, ritualistic, 129–130
Worry imagery exposure, for GAD, 84–
      85, 104–106, 117
Worrying
  beliefs about, 102, 104, 110
  in GAD, 101–102, 115–116
  metacognitive process underlying, 96